Bethesda Handbook
of Clinical Oncology

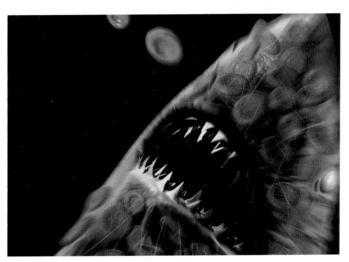

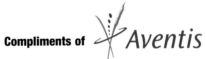

Compliments of *Aventis*

Aventis Pharmaceuticals
Bridgewater, NJ 08807

LOV-LB-10650-1

Bethesda Handbook of Clinical Oncology

Editors

Jame Abraham, M.D.
Division of Clinical Sciences
National Cancer Institute
National Institutes of Health
Bethesda, Maryland

Carmen J. Allegra, M.D.
Chief of Medicine Branch
National Cancer Institute
National Institutes of Health
Bethesda, Maryland

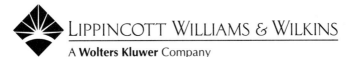

LIPPINCOTT WILLIAMS & WILKINS

A **Wolters Kluwer** Company

Philadelphia · Baltimore · New York · London
Buenos Aires · Hong Kong · Sydney · Tokyo

Acquisitions Editor: Stuart Freeman
Developmental Editor: Will Wiebalck
Production Editor: Jeff Somers
Manufacturing Manager: Benjamin Rivera
Cover Designer: Kevin Kall
Compositor: Lippincott Williams & Wilkins Desktop Division
Printer: R.R. Donnelley–Crawfordsville

Library of Congress Cataloging-in-Publication Data

Bethesda handbook of clinical oncology / [edited by] Jame Abraham, Carmen Allegra.
    p. ; cm.
Includes bibliographical references and index.
ISBN 0-7817-2300-0 (alk. paper)
    1. Cancer—Handbooks, manuals, etc. 2. Oncology—Handbooks, manuals, etc. I. Title:
Handbook of clinical oncology. II. Abraham, Jame. III. Allegra, Carmen.
    [DNLM: 1. Neoplasms—therapy—Handbooks. QZ 39 B562 2001]
RC261 .B624 2001
616.99′4—dc21

Care has been taken to confirm the accuracy of the information presented and to describe generally accepted practices. However, the editors, authors, and publisher are not responsible for errors or omissions or for any consequences from application of the information in this book and make no warranty, expressed or implied, with respect to the currency, completeness, or accuracy of the contents of the publication. Application of this information in a particular situation remains the professional responsibility of the practitioner.

The editors, authors, and publisher have exerted every effort to ensure that drug selection and dosage set forth in this text are in accordance with current recommendations and practice at the time of publication. However, in view of ongoing research, changes in government regulations, and the constant flow of information relating to drug therapy and drug reactions, the reader is urged to check the package insert for each drug for any change in indications and dosage and for added warnings and precautions. This is particularly important when the recommended agent is a new or infrequently employed drug.

Some drugs and medical devices presented in this publication have Food and Drug Administration (FDA) clearance for limited use in restricted research settings. It is the responsibility of the health care provider to ascertain the FDA status of each drug or device planned for use in their clinical practice.

10 9 8 7 6 5 4

To the courage and dedication of our patients, whose today is filled
with anxiety, and whose tomorrow is unpredictable.

"May I never forget that the patient is a fellow creature in pain.
May I never consider him merely a vessel of disease."
— Maimonides
(*12th century philosopher–physician*)

Contents

SECTION 4: BREAST

SECTION 5: GENITOURINARY

SECTION 6: GYNECOLOGIC

SECTION 7: MUSCULOSKELETAL

SECTION 8: SKIN CANCER

SECTION 9: HEMATOLOGIC MALIGNANCIES

SECTION 10: OTHER MALIGNANCIES

SECTION 11: SUPPORTIVE CARE

SECTION 12: COMMON THERAPEUTIC PROCEDURES

APPENDIX

Contributing Authors

Jame Abraham, M.D. *Medicine Branch, DCS, National Cancer Institute, National Institutes of Health, Bethesda, Maryland*

Carmen J. Allegra, M.D. *Chief of Medicine Branch, National Cancer Institute, National Institutes of Health, Bethesda, Maryland*

Susan Bates, M.D. *Medicine Branch, DCS, National Cancer Institute, National Institutes of Health, Bethesda, Maryland*

Michael R. Bishop, M.D. *Medicine Branch, DCS, National Institutes of Health, Bethesda, Maryland*

Philippe C. Bishop, M.D. *Food and Drug Administration, Center for Biologics Evaluation and Research, Division of Clinical Trial Design and Analysis, Rockville, Maryland*

Oscar S. Breathnach, M.D., M.R.C.P.I. *Dana Farber Cancer Institute, Lowe Center for Thoracic Oncology, Harvard Medical School, Boston, Massachusetts*

June Cai, M.D. *National Institute of Mental Health, National Institutes of Health, Bethesda, Maryland*

Jane Carter, R.N. *Nursing Department, Clinical Center, National Institutes of Health, Bethesda, Maryland*

Usha Chaudhry, M.D. *Department of Rehabilitation Medicine, National Institutes of Health, Bethesda, Maryland*

John Chute, M.D. *National Naval Medical Center, National Institutes of Health, Bethesda, Maryland*

William Dahut, M.D. *Medicine Branch, DCS, National Cancer Institute, National Institutes of Health, Bethesda, Maryland*

Suzanne G. Demko, P.A. *Medicine Branch, DCS, National Cancer Institute, National Institutes of Health, Bethesda, Maryland*

Marnie Dobbin, M.S., R.D. *Nutrition Department, National Institutes of Health, Bethesda, Maryland*

Peter Q. Eichacker, M.D. *Vascular Access Device Service, Critical Care Medicine Department, Warren Magnuson Clinical Center, National Institutes of Health, Bethesda, Maryland*

Bruno Fang, M.D. *Medicine Branch, DCS, National Cancer Institute, National Institutes of Health, Bethesda, Maryland*

Tito Fojo, M.D., Ph.D. *Medicine Branch, DCS, National Cancer Institute, National Institutes of Health, Bethesda, Maryland*

Arlene Forastiere, M.D. *Johns Hopkins Oncology Center, Johns Hopkins University School of Medicine, Baltimore, Maryland*

Alison G. Freifeld, M.D. *National Cancer Institute, National Institutes of Health, Bethesda, Maryland*

Barry Gause, M.D. *Medicine Branch, DCS, National Cancer Institute, National Institutes of Health, Bethesda, Maryland*

Barry R. Goldspiel, Pharm.D. *Pharmacy Department, National Institutes of Health, Clinical Center, Bethesda, Maryland*

Jean Grem, M.D. *Medicine Branch, DCS, National Cancer Institute, National Naval Medical Center, National Institutes of Health, Bethesda, Maryland*

Louise Grochow, M.D. *Investigational Drug Branch, Cancer Therapy and Evaluation Program, National Cancer Institute, National Institutes of Health, Bethesda, Maryland*

Deborah C. Guiterrez, R.N., B.S.N. *Vascular Access Device Service, Critical Care Medicine Department, Warren Magnuson Clinical Center, National Institutes of Health, Bethesda, Maryland*

Martin Guitierrez, M.D. *Medicine Branch, DCS, National Cancer Institute, National Institutes of Health, Bethesda, Maryland*

James Gulley, M.D., Ph.D. *Medicine Branch, DCS, National Cancer Institute, National Institutes of Health, Bethesda, Maryland*

J. Michael Hamilton, M.D. *National Cancer Institute, National Institutes of Health, Bethesda, Maryland*

Upendra Hegde, M.D. *Medicine Branch, DCS, National Cancer Institute, National Institutes of Health, Bethesda, Maryland*

Lee Helman, M.D. *Pediatric Branch, DCS, National Cancer Institute, National Institutes of Health, Bethesda, Maryland*

William Jawien, M.D. *National Naval Medical Center, National Institutes of Health, Bethesda, Maryland*

Kenneth B. Johnson, M.D. *Division of Hematology and Medical Oncology, Department of Medicine, Uniformed Services University of the Health Sciences, National Naval Medical Center, Bethesda, Maryland*

Frederic Kaye, M.D. *Medicine Branch, DCS, National Cancer Institute, National Naval Medical Center, National Institutes of Health, Bethesda, Maryland*

Samir Khleif, M.D. *Medicine Branch, DCS, National Cancer Institute, National Institutes of Health, Bethesda, Maryland*

Hung T. Khong, M.D. *Surgery Branch, DCS, National Cancer Institute, National Institutes of Health, Bethesda, Maryland*

George P. Kim, M.D. *Medicine Branch, National Cancer Institute, National Institutes of Health, Bethesda, Maryland*

Kevin Knopf, M.D., M.P.H. *Medicine Branch, DCS, National Cancer Institute, National Institutes of Health, Bethesda, Maryland*

David R. Kohler, Pharm.D. *National Institutes of Health, Clinical Center Pharmacy, Bethesda, Maryland*

Elise Kohn, M.D. *National Cancer Institute, National Institutes of Health, Bethesda, Maryland*

Barnett S. Kramer, M.D. *Division of Cancer Prevention and Control, National Cancer Institute, National Institutes of Health, Bethesda, Maryland*

Stan Lipkowitz, M.D., Ph.D. *Medicine Branch, DCS, National Institutes of Health, National Naval Medical Center, Bethesda, Maryland*

Richard F. Little, M.D. *HIV and AIDS Malignancy Branch, National Cancer Institute, National Institutes of Health, Bethesda, Maryland*

Johnson M. Liu, M.D. *National Heart, Lung, and Blood Institute, National Institutes of Health, Bethesda, Maryland*

Jennifer Loud, M.S.N., C.R.N.P. *Medicine Branch, DCS, National Cancer Institute, National Institutes of Health, Bethesda, Maryland*

Patrick J. Mansky, M.D. *National Cancer Institute, National Institutes of Health, Bethesda, Maryland*

Nicole McCarthy, M.D. *Medicine Branch, DCS, National Cancer Institute, National Institutes of Health, Bethesda, Maryland*

Ian T. McGrath, M.D., F.R.C.P. *INCTR at the Institut Pasteur, Rue Engeland 642, B-1180 Brussels, Belgium*

Richard A. Messmann, M.D., M.S. *Medicine Branch, DCS, National Cancer Institute, National Institutes of Health, Bethesda, Maryland*

Brian P. Monahan, M.D. *Division of Hematology and Medical Oncology, Department of Medicine, Uniformed Services University of the Health Sciences, National Naval Medical Center, Bethesda, Maryland*

Sattva Neelapu, M.D. *Medicine Branch, DCS, National Cancer Institute, National Institutes of Health, Bethesda, Maryland*

V. Koneti Rao, M.D. *Medicine Branch, DCS, National Cancer Institute, National Institutes of Health, Bethesda, Maryland*

Donald L. Rosenstein, M.D. *National Institute of Mental Health, National Institutes of Health, Bethesda, Maryland*

Muhammad Wasif Saif, M.D. *Medicine Branch, DCS, National Cancer Institute, National Institutes of Health, Bethesda, Maryland*

Nishaat Saini, Pharm.D. *Pharmacy Department, University College Hospital, London, England*

Yogen Saunthararajah, M.D. *National Heart Lung and Blood Institute, National Institutes of Health, Bethesda, Maryland*

Jay P. Shah, M.D. *Department of Rehabilitation Medicine, National Institutes of Health, Bethesda, Maryland*

Ramaprasad Srinivasan, M.D., Ph.D. *Medicine Branch, DCS, National Cancer Institute, National Institutes of Health, Bethesda, Maryland*

Chris H. Takimoto, M.D., Ph.D. *Medicine Branch, National Cancer Institute, National Institutes of Health, Bethesda, Maryland*

Rebecca Thomas, M.D. *Medicine Branch, DCS, National Cancer Institute, National Institutes of Health, Bethesda, Maryland*

Helgi Van de Velde, M.D., Ph.D. *Janssen Pharmaceutica N.V, Turnhoutseweg 30, B-2340, Beerse, Belgium*

Wyndham H. Wilson, M.D., Ph.D. *Medicine Branch, DCS, National Cancer Institute, National Institutes of Health, Bethesda, Maryland*

Margaret Wojtowicz, M.D. *Medicine Branch, DCS, National Cancer Institute, National Institutes of Health, Bethesda, Maryland*

JoAnne Zujewski, M.D. *Medicine Branch, DCS, National Cancer Institute, National Institutes of Health, Bethesda, Maryland*

Preface

The Bethesda Handbook of Clinical Oncology is a clear, concise, and comprehensive reference book for the busy clinician to use in his or her daily patient encounters. The book has been compiled by clinicians at the National Cancer Institute and National Naval Medical Center and scholars from other academic institutions. To limit the size of the book, less space is dedicated to etiology, pathophysiology, and epidemiology and greater emphasis is placed on practical clinical information. For easy accessibility to the pertinent information, long descriptions are avoided, and more tables, pictures, algorithms, and phrases are included.

The Bethesda Handbook of Clinical Oncology is not intended as a substitute for the many excellent oncology reference textbooks essential for a more complete understanding of the pathophysiology and management of complicated oncology patients. We hope that the reader-friendly format of this book, with its comprehensive review of the management of each disease with treatment regimens including dosing and schedule, will make this book unique and useful for oncologists, oncology fellows, residents, students, oncology nurses, and allied health professionals.

Acknowledgments

We thank all of our friends and colleagues who worked hard to make this book possible. We are particularly indebted to Dave Kohler, Pharm.D., the Clinical Pharmacy Specialist at the National Institutes of Health, for careful review of each treatment regimen. We also thank Hung Khong, M.D., and Richard Messmann, M.D., for their excellent comments.

This book would not be possible without the strong and continued support of J. Stuart Freeman Jr., the Senior Oncology editor at Lippincott Williams and Wilkins. We also thank William Wiebalck, who was responsible for coordinating and organizing this effort.

Finally, we thank our wives, Shyla and Linda, for their encouragement and support in this endeavor.

SECTION 1

Head and Neck

1

Head and Neck Cancer

Bruno Fang[*] and Arlene Forastiere[**]

[*]*Medicine Branch, DCS, National Cancer Institute, National Institutes of Health, Bethesda, Maryland;* [**]*Johns Hopkins Oncology Center, Baltimore, Maryland*

Extracranial tumors of the head and neck rank as the sixth most common malignancy in the United States, with an incidence of 50,000 cases and a mortality of 12,000 cases per year. Squamous cell carcinoma is the most common histologic type (90% of cases) in tumors originating from the oral and nasal cavities, pharynx, larynx, and paranasal sinuses. Hence the term head and neck cancer is frequently used to imply squamous cell carcinoma of these anatomic sites. Sarcoma, lymphoma, melanoma, and thyroid and salivary gland malignancies are less common tumors found in this location.

EPIDEMIOLOGY

The incidence of head and neck cancer worldwide is greater than 500,000 cases per year, constituting a significant public health problem in many Third World countries. In the U.S., head and neck cancer is a relatively rare disease, accounting for approximately 5% of all new cases of cancer and 2% of all cancer deaths (12,000 per year). Most patients are older than 50 years, and the incidence increases with age. The male-to-female ratio is 2.5:1. However, with the increasing smoking and alcohol-intake pattern in women, the ratio is shifting toward equilibrium. The age-adjusted incidence is higher among black men, and the survival among African-Americans is lower overall and stage by stage.

RISK FACTORS

Tobacco and alcohol are the major risk factors for head and neck cancers. The relative risk of a heavy drinker is estimated to be twofold to sixfold, whereas smoking increases the risk fivefold to 25-fold, depending on gender, race, and the amount of smoking. The presence of both risk factors increases the risk overproportionately to a 15- to 40-fold risk. The use of smokeless tobacco and snuff is especially associated with increased incidence of oral cavity cancers. A case–control study done in the 1980s in North Carolina showed that among long-term users, the relative risk reached nearly 50 for tumors arising in the cheek and gum, tissues in contact with snuff powder.

Alcohol and tobacco affect the respiratory mucosa in its entirety, leading to multifocal mucosal abnormalities known as field cancerization. The risk for a second head and neck cancer in patients with a history of cancer in this area is considered to be around 4% to 6% per year.

Other risk factors include sun exposure (lip cancer), occupational exposure to substances such as nickel (nose, ethmoids), radium (antrum), mustard gas (sphenoid), chromium (sinuses, nose), leather (ethmoids, nasal cavity), wood dust (ethmoids, nasal cavity), radiation exposure (thyroid and salivary glands cancer), and possibly vitamin A deficiency and marijuana.

PREVENTION AND CHEMOPREVENTION

The most important recommendation for the prevention of head and neck cancer is to avoid smoking and to limit alcohol intake.

Chemoprevention has been extensively studied in patients with premalignant lesions and previously treated head and neck cancers, who constitute the group with the highest risk of new tumors in this location. Among the drugs that have been tested to prevent oral malignancies, the most promising are the retinoids. Isotretinoin (13-*cis*-retinoic acid) is effective in reversing premalignant lesions, although this effect ceases after termination of treatment. This observation led to a small randomized placebo-controlled trial in patients treated for a head and neck cancer at high risk for recurrence. Isotretinoin decreased the incidence of second primary tumors, but survival was not changed at 55 months' median follow-up. A larger definitive randomized trial is in progress. Other studies are ongoing to evaluate new agents with potential for chemoprevention.

PATHOLOGY

In adults, more than 90% of tumors of the head and neck are squamous cell carcinomas. The grading system is histologic and is based on the morphologic parameters of tumor dif-

TABLE 1. *Premalignant lesions*

Premalignant lesion	Leukoplakia	Erythroplakia	Dysplasia
Clinical features	White patch or plaque occurring in surface of mucous membrane that does not rub off, once ruled out other oral disease	Bright red velvety plaques that cannot be characterized clinically or pathologically as being due to any other condition	Can present as leukoplakia, erythroplakia, or without obvious macroscopic findings
Probability of progression to malignant lesions	4%	15–30% of dysplastic lesions	15–30%
Histopathology	Hyperkeratosis associated with variable histologic findings. Rarely contain dysplasia or carcinoma. (Invasive or in situ carcinoma found in only 6% of cases)	Mild to moderate dysplasia in 10%; severe dysplasia, in situ or invasive carcinoma in 90% of cases	True histologic diagnosis: pleomorphic changes, increased number of nucleoli, prominent nucleoli

From McFarland M, Abaza NA, El-Mofty S. In: Damjanov I, Linder J, eds. *Anderson's pathology.* St. Louis: Mosby, 1996, with permission.

ferentiation such as the degree of keratinization. The tumors are graded as well differentiated, moderately differentiated, or poorly differentiated.

Leukoplakia, erythroplakia, and dysplasia are premalignant lesions observed in the mucosa. Whereas the first two are clinical findings, the latter represents a true histopathologic diagnosis (Table 1).

The pathology of salivary gland tumors is discussed in the respective sections later.

ANATOMY

The extracranial head and neck anatomy is complex. A simplified depiction is presented in Fig. 1.

The patterns of lymphatic drainage divide the neck into five levels (Fig. 2). Knowledge of the lymphatic drainage of the neck is critical in planning the extent of neck resection for each primary site, and assists the clinician in locating a primary tumor when a palpable involved lymph node is the initial presentation.

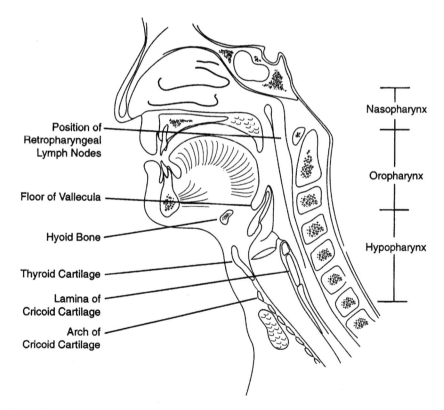

FIG. 1. Sagittal section of the upper aerodigestive tract. From *AJCC Staging Manual 5e*. New York: Lippincott-Raven, 1997. Fig. 4-1, p. 32, with permission.

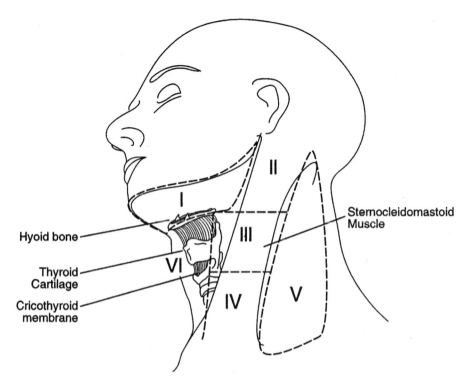

FIG. 2. Diagram of the neck showing levels of lymph nodes. Level I, submandibular; level II, high jugular; level III, midjugular; level IV, low jugular; level V, posterior jugular; level VI, tracheoesophageal; level VIII (superior mediastinal) is not shown. From *AJCC Staging Manual 5e*. New York: Lippincott-Raven, 1997. Fig. 1, p. 22.

STAGING SYSTEM

The American Joint Committee for Cancer (AJCC) and International Union Against Cancer (UICC) staging system (TNM) is used for head and neck cancers, and different classifications and grouping systems were developed for different primary sites.

The T classification indicates the extent of the primary tumor. It differs for each site because of anatomic considerations. For oral cavity, hypopharynx, and oropharynx primary tumors, lesions greater than 4 cm are T3, and those with local invasion of adjacent structures are T4. Vocal cord paralysis with a larynx or hypopharynx primary indicates a T stage no less than T3.

The N classification for cervical lymph nodes is uniform for all sites, except the nasopharynx. The nodal classification for nasopharyngeal carcinoma is different because of the distinctive behavior and prognosis of this tumor. For all sites except the nasopharynx, the following rules apply: clinical lymph node involvement indicates an overall stage no less than III, and the presence of nodal disease more extensive than a single 3-cm ipsilateral node indicates stage IV disease, regardless of T stage.

The presence of distant metastases indicates stage IV disease. Mediastinal lymph node involvement is considered a distant metastasis.

The grade of tumor is not considered when staging head and neck cancers.

The TNM definitions and stage grouping are shown in Table 2.

TABLE 2. TNM staging of head and neck tumors

Primary Tumor (T)

Lip and oral cavity
- TX Primary tumor cannot be assessed
- T0 No evidence of primary tumor
- Tis Carcinoma in situ
- T1 Tumor ≤2 cm in greatest dimension
- T2 Tumor >2 cm but ≤4 cm in greatest dimension
- T3 Tumor >4 cm in greatest dimension
- T4 (Lip) Tumor invades adjacent structures (e.g., through cortical bone, inferior alveolar nerve, floor of mouth, skin of face)
- T4 (Oral cavity) Tumor invades adjacent structures (e.g., through cortical bone, into deep [extrinsic] muscle of tongue, maxillary sinus, skin. Superficial erosion alone of bone/tooth socket by gingival primary is not sufficient to classify as T4)

Pharynx, including base of tongue, soft palate, and uvula
- TX Primary tumor cannot be assessed
- T0 No evidence of primary tumor
- Tis Carcinoma in situ

Nasopharynx
- T1 Tumor confined to the nasopharynx
- T2 Tumor extends to soft tissue of oropharynx and/or nasal fossa
  - T2a Without parapharyngeal extension
  - T2b With parapharyngeal extension
- T3 Tumor invades bony structures and/or paranasal sinuses
- T4 Tumor with intracranial extension and/or involvement of cranial nerves, infratemporal fossa, hypopharynx, or orbit

Oropharynx
- T1 Tumor ≤2 cm in greatest dimension
- T2 Tumor >2 cm but ≤4 cm in greatest dimension
- T3 Tumor >4 cm in greatest dimension
- T4 Tumor invades adjacent structures [e.g., pterygoid muscle(s), mandible, hard palate, deep muscle of tongue, larynx]

Hypopharynx
- T1 Tumor limited to one subsite of hypopharynx and ≤2 cm in greatest dimension
- T2 Tumor involves more than one subsite of hypopharynx or an adjacent site, or measures >2 cm but ≤4 cm in greatest dimension without fixation of hemilarynx
- T3 Tumor measures >4 cm in greatest dimension or with fixation of hemilarynx
- T4 Tumor invades adjacent structures (e.g., thyroid/cricoid cartilage, carotid artery, soft tissues of neck, prevertebral fascia/muscles, thyroid, and/or esophagus)

Larynx
- TX Primary tumor cannot be assessed
- T0 No evidence of primary tumor
- Tis Carcinoma in situ

Supraglottis
- T1 Tumor limited to one subsite of supraglottis with normal vocal cord mobility
- T2 Tumor invades mucosa of more than one adjacent subsite of supraglottis or glottis or region outside the supraglottis (e.g., mucosa or base of tongue, vallecula, medial wall of pyriform sinus) without fixation of the larynx
- T3 Tumor limited to larynx with vocal cord fixation and/or invades any of the following: postcricoid area, preepiglottic tissues
- T4 Tumor invades through the thyroid cartilage, and/or extends into soft tissues of the neck, thyroid, and/or esophagus

Glottis
- T1 Tumor limited to vocal cord(s) (may involve anterior or posterior commissure) with normal mobility
  - T1a Tumor limited to one vocal cord
  - T1b Tumor involves both vocal cords
- T2 Tumor extends to supraglottis and/or subglottis, and/or with impaired vocal cord mobility
- T3 Tumor limited to the larynx with vocal cord fixation
- T4 Tumor invades through the thyroid cartilage and/or to other tissues beyond the larynx (e.g., trachea, soft tissues of neck, including thyroid, pharynx)

continued on next page

TABLE 2. *Continued*

Subglottis

T1	Tumor limited to subglottis
T2	Tumor extends to vocal cord(s) with normal or impaired mobility
T3	Tumor limited to larynx with vocal cord fixation
T4	Tumor invades through cricoid or thyroid cartilage and/or extends to other tissues beyond the larynx (e.g., trachea, soft tissues of neck, including thyroid, esophagus)

Paranasal sinuses

Maxillary sinus

TX	Primary tumor cannot be assessed
T0	No evidence of primary tumor
Tis	Carcinoma in situ
T1	Tumor limited to the antral mucosa with no erosion or destruction of bone
T2	Tumor causing bone erosion or destruction, except for the posterior antral wall, including extension into the hard palate and/or the middle nasal meatus
T3	Tumor invades any of the following: bone of the posterior wall of maxillary sinus, subcutaneous tissues, skin of cheek, floor or medial wall of orbit, infratemporal fossa, pterygoid plates, ethmoid sinuses
T4	Tumor invades orbital contents beyond the floor or medial wall including any of the following: the orbital apex, cribriform plate, base of skull, nasopharynx, sphenoid, frontal sinuses

Ethmoid sinus

T1	Tumor confined to the ethmoid with or without bone erosion
T2	Tumor extends into the nasal cavity
T3	Tumor extends into the anterior orbit and/or maxillary sinus
T4	Tumor with intracranial extension, orbital extension including apex, involving sphenoid, and/or frontal sinus and/or skin of external nose

Major salivary glands (parotid, submandibular, and sublingual)

TX	Primary tumor cannot be assessed
T0	No evidence of primary tumor
T1	Tumor ≤2 cm in greatest dimension without extraparenonimal extension
T2	Tumor >2 cm but ≤4 cm in greatest dimension without extraparenonimal extension
T3	Tumor having extraparenonimal extension without seventh nerve involvement and/or >4 cm but ≤6 cm in greatest dimension
T4	Tumor invades base of skull, seventh nerve, and/or >6 cm in greatest dimension

Regional nodes (N)

All sites, except nasopharynx

NX	Regional nodes cannot be assessed
N0	No regional lymph node metastasis
N1	Metastasis in a single ipsilateral lymph node, ≤3 cm in greatest dimension
N2	Metastasis in a single ipsilateral lymph node, >3 cm but ≤6 cm in greatest dimension; or in multiple ipsilateral lymph nodes, none >6 cm in greatest dimension; or in bilateral or contralateral lymph nodes, none >6 cm in greatest dimension
	N2a Metastasis in single ipsilateral lymph node >3 cm but ≤6 cm in greatest dimension
	N2b Metastasis in multiple ipsilateral lymph nodes, none >6 cm in greatest dimension
	N2c Metastasis in bilateral or contralateral lymph nodes, none >6 cm in greatest dimension
N3	Metastasis in a lymph node >6 cm in greatest dimension

continued on next page

TABLE 2. *Continued*

Nasopharynx
NX   Regional nodes cannot be assessed
N0   No regional lymph node metastasis
N1   Unilateral metastasis in lymph node(s), ≤6 cm in greatest dimension, above the
         supraclavicular fossa
N2   Bilateral metastasis in lymph node(s), ≤6 cm in greatest dimension, above the
         supraclavicular fossa
N3   Metastasis in a lymph node(s)
         N3a   >6 cm in dimension
N3b Extension to the supraclavicular fossa

Distant metastasis (M)
All sites, including nasopharynx
MX   Distant metastasis cannot be assessed
M0   No distant metastasis
M1   Distant metastasis

Stage grouping
Lip, oral cavity, oropharynx, hypopharynx, larynx

Stage 0	Tis	N0	M0
Stage I	T1	N0	M0
Stage II	T2	N0	M0
Stage III	T3	N0	M0
	T1	N1	M0
	T2	N1	M0
	T3	N1	M0
Stage IVA	T4	N0	M0
	T4	N1	M0
	Any T	N2	M0
Stage IVB	Any T	N3	M0
Stage IVC	Any T	Any N	M1

Nasopharynx

Stage 0	Tis	N0	M0
Stage I	T1	N0	M0
Stage IIA	T2a	N0	M0
Stage IIB	T1	N1	M0
	T2	N1	M0
	T2a	N1	M0
	T2b	N0	M0
	T2b	N1	M0
Stage III	T1	N2	M0
	T2a	N2	M0
	T2b	N2	M0
	T3	N0	M0
	T3	N1	M0
	T3	N2	M0
Stage IVA	T4	N0	M0
	T4	N1	M0
	T4	N2	M0
Stage IVB	Any T	N3	M0
Stage IVC	Any T	Any N	M1

continued on next page

TABLE 2. *Continued*

Paranasal sinuses			
Stage 0	Tis	N0	M0
Stage I	T1	N0	M0
Stage II	T2	N0	M0
Stage III	T3	N0	M0
	T1	N1	M0
	T2	N1	M0
	T3	N1	M0
Stage IVA	T4	N0	M0
	T4	N1	M0
Stage IVB	Any T	N2	M0
	Any T	N3	M0
Stage IVC	Any T	Any N	M1
Major salivary glands			
Stage I	T1	N0	M0
	T2	N0	M0
Stage II	T3	N0	M0
Stage III	T1	N1	M0
	T2	N1	M0
Stage IV	T4	N0	M0
	T3	N1	M0
	T4	N1	M0
	Any T	N2	M0
	Any T	N3	M0
	Any T	Any N	M1

PRESENTATION

Signs and symptoms are usually secondary to mass effect created by the tumor or involved lymph nodes and invasion of adjacent structures (Table 3).

Adult patients (especially the elderly) with any of these symptoms for more than 2 to 4 weeks should be referred to an otolaryngologist. Delay in diagnosis is not uncommon, as many patients are treated with repeated courses of antibiotics for otitis media or a sore throat, for example. A lateralized firm cervical mass in an elderly smoker is highly suggestive of metastatic squamous cell carcinoma.

TABLE 3. *Common presenting signs and symptoms of head and neck cancer*

Painless neck mass
Odynophagia
Dysphagia
Hoarseness
Hemoptysis
Trismus
Otalgia
Otitis media
Loose teeth
Ill-fitting dentures
Cranial nerve deficits
Nonhealing oral ulcers

With the exception of hypopharynx and nasopharynx cancers, distant metastases are uncommon at presentation. The most common sites of distant metastases are lung and bone; liver involvement is less common.

DIAGNOSIS

A detailed history should be obtained, including exposure to the risk factors mentioned earlier, as well as questioning about the signs and symptoms listed in Table 3. The physical examination should include careful inspection of the scalp, ears, nose, and mouth; palpation of the neck and mouth; and bimanual palpation of the base of the tongue and floor of the mouth. Special attention should be given to the examination of cranial nerves. Abnormalities are suggested by asymmetry in the physical examination.

Friability (easy bleeding) is the most significant indicator of an early malignant process involving the mucosa. Erythroplakia, which refers to red friable areas in the mucosa, is frequently associated with severe dysplasia or carcinoma in situ, and therefore, is more worrisome than leukoplakia (white mucosal patches). Biopsies should be performed on such mucosal abnormalities. Table 1 lists the different characteristics of these premalignant lesions.

When the first presentation of cancer is a neck mass (lymph node metastasis), a detailed physical examination by an otolaryngologist usually reveals the primary site, on which a biopsy can be performed (in approximately 80% of cases). If the primary site is not obvious by examination, histopathology can be obtained by fine-needle aspiration (FNA) of the neck mass. This is the most frequently used method for obtaining a tissue diagnosis. FNA is inexpensive and fast, and causes little discomfort to the patient. Its sensitivity and specificity for squamous cell carcinoma approaches 99% in trained hands. In many centers, a cytopathologist performs the FNA. This is important because most of the nondiagnostic tests are caused by poor tissue sampling, frequently due to inexperience on the part of the operator. A nondiagnostic FNA does not rule out the presence of tumor.

The anatomic location of the involved lymph node may suggest the location of the primary tumor. Computed tomography (CT) scan remains the primary imaging study for evaluation of metastatic adenopathy. Magnetic resonance imaging (MRI) may complement the CT scan (see later). Panendoscopy (laryngoscopy, bronchoscopy, esophagoscopy, and nasopharyngoscopy) should be performed with directed biopsies of the nasopharynx, tonsil, base of tongue, and pyriform sinus. These are the most likely sites to harbor an occult primary tumor (Fig. 3).

Surgical biopsy of a neck mass is contraindicated if a squamous cell carcinoma is suspected (as opposed to lymphoma, for example). Retrospective studies show that open biopsy may worsen local control, increase the rate of distant metastases, and decrease overall survival, possibly by spreading of disease at the time of the biopsy. Finally, if squamous cell carcinoma is diagnosed, an open biopsy does not provide any additional information to that from FNA.

WORK-UP AND STAGING EVALUATION

Once the diagnosis of cancer is established, the patient should be evaluated for extension of tumor, lymph node involvement, presence of metastasis, and secondary tumors to determine the clinical stage. In general, besides a thorough physical examination, CT scan and/or MRI of the primary tumor and neck are indicated. CT scan is cheaper and faster, has better definition for cortical bone, and is better than MRI for evaluating metastatic adenopathy. MRI has superior soft tissue contrast, does not involve radiation, and may be better than CT scan for primary tumor staging. A chest radiograph is indicated for all patients, mostly because of the risk of a second malignancy in this high-risk population. Additional studies will vary according to the primary site.

PROGNOSIS

The most important determinant of prognosis is stage at diagnosis. The 5-year survival for patients with stage I tumors in many sites exceeds 80%, decreasing to less than 40% in stage

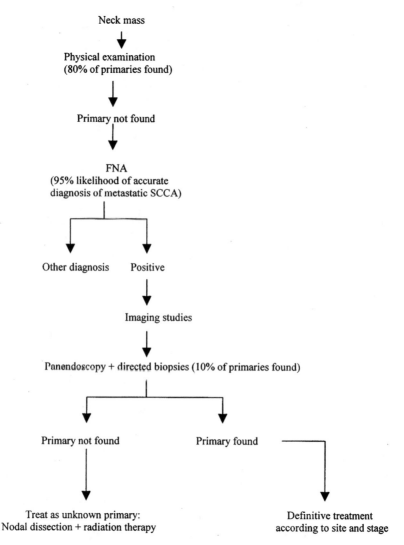

FIG. 3. Evaluation of cervical adenopathy when a primary cancer of the head and neck is suspected.

III and IV disease. Most patients initially seen with head and neck tumors have advanced-stage disease.

The majority of relapses occur locoregionally in the head and neck area. Distant metastases are more commonly seen later in the course of the disease, and predominantly involve lung, bone, and liver. The lifetime risk of developing a new cancer for a patient with head and neck cancer is 20% to 40%. Over time, the risk of relapse from the primary cancer decreases, and the development of a new cancer represents the greatest risk. See Tables 4 to 6 for site-specific prognoses.

TABLE 4. *Head and neck cancer: Oral cavity*

Site	Epidemiology	Natural history and common presenting symptoms	Nodal involvement	Prognosis (5-yr survival)
Lip	Risk factors: sun exposure and tobacco 3,600 new cases a year 10 to 40 times more common in white men than in black men or women (black or white)	Exophytic mass or ulcerative lesion More common in lower lip (92%) Slow growing Pain, bleeding	5–10% Midline tumors spread bilaterally Level I more common (submandibular and submental) Upper lip lesions metastasize earlier: Level I and also preauricular	T1, 90% T2, 84% With LN involvement, 50%
Alveolar ridge and retromolar trigone	10% of all oral cancers M:F, 4:1	Exophytic mass or infiltrating tumor, may invade bone Bleeding, pain exacerbated by chewing, loose teeth, ill-fitting dentures	30% (70% if T4) Levels I and II more common	T1, 85% T2, 80% T3, 60% T4, 20%
Floor of mouth	10–15% of oral cancers, (0.6/100,000) M:F, 3:1 Median age, 60 yr	Painful infiltrative lesions, may invade bone, muscles of floor of mouth, tongue	T1, 12%; T2, 30%; T3, 47%; T4, 53% Levels I and II more common	By stage: I, 85–90% II, 80% III, 66% IV, 32%
Tongue (anterior two thirds)	6,200 new cases per year Median age, 60 yr M:F, 3:1	Exophytic or infiltrative Pain, occasionally difficulty in speech and deglutition	Greatest propensity for lymph node metastasis of oral cavity sites Bilateral involvement, 25% Level II more common, followed by I, III, and IV Less frequently: 6–29%	Early stage node negative, 74% Advanced stage, 30%
Hard palate	0.4 cases/100,000 (5% of oral cavity) M:F, 8:1 50% cases squamous, 50% salivary glands	Deeply infiltrating or superficially spreading Pain	10% at diagnosis	By stage: I, 75% II, 46%, III, 36%, IV, 11%
Buccal mucosa	8% of oral cavity cancers in U.S. Women > men	Exophytic more often, silent presentation Pain, bleeding, difficulty chewing	10% at diagnosis Levels I and II more common	18–77% all stages

TABLE 5. *Head and neck cancer: Oropharynx and larynx*

Site	Epidemiology	Natural history and common presenting symptoms	Nodal involvement	Prognosis (5-yr survival)
Base of tongue	4,000 new cases annually in the U.S. Male: female ratio, 3 to 5:1.	Advanced at presentation (silent location, aggressive behavior) Pain, dysphagia, weight loss, otalgia (from cranial nerve involvement) Neck mass is frequent presentation	All stages: 70 (T1) to 80% (T4) Level II and III more common, also IV, V, VI	By stage: I, 60% II, 40% III, 30% IV, 15%
Tonsil, tonsillar pillar, soft palate	Tobacco and alcohol are the most significant risk factors	Tonsillar fossa: more advanced at presentation: 75% stage III or IV, pain, dysphagia, weight loss, and neck mass Soft palate: More indolent, may present as erythroplakia	Tonsilar pillar T2, 38% Tonsilar fossa T2, 68% (55% present with N2 or N3 disease)	Tonsilar fossa, 93% (stage I) to 17% (stage IV) Soft palate, 85% (stage I) to 21% (stage IV)
Posterior pharyngeal wall		Advanced at diagnosis (silent location) Pain, bleeding, weight loss Neck mass common initial symptom	Clinically palpable nodes T1, 25% T2, 30% T3, 66% T4, 75% Bilateral involvement is common	By stage: I, 75% II, 70% III, 42% IV, 27%
Supraglottis	35% of laryngeal cancers	Most arise in epiglottis Early lymph node involvement due to extensive lymphatic drainage 2/3 have nodal metastases at diagnosis	Overall rate: T1, 63%; T2, 70%; T3, 79%; T4, 73% Levels II, III and IV more common	By stage: I, 70–100% II, 50–90% III, 45–70% IV, 20–60%
Glottis	Most common laryngeal cancer	Most favorable prognosis Late lymph node involvement Usually well differentiated, but with infiltrative growth pattern Hoarseness is an early symptom, 70% have localized disease at diagnosis	Sparse lymphatic drainage, early lesions rarely metastasize to lymph nodes. Clinically positive: T1, T2 <2% Levels II, III, and IV more common T3, T4, 20–25%	T1, 74–86% T2, 67–75% T3, 55% T4, 50%
Subglottis	Rare, 1–8% of laryngeal cancers	Poorly differentiated, infiltrative growth pattern unrestricted by tissue barriers Rarely causes hoarseness, may cause dyspnea from airway involvement 2/3 of patients have metastatic disease at presentation	20–30% overall Pretracheal and paratracheal nodes more commonly involved	26% overall

TABLE 6. *Head and neck cancer: Hypopharynx, nasal cavity, paranasal sinuses, and nasopharynx*

Site	Epidemiology	Natural history and common presenting symptoms	Nodal involvement	Prognosis (5-yr survival)
Hypopharynx	2,500 new cases yearly in U.S. Etiology: tobacco, alcohol, nutritional abnormalities	Aggressive, diffuse local spread, early lymph node involvement Occult metastases to thyroid and paratracheal node chain Pain, neck stiffness (retropharyngeal nodes), otalgia (cranial nerve X), irritation and mucus retention 50% present as neck mass High risk of distant metastases	Abundant lymphatic drainage Up to 60% have clinically positive lymph nodes at diagnosis	Survival varies between sites within hypopharynx T1, T2, 40% T3–T4, 16–37%
Nasal cavity and paranasal sinuses	Rare 0.75/100,000 in U.S. Nasal cavity and maxillary sinus, 4/5 of all cases M:F, 2:1 Increased risk with exposure to: furniture, shoe, textile industries; nickel, chromium, mustard gas, isopropyl alcohol, and radium	Nonhealing ulcer, occasional bleeding, unilateral nasal obstruction, dental pain, loose teeth, ill-fitting dentures, trismus, diplopia, proptosis, epiphora, anosmia, and headache, depending of site of invasion Usually advanced at presentation	10–20% clinically positive nodes Levels I and II more common	60% all sites all stages, 30% for T4 Principal determinant for survival is local recurrence
Nasopharynx	Rare (less than 1/100,000) except in North Africa, southeast Asia, and China, far northern hemisphere Associated with EBV, diet, genetic factors	Most common initial presentation: neck mass Other presentations: otitis media, nasal obstruction, tinnitus, pain, cranial nerve involvement	Clinically positive: WHO I, 60% WHO II and III, 80–90%	T1, 37–60% T2, 46–68% T3, 16–25% T4, 11–40%

EBV, Epstein–Barr virus.

15

SCREENING

Careful routine examination of the head and neck area is warranted in older individuals with risk factors, particularly a history of smoking and alcohol abuse. Biopsies should be performed of mucosal abnormalities, as well as palpable neck masses (see Diagnosis).

The United States Preventive Task Force does not recommend regular screening for oral cancer in the general population, but recommends counseling for tobacco-use cessation and limitation of alcohol intake. The American Cancer Society recommends a cancer check-up that includes oral examination every 3 years for persons older than 20 years and annually for those older than 40 years. Any of the complaints described earlier require evaluation, especially if symptoms are persistent for more than 2 weeks in patients older than 60 years.

TREATMENT

The management of patients with head and neck cancer is complex. The choice of treatment will depend not only on the stage, but also on the specific site of disease (see later). Patients with locally advanced disease should be evaluated by a multidisciplinary team including surgeons, radiation therapists, oncologists, and personnel involved in rehabilitation (prosthodontics, speech, and swallowing) before treatment is initiated.

In general, surgery and radiation are equally effective as single-modality therapy for patients with early-stage disease (stage I or II). The choice of modality is dependent on local expertise, patient preference, and functional result. For the 60% of patients seen with locally advanced disease (M0) at diagnosis, combined modality therapy is generally indicated.

Surgery

Different surgical options are available for each specific site of head and neck cancer; the nature of the procedure is determined primarily by the size of the tumor and the structures involved.

Resectability in head and neck cancer is a controversial issue. It will depend on the experience of the surgeon and the team involved in rehabilitation. In general, a tumor is considered unresectable if the surgeon does not believe that all gross tumor can be removed on anatomic grounds, or that local control will not be achieved after an operation even with the addition of radiation therapy.

Cervical lymph node dissections are classified as radical, modified radical, or selective. The radical dissection includes removal of all lymph nodes in the neck from levels I to V (see Fig. 2), with removal of the internal jugular vein, spinal accessory nerve, and sternocleidomastoid muscle. This surgery is now rarely performed because of excessive morbidity, especially loss of shoulder function. The modified radical dissection preserves one or more of the nonlymphatic structures. In selective neck dissections, only certain levels of lymph nodes are removed, based on the specific lymphatic drainage from the primary site. With no clinical nodal involvement from a squamous cancer of the head and neck, nodal metastases will be present beyond the confines of an appropriate selective neck dissection less than 10% of the time.

The findings of T4 tumor, perineural/perilymphatic or vascular invasion, multiple positive nodes, and extracapsular lymph node invasion indicate higher risk of local recurrence after surgery.

Radiation Therapy

Radiation therapy is used in the management of head and neck cancer as single therapy in early-stage tumors (T1, T2) with cure rates comparable to those of surgery. The choice of therapy will depend on factors such as expected quality of life, functional outcome, sequelae of therapy, and options for treatment in case of recurrence.

In locally advanced tumors (T3, T4), radiation therapy is combined with surgery. In general, postoperative is preferred over preoperative radiation. This approach is based on the results of two randomized prospective studies. The first one showed increased survival in the postoperative radiation arm in patients with hypopharyngeal cancer. The most recent study showed superior local control in the postoperative radiation arm, particularly in the subgroup of patients with supraglottic disease.

Postoperative radiotherapy is recommended for patients at high risk of local recurrence. Risks factors include T4 tumor, close or positive margins, perineural/perilymphatic/vascular invasion by the tumor, multiple positive nodes, and extracapsular invasion.

The type of radiation therapy (dose, fractionation regimen, and indication for brachytherapy) varies for specific sites. The standard fractionation regimen in the U.S. is 200 cGy once daily, 5 days per week. Recent large randomized trials have shown improved local control with twice-daily fractionation, particularly in intermediate-stage oropharyngeal carcinoma, but no improvement in overall survival. A number of altered fractionation schemes that compress the treatment time are under investigation. It is well established that treatment breaks or prolonged treatment time adversely affects outcome.

Acute radiation toxicity includes epidermitis, mucositis, loss of taste, xerostomia, and hair loss. All patients should be evaluated by a dentist before initiation of radiotherapy and given prophylactic fluoride. Patients receiving radiation therapy are at high risk for tooth decay due to the xerostomia caused by injury to the salivary glands as well as mucosal damage. Dental extractions should be performed before radiation, because it has been shown that dental extractions in a radiated mandible can lead to osteonecrosis. The drug amifostine has been shown in a randomized trial to decrease the incidence of radiation-induced xerostomia in patients receiving postoperative radiation to a maximal dose of 6,000 cGy.

Brachytherapy can be used as a definitive treatment for early-stage tumors or combined with external beam radiation in more advanced lesions in selected tumors (tongue, floor of mouth, tonsil, and nasopharynx) with excellent results. Brachytherapy is another option for recurrent cancers of the head and neck, particularly in previously irradiated patients.

Chemotherapy

Traditionally, the use of chemotherapy in the management of head and neck cancer was limited to patients with locally recurrent or disseminated disease. In this setting, chemotherapy is given as a single-modality therapy with palliative intent. Combination chemotherapy yields higher response rates but increased toxicity when compared with single-agent chemotherapy. The choice of single-agent or combination chemotherapy will depend on patient preference and performance status. The use of chemotherapy (or any other therapy) in this setting has not been shown to increase survival.

Single agents with greater than 15% response activity are listed in Table 7. Several combination regimens have been developed to improve response rates. The best results were reported in 1984 by researchers at Wayne State University by using a combination of cisplatin and infusional 5-fluorouracil (5-FU): 70% response and 27% complete remission (CR). The addition of other drugs to this regimen resulted in increased toxicity with no survival improvement.

A meta-analysis of randomized trials published between 1980 and 1992 demonstrated improved response for cisplatin when compared with methotrexate, improved response of cisplatin plus 5-FU when compared with single drugs, and improved response of cisplatin plus 5-FU when compared with other regimens. A randomized trial demonstrated superiority of continuous-infusion 5-FU plus cisplatin when compared with bolus 5-FU plus cisplatin. Based on results from multicenter trials evaluating cisplatin plus infusional 5-FU, the response

TABLE 7. *Single agents of demonstrated benefit in advanced head and neck cancer*

Drug	Schedule	Cycle duration	Response rate	Reference
Methotrexate	40 mg/m² /wk i.v. to be escalated weekly by 10 mg/m² increments to 60 mg/m² or until dose-limiting toxicity or an objective response is achieved. (total dose/week, 40, 50, or 60 mg/m²)	7 days	15–31%	*Cancer* 1983; 52(2):206–210
Cisplatin	80–100 mg/m² i.v. (total dose/cycle, 80–100 mg/m²)	21–28 days	14–41%	*J Clin Oncol* 1992;10(2):257–263
Carboplatin	Dosage is calculated by the Calvert formula to achieve a target AUC = 6 mg/ml/min i.v.[a]	21 days	14–30%	*Semin Oncol* 1992; 19(1 Suppl 2):60–65
Paclitaxel	175–220 mg/m² i.v. infusion over 3 h (total dose/cycle = 175–220 mg/m²)	21 days	30–40%	*Br J Cancer* 1995;72(4):1016–1019 *Cancer* 1998;82(11): 2270–2274
Fluorouracil	1,000 mg/m² per day continuous i.v. infusion for 4 days (d 1–4; total dose/cycle = 4,000 mg/m²); OR 1,000 mg/m² per day i.v. bolus for 5 days (d 1–5; total dose/cycle = 5,000 mg/m²)		0–33%	*J Clin Oncol* 1992; 10(2):257–263
Gemcitabine	800–1,250 mg/m² per week i.v. for 3 weeks (d 1, 8, & 15; total dose/cycle = 2,400–3,750 mg/m²)	28 days	13%	*Ann Oncol* 1994;5(6): 543–547
Docetaxel	75–100 mg/m² i.v. bolus every 3 weeks	21 days	30–40%	*J Clin Oncol* 1996;14:1672–1678

[a]Calvert formula: Total dose (mg) = [Target AUC (mg/ml/min)] × [GFR (mL/min) + 25]. From Calvert AH, Newell DR, Gumbrell LA, et al. Carboplatin dosage: prospective evaluation of a simple formula based on renal function. *J Clin Oncol* 1989;7:1748–1756, with permission.

AUC, Graphically represented area under the plasma concentration versus time curve for carboplatin; GFR, glomerular filtration rate. In clinical application, urinary creatinine clearance during 24 h approximates the GFR; i.v., intravenously.

TABLE 8. *Combination chemotherapy regimens*[a]

Drugs	Schedule	Cycle duration	Reference
Cisplatin + 5-FU (previously untreated patients)	Cisplatin, 100 mg/m² i.v., day 1 (total dose/cycle = 100 mg/m²) Fluorouracil, 1,000 mg/m² per day continuous-infusion i.v. for 5 days (total dose/cycle, 5,000 mg/m²)	21 days	*N Engl J Med* 1991; 324(24): 1685–1690
Cisplatin + 5-FU (palliation of recurrent disease)	Cisplatin, 100 mg/m² i.v., day 1 Fluorouracil, 1,000 mg/m² per day continuous-infusion i.v. for 4 days (total dose/cycle, 4,000 mg/m²)	21 days	*Cancer* 1984;53: 1819–1824
Paclitaxel + cisplatin	Paclitaxel, 175 mg/m² i.v. infusion over 3 h (total dose/cycle, 175 mg/m²) Cisplatin, 75 mg/m² i.v., day 1 (total dose/cycle, 75 mg/m²)	21 days	*Semin Oncol* 1997; 24(6):S19–24
Docetaxel + cisplatin	Docetaxel, 75 mg/m² i.v., day 1 (total dose/cycle, 75 mg/m²) Cisplatin, 75 mg/m² i.v., day 1 (total dose/cycle, 75 mg/m²)	21 days	*Ann Oncol* 1999; 10(1):119–122

[a]Carboplatin should be substituted for cisplatin in patients with creatinine clearance of <50 ml/min or preexisting peripheral neuropathy.
5-FU, 5-fluorouracil; i.v. intravenously.

rate is approximately 30% to 40%, and CRs are observed in fewer than 10% of patients. This regimen is described in Table 8.

The role of chemotherapy has expanded significantly over the past decade, based on the results of clinical trials incorporating chemotherapy in multimodality regimens for previously untreated disease.

Studies have evaluated the use of chemotherapy administered before (neoadjuvant or induction chemotherapy), during (concomitant chemotherapy), or after (adjuvant chemotherapy) radiation therapy or surgery.

Induction Chemotherapy

Induction chemotherapy followed by definitive radiation therapy in chemotherapy responders is indicated for patients with locally advanced cancers of the larynx and hypopharynx who wish to preserve their larynx. No significant difference in overall survival has been demonstrated with the use of induction chemotherapy followed by radiotherapy compared with surgery. However, the local failure rate was higher with chemotherapy/radiation; therefore close follow-up is required so that salvage surgery may be performed if indicated. There is no evidence at this point that induction chemotherapy followed by radiation therapy is more efficacious than radiation therapy alone. An ongoing large multicenter randomized study is evaluating this issue.

Cisplatin, 100 mg/m² i.v., on day 1, and 5-FU, 1,000 mg/m² per day as continuous i.v. infusion for 5 consecutive days (days 1–5), repeated every 3 weeks, is the most active regimen in use as induction therapy in previously untreated patients. The overall response rate is 85%, with a 40% CR rate; two thirds of clinical CRs are found to be pathologic CRs in resected specimens. Response varies by site, with the larynx and nasopharynx the most responsive, and the oral cavity the least responsive.

Response to chemotherapy after two to three courses of treatment predicts sensitivity to radiation therapy and correlates with survival prognosis. Induction chemotherapy does not increase surgical or radiation therapy complications. Other prognostic factors for survival are performance status, tumor site, and stage.

Adjuvant Chemotherapy

Adjuvant chemotherapy (given after the patient is rendered disease free) has the advantage of not delaying definitive surgery. A large randomized study in resected patients with stages III or IV disease compared adjuvant radiation therapy with adjuvant chemotherapy plus radiation. The results of this trial showed improved local control and overall survival that approached statistical significance in a subset of patients at high risk of local recurrence treated with chemotherapy. Patients with low-risk disease (negative resection margins, one or no positive nodes, and no extracapsular spread of tumor) did not benefit from adjuvant chemotherapy. There is now no indication for the use of adjuvant chemotherapy outside the setting of a clinical trial.

A study of adjuvant concomitant chemoradiation in patients at high risk of recurrence demonstrated significantly better median survival (40 months vs. 22 months) and 5-year survival (13% vs. 36%) for the chemoradiation group compared with the group of patients receiving radiation alone. A large multicenter randomized trial testing concomitant cisplatin and radiotherapy in high-risk surgically resected patients is under way to confirm these results.

Concomitant Chemoradiation

The rationale for concomitant chemoradiation is based on experimental evidence of synergism between chemotherapy and radiation to kill tumor cells. This effect is theoretically mediated by interference of chemotherapy with cell repair after sublethal or potentially lethal damage from radiation therapy or interference with tumor cell synchronization. The experimental finding that certain chemotherapy agents (e.g., cisplatin, 5-FU) can add to this effect by inducing radiosensitivity and increasing the log cell kill for a given dose of radiation further supports this treatment strategy. Cisplatin also has the advantage of not having mucositis as toxicity, although as a radiation enhancer, it does increase radiation-induced mucositis. Cisplatin has been the drug of choice in recent large randomized trials evaluating this question.

As expected, this regimen is associated with an increase in toxicity compared with sequential chemoradiation (neoadjuvant or adjuvant), which may be decreased in part by the use of alternating instead of synchronous regimens.

Several controlled randomized trials have evaluated the use of concomitant chemoradiation for advanced unresectable head and neck cancer, using single-agent or combination chemotherapy and conventional or altered fractionation radiation treatments. Concomitant chemoradiation was shown in several of these studies to be superior to sequential chemotherapy and to radiation alone in terms of improved local control, as well as increased disease-free and overall survival. It has become standard therapy for patients with unresectable advanced head and neck cancer with good performance status.

The use of concomitant chemotherapy and radiation therapy in patients with stage III and IV nasopharyngeal carcinoma was shown to confer superior local control and improved overall survival when compared with radiation therapy alone. It is now the standard of care for this group of patients (see later). Chemoradiation is also an acceptable standard of care for treating locally advanced oropharyngeal cancer when a nonsurgical approach is preferred.

Simultaneous chemoradiotherapy is the only multimodality strategy that has been shown to increase survival significantly when compared with surgery and/or radiation therapy in patients with head and neck cancer. Meta-analyses indicate that this is the best way to combine radiation therapy and chemotherapy.

SITE-SPECIFIC HEAD AND NECK TUMORS

Oral Cavity

The oral cavity includes the lip, anterior two thirds of the tongue, floor of the mouth, buccal mucosa, gingiva, hard palate, and retromolar trigone. Approximately 30,000 new cases are diagnosed annually in the U.S. In addition to tobacco (in the form of cigarette, cigar, pipe, or smokeless tobacco) and alcohol, other risk factors include vitamin A deficiency and genetic susceptibility (DNA repair defect syndromes such as xeroderma pigmentosum, Fanconi's anemia, and ataxia–telangiectasia).

Squamous cell carcinoma is the histologic type observed in the vast majority of the cases.

The epidemiology, natural history, common presenting symptoms, risk of nodal involvement, and prognosis for specific subsites are shown in Table 4. Treatment for oral cavity cancers follows the general guidelines for head and neck cancers. Early lesions (stages I and II) can be treated with surgery or radiation therapy as single-modality therapy, depending on physician and patient preferences (as discussed earlier). For resectable locally advanced disease (stages III and IV, M0), surgery followed by radiation therapy is indicated (Fig. 4). Defin-

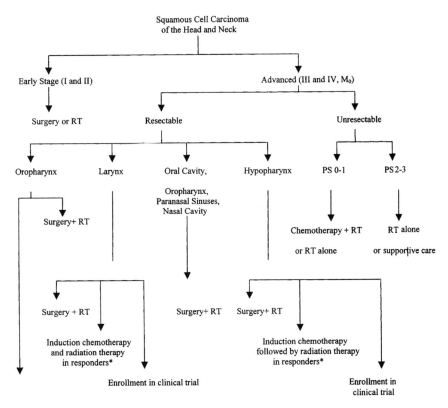

FIG. 4. Treatment for head and neck squamous cell carcinomas, M0.

itive radiation therapy is an option for patients with resectable disease of any stage who are considered a poor medical or surgical risk, or depending on patient preference (based on discussions about quality of life, functional outcome, and toxicity profile of each treatment). Treatment for locally advanced and metastatic disease is discussed later.

Oropharynx

The oropharynx includes the base of the tongue, tonsils, posterior pharyngeal wall, and the soft palate.

The epidemiology, natural history, common presenting symptoms, risk of nodal involvement, and prognosis for specific subsites of the oropharynx are shown in Table 5. Treatment for oropharyngeal cancers may include primary surgery and postoperative radiotherapy or primary radiation therapy, reserving surgery for management of regional node metastases or for salvage of persistent disease. In patients with locally advanced disease, randomized trials have shown concurrent chemotherapy and radiotherapy to be superior (significantly improved locoregional control and survival) compared with radiotherapy and it is preferred when organ-function conservation is the goal. However, because of the increased complexity and toxicity of this combined-modality approach, the success of this approach depends on the patient's adequate performance status and psychosocial resource availability.

Larynx

More than 12,500 cases of laryngeal cancer were diagnosed in the U.S. in 1994, and more than 10,000 of these were in men. Laryngeal cancer more commonly affects middle-aged or older men with a history of tobacco and/or alcohol intake. It is 50% more common in African-Americans than in whites and twice as common among whites as among Hispanics and Asians. It has a male-to-female ratio of 4.5:1, with a peak incidence in the sixth decade of life. In addition to tobacco (cigarette, cigar, pipe), certain dietary factors and exposure to wood dust, nitrogen mustard, asbestos, and nickel have been implicated as etiologic factors. More than 95% of cancers are squamous cell carcinomas.

Laryngeal cancers are divided into supraglottic, glottic, and subglottic. The epidemiology, natural history, common presenting symptoms, risk of nodal involvement, and prognosis for specific subsites of the larynx are shown in Table 5.

Early cancers not requiring laryngectomy (most T1–T2) can be treated with surgery or radiation therapy depending on physician and patient preferences (as discussed earlier). If lymph node involvement is present, neck dissection and/or radiation to the neck is indicated.

Locally advanced resectable tumors (T3–T4) may be treated with surgery followed by radiation if locoregional risk factors are present (close or positive margins, T4 tumor, lymphatic/vascular/perineural involvement, vascular invasion, multiple positive nodes, extracapsular invasion, subglottic extension, or prior tracheostomy). An alternative for patients who are interested in preserving laryngeal function is the use of combined radiation and chemotherapy. Two cycles of induction chemotherapy (Table 5) are given, and response is evaluated. Patients with CR receive definitive radiation therapy. In case of less than a partial response (<50% reduction in tumor dimensions), surgery is performed. Patients with a partial response (50% or more reduction in tumor dimensions) receive an additional cycle of chemotherapy followed by radiation therapy if CR is achieved; otherwise, salvage surgery is performed.

A large multicenter trial with long follow-up showed that this strategy could lead to laryngeal preservation without compromising survival as compared with surgery and radiation. Patients treated with chemotherapy had a higher rate of local recurrence requiring salvage laryngectomy. The group of patients with N2 and N3 disease was the most likely to have regional failure; therefore, close follow-up by a head and neck surgical oncologist is critical if larynx-preservation therapy is to be undertaken.

It is unclear if the addition of induction chemotherapy adds any benefit to radiation alone. The standard of care in Europe and Canada is radiation alone, and similar rates of survival (50%) and larynx preservation (65%) are reported from nonrandomized trials as for the previously mentioned American trial. An ongoing randomized trial in the U.S. is evaluating this question.

Speech rehabilitation is critically important for patients with advanced laryngeal cancer undergoing total laryngectomy (as primary treatment or salvage therapy). Phonation options include a mechanical electrolarynx, esophageal speech, and tracheoesophageal puncture. Each has advantages and disadvantages; however, most patients can obtain satisfactory communication through one of these techniques.

Whenever possible, these patients should be encouraged to enroll in clinical trials. Patients who are considered poor surgical or medical risks are candidates for definitive radiation therapy. The treatment for a patient with metastatic disease is discussed later.

Hypopharynx

The epidemiology, natural history, common presenting symptoms, risk of nodal involvement, and prognosis for specific subsites of the hypopharynx are shown in Table 6.

Early cancers not requiring laryngectomy (most T1, N0–1; small T2, N0) can be treated with surgery or radiation therapy depending on physician and patient preferences (as discussed earlier). Locally advanced resectable tumors (T3–T4, any N) may be treated with surgery followed by radiation. Surgery in these cases involves total laryngectomy and partial or total pharyngectomy and neck dissection. Despite this radical surgery and the consequent functional impairment experienced by patients, the prognosis for survival is poor. In the face of these facts, participation in clinical trials is emphasized for locally advanced cancers of the hypopharynx.

Combined-modality treatment with chemotherapy and radiation therapy is accepted as an alternative to resection in locally advanced resectable cancers (T2, T4, any N). This approach allows organ function preservation with survival equivalent to that after surgery. Two to three cycles of induction chemotherapy (see Table 6) are given, and this response is evaluated. Patients who achieve a CR receive definitive radiation therapy, whereas those achieving less than CR at the primary site undergo surgery.

Patients with poor medical or surgical risks can be treated with radiation therapy. The management of metastatic disease is discussed later.

Nasal Cavity and Paranasal Sinuses

The epidemiology, natural history, common presenting symptoms, risk of nodal involvement, and prognosis for carcinomas of the nasal cavity and paranasal sinuses are shown in Table 6.

The majority of the tumors are squamous cell carcinomas and are usually slow growing with low incidence of metastasis.

Patients with carcinomas of the nasal cavity and paranasal sinuses usually are first seen at advanced stages because of the relatively silent location of the tumor. The treatment of nasal cavity and paranasal sinus cancers follows the same general guidelines as those for oral cancer. If feasible, surgery is the preferred primary management.

Nasopharynx

Nasopharyngeal cancer differs from other head and neck cancers. The epidemiology, natural history, common presenting symptoms, risk of nodal involvement, and prognosis are shown in Table 6. It is extremely rare in most parts of the world, with an incidence of less than 1/100,000. However, it is endemic in certain areas, including North Africa, southeast Asia,

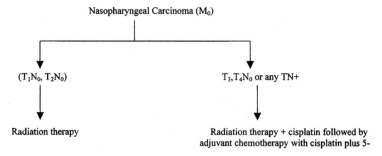

FIG. 5. Treatment of nasopharyngeal carcinoma (M0).

China, and the far northern hemisphere. Epstein–Barr virus (EBV) is strongly associated with nasopharyngeal carcinoma. This association has been demonstrated by serologic studies and by the detection of the viral genome in tumor samples. EBV induces malignant transformation in cell lines and is associated with other malignancies, including lymphoma and Hodgkin's disease.

Diet (salt-cured fish and meat) and genetic susceptibility are other probable risk factors; tobacco and alcohol are not, except in a minority of cases.

The World Health Organization (WHO) classification divides nasopharyngeal carcinoma into three types: type I, keratinizing squamous cell carcinoma; type II, nonkeratinizing squamous cell carcinoma; and type III, undifferentiated carcinoma. The latter, the most common type of nasopharyngeal carcinoma, is also known as lymphoepithelioma because of the characteristic exuberant lymphoid infiltrate accompanying the malignant epithelial cells.

The most common initial presentation of nasopharyngeal carcinoma is a neck mass. Other presenting signs and symptoms are related to tumor growth, with resulting compression or infiltration of neighboring organs. These include serous otitis media, nasal obstruction, tinnitus, pain, and cranial nerve involvement.

Nasopharyngeal carcinoma has a high metastatic potential to the regional nodes and to distant sites. WHO type I has the greatest propensity for uncontrolled local tumor growth and the lowest propensity for metastatic spread (60% clinically positive nodes) compared with WHO types II and III cancers (80–90% clinically positive nodes). Even though type I WHO cancers are associated with a lower incidence of lymphatic and distant metastases than are types II and III, its prognosis is worse because of a higher incidence of deaths from uncontrolled primary tumors and nodal metastases.

The prognoses for different stages of nasopharyngeal carcinoma are shown in Table 6.

General treatment guidelines are shown in Fig. 5. Surgery is usually not feasible because of anatomic considerations and is not recommended. Radiation has been the standard treatment, with good results (local control rates: T1–T2, 70–90%; T3–T4, 30–65%) and remains the standard of care for early (stages I and II) cancer.

The addition of chemotherapy to radiation in advanced cases was shown to prevent locoregional node recurrence and distant metastasis, and to improve overall survival (76% vs. 46% for radiation alone). Based on this study, concurrent chemoradiation is considered standard treatment for locally advanced nonmetastatic (stages III and IV) nasopharyngeal cancer in the U.S.

ADVANCED HEAD AND NECK TUMORS: UNRESECTABLE, RECURRENT, AND METASTATIC DISEASE

Radiation therapy has been considered the standard treatment for patients with newly diagnosed locally advanced disease that is deemed unresectable. However, combined-modality treatment with radiation therapy was shown in several recent trials to improve the overall survival, disease-free survival, and/or local control when compared with radiation therapy alone and is now considered an option depending on patient preference and performance.

Local or regional recurrences can be salvaged in some situations by radiation therapy or surgery, depending on the initial treatment. In patients with nasopharyngeal carcinoma, a second course of radiation may be delivered. If salvage is not possible, palliative treatment will be guided by the performance status of the patient.

Single-agent or combination chemotherapy is indicated for palliation of patients with local or distant recurrence and those who are first seen with distant metastasis. Combination chemotherapy achieves higher response rates at the cost of increased toxicity when compared with single-agent chemotherapy. The most active agents are listed in Table 7. Cisplatin plus infusional fluorouracil (Table 8) is the most commonly used combination-chemotherapy regimen in this setting. The choice of single-agent or combination chemotherapy will depend on patient preference and performance status. Patients with good performance status, no prior chemotherapy for treatment of recurrent disease, and minimal tumor burden may benefit most from combination chemotherapy. A subset of these patients may achieve durable CR and prolonged survival.

The median survival for patients with locally recurrent or disseminated disease is 6 months, and only 20% are alive at 1 year. No therapy has been shown to affect survival in this group of patients. Therefore whenever possible, patients should be encouraged to enroll in clinical trials evaluating new agents or new combination regimens.

Cancer of Unknown Primary (of the Head and Neck)

The work-up of a patient with a neck mass is shown in Fig. 3. In 10% of cases, a primary tumor is not found, and the term "cancer of unknown primary site" is used.

Cervical lymph node involvement (except supraclavicular) by carcinoma indicates a primary tumor in the head and neck. The unknown primary tumor of the head and neck is usually treated with neck dissection and radiation. The prognosis is roughly equivalent to cancers with the same N (nodal) status. Five-year survival ranges from 30% to 50% in patients treated definitively.

A supraclavicular mass usually represents spread from an infraclavicular (thoracic or abdominal) cancer, and the work-up and treatment of these cancers is discussed elsewhere in this book.

Salivary Gland Cancer

Salivary cancers make up about 3% of all head and neck cancers diagnosed in the U.S. every year. Tobacco and alcohol consumption are not considered risk factors, except possibly in women. Ionizing radiation and certain occupational exposures (rubber and automotive industries, wood and farm workers) have been associated with the development of salivary gland cancer.

The salivary glands are classified as major (parotid, submandibular, and sublingual) and minor (distributed along upper aerodigestive tract, predominantly in the oral and nasal cavities and the paranasal sinuses). Most of the salivary gland cancers arise from the parotid glands; sublingual and minor salivary gland cancers are rare.

Most salivary gland tumors are benign, and of these the most common histology is pleomorphic adenoma. It is characterized by slow growth and few symptoms, and is most frequently seen in the parotid gland. The most common presentation of benign salivary gland tumors is asymptomatic swelling of the lip, the parotid, or the submandibular or the sublingual glands. Persistent pain or neurologic involvement (mucosal or tongue numbness, facial nerve weakness) suggests malignant disease. The benign salivary gland tumors are listed in Table 9.

The clinical characteristics and prognosis of specific malignant salivary gland tumors are shown in Table 10.

TABLE 9. *Salivary gland benign tumors*

Pleomorphic adenoma (benign mixed tumor)
Warthin's tumor (papillary cystadenoma lymphomatosum)
Monomorphic adenoma
Benign lymphoepithelial lesion
Oncocytoma
Ductal papilloma
Sebaceous lymphadenoma

TABLE 10. *Salivary gland malignant tumors: clinical characteristics and prognosis*

Histology	Clinical characteristics	Prognosis
Mucoepidermoid carcinoma	Most common malignant tumor in major salivary glands. Most common in parotid (32%) Low grade: Local problems, long history, cure with aggressive resection. Rarely metastasizes High grade: locally aggressive, invades nerves and vessels and metastasizes early	Low grade: 76–95% 5-yr survival High grade: 30–50% 5-yr survival
Adenocarcinoma	16% of parotid and 9% of submandibular malignant tumors Grade correlates with survival	76–85% 5-yr survival 34–71% 10-yr survival
Squamous cell carcinoma	Uncommon: 7% of parotid gland and 10% of submandibular gland malignant tumors Grade correlates with survival Squamous cell carcinoma of temple, auricular and facial skin can metastasize to parotid nodes and can be confused with primary parotid tumor	24% 5-yr survival 18% 10-yr survival
Acinic cell carcinoma	Less than 10% of all salivary gland malignant tumors Low grade with slow growth, infrequent facial nerve involvement, infrequent and late metastases (lungs) Regional metastasis in 5–10% of patients	82% 5-yr survival 68% 10-yr survival
Adenoid cystic carcinoma	Most common malignant tumor in submandibular gland (41%), 11% of parotid gland High incidence of nerve invasion, which compromises local control 40% of patients develop metastases. Most common site of metastases is the lung. Patients may live many years with lung metastasis, but visceral or bone metastases indicate poor prognosis	50–90% 10 yr: 30–67% 15 yr: 25%
Malignant mixed tumor	14% of parotid gland and 12% of submandibular gland cancers May originate in previous pleomorphic adenoma Lymph node involvement in 25% of cases 26–32% of patients develop metastases	31–65% 10 yr; 23–30%

Surgery is the mainstay of treatment for all stages of salivary gland tumors. Postoperative radiation therapy is indicated for tumors that are of high-grade histology, large, with close or positive margins, and/or positive regional lymph nodes. Radiation therapy is the primary form of treatment for unresectable tumors. The role of chemotherapy is limited to the management of tumors that are either locally recurrent and unresectable or metastatic. There is no established standard chemotherapy for the treatment of salivary gland cancer because of the lack of formal trials with adequate numbers of patients. Regimens such as cisplatin + 5-FU or cisplatin + doxorubicin + cyclophosphamide result in transient responses in 20% to 30% of patients.

Follow-up

Patients with head and neck cancer treated with curative intent should be followed with a comprehensive head and neck physical examination every 1 to 3 months during the first year after treatment, every 2 to 4 months during the second year, every 3 to 6 months from years 3 to 5, and every 6 to 12 months after year 5. The thyroid-stimulating hormone (TSH) level should be checked every 12 months if the thyroid was irradiated. The recommendation for annual chest radiograph is controversial.

The first 2 years after the treatment of a head and neck cancer represent the period of highest risk of relapse. At 3 years and beyond, a second primary tumor in the lung or head and neck becomes the most important cause of morbidity or mortality. Because some recurrences, as well as second primaries, can be treated with curative intent, these patients should be followed closely with physical examinations, including laryngoscopies if indicated.

REFERENCES

1. *Cancer epidemiology and prevention.* 2nd ed. New York: Oxford University Press, 1996.
2. Browman GP, Cronin L. Standard chemotherapy in squamous cell head and neck cancer: what we have learned from randomized trials. *Semin Oncol* 1994;21:311–319.
3. Schrijvers D, Vermorken JB. Update on the taxoids and other new agents in head and neck cancer therapy. *Curr Opin Oncol* 1998;10:233–241.
4. Jacobs C, Lyman G, Velez-Garcia E, et al. A phase III randomized study comparing cisplatin and fluorouracil as single agents and in combination for advanced squamous cell carcinoma of the head and neck. *J Clin Oncol* 1992;10:257–263.
5. Forastiere A, Metch B, Schuller D, et al. Randomized comparison of cisplatin and 5-fluorouracil versus carboplatin + 5-FU versus methotrexate in advanced squamous cell carcinoma of the head and neck. *J Clin Oncol* 1992;10:1245–1251.
6. Kish JA, Ensley JF, Jacobs J, et al. A randomized trial of cisplatin (CACP) + 5-fluorouracil (5-FU) infusion and CACP + 5-FU bolus for recurrent and advanced squamous cell carcinoma of the head and neck. *Cancer* 1985;56:2740.
7. Department of Veterans Affairs Laryngeal Study Group. Induction chemotherapy plus radiation compared with advanced laryngeal cancer. *N Engl J Med* 1991;324:1685–1690.
8. Lefebvre JL, Chevalier D, Lubomski B, et al. Larynx preservation in hypopharynx and lateral epilarynx cancer: preliminary results of EORTC randomized phase III trial 24891. *J Natl Cancer Inst* 1996;88:890–899.
9. Adelstein DJ. Induction chemotherapy in head and neck cancer. *Hematol Oncol Clin North Am* 1999;13:689–698.
10. Laramore G, Scott C, Al-Sarraf M, et al. Adjuvant chemotherapy for resectable squamous cell carcinomas of the head and neck: report on Intergroup study 01034. *Int J Radiat Oncol Biol Phys* 1992;23:705–713.
11. Cooper JS, Pajak TF, Forastiere A, et al. Precisely defining high-risk operable head and neck tumors based on RTOG #85-03 and #88-24: targets for postoperative radiochemotherapy? *Head Neck* 1998;20:588–594.
12. Brizel DM. Radiotherapy and concurrent chemotherapy for the treatment of locally advanced head and neck squamous cell carcinoma. *Semin Radiat Oncol* 1998;8:237–246.
13. Bachaud JM, Choen-Jonathan E, Alzieu C, et al. Combined postoperative radiotherapy and weekly

cisplatin infusion for locally advanced head and neck carcinoma: final report of a randomized trial. *Int J Radiat Oncol Biol Phys* 1996;36:999–1004.

14. Pignon JP, Bourhis J, Domenge C, et al. Chemotherapy as an adjunct to definitive locoregional treatment for head and neck squamous cell carcinoma: results of three meta-analyses using updated individual data. *Lancet* (in press).

15. Al-Sarraf M, LeBlanc M, Giri PG, et al. Chemoradiotherapy versus radiotherapy in patients with advanced nasopharyngeal cancer: Phase III Randomized Intergroup Study 0099. *J Clin Oncol* 1998; 16:1310–1317.

16. Calais G, Alfonsi M, Bardet E, et al. Randomized trial of radiation therapy versus concomitant chemotherapy and radiation therapy for advanced-stage oropharynx carcinoma. *J Natl Cancer Inst* 1999;91:2081–2086.

17. Wendt TG, Grabenbauer GG, Rodel CM, et al. Simultaneous radiochemotherapy versus radiotherapy alone in advanced head and neck cancer: a randomized multicenter study. *J Clin Oncol* 1998:16:1318–1324.

18. Brizel DM, Albers ME, Fisther SR, et al. Hyperfractionated irradiation with or without concurrent chemotherapy for locally advanced head and neck cancer. *N Engl J Med* 1998;42:145.

19. Khuri FR, Lippman SM, Spitz MR, et al. Molecular epidemiology and retinoid chemoprevention of head and neck cancer. *J Natl Cancer Inst* 1997;89:199–211.

SECTION 2

Thorax

2

Non–Small Cell Lung Cancer

Oscar S. Breathnach

Lowe Center for Thoracic Oncology, Department of Adult Oncology, Dana Farber Cancer Institute, Harvard Medical School, Boston, Massachusetts 02115

Primary carcinoma of the lung was an uncommon cancer until the 1930s. The dramatic increase since then in the incidence of lung cancer has not yet abated. Lung cancer now is the most common cause of cancer mortality in both male and female patients in the United States of America. The long period between the initial exposure to tobacco carcinogens and the development of clinical lung cancer suggests that multiple steps are required to express the malignant phenotype. Prevention, through smoking prevention, will have the greatest impact on curbing lung cancer and prolonging survival.

CLINICAL FEATURES

Epidemiology

- 178,000 new cases and 158,000 deaths from non–small cell lung cancer (NSCLC) were expected for 1999.
- Peak frequency in sixth decade.
- Male > female patients.
- Only 13% of all patients with lung cancer are expected to live 5 years. Unfortunately these survival rates have been stationary over the past two decades, despite new therapeutic agents.

Risk Factors

Smoking

- 90% of patients with lung cancer have a smoking history.
- The cumulative probability of developing lung cancer in the general population for individuals up to age 74 years is 10% to 15% among those who smoke one or more packs of cigarettes per day.
- The risk of lung cancer after smoking cessation appears to be related to the level of consumption. The risk in persons who have smoked 1 to 20 cigarettes per day decreases to 1.6 at 16 years after stopping smoking. In those who have smoked 21 or more cigarettes per day, the risk of developing lung cancer at 16 years after quitting smoking remains fourfold that of a never-smoker.
- Sidestream smoke emitted from a smoldering cigarette between puffs contains virtually all of the carcinogenic compounds that have been identified in the mainstream smoke inhaled by smokers. The risk of dying of lung cancer is 30% higher for a nonsmoker living with a smoker compared with a nonsmoker living with a nonsmoker.

Occupational

- Exposure to agents such as arsenic, asbestos, beryllium, chloromethylethers, chromium, hydrocarbons, mustard gas, nickel, and radiation (including radon) has been linked with development of lung cancer.

Residential

- The exact risk of indoor exposure to radon remains uncertain.

Dietary

- Two recent studies have suggested an adverse effect on the incidence of lung cancer and overall mortality with the use of supplemental β-carotene and retinol administration in high-risk groups.

Familial/genetic

- The contributions of hereditary factors to the development of lung cancer are probably less well understood than those for any of the common forms of solid tumors in humans. Table 1 outlines a summary of known genetic changes in NSCLC.

Symptoms and Signs of Lung Cancer

- A minority of patients have an asymptomatic lesion that is discovered incidentally on a chest radiograph (Table 2).
- Most lung cancers, however, are discovered because of the development of a new or worsening existing symptom or sign.
- The clinical signs and symptoms of lung cancer may be divided into four categories: those resulting from local tumor growth, those from regional spread, those due to distant metastases, and those related to paraneoplastic syndromes. Table 3 outlines the characteristic symptoms or signs.

TABLE 1. *Genetic mutations in non–small cell lung cancers*

	NSCLC
Recessive oncogene (tumor-suppressor gene) and allelotype abnormalities	
Rb Mutations (13q14)	~20%
p16/CDKN2 mutations (9p21)	~50%
p53 mutations (17p13)	>50%
3p deletions	>80%
Microsatellite alterations	Present
Dominant oncogene abnormalities	
ras mutations	~30%
Her-2/neu overexpression	~30%
myc family amplification	>50%
bcl-2 overexpression	>50%
Telomerase expression	>90%

TABLE 2. *WHO classification of non–small cell lung cancer*

I. Squamous cell carcinoma
  a. Epidermoid
  b. Spindle cell variant
II. Adenocarcinoma
  a. Acinar
  b. Papillary
  c. Bronchioloalveolar
  d. Solid carcinoma with mucin
III. Large cell
  a. Giant cell
  b. Clear cell
IV. Adenosquamous

TABLE 3. *Symptoms and signs of lung cancer*

Primary disease
Central or endobronchial tumor growth
  Cough
  Sputum production
  Hemoptysis
  Dyspnea
  Wheeze (classically unilateral)
  Stridor
  Pneumonitis, with fever and productive cough (secondary to obstruction)
Peripheral tumor growth
  Pain, from pleural or chest wall involvement
  Cough
  Dyspnea
  Pneumonitis
Regional involvement (either direct or metastatic spread)
  Hoarseness (recurrent larnygeal nerve paralysis)
  Tracheal obstruction
  Dysphagia (esophageal compression)
  Dyspnea (pleural effusion, tracheal/bronchial obstruction, pericardial effusion, phrenic nerve palsy, lymphatic infiltration, superior vena cava obstruction)
  Horner's syndrome (sympathetic nerve palsy)
Metastatic involvement (common sites)
Bone involvement
  Pain, exacerbated by movement or weight bearing. Often worse at night
  Fracture
Liver metastases
  Right hypochondrial pain
  Icteris
  Altered mentation
Brain metastases
  Altered mental status
  Seizures
  Motor and sensory deficits
Paraneoplastic syndromes
  Clubbing
  Hypertrophic pulmonary osteoarthropathy
  Hypercalcemia
  Dermatomyositis
  Eaton–Lambert syndrome
  Hypercoagulable state
  Gynecomastia

MAKING THE DIAGNOSIS/PLANNING THERAPY

Goals

- Once a suspected tumor is identified, it is then necessary to obtain a histologic diagnosis and to stage the tumor accurately.
- The stage of the disease provides an index of the prognosis and allows selection of an appropriate therapeutic approach.
- In some cases, such as a patient with an asymptomatic, solitary pulmonary nodule, tissue diagnosis may not be established until the time of definitive surgical resection.
- Since 30% to 50% of all patients have metastatic disease at the time of presentation, clues to the clinical stage will often be evident on the clinical history and physical examination.
- Sputum cytology is the noninvasive pathologic technique for the diagnosis of NSCLC. It is most sensitive for centrally located tumors.
- Other noninvasive methods of tumor evaluation include chest radiographs, computed tomography (CT) of the chest (including the liver and adrenals), magnetic resonance imaging (MRI; in particular for superior sulcus tumors), and PET (positron emission tomography) scanning. These tests can only infer the presence of cancer.
- CT and MRI can provide information regarding hilar and mediastinal nodal involvement by tumor. Size is the criterion used to distinguish normal from abnormal nodes, with a short-axis nodal diameter of 1 cm typically used as the upper limit of normal. However, nodal enlargement may relate to hyperplastic reactive nodes, particularly after obstructive pneumonia.
- The accuracy of CT and MRI for detecting metastatic hilar (N1) or mediastinal disease is only 62% to 68% and 68% to 74%, respectively. Thus mediastinoscopy remains an important staging procedure.
- MRI is the investigation method of choice in evaluating superior sulcus tumors, because CT is limited by axial plane and streak artifact from the shoulders.

Pathologic Evaluation

- Invasive techniques are usually required to obtain the tissue sample(s) to make a conclusive histologic diagnosis.
- These procedures include bronchoscopy (with brushings, washings), transthoracic bronchial biopsy, CT-guided transthoracic biopsy, thoracocentesis (for pleural effusions), and mediastinoscopy with mediastinal node biopsy.
- Common sites of metastatic disease from NSCLC are lymph nodes, brain, bone, liver, and adrenal glands.
- Table 2 outlines the World Health Organization (WHO) classification of NSCLC.
- Adenocarcinoma is the most frequently diagnosed form of NSCLC in both men and women, having replaced squamous cell carcinoma.
- Bronchioloalveolar carcinoma, although currently classified as a subtype of adenocarcinoma, demonstrates clinical features that suggest it represents a distinct histologic form of NSCLC. These features are manifested as a greater tendency to occur in women and in non-smokers; the development of bilateral, multifocal pulmonary involvement, with a lesser tendency for extrathoracic metastases; and a better survival rate than similar stage NSCLC.

Staging

- Once a tissue diagnosis is securely made, the next step is to define the patient's disease stage.
- The current TMN staging system was revised in June 1997 (see Table 4 and Figure 1).

TABLE 4. *Lung cancer staging: TMN classification*

TX	Primary tumor cannot be assessed or tumor proven by the presence of malignant cells in sputum or bronchial washings but not visualized by imaging or bronchoscopy
T0	No evidence of primary tumor
Tis	Carcinoma in situ
T1	Primary tumor <3 cm in greatest dimension, surrounded by lung or visceral pleura, without bronchoscopic evidence of invasion more proximal than the lobar bronchus (i.e., not in the main bronchus)
T2	Tumor with any of the following features: >3 cm in greatest dimension Involves main bronchus, ≥2 cm from carina Invades the visceral pleura Associated with atelectasis or obstructive pneumonitis that extends to the hilar region but does not involve the entire lung
T3	Tumor of any size that directly invades any of the following: Chest wall (including superior sulcus tumors) Diaphragm Mediastinal pleura Parietal pericardium Involves main bronchus <2 cm from the carina Associated atelectasis/obstructive pneumonitis of the whole lung
T4	Tumor of any size that directly invades Mediastinum, trachea or carina, esophagus Vertebral body, heart, great vessels Malignant pleural/pericardial effusion Satellite tumor within the ipsilateral primary-tumor lobe of the lung
N1	Ipsilateral: peribronchial and/or hilar lymph nodes, intrapulmonary nodes by direct extension of primary
N2	Ipsilateral: mediastinal and/or subcarinal lymph nodes
N3	Contralateral: mediastinal, hilar, scalene, supraclavicular lymph nodes Ipsilateral: scalene, supraclavicular lymph nodes
M1	Presence of distant metastases

Stage I	T1–T2	N0	M0
Stage II	T1–T2,	N1 (T1–T2)	T3 N0	M0
Stage IIIA	T3 N1 M0,	N2 (T1–T3)	M0
Stage IIIB	N3 (T1–T4)	T4 (N0–N3)	M0
Stage IV	Any T	Any N	M1

Adapted from Mountain et al, 1997, with permission.

- The revised staging divides stage I and stage II into A and B categories, and modifies stage IIIA to more accurately represent the prognostic implications of the anatomic extent of disease. The T1 N0 M0, T2 N0 M0, and T1 N1 M0 anatomic subsets are designated as separate entities, and the T3 N0 M0 category is placed in stage IIB, to more accurately reflect the differences in clinical outcome.
- Stages IIIB and IV categories remained unchanged, with two exceptions: satellite tumor nodule(s) in the primary tumor lobe are designated T4, and separate metastatic tumor nodule(s) in the ipsilateral nonprimary tumor lobe(s) of the lung are designated M1.
- Despite very different clinical outcomes, no distinction has been made between stage IIIB disease with and without malignant effusion.
- Tables 4 through 6 give TMN descriptions and stages, the prognosis per clinical and pathologic stage, and the description of mediastinal nodal status, respectively.

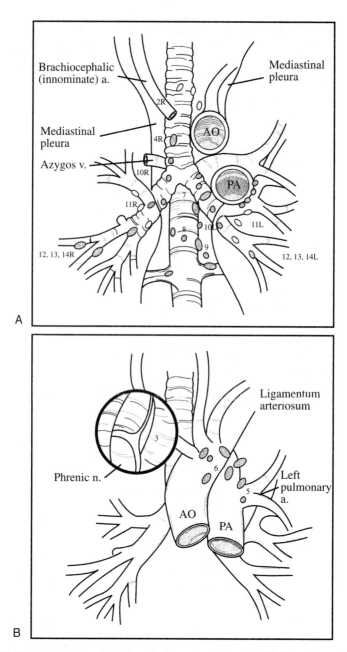

FIG. 1. A: Regional lymph node stations for lung cancer staging. C.F. Mountain and C.M. Dresler modifications from Naruke/ATS-LCSG Map. **B:** Legend for lymph node map.

TABLE 5. *Prognosis for clinical and pathologic stage of disease*

Stage		Clinical stage 5-yr survival (%)	Pathologic stage 5-yr survival (%)
T1 N0 M0	(IA)	61	67
T2 N0 M0	(IB)	38	57
T1 N1 M0	(IIA)	34	55
T2 N1 M0	(IIB)	24	39
T3 N0 M0	(IIB)	22	38
T3 N1 M0	(IIIA)	9	25
T1–3 N2 M0	(IIIA)	13	23
T4 N0–2 M0	(IIIB)	7	—
T1–4 N3 M0	(IIIB)	3	—
T1–4 N0–3 M1	(IV)	1	—

Adapted from Mountain et al, 1997, with permission.

TABLE 6. *Nodal stations for intrapulmonary, hilar, and mediastinal adenopathy*

N2 nodes (lie within the mediastinal pleural envelope)
  Superior mediastinum
    1. Highest mediastinal nodes
    2. Upper paratracheal nodes
    3. Prevascular/Retrotracheal nodes
    4. Lower paratracheal nodes
  Aortic nodes
    5. Subaortic nodes (aortopulmonary window)
    6. Paraaortic nodes (ascending aorta or phrenic nerve)
  Inferior mediastinum
    7. Subcarinal nodes
    8. Paraesophageal nodes (below carina)
    9. Pulmonary ligament nodes
N1 nodes (lie distal to the mediastinal pleural reflection and within the visceral pleura)
    10. Hilar nodes
    11. Interlobar nodes
    12. Lobar nodes
    13. Segmental nodes
    14. Subsegmental nodes

Adapted from Mountain et al, 1997, with permission.

Pretreatment Evaluation

- Preexisting medical conditions are evaluated, and the required therapeutic interventions instituted to maximize the patient's condition. This is particularly important in relation to the cardiopulmonary status.
- Pulmonary function tests help guide the feasibility of resection and the extent of possible resection. A minimal preresection FEV_1 (forced expiratory volume in 1 s) of 2 L, 1 L, and 0.6 L is required before considering a pneumonectomy, lobectomy, or segmentectomy, respectively. The FVC (forced vital capacity) should be at least 1.7 to 2 L as a general cut-off for resection candidates.
- Cigarette smoke acts as an irritant to the bronchial tree, contributing to excess mucus secretion and airway hyperactivity. Patients should be encouraged to stop smoking at least 8 weeks before the surgical resection.

Prognostic Features

- The patient's performance status (PS) is a key factor in predicting not only the patient's ability to receive therapy, but also the prognosis. Recognized prognostic factors are:

1. PS: Patients with PS 3–4 would not be regarded as appropriate candidates for either surgical resection or chemotherapy. Radiation therapy may be appropriate for specific issues, such as relief of bone pain resulting from bone metastases.
2. Stage of disease: The higher the stage, the worse the prognosis, as outlined in Table 5.
3. Weight loss: A documented weight loss of 10% in the 6 months before diagnosis is associated with a poor prognosis.
4. Presence of systemic symptoms: These symptoms usually reflect advanced-stage disease.
5. Histology: Patients with large cell carcinoma, followed by those with adenocarcinoma, are reported to have a poorer prognosis than those with either squamous cell or bronchioloalveolar carcinoma of the lung.
6. Sex: Women tend to have a better prognosis than men.
7. Gene mutations: p53 expression, K-*ras* mutations at codon 12, and lack of h-*ras* p21 expression are associated with a poor outcome.

MANAGEMENT

Treatment Modalities According to Stage of Disease

Early-Stage Disease (Stage I,II)

- Surgical resection is the treatment of choice in patients with stage I/II NSCLC, provided they are medically fit for the procedure.
- Lobectomy is the operation of choice in patients with adequate pulmonary reserves, based on results from the Lung Cancer Study Group (LCSG). The LCSG performed a randomized controlled trial comparing lobectomy with wedge resection in patients with T1 N0 M0 NSCLC. The rate of local recurrence was threefold greater in the patients receiving limited resection, although no statistical difference in survival was detected.
- For patients who are medically unfit for surgery, radiation therapy is the therapy of choice.
- Although no randomized trial has compared surgical resection with radiation therapy, results from retrospective comparisons favor surgery in long-term survival. However, one must remember that patients who are unfit for surgery, thus receiving radiation therapy, also are more likely to do less favorably.
- Various authors have reported on the rates of local and distal failure after surgical resection (see Table 7).
- The major causes of mortality in these patients were distal disease and second primary cancers.
- Data from the meta-analysis performed by the Non–Small Cell Lung Cancer Collaborative Group of 14 trials comparing surgical resection ± chemotherapy involved 4,357 patients with early-stage disease. Five of the trials used long-term alkylating agents. Eight more recent trials were cisplatin based, using either cyclophosphamide/doxorubicin/cisplatin (t = 3), cisplatin/vindesine (t = 3), or cisplatin/doxorubicin (t = 2). Alkylating agent–based therapy was associated with a 15% increase in the risk of death (p = 0.005). Cisplatin-based therapy was not associated with a statistically significant survival advantage. They also assessed data from seven trials comparing surgery with radiation therapy ± chemotherapy involving 807 patients with early-stage disease. Six of the trials involved cisplatin-based regimens. The overall hazard ratio of 0.98 was not statistically significant.
- Although neither adjuvant chemotherapy nor radiation therapy can be recommended as the standard of care, patients should be encouraged to participate in clinical trials evaluating

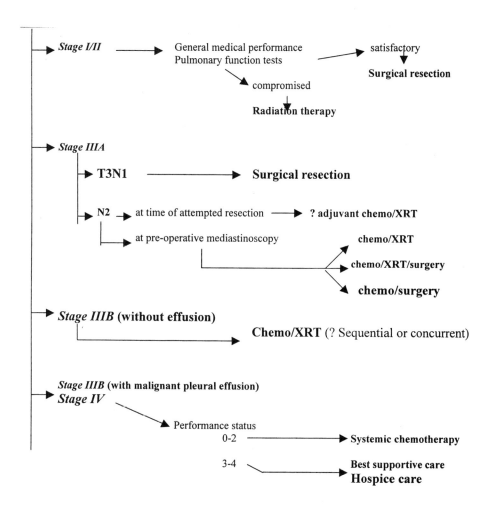

FIG. 2. An overview of current approaches in the treatment of patients with non–small cell lung cancer.

new approaches. As these patients are at increased risk of second primary tumors or recurrent disease, close follow-up is recommended (see Figure 2).

Stage IIIA Disease

• The best treatment for patients with stage IIIA disease is unclear, and the therapeutic approach remains an area of active investigation. Randomized trials and institutional series

TABLE 7. *Summary of recurrence rates after surgical resection in patients with early stage non–small cell lung cancer*

Author	Stage	No.	Thorax (%)	Distal (%)
Pairolero	T1 N0	170	6	15
	T2 N0	158	6	23
	T1 N1	18	28	39
Mountain	T3 N0/1	69	12	25
	T1/3 N2	92	1	32
Martini	T1 N1	17	0	47
	T2 N1	58	14	36
Iascone	T1 N0	16	19	6
	T2 N0	20	25	5

have sought several different treatment strategies for potentially resectable stage IIIA (N2) disease, including preoperative chemotherapy and radiation therapy, or chemotherapy and radiation therapy with no surgery.

- Surgical resection is the therapy of choice, but requires an experienced and skilled thoracic surgeon.
- Patients with clinical (preoperative) N0 or N1 disease but microscopic pathologic (postresection) N2 disease survive longer than do patients with clinical N2 disease, with 5-year survival rates of 34% and 9%, respectively.
- Neoadjuvant chemotherapy has the theoretic advantage of diminishing nodal involvement, thus making surgical intervention less difficult, more likely to have an impact on survival, and more likely to provide immediate systemic therapy in patients at high risk for distal relapse. However, local treatment is delayed, and the tumor volume, if it does not respond adequately to the chemotherapy, may become unresectable. The continued presence of N2 nodal involvement after neoadjuvant chemotherapy is associated with a poor prognosis.
- Two prospective randomized phase III trials assessing the role of neoadjuvant chemotherapy showed a statistically significant survival advantage in favor of the chemotherapy arm (see Table 8). However, there were a number of potential flaws in these trials. Both trials were terminated prematurely because of strong statistical significance at the interval evaluation, and so only a limited number of patients were treated per arm in each trial. In one of the trials (13), both treatment arms received radiation therapy after the surgery. There was also stage heterogeneity in the Rosell study, since patients with stage T3 N0 N0 were included, who would be considered as having stage II disease under the new staging clas-

TABLE 8. *Summary of selected phase III trials in patients with stage IIIA NSCLC comparing surgical resection with neoadjuvant chemotherapy and resection showing a statistically significant difference in survival*

Author	No.	Chemotx.	Schedule	Median surv.	Actuarial surv.
Roth et al.	26	CEP	CEP->Surg.	64	56% @ 3yr
	32	—	Surg. alone	11	15% @ 3 yr
Rosell et al.	30	MIC	MIC->Surg. Postop XRT (50 Gy)	26	25% @ 2 yr
	30	—	Surg. alone Postop XRT (50 Gy)	8	0 @ 2 yr

CEP, Cyclophosphamide, etoposide, and cisplatin; MIC, mitomycin C, ifosfamide, and cisplatin; Postop. XRT, postoperative mediastinal radiation therapy.

sification. None of the patients in the control arm in this study were alive at 2 years, which is unexpected and would not reflect the usual survival rates of stage IIIA disease. In addition, there was a disproportionate number of patients with K-*ras* mutations within the control group, potentially biasing the results. This higher proportion of patients with K-*ras* mutations in the "surgery alone" arm may have contributed to the poor outcome observed in this group.

Stage IIIB Disease (in Absence of Malignant Pleural Effusions)

- Patients with T4 lesions, bulky multilevel N2, or N3 involvement are not eligible for curative surgical resection.
- Traditionally radiation therapy alone was the standard therapy. However, this was associated with 5-year failure rates within the ipsilateral chest and systemically of 90% and 50% to 70%, respectively. Chemotherapy was added in an attempt to overcome these high relapse rates and poor outcomes with radiation therapy alone.
- The most appropriate scheduling of the chemotherapy and radiation therapy is still under evaluation, as is the most efficacious fractionation of the radiation therapy. The various options are concurrent, sequential, or alternating schedules.

1. Sequential scheduling aims to avoid the interactions between the two modalities, thereby limiting toxicity.
2. Concurrent scheduling aims to maximize the therapeutic effect from chemosensitization, but also results in potentiation of toxicity.
3. Rapidly alternating schedules allow time for recovery from the acute toxicity of each modality.

- The various forms of radiation fractionation are standard, hyperfractionated, accelerated, continuous hyperfractionated accelerated radiation therapy (CHART), and hypofractionated split-course therapy.
- Data from the Non–Small Cell Lung Cancer Collaborative Group's meta-analysis included 22 trials, with 3,033 patients, assessing radical radiation therapy ± chemotherapy. Five trials included long-term alkylating agents. Eleven trials (1,780 patients) included cisplatin-based therapy. Chemotherapy showed a significant overall benefit, with a hazard ratio of 0.90 ($p = 0.006$), a 10% reduction in the risk of death, which translates into an absolute benefit of 3% at 2 years and 2% at 5 years.
- Trials using cisplatin-based therapy yielded the strongest evidence for a positive chemotherapy effect, with a hazard ratio of 0.87 ($p = 0.005$).
- Two phase III trials comparing sequential chemoradiation and one phase III trial evaluating concurrent chemoradiation therapy with radiation alone showed statistically significant increases in survival over radiation therapy alone (Table 9). The chemotherapy regimens tested in these settings have been predominantly cisplatin based.
- The sequential schedule was associated with similar local control in both groups, but lower rates of distal metastases, which may be responsible for the prolonged survival in the combined-modality arms of the trials.
- The concurrent schedule was associated with improved local control, with no influence on systemic metastases.
- A recent phase III study in patients with unresectable stage III NSCLC comparing concurrent and sequential radiation therapy, in association with mitomycin, vindesine, and cisplatin chemotherapy, reported a significantly increased response rate and enhanced median survival duration in favor of the concurrent approach.
- The role of triple therapy (chemotherapy, radiation therapy, and surgical resection) over combination chemoradiation is also under evaluation in phase III trials.

TABLE 9. *Summary of selected phase III trials showing a statistically significant difference in survival in patients with locally advanced NSCLC*

	No. of pts	Chemo	XRT (Gy)	MST (mo.)	Survival % 1 yr	3 yr	p Value
Sequential therapy							
Dillman et al.	78	PV	60c	13.8	55	23	0.007
	77		60c	9.7	40	11	
Le Chevalier et al.	176	VCPC	65c	12.0	50	11	0.02
	177		65c	10.0	41	5	
Concurrent therapy							
Schaake-Koning et al.	107	P daily	55s	NR	54	16	0.009
	110	P weekly	55s	NR	44	13	
	114		55s	NR	46	2	
Concurrent versus sequential therapy							
Furuse et al.							
Concurrent	156	MVC	56	16.5	NR	22	0.04
Sequential	158	MVC	56	13.3	NR	15	

The trials compared sequential or concurrent chemoradiation therapy with radiation alone, and sequential chemoradiation with concurrent therapy.

Pancoast Tumor/Superior Sulcus Tumor

- The syndrome described by Pancoast in 1924 comprises the characteristic and constant clinical phenomenon of pain in the distribution of the eighth cervical and first and second thoracic spinal nerves, a Horner's syndrome, with radiologic evidence of a small homogeneous radiologic density at the apex of the lung, and minor or major destruction of the ribs and vertebral infiltration.
- Superior sulcus tumors are at least T3, and may be T4, as per the TMN staging classification.
- Nodal involvement is a prognostic indicator of poor outcome, as are positive resection margins and metastatic disease.
- Sixty percent of patients have adenocarcinoma.
- Untreated patients have an average survival of 10 to 14 months after diagnosis.
- Several early reports suggested that external beam radiation therapy could produce long-term survivals.
- Combination radiation therapy and surgical resection appears most advantageous, if possible, and represents the standard of care. Five-year survival rates of up to 15% to 50% have been reported with this approach.
- No direct randomized clinical trial comparing sequencing of radiation and surgery in these patients has been performed.
- Indirect evidence from Ginsberg et al. (8) suggests similar results with either pre- or post-surgical radiation therapy.
- Patients with T4 lesions (invasion of vertebral bodies, subclavian vessel) have a poorer prognosis, with 5-year survival rates of 9% to 11%. In those with suspected subclavian vessel involvement, an anterior approach is critical to facilitate resection.
- Rib involvement may have no impact on survival rates in resectable cases (5-year survival, 45–56%), although one study with 23 such patients revealed a statistically significant disadvantage [2-year pulmonary function score (PFS), 37% vs. 25%] on PFS. Of 75 patients, from six studies, with resected N2, N3 disease, the 4-year survival was 8%.

- Ipsilateral supraclavicular nodal involvement (N3) seems to have a better prognosis than does ipsilateral mediastinal nodes (N2).
- In a nonrandomized review of 100 patients with resected superior sulcus tumors, patients treated with lobectomy had twice the 5-year survival of patients treated with wedge resections (65% vs. 30%, respectively; $p = 0.06$). All patients had chest wall resection in addition to the pulmonary resection. The local recurrence rates were similar (23% vs. 38%, respectively).
- Most common sites of residual disease are the brachial plexus, the neural foramina, the vertebral bodies, and the subclavian veins.
- The most common sites of metastases are brain and bone.
- Patients with incomplete resections have similar overall survival rates to those who were not resected. There appears to be no survival benefit to postoperative irradiation in patients with incompletely resected disease.

Advanced Disease (Stage IIIB with Malignant Pleural Effusions, and Stage IV)

- The survival of patients with advanced stage (stage IIIB with malignant effusions, and stage IV) NSCLC is extremely poor.
- The therapeutic approach includes consideration of systemic chemotherapy or supportive therapy alone if the patient's general condition is not suitable for systemic chemotherapy.
- Best supportive care (BSC) produces median survival rates of 16 to 17 weeks, and 1-year survival rates of 10% to 15%.
- Data evaluated from the meta-analysis performed by Non–Small Cell Lung Cancer Collaborative Group included 1,190 patients with NSCLC from 11 trials, comparing supportive care with supportive care plus chemotherapy. Eight of the trials included cisplatin-based regimens. The majority of the trials, however, included patients with both unresectable locally advanced and advanced disease. Therapy with alkylating agents had a negative impact on survival (hazard ratio, 1.26), but the result was based on only two trials. The cisplatin-based trials showed a benefit of chemotherapy with a hazard ratio of 0.73 ($p < 0.0001$), equivalent to an absolute improvement in survival of 10% (5–15%) at 1 year, or an increase in median survival of 1½ months (1–2½ months).
- Completed prospective randomized trials including quality-of-life analyses show that cisplatin-based therapeutic regimens also improve quality of life in these patients.
- On the basis of these collective data, the American Society of Clinical Oncology guidelines on advanced NSCLC recognize the survival and quality-of-life advantages that chemotherapy can impart to patients with advanced-stage NSCLC.
- However, the greatest benefit is associated with patients with good performance status (ECOG PS 0–1). Treatment-related toxicity is increased in patients with lower performance status (ECOG PS 3,4).
- Agents in phase III trials in patients with advanced NSCLC include the taxanes (paclitaxel and docetaxel), vinca alkaloid (vinorelbine), antimetabolite (gemcitabine), and camptothecin (irinotecan). These agents have shown promise in both phase I and II trials, both as single agents and in combination with a platinum agent. One-year survival rates of up to 40% have been commonly reported.
- Trials using two of these more recent agents in combination are under way, in an effort to avoid platinum-related toxicities and to increase survival. Nonetheless, few if any patients with advanced-stage disease live up to 5 years.
- Because of the modest results from chemotherapy, predictable toxicity, and high costs of new chemotherapy agents, there has been concern about the clinical benefits and economic value of chemotherapy in these patients.
- However, data from Canada, which compared patients with advanced-stage NSCLC treated either with BSC or platinum-based chemotherapy, confirmed that systemic chemotherapy is more cost-effective than BSC.

- More recent economic comparisons have focused on comparing newer agents with older regimens, and have reported favorable findings.
- Patients should receive between two and eight cycles of chemotherapy, with six cycles being the usual practice, in stable or responsive disease.
- Prolonged or maintenance chemotherapy is associated with cumulative toxicities with limited additional clinical benefit.
- Patients who progress on or after first-line chemotherapy may be offered second-line chemotherapy, provided their PS remains good (ECOG 0–2).

Best Supportive Care

- At all stages of disease, it is important to attend to the symptoms experienced by patients. These include therapy-related factors such as nausea, vomiting, anemia, and disease-related issues such as pain, dyspnea (from either parenchymal involvement or effusions), ataxia (cerebral involvement or peripheral neuropathy), and confusion (metabolic effects).
- Adequate antiemetic coverage before and after chemotherapy is essential and should be based on the emetogenic potential of the chemotherapeutic agent(s) prescribed for the individual patient.
- Anxiety is a common problem in patients with cancer and can be debilitating.
- Patients who stop smoking on their diagnosis of lung cancer are prone to develop depression; a high level of awareness of this potential issue should be maintained by the treating physician.
- By addressing these issues early, quality of life of patients can be maintained at the maximal possible level.
- When chemotherapy no longer has a role, extra support for the patient and family is available through hospice services.

NOVEL THERAPEUTIC APPROACHES

Several of the current directions in new treatment approaches follow.

- Photodynamic therapy.
- Endobronchial implants.
- Hypoxic cytotoxins (e.g., tirapazamine).
- Monoclonal antibodies to tumor factor receptors (e.g., trastuzumab).
- Signal-transduction modulators (e.g., bryostatin, UCN-01, farnesyl transferase inhibitors).
- Matrix metalloproteinase inhibitors/antiangiogenesis agents (e.g., marimastat, antiVEGF, endostatin).
- Gene replacement therapy (e.g., Ad-p53).
- Vaccine-based therapy.
- Immunotherapy

Screening

- Screening for lung cancer remains an issue of great debate, in terms of both the most appropriate approach and the expected impact.
- Four prospective randomized trials evaluating early detection of NSCLC by chest radiograph have failed to demonstrate a significant reduction in lung cancer mortality resulting from screening. They included 37,724 male cigarette smokers. No women were included.
- Two of the studies, the Memorial–Sloan Kettering Lung Project (MSKLP) and the Johns Hopkins Lung Project (JHLP), were designed to assess the impact of the addition of four monthly sputum cytologies to annual chest radiograph evaluations. They concluded that sputum cytology added no benefit over chest radiograph alone. The long-term survival rates

in the experimental and control groups in the MSKLP and JHLP were superior to the Surveillance Epidemiology and End Results (SEER) data during the same period.
- The other two studies, the Mayo Lung Project (MLP) and the Czechoslovakia study (CS), compared regular screening with chest radiographs in the experimental group, and infrequent or no rescreening in the control group. Both studies found advantages favoring the experimental population with regard to stage distribution, resectability, and survival.
- In view of the lack of significant reduction in mortality, screening for the detection of early-stage lung cancer is not recommended by any major public policy advisory organization.
- There is renewed interest in defining the role of screening in those persons at high risk for lung cancer.
- Retrospective data show an increased risk of second lung cancer after a diagnosis of prior lung cancer. In those with NSCLC, 1% to 2% of patients per year will develop a second primary.
- New techniques such as low-dose spiral CT scan, autofluorescent bronchoscopy, and molecular markers in sputum cytology must be evaluated.

Chemoprevention

- No strategy has been proven effective for preventing NSCLC in at-risk individuals.
- Two large trials using development of lung cancer as a primary end point have now been completed. Both demonstrated an adverse risk of lung cancer with β-carotene.
- The first study involved 29,133 men aged 50 to 69 years from Finland, who were heavy cigarette smokers at entry (average, one pack/day for 36 years). The study randomized participants to receive either supplemental β-carotene, α-tocopherol, the combination, or placebo for 5 to 8 years. Unexpectedly, participants receiving β-carotene (alone or in combination with α-tocopherol) had a statistically significant 18% increase in lung cancer incidence [relative risk (RR), 1.18; 95% confidence interval (CI), 1.03–1.36] and an 8% increase in total mortality (RR, 1.08; 95% CI, 1.01–1.16) relative to participants receiving placebo. Supplemental β-carotene did not appear to affect the incidence of other major cancers occurring in this population.
- The finding of an increased incidence of lung cancer in β-carotene–supplemented smokers was replicated in the CARET (Carotene and Retinol Efficacy Trial). CARET was a multicenter lung cancer prevention trial of supplemental β-carotene plus retinol, versus placebo in asbestos workers and smokers. This trial was terminated prematurely because interim analyses of the data indicated that the supplemented group was developing more lung cancer, not less, consistent with the results of the Finnish trial. Overall, lung cancer incidence was increased by 28% in the supplemented subjects (RR, 1.28; 95% CI, 1.04–1.57), and total mortality was also increased (RR, 1.17; 95% CI, 1.03–1.33). The increase in lung cancer after supplementation with β-carotene and retinol was observed for current but not former smokers.
- *Cis*-retinoic acid has been shown to have benefit in patients with leukoplakia and head/neck cancer. The chemopreventive potential of 13-*cis*-retinoic acid in patients with stage I NSCLC after resection has been assessed. The trial closed in April 1997, and the mature data are awaited. Continued research and patient participation are required to define the best approach toward chemoprevention.

Suggested Therapeutic Chemotherapy Regimens
Paclitaxel + Carboplatin (per CALGB 9730)

Premedication (see Table 10)

1. Dexamethasone, 20 mg p.o., for two doses, 12 and 6 hours before starting paclitaxel on day 1.

TABLE 10. *Dose modifications of paclitaxel and carboplatin*

ANC (cells/mm³)	Platelets (/mm³)	Paclitaxel and carboplatin dosages
≥1,500	>100,000	100%
<1,500	<100,000	0[a]

[a]Repeat counts weekly; recommence therapy after counts are adequate.

2. Diphenhydramine, 50 mg i.v., 0.5 hour before starting paclitaxel on day 1.
3. Ranitidine, 50 mg i.v., 0.5 hour before starting paclitaxel on day 1.

Chemotherapy

1. Paclitaxel, 225 mg/m² i.v. over 3 hours on day 1 (total dose/cycle = 225 mg/m²).
2. Carboplatin, i.v., over 60 minutes on day 1, after paclitaxel; dosage is calculated by the Calvert formula to achieve a target area under the curve (AUC) of 6 mg/mL/min.
   • Treatment cycle repeats every 21 days.
   • Treatment duration is a total of six cycles.
   Calvert formula: Total dose [mg] = (Target AUC [mg/mL/min]) × (GFR [ml/min] + 25)
   • For intracycle fever and neutropenia (F/N), add to subsequent cycles primary hematopoietic growth factor support with filgrastim, 5 µg/kg/day s.c., starting on cycle day 3.
   • Continue filgrastim until absolute neutrophil count (ANC) > 1,000/mm³ for 3 consecutive days after ANC nadirs.
   • For patients who experience F/N or grade IV neutropenia in spite of filgrastim prophylaxis, reduce all antineoplastic chemotherapy doses by 20% during subsequent cycles (i.e., 80% of the previous cycle dosage).
   • For patients who experience platelet nadir counts <25,000/mm³, decrease carboplatin target dosage to AUC = 5 mg/mL/min for all subsequent cycles.
   • If platelet nadir counts remain <25,000/mm³ after decreasing the carboplatin target AUC to 5 mg/mL/min, decrease the target dosage to AUC = 4 mg/mL/min during subsequent cycles.
   • Discontinue therapy with evidence of disease progression or excessive toxicity or at a patient's request.

Vinorelbine + Cisplatin (per SWOG 93-08)

Pretreatment (see Tables 11 and 12)

1. Start intravenous hydration with ≥1,000 to 2,000 mL over 4 hours before starting cisplatin.
2. Give mannitol diuresis, and continue hydration after cisplatin administration.

TABLE 11. *Dose modifications of vinorelbine and cisplatin*

ANC (cells/mm³)	Platelets (/mm³)	Dosage modifications
≥1,500	>100,000	100%
1,000–1,499	75,000–99,999	50%
<1,000	<75,000	0[a]

[a]Repeat counts weekly; recommence therapy after counts are adequate.

TABLE 12. *Pretreatment with vinorelbine*

Serum biliburin	Dosage modification
2.1–3 mg/dL	Reduce vinorelbine by 50%
>3 mg/dL	Reduce vinorelbine dose by 75%

3. Give antiemetic primary prophylaxis with a serotonin receptor antagonist and dexamethasone ± lorazepam.

Chemotherapy

1. Vinorelbine, 25 mg/m^2/dose i.v. infusion over 30 minutes for four doses, days 1, 8, 15, and 22 (total dose/cycle = 100 mg/m^2).
2. Cisplatin, 100 mg/m^2 i.v., day 1 (total dose/cycle = 100 mg/m^2).
   - Treatment cycle repeats every 28 days.
   - Treatment duration is a total of six cycles.
   - For treatment delays longer than 2 weeks but ≤3 weeks or for an F/N episode in a prior cycle, reduce the dosage of both drugs by 50% (i.e., 50% of the previous cycle's dosage).
   - For an ANC nadir <500/mm^3 and/or platelet nadir <50,000 in a prior cycle, reduce the cisplatin dosage by 50%.
   - Dose reductions for vinorelbine are based on the weekly cycle as previously outlined.
   - Serum creatinine ≥1.6 mg/dL or creatinine clearance ≥50 mL/min, decrease the cisplatin dosage by 50%.
   - For day 1 creatinine clearance <50 mL/min, withhold cisplatin.
   - If creatinine clearance has not improved after 1-week delay, retreat at a 50% dose level.
   - Discontinue therapy if evidence of disease progression or excessive toxicity or at a patient's request.

Gemcitabine + Cisplatin

Pretreatment (Table 13)

1. Start intravenous hydration with ≥1,000 to 2,000 mL over 4 hours before starting cisplatin.
2. Give mannitol diuresis and continue hydration after cisplatin administration.
3. Give antiemetic primary prophylaxis with a serotonin receptor antagonist and dexamethasone ± lorazepam.

Chemotherapy

1. Gemcitabine, 1,000 mg/m^2 per dose i.v. infusion over 30 minutes for four doses, days 1, 8, and 15 (total dose/cycle, 3,000 mg/m^2).

TABLE 13. *Modifications of gemcitabine and cisplatin*

ANC (cells/mm^3)	Platelets (/mm^3)	Dosage modifications
≥1,000	>100,000	100%
500–999	50,000–99,999	75%
<500	<50,000	0[a]

ANC, absolute neutrophil count.
[a]Repeat counts weekly; recommence therapy after counts are adequate.

2. Cisplatin, 100 mg/m^2 i.v., day 1 (total dose/cycle, 100 mg/m^2).
   - Treatment cycle repeats every 28 days.
   - Treatment duration is a total of six cycles.
   - If ANC nadir count was <500 cells/mm^3 and/or platelet nadir counts were <50,000/mm^3 during the prior cycle, omit the next dose.
   - For a creatinine clearance <40 mL/min, withhold cisplatin and decrease gemcitabine dosage by 25% (i.e., 75% of the previous cycle dosage).
   - For a creatinine clearance of 40 to 60 mL/min, decrease the cisplatin dose by 40% (i.e., 60% of the previous cycle dosage), and decrease the gemcitabine dose by 25% (i.e., 75% of the previous cycle dosage).
   - Discontinue therapy if evidence of disease progression or excessive toxicity or at a patient's request.

REFERENCES

1. Landis SH, Murray T, Bolden S, et al. Cancer statistics, 1999. *CA Cancer J Clin* 1999;49:8–31.
2. Villeneuve PJ, Mao Y. Lifetime probability of developing lung cancer, by smoking status, Canada. *Can J Publ Health* 1994;85:385–388.
3. Wiencke JK, Thurston SW, Kelsey KT, et al. Early age at smoking initiation and tobacco carcinogen DNA damage in the lung. *J Natl Cancer Inst* 1999;91:614–619.
4. Garfinkel L, Silverberg E. Lung cancer and smoking trends in the United States over the past 25 years. *CA Cancer J Clin* 1991;41:137–145.
5. Wingo PA, Ries LA, Giovino GA, et al. Annual report to the nation on the status of cancer, 1973-1996, with a special section on lung cancer and tobacco smoking. *J Natl Cancer Inst* 1999;91: 675–690.
6. Salgia R, Skarin A. Molecular abnormalities in lung cancer. *J Clin Oncol* 1998;16:1207–1217.
7. The World Health Organization. Histological typing of lung tumors. *Am J Clin Pathol* 1982;77: 123–136.
8. Ginsberg RJ, Rubenstein LV. Randomized trial of lobectomy versus limited resection for T1 N0 non-small cell lung cancer. *Ann Thorac Surg* 1995;60:615–623.
9. Group N-SCLCC. Chemotherapy in non-small cell lung cancer: a meta-analysis using updated data on individual patients from 52 randomized clinical trials. *Br Med J* 1995;311:899–909.
10. Souquet PJ, Chauvin F, Boissel JP, et al. Polychemotherapy in advanced non small cell lung cancer: a meta-analysis. *Lancet* 1993;342:19–21.
11. PORT Meta-analysis Trialists Group. Postoperative radiotherapy in non-small-cell lung cancer: systematic review and meta-analysis of individual patient data from nine randomised controlled trials. *Lancet* 1998;352:257–263.
12. Roth JA, Fossella F, Komaki R, et al. A randomized trial comparing perioperative chemotherapy and surgery with surgery alone in resectable stage IIIA non-small-cell lung cancer. *J Natl Cancer Inst* 1994;86:673–680.
13. Rosell R, Gomez-Codina J, Camps C, et al. A randomized trial comparing preoperative chemotherapy plus surgery with surgery alone in patients with non-small-cell lung cancer. *N Engl J Med* 1994;330:153–158.
14. Dillman RO, Seagren SL, Propert KJ, et al. A randomized trial of induction chemotherapy plus high-dose radiation versus radiation alone in stage III non-small-cell lung cancer. *N Engl J Med* 1990;323:940–945.
15. LeChevalier T, Arriagada R, Quoix E, et al. Radiotherapy alone versus combined chemotherapy and radiotherapy in nonresectable non-small-cell lung cancer: first analysis of a randomized trial in 353 patients. *J Natl Cancer Inst* 1991;83:417–423.
16. Schaake-Koning C, Van dan Bogaert W, Dalesio O, et al. Effects of concomitant cisplatin and radiotherapy on inoperable non-small-cell lung cancer. *N Engl J Med* 1992;326:524–530.
17. Albain KS, Rusch VW, Crowley JJ, et al. Concurrent cisplatin/etoposide plus chest radiotherapy followed by surgery for stages IIIA (N2) and IIIB non-small-cell lung cancer: mature results of Southwest Oncology Group phase II study 8805. *J Clin Oncol* 1995;13:1880–1892.
18. Furuse K, Fukuoka M, Kawahara M, et al. Phase III study of concurrent versus sequential thoracic radiotherapy in combination with mitomycin, vindesine, and cisplatin in unresectable stage III non-small cell lung cancer. *J Clin Oncol* 1999;17:2692–2699.

19. Bunn PA, Kelly K. New chemotherapeutic agents prolong survival and improve quality of life in non-small cell lung cancer: a review of the literature and future directions. *Clin Cancer Res* 1998;5: 1087–1100.
20. Clinical practice guidelines for the treatment of unresectable non- small-cell lung cancer: adopted on May 16, 1997 by the American Society of Clinical Oncology. *J Clin Oncol* 1997;15:2996–3018.
21. Ettinger DS, Cox JD, Ginsberg RJ, et al. NCCN Non-Small-Cell Lung Cancer Practice Guidelines: the National Comprehensive Cancer Network. *Oncology (Huntingt)* 1996;10:81–111.
22. Johnson BE. Second lung cancers in patients after treatment for an initial lung cancer. *J Natl Cancer Inst* 1998;90:1335–1345.
23. Strauss GM, Gleason RE, Sugarbaker DJ. Chest x-ray screening improves outcome in lung cancer: a reappraisal of randomized trials on lung cancer screening. *Chest* 1995:107:270S–279S.
24. Henschke CI, McCauley DI, Yankelevitz DF, et al. Early Lung Cancer Action Project: overall design and findings from baseline screening. *Lancet* 1999;354:99–105.
25. Calvert AH, Newell DR, Gumbrell LA, et al. Carboplatin dosage: prospective evaluation of a simple formula based on renal function. *J Clin Oncol* 1989;7:1748–1756.

3

Small Cell Lung Cancer

Ramaprasad Srinivasan and Frederic Kaye

*Medicine Branch, DCS, National Cancer Institute,
National Institutes of Health, Bethesda, Maryland*

Small cell lung cancer (SCLC) constitutes approximately 15% to 25% of all lung cancers. SCLC has an aggressive natural history, with a much greater propensity for regional and distant metastases than the other major types of lung cancer. SCLC also differs from non–small cell lung cancer (NSCLC) in being highly sensitive to initial chemotherapy and radiation therapy. The principles of management of this class of tumors are hence significantly different from those pertaining to NSCLC.

EPIDEMIOLOGY AND ETIOLOGY

Approximately 35,000 to 40,000 new cases of SCLC are diagnosed in the United States every year, comprising 18% of all lung cancers as assessed by the National Cancer Institute's Surveillance, Epidemiology, and End Results data. Epidemiologic data suggest that SCLC is increasing in incidence, particularly in women.

Risk factors implicated in the development of SCLC include

- Cigarette smoking, by far the most important risk factor.
- Exposure to uranium, as in uranium miners.
- Exposure to radon gas.

SCLC is distinguished from all other human cancers by its high incidence of tumor-suppressor gene inactivation.

- More than 90% of SCLCs inactivate p53 function, which is an important sensor of DNA damage and regulates progression through cell-cycle checkpoints.
- More than 90% inactivate Rb function, a major determinant of the G_1/S cell-cycle checkpoint.
- More than 90% show deletions on the short arm of chromosome 3, suggesting the presence of additional important candidate tumor-suppressor genes for SCLC.

SCLC shows overexpression of many dominant oncogenes including the following.

- *Myc*, a family of nuclear phosphoproteins that regulate transcription.
- KIT, growth factor receptor with tyrosine kinase activity.
- KIT ligand (stem cell factor).
- Telomerase, which is believed to block senescence by preventing telomeric shortening.

PATHOLOGY

An accurate pathologic diagnosis is essential for treatment planning. This is aided by obtaining tissue blocks wherever possible, because crush artifacts in needle aspirations or bronchoscopy can lead to mistaken diagnoses of SCLC. The older term, "oat-cell," is believed to reflect the morphology of crush artifact.

The cell of origin of SCLC is undefined but is believed to be the peptide hormone–secreting basal neuroendocrine or Kulchitsky's cell. These cells often stain with silver and have demonstrable neurosecretory granules.

The current pathologic classification of SCLC recognizes three classes:

1. Small cell carcinoma (commonest, comprising more than 90% of all SCLCs);
2. Mixed small and large cell variant; and
3. Combined small and non–small cell carcinoma.

No consistent clinical or prognostic differences have been identified among these groups. Atypical neuroendocrine carcinoid tumors and NSCLCs with neuroendocrine differentiation exhibit a genetic pattern and clinical course distinct from those of SCLC.

CLINICAL FEATURES

Most SCLCs have an identifiable pulmonary lesion, although approximately 4% may be in solely extrapulmonary sites (cervix, head and neck, esophagus, colon, and others). Approximately two thirds of patients have distant metastases at diagnosis. Common sites of extranodal metastases include the bone, the liver, the central nervous system (CNS), and bone marrow. A significant number of metastases to endocrine organs are also seen. Signs and symptoms relate to

1. The primary tumor and local spread
   Most tumors begin in a central, endobronchial location and have:
   • Cough, dyspnea, wheezing, hemoptysis.
   • Postobstructive pneumonitis.
   • Hilar adenopathy.
   • Superior vena cava syndrome (≤10% of patients).
   • Compression of other mediastinal structures: recurrent laryngeal nerve (hoarseness), esophagus (dysphagia).
2. Distant metastases
   • Headache, seizures, visual disturbances.
   • Jaundice, asymptomatic elevations in liver enzymes.
   • Bone marrow involvement with resultant anemia, leukopenia, or thrombocytopenia.
   • Weight loss, anorexia.
3. Paraneoplastic syndromes, often a result of secreted polypeptide hormones.
   • Hyponatremia (SIADH, secretion of excess atrial natriuretic peptide).
   • Cushing's syndrome due to ectopic adrenocorticotropic hormone (ACTH).
   • Eaton–Lambert myasthenic-like syndrome.
   • Cerebellar ataxia, subacute sensory neuropathy, and other neurologic syndromes.

STAGING

The intensity of treatment regimens currently recommended (treatment-related mortality of up to 5%) dictates the need for accurate staging. The main goal of staging is to identify those patients who may benefit from combined-modality treatment (combination chemotherapy with concurrent thoracic radiation).

The most frequently used staging system is that devised by the Veterans Administration Lung Group (Table 1).

TABLE 1. *VA Lung Cancer Study Group staging of SCLC and prognosis*

			Survival	
Stage	%	Untreated	Combination chemotherapy
Limited-stage disease	30–40	12 wk	12–20 mo
Tumor confined to one hemithorax and regional lymph nodes that can be encompassed within a radiotherapy port[a]			
Extensive-stage disease			
Disease extending beyond the limits described for limited-stage disease[b]	60–70	5 wk	7–11 mo

[a]Contralateral hilar, mediastinal, or supraclavicular nodes usually included in limited-stage disease.
[b]Ipsilateral malignant pleural effusion is considered extensive disease.

The TNM classification suggested by the American Joint Commission for Cancer (AJCC) is used rarely, primarily to select the exceedingly small population of patients (stage I) that may benefit from surgical resection in addition to combination chemotherapy:
Necessary components of an adequate staging evaluation include:

- Complete history and physical examination.
- Chest imaging: a chest radiograph; chest computed tomography (CT) scan, particularly if thoracic radiotherapy is planned; bronchoscopy if no evaluable tumor is found on chest radiograph/CT scan.
- Liver function tests, with abnormal tests prompting CT imaging.
- Alkaline phosphatase, with a bone scan if abnormal.
- Complete blood count, followed by bilateral bone marrow biopsy if results are abnormal.
- CT scan of the brain if indicated by an appropriate history or the presence of neurologic deficits, for extensive stage. CT scan of the brain in limited stage.

The most important physiologic factors that portend a favorable outcome are limited stage of disease, good performance status, and good cardiopulmonary, hepatic, and renal function.

TREATMENT

Limited-Stage Disease

Combined chemotherapy with concurrent thoracic irradiation is generally recommended (Table 2). Toxicities of therapy, including dysphagia, esophagitis, pneumonitis, myelosup-

TABLE 2. *Stage-dependent treatment of SCLC*

Stage	Treatment
Limited-stage disease	Combination chemotherapy
	Thoracic radiation recommended
	Prophylactic cranial irradiation may be considered in complete responders
Extensive-stage disease	Combination chemotherapy
	Referrals to clinical trials or single-agent chemotherapy are acceptable alternatives in selected patients

pression, and fatigue, may be observed more frequently in patients receiving concurrent treatments. Some stage I patients may be candidates for surgical resection combined with multiagent chemotherapy.

Chemotherapy

Although several single agents show activity against SCLC, significantly superior response rates and survival with multiagent therapy have made combination chemotherapy the standard approach in initial treatment. Optimal regimens yield 80% to 90% response rates, 50% to 60% complete response rates, and 2-year survival rates of 15% to 40%.

Several combinations have been used successfully (Table 3). The most commonly used regimen currently is etoposide + cisplatin (EP) because of its favorable toxicity profile and reports of activity in tumors initially treated with cyclophosphamide-containing regimens.

The optimal duration of chemotherapy is four to six cycles (or two cycles beyond best response). Longer duration of treatment has not been shown to be of any benefit. High-dose chemotherapy with autologous stem cell reinfusion has not been demonstrated in phase III trials to be superior to conventional therapy and is currently used only in clinical trials.

Radiotherapy

Thoracic radiation provides a marginal survival advantage and reduced local recurrence rates when added to chemotherapy in limited-stage disease.

Most regimens incorporating radiation therapy use a total dose of 45 to 50 Gy. The optimal timing of radiotherapy is unclear, but administration either concurrent or interdigitating with chemotherapy is favored over sequential regimens.

Radiation therapy is also used in local control of disease (CNS, other isolated metastatic sites not responding to systemic chemotherapy).

TABLE 3. *Summary of commonly used chemotherapeutic regimens*

Regimen	Dose	Duration
EP		
Etoposide	100 mg/m^2 i.v. days 1–3	
Cisplatin	25 mg/m^2 i.v. days 1–3	
Etoposide	80 mg/m^2 i.v. days 1–3	
Cisplatin	80 mg/m^2 i.v. day 1	Cycles repeated every 3 weeks, for 4 cycles
CAV		
Cyclophosphamide	1,000 mg/m^2 i.v. day 1	
Doxorubicin	45 mg/m^2 i.v. day 1	
Vincristine	2 mg i.v. day 1	Cycles repeated every 3 weeks, continued for 4–6 cycles
CAE		
Cyclophosphamide	1,000 mg/m^2 i.v. day 1	
Doxorubicin	45 mg/m^2 i.v. day 1	
Etoposide	50 mg/m^2 i.v. days 1–5	
CAVE		
Cyclophosphamide	1,000 mg/m^2 i.v. day 1	
Doxorubicin	50 mg/m^2 i.v. day 1	
Vincristine	1.5 mg/m^2 i.v. day 1	
Etoposide	60 mg/m^2 i.v. days 1–5	
CAV alternating with EP	Cycles as above with one cycle of CAV alternating every 3 weeks with a cycle of EP	

Use of prophylactic cranial irradiation (PCI) has received considerable attention, as the risk of developing CNS metastases in 2-year survivors approaches 50% to 60%. Although PCI reduces the frequency of brain metastases, no significant survival advantage was observed in earlier randomized studies. In addition, possible toxicities (neurologic, mental, and psychometric) argue against its routine use. A recent international cooperative randomized trial, however, reported that PCI improved both overall survival and disease-free survival among patients with SCLC in complete remission. The use of PCI, therefore, may be indicated in selected patients with SCLC in complete remission.

Extensive-Stage Disease

Combination chemotherapy without thoracic irradiation is the cornerstone of therapy. Combination chemotherapies identical to those used in limited-stage disease are used with overall response rates of 60% to 80%, complete response rates of 15% to 20%, and median survival of 7 to 11 months. Two-year survival is uncommon with current therapy.

Because of the poor performance status commonly encountered in this stage and the low cure rate with standard treatment, single-agent chemotherapy with oral VP-16 or referral to clinical trials is appropriate in selected patients.

Recurrent Disease or Disease Progressing on Initial Therapy

Recurrent disease or disease progressing on initial therapy has an extremely poor prognosis, with a median survival of 2 to 3 months. Treatment options in this group are limited. Thoracic irradiation should be considered in those patients whose recurrence is confined to the thorax and who have not previously received irradiation. Patients who have not received a platinum-containing regimen may benefit from combinations containing cisplatin. Taxol and topotecan as single agents have also been shown to have some activity in this setting. Patients may be referred to clinical trials testing new pharmacologic agents that target oncogenes, signaling pathways, or blood supply and that are currently under development.

Long-Time Survivors of SCLC Are at a High Risk of Developing Second Primary Tumors of NSCLC in Addition to Recurrent SCLC

Patients who are able to quit smoking seem to do better than patients who continue to smoke. These patients should be considered for chemoprevention strategies.

SUGGESTED READINGS

1. Ihde DC, Pass HI, Glatstein E. Small cell lung cancer. In: De Vita VT, Hellman S, Rosenberg SA, eds. *Cancer: principles and practice of oncology.* 5th ed. Philadelphia: Lippincott-Raven, 1997: 911–949.
2. Adjei AA, Marks RS, Bonner JA. Current guidelines for the management of small cell lung cancer. *Mayo Clin Proc* 1999;74:809–816.
3. Kelly K, Mikhaeel-Kamel N. Medical treatment of lung cancer. *J Thorac Imaging* 1999;14:257–265.
4. Sandler AB. Current management of small cell lung cancer. *Semin Oncol* 1997;244:463–476.
5. Demetri G, Elias A, Gershenson D, et al. NCCN small-cell lung cancer practice guidelines. *Oncology* 1996;10(suppl 11):179–194.
6. Teng M, Choy H, Ettinger D. Combined chemoradiation therapy for limited-stage small-cell lung cancer. *Oncology* 1999;13(10 suppl 5):107–115.
7. Auperin A, et al. Prophylactic cranial irradiation for patients with small-cell lung cancer in complete remission: Prophylactic Cranial Irradiation Overview Collaborative Group. *N Engl J Med* 1999; 341(7):476–484.

SECTION 3

Digestive System

4

Esophageal Cancer

Nicole McCarthy and Jean Grem

Medicine Branch, DCS, National Cancer Institute,
National Institutes of Health, Bethesda, Maryland

Esophageal cancer is the ninth most common cancer worldwide. It is highly curable in its earliest stages; however, it usually presents as advanced disease. Despite the last two decades of clinical research, the median survival time for the patient with symptoms of a primary esophageal cancer is less than 18 months.

EPIDEMIOLOGY

In the United States:

- Esophageal cancer constitutes 1.5% of all malignancies and 7% of all gastrointestinal malignancies.
- Approximately 12,500 new cases and 12,200 deaths are estimated for 1999.
- The median age at diagnosis is 67 years, rarely occurring in people younger than 25 years.
- Esophageal cancer occurs 2 to 4 times more frequently in men than in women.
- Rates are approximately threefold higher among blacks than among whites.
- Squamous cell carcinoma is 6 times more common in black male than white male subjects.
- Adenocarcinoma occurs at a frequency 3 times greater in white male than black male subjects.

In the rest of the world:

- There is substantial geographic variation in the incidence of esophageal cancer. Regions with clusters of high rates include China (e.g., Linxian), Iran, France, and South Africa.
- In the 1970s, approximately 90% of esophageal cancers were squamous cell carcinomas. The incidence of adenocarcinomas has increased dramatically and currently accounts for about 50% of new cases, a rate of acceleration greater than that of any other cancer in the United States.

ETIOLOGY

- Tobacco.
- Alcohol.
- Predisposing conditions:
    Barrett's esophagus/gastroesophageal reflux (adenocarcinoma).
    Tylosis (squamous cell carcinoma).
    Achalasia.
    Strictures after caustic injury.

Esophageal diverticula and webs (squamous cell carcinoma).
Plummer–Vinson syndrome.
Celiac disease.
Obesity (adenocarcinoma).
- Environmental exposure.
  Asbestos.
  Radiation.
  Nitrosamines.
  Perchloroethylene.
- Dietary factors.
  Low intake of fruit and vegetables.
  Low intake of vitamin B, vitamin C, magnesium, zinc, β-carotene.

BARRETT'S ESOPHAGUS

Barrett's esophagus is the single most important risk factor for adenocarcinoma. Prospective data quantifying the risk of carcinoma developing from Barrett's esophagus are awaited.

- Screening recommendations (no randomized trial data for surveillance practices)
- No dysplasia: endoscopy every 2 to 3 years.
- Low-grade dysplasia: endoscopy every 6 months for 12 months and then yearly.
- High-grade dysplasia: esophagectomy or three monthly endoscopies.

Clinical Presentation

Other clinical presentations include hematemesis or melena, regurgitation of undigested food, aspiration pneumonia, superior vena cava syndrome, adenopathy, and very rarely, hemoptysis or malignant hypercalcemia due to metastases to bone. The most common clinical presentations are listed in Table 1.

DIAGNOSIS AND STAGING

Staging is based on the TNM system, which defines the anatomic extent of disease. The American Joint Commission for Cancer (AJCC) has designated staging by TNM classification (Table 2).

- Physical examination may reveal malignant adenopathy, Horner's syndrome, or evidence of metastatic disease, especially to liver and/or lungs.
- Upper gastrointestinal endoscopy with biopsy is the primary method for diagnosis of esophageal cancer. The combination of endoscopic biopsies and brush cytology has an accuracy of virtually 100% in obtaining a tissue diagnosis of esophageal cancer.

TABLE 1. *Clinical presentation of esophageal cancer*

Symptoms	Patients with symptoms (%)
Dysphagia (solids usually before liquids)	80–96
Weight loss	42–46
Odynophagia	≤50
Epigastric or retrosternal pain	≤20
Cough/hoarseness	≤5
Tracheocsophageal fistula	1–13

TABLE 2. *Definition of TNM and stage grouping*

Primary tumor (T)	
TX:	Primary tumor cannot be assessed
T0:	No evidence of primary tumor
Tis:	Carcinoma in situ
T1:	Tumor invades lamina propria or submucosa
T2:	Tumor invades muscularis propria
T3:	Tumor invades adventitia
T4:	Tumor invades adjacent structures
Regional lymph nodes (N)	
NX:	Regional lymph nodes cannot be assessed
N0:	No regional lymph node metastasis
N1:	Regional lymph node metastasis
Distant metastasis (M)	
MX:	Distant metastasis cannot be assessed
M0:	No distant metastasis
M1:	Distant metastasis
Tumors of the lower thoracic esophagus	
M1a:	Metastasis in celiac lymph nodes
M1b:	Other distant metastasis
Tumors of the midthoracic esophagus	
M1a:	Not applicable
M1b:	Other distant metastasis
Tumors of the upper thoracic esophagus	
M1a:	Metastasis in cervical nodes
M1b:	Other distant metastasis

Stage Grouping			
Stage 0	Tis	N0	M0
Stage 1	T1	N0	M0
Stage IIA	T2	N0	M0
	T3	N0	M0
Stage IIB	T1	N1	M0
	T2	N1	M0
Stage III	T3	N1	M0
	T4	Any N	M0
Stage IV	Any T	Any N	M1
Stage IVA	Any T	Any N	M1a
Stage IVB	Any T	Any N	M1b

For tumors of midthoracic esophagus, use only M1b, because these tumors with metastasis in nonregional lymph nodes have an equally poor prognosis as those with metastasis in other distant sites.

- Barium contrast radiography can document contour and motility abnormalities and unexpected airway fistula and may be useful when the entire esophagus has not been visualized endoscopically.
- Chest radiograph may identify mediastinal or pulmonary disease.
- Computed tomography (CT) of the chest and abdomen may demonstrate evidence of local extension of the tumor or metastases to the liver, lungs, adrenals, and adjacent organs. CT scanning may underestimate the depth of tumor invasion and periesophageal lymph node involvement in up to 50% of cases.
- Endoscopic ultrasound has the advantage of being able to image distinct wall layers. In experienced hands, the accuracy of staging the depth of invasion and involvement of

regional lymph nodes is 85% and 75%, respectively, when compared with surgical pathology.
- Laparoscopy can document small liver metastases and/or intraperitoneal metastases before aggressive surgical therapy.
- Bronchoscopy should be performed in tumors involving the upper two thirds of the esophagus to exclude invasion of the posterior membranous trachea or tracheoesophageal fistula.

TREATMENT
Surgery

- Surgery remains the mainstay of treatment of esophageal cancer with resectable local or locoregional disease and represents the best chance for cure, palliation of dysphagia, and local control.
- The overall 5-year survival in cases amenable to surgery ranges from 5% to 20%.
- Surgical principles include a wide resection of the primary tumor, including more than 5-cm resection margins plus regional lymphadenectomy.
- One of the major recent developments has been the marked improvement in surgical morbidity and mortality as a result of improved staging techniques, patient selection, and support systems. Operative mortality rates have fallen to less than 10%.
- Age alone is not a contraindication to surgery.
- In general, patients with cervical carcinoma of the esophagus are not considered candidates for surgical resection.

Surgical approaches include:

- Transthoracic esophagectomy: laparotomy and right thoracotomy with reanastomosis of gastric conduit in the chest.
- Transhiatal esophagectomy: laparotomy and cervical anastomosis—avoids thoracotomy.
- Total thoracic esophagectomy: laparotomy, right thoracotomy, and cervical anastomosis of the stomach or colonic conduit.
- Radical en bloc esophagectomy: laparotomy, thoracoabdominal exploration with en bloc resection.
- Endothoracic endoesophageal resection.
- Laryngoesophagectomy for cancer of cervical esophagus.

Primary Radiation Therapy

The survival of patients with esophageal cancer treated with radiation alone has not changed significantly in the last two decades. Five-year survival ranges from 0 to 10%, and median survival is typically about 12 months. These series usually include patients with unfavorable features including T4 disease, positive lymph nodes, and medically unfit patients. Radiation therapy as a potentially curative modality requires at least 50 Gy at 1.8 to 2.0 Gy per fraction. Larger unresectable tumors probably require doses of 60 Gy or higher. Reviews of clinical failure patterns indicate persistence or recurrence of tumor at the primary site in 56% to 85% of cases. Intraluminal radiation therapy (brachytherapy) has been tried, but its benefits remain unproven.

Preoperative Radiation Therapy

The potential advantages include:

- Increased resectability.
- Decreased tumor seeding at the time of surgery.

TABLE 3. *Results of meta-analysis of preoperative radiation therapy*

Surgery	Radiation therapy	No radiation therapy
All patients	573	574
Deaths	83.8%	85.5%
Hazard ratio	0.89 ($p = 0.06$)	
2-yr survival	34%	30%
5-yr survival	18%	15%

- Increased radiosensitivity due to more oxygenated cells.

A recent meta-analysis reviewed data on 1,147 patients from five randomized preoperative radiotherapy trials (2).

- Patients received 20 to 40 Gy in 10 to 20 fractions (1–4 weeks), and in one trial half the patients received bleomycin and cisplatin.
- The time interval between the completion of radiation therapy and surgery ranged between 1 and 4 weeks (Table 3).
- Resectability appeared to be unaffected by preoperative radiotherapy.
- At a median follow-up of nine years, an overall reduction in the risk of death of 11% and an absolute survival benefit of 3% at 2 years and 4% at 5 years is not statistically significant (p = 0.062).
- Preoperative radiation therapy cannot currently be recommended outside of controlled clinical trials.

Postoperative Radiation Therapy

Postoperative radiation therapy provides the advantages of accurate pathologic staging and directing treatment to areas of high risk of recurrence. Of three randomized studies, only one (see later) showed a significant reduction in locoregional failure from 35% to 10% with postoperative radiation therapy in a subgroup of patients with negative nodes after curative resection.

In a multicenter French study (13), of 221 patients who underwent curative resections, 119 patients were randomized to surgery alone, and 102 patients to postoperative radiation therapy (1.8 Gy per fraction; total dose, 45–55 Gy). The results are shown in Table 4.

A single-institution study by Fok et al. (7) randomized 130 patients, of whom 60 patients had curative resections. The authors concluded that postoperative radiation therapy:

- May decrease local recurrence after palliative resection (20% vs. 46%; $p = 0.04$).
- Increases toxicity and decreases survival (median survival, 8.7 vs. 15.2 months; $p = 0.02$).

Postoperative radiation therapy is frequently given if the surgical resection is incomplete or the surgical margins are positive to prevent morbidity from locoregional relapse.

TABLE 4. *Results of postoperative radiation therapy*

Outcome	Radiation therapy	No radiation therapy
RT complications	23%	N/A
Locoregional failure (5 yr)		
All patients	15%	30%
Node negative	10%	35% (p < 0.02)

Chemotherapy

Cisplatin has been considered one of the more active agents, with a single-agent response rate consistently in the range of approximately 20%, with no associated survival advantage. Other active agents include 5-fluorouracil (5-FU), mitomycin, and bleomycin; more recent studies suggest that paclitaxel, vinorelbine, and gemcitabine are all active agents. The combination of cisplatin and 5-FU has been the most frequently used regimen, with response rates of between 20% and 50% in the neoadjuvant setting or combined with radiation. New combinations continue to be investigated. Although squamous cell carcinoma is thought to be more sensitive to chemotherapy, chemoradiation, or radiation therapy alone, there is no difference in long-term outcome of patients with either histologic subtype.

Preoperative Chemotherapy

The poor survival, even for patients with clinically localized carcinoma of the esophagus, suggests that occult metastases are present at diagnosis and hence the impetus to add systemic therapy. An intergroup trial conducted in the United States evaluated the potential benefit of preoperative chemotherapy to surgery (9).

The 467 patients (94% eligible) were randomized to chemotherapy followed by surgery OR surgery alone.

Cisplatin, 100 mg/m^2 i.v., day 1 (total dose/cycle, 100 mg/m^2);
Fluorouracil, 1,000 mg/m^2 per day by continuous i.v. infusion for 5 days, days 1–5 (total dose/cycle, 5,000 mg/m^2).

- Treatment cycle duration is 28 days.
- Three complete cycles given before surgery.
- Chemotherapy may be repeated for two postoperative cycles if patient achieves a response or stable disease.

Postoperative radiation therapy was given for a positive margin or residual disease at the discretion of the investigator (Table 5).

Despite the theoretic potential benefits of preoperative chemotherapy, the intergroup trial did not show any survival advantage for patients with potentially resectable carcinoma of the esophagus of either histologic subtype. Distant failure rate was significantly reduced in the chemotherapy arm, but local failure was unchanged.

Similarly, randomized trials have shown no benefit with postoperative adjuvant chemotherapy in patients who have undergone curative resection and have negative nodes in terms of either disease-free or overall survival.

TABLE 5. *Results of preoperative chemotherapy*

Results	No preop chemotherapy	Preop chemotherapy
Number of patients	227	213
Histology		
Squamous	47%	46%
Adenocarcinoma	53%	54%
Response	N/A	19%
Surgery	96%	80%
Curative	59%	62%
Positive margins	15%	4% ($p = 0.001$)
Postoperative deaths	6%	6%
Median survival	16.1 mo	14.9 mo
DFS (3 yr)	20%	20%

DFS, disease-free survival.

Multimodality Therapy

Whereas no large prospective randomized trials have directly compared primary chemoradiation with surgery, definitive chemoradiation for locoregional carcinoma of the esophagus is considered an alternative to surgery.

RTOG 85-01 **multiinstitution study** (123 patients eligible) randomized to:

- Chemotherapy *PLUS* radiation therapy *OR* radiation therapy alone:
  Fluorouracil, 1,000 mg/m^2 per day by continuous i.v. infusion for 4 consecutive days, weeks 1, 5, 8, and 11 (total dose/4-day cycle, 4,000 mg/m^2)
  Cisplatin, 75 mg/m^2 i.v., day 1 of weeks 1, 5, 8, and 11 (total dose/cycle, 100 mg/m^2)
  Radiation therapy, 2 Gy/fraction for five fractions per week, weeks 1–5 (total dose/course, 50 Gy)

  OR

- Radiation therapy, 2 Gy/fraction for five fractions per week, weeks 1–6.4 (total dose/course, 64 Gy).

This trial was stopped early after an interim analysis demonstrated a 4-month median survival advantage for patients receiving combined-modality therapy compared with those given radiation alone. Seventy-three additional patients were then registered directly to receive chemoradiation. Long-term follow-up indicated that the median survival was 14.1 months versus 9.3 months, in favor of the combined-modality arm. At 5 years, no patient who received radiation therapy alone was alive compared with 26% who received chemoradiation ($p <$ 0.001).

Combined Preoperative Chemotherapy and Radiotherapy

Nonrandomized studies using 5-FU and cisplatin-based regimens given concurrently with radiotherapy showed pathologic complete response (CR) rates of 25% and a possible survival advantage in this group. The results of selected phase III studies (Tables 6–8) are varied. These data do not support the routine use of preoperative chemoradiation; however, this approach is being addressed further in large randomized studies.

University of Michigan Trial (15): 100 Patients with Squamous Cell Carcinoma or Adenocarcinoma

Treatment Strata

Chemotherapy *PLUS* radiation *PLUS* surgery *OR* surgery alone (Table 6).

- Fluorouracil, 300 mg/m^2 per day by continuous i.v. infusion for 21 days, days 1–21 (total dose/cycle, 6,300 mg/m^2);

TABLE 6. *Results of combined preoperative chemotherapy and radiotherapy (University of Michigan Trial)*

	Chemo/radiotherapy/surgery	Surgery alone
Pathologic CR	28%	
Median survival	1.41 yr	1.46 yr
3-yr survival	32% ($p = 0.073$)	15%
Locoregional failure (1st site)	19% ($p = 0.039$)	39%

CR, complete response.

TABLE 7. *Results of combined preoperative chemotherapy and radiotherapy (Dublin Trial)*

	Chemo/radiotherapy/surgery	Surgery alone
Pathologic CR	25%	
Median survival	16 mo ($p = 0.01$)	11 mo

CR, complete response.

- Cisplatin, 20 mg/m^2 per day by continuous i.v. infusion for 10 days, days 1–5 and 17–21 (total dose/cycle, 200 mg/m^2);
- Vinblastine, 1 mg/m^2 per day i.v. bolus for 8 days, days 1–4 and 17–20 (total dose/cycle, 8 mg/m^2);
- Radiation therapy, 1.5 Gy twice daily, days 1–5, 8–12, and 15–19;
- Surgery on day 42.

Dublin Trial (16): 113 Patients with Adenocarcinoma

Treatment Strata

Chemotherapy *PLUS* radiation *PLUS* surgery *OR* surgery alone (Table 7).

- Fluorouracil, 15 mg/kg body weight per day by i.v. infusion, 16 hours/day for 10 days, days 1–5 and 35–39 (total dose/cycle, 150 mg/kg);
- Cisplatin, 75 mg/m^2 per dose i.v. for two doses, days 7 and 41 (total dose/cycle, 150 mg/m^2);
- Radiation therapy, 15 fractions, days 1–5, 8–12, and 15–19 (total dose/course, 40 Gy);
- Surgery.

European Trial (5): 282 Patients with Squamous Cell Carcinoma

Treatment Strata

Chemotherapy *PLUS* radiation *PLUS* surgery *OR* surgery alone (Table 8).

- Cisplatin, 80 mg/m^2 i.v. for 1 dose, day 2 or 1 before or the same day as radiation therapy (total dose/cycle, 80 mg/m^2);
- Radiation therapy, 3.7 Gy per fraction, five fractions, days 1–5, (total dose/course, 18.5 Gy); repeat in two weeks.
- Surgery, 2–4 weeks after radiotherapy.

Palliation

External beam radiation either alone or in combination with chemotherapy offers palliation of dysphagia in approximately 80% of patients; approximately half have ongoing palliation

TABLE 8. *Results of combined preoperative chemotherapy and radiotherapy (European Trial)*

	Chemo/radiotherapy/surgery	Surgery alone
Pathologic CR	26%	
3-yr disease-free survival	40% ($p = 0.003$)	25%
Median survival	18.6 months	18.6 mo

CR, complete response.

until time of death. If a patient requires rapid palliation, laser or stenting is recommended. Brachytherapy also should be considered if external beam radiation therapy is not possible.

Current methods of endoscopic palliation include balloon dilatation or bougienage, thermocoagulation (laser), photodynamic therapy, intracavitary irradiation, and placement of expandable metal stents or hollow plastic tubes. The placement of a gastrostomy or jejunostomy tube may improve the patient's nutritional status.

TREATMENT FOR ESOPHAGEAL CANCER

Stage I

Surgical resection

Most common procedures:

- Transthoracic esophagectomy.
- Transhiatal esophagectomy.

Stage IIa

Surgical resection[1]

- If surgical margins are positive, postoperative radiation therapy is often used to improve locoregional control.
- Postoperative chemotherapy + radiation therapy may be considered, but the benefit of this approach has not been tested in randomized trials.

Primary chemotherapy plus radiation (as per RTOG 85-01[2] or INT 0123[3]).

- Surgery may be considered after recovery from chemoradiation, but the benefit of this approach has not yet been proven in multiinstitutional phase III trials.

Stage IIb

Surgical resection

Outcome is poor in patients with nodal involvement with esophagectomy alone.
Primary chemotherapy plus radiation (as per RTOG 85-01[2] or INT 0123[3]).

- Surgery may be considered after recovery from chemoradiation, but the benefit of this approach has not yet been proven in multiinstitutional phase III trials.

---

[1]In patients selected for primary surgery, there is no clear survival advantage with pre- or postoperative radiation alone or chemotherapy alone.

[2]RTOG 85-01
- Radiation therapy, 2 Gy/fraction (total dose/course, 50 Gy).
- Cisplatin, 75 mg/m^2 i.v., day 1 of weeks 1, 5, 8, and 11 (total dose/cycle, 75 mg/m^2).
- Fluorouracil, 1,000 mg/m^2/day by continuous i.v. infusion for 4 days, days 1 to 4 during weeks 1, 5, 8, and 11 (total dose/4-day course, 4,000 mg/m^2).

[3]INT 0123
- Radiation therapy, 1.8 Gy/fraction (total dose/course, 50.40 Gy).
- Cisplatin, 75 mg/m^2 i.v., day 1 of weeks 1, 5, 9, and 13 (total dose/cycle, 75 mg/m^2).
- Fluorouracil, 1,000 mg/m^2/day by continuous i.v. infusion for 4 days, days 1 to 4 during weeks 1, 5, 9, and 13 (total dose/4-day course, 4,000 mg/m^2).

Stage III

Palliative surgical resection may be considered for T3 lesions
Primary chemotherapy plus radiation (as per RTO G 85-01[2] or INT 0123[3]).

- Surgery may be considered after recovery from chemoradiation, but the benefit of this approach has not yet been proven in multiinstitutional phase III trials.

Stage IV

Local palliation options

1. Radiation therapy, 2 Gy/fraction, days 1–5, weeks 1–3 (total dose/course, 30 Gy).
2. Intraluminal intubation and dilatation.
3. Intraluminal brachytherapy.
4. Endoluminal tumor destruction.
   - Laser (Nd:YAG[4]).
   - Electrocoagulation.
5. Photodynamic therapy.
   Porfimer sodium, 2 mg/kg body weight by slow i.v. injection over 3–5 minutes, followed by
   Laser light (630 ± 3 nm wavelength) with a fiberoptic probe 40 to 50 h after porfimer sodium injection.
   - FDA-approved laser light dose, 300 joules/cm of tumor length.
   - Total power output is set to deliver the appropriate light dose with exposure times equal to 12 minutes, 3 seconds.
   - Laser treatment may be repeated, typically within 96 to 120 hours after porfimer sodium injection.

METASTATIC DISEASE

Palliative chemotherapy may be considered in patients with a good performance status.

1. Cisplatin, 75 to 100 mg/m^2 i.v. day 1 (total dose/cycle, 75–100 mg/m^2), *PLUS*
   Fluorouracil, 1,000 mg/m^2/day by continuous i.v. infusion for 4 to 5 days, days 1 to 4 or 1 to 5 (total dose/cycle, 4,000–5,000 mg/m^2).
   - The most commonly used regimen for all histologies.
   - Treatment cycle duration is 28 days.
2. May consider epirubicin, cisplatin, and 5-FU for adenocarcinomas.
3. Taxane-based regimens are undergoing clinical testing.

FOLLOW-UP FOR PATIENTS WITH LOCOREGIONAL DISEASE

- History and physical examination, CBC, urea, and electrolytes, liver function tests every 3 months for 2 years and then every 6 months.
- Chest radiograph every 6 months for 2 years and then every 12 months.
- CT chest/abdomen as clinically indicated.
- Upper gastrointestinal endoscopy as clinically indicated.

---

[4]Neodymium:yttrium-aluminum-garnet laser.

REFERENCES

1. Ajani JA, Eisenberg B, Emanuel P, et al. NCCN practice guidelines for upper gastrointestinal carcinomas. *NCCN Proc Oncol Am* 1999;11:179–223.
2. Arnott SJ, Duncan W, Gignoux M, et al. Pre-operative radiotherapy in esophageal carcinoma: a meta-analysis using individual patient data (Oesophageal Cancer Collaborative Group). *Int J Radiat Oncol Biol Phys* 1998;14:579–583.
3. Blot WJ, Devesa SS, Kneller RW, et al. Rising incidence of adenocarcinoma of the esophagus and gastric cardia. *JAMA* 1991;265:1187–1212.
4. Blot WJ. Esophageal cancer trends and risk factors. *Semin Oncol* 1994;21:403–410.
5. Bosset JF, Gignoux M, Triboulet JP, et al. Chemoradiotherapy followed by surgery compared with surgery alone in squamous cell cancer of the esophagus. *N Engl J Med* 1997;337:161–167.
6. Cooper JS, Guo MD, Herskovic A, et al. Chemoradiotherapy of locally advanced esophageal cancer long-term follow-up of a prospective randomized trial (RTOG 85-01). *JAMA* 1999;281:1623–1627.
7. Fok M, Sham JS, Choy D, et al. Postoperative radiotherapy for carcinoma of esophagus: a prospective, randomized controlled study. *Surgery* 1993;113:138–147.
8. Herskovic A, Martz L, Al-Sarraf M, et al. Combined chemotherapy and radiotherapy compared with radiotherapy alone in patients with cancer of the esophagus. *N Engl J Med* 1992;326:1593–1598.
9. Kelsen DP, Ginsberg R, Pajak TF, et al. Chemotherapy followed by surgery compared with surgery alone for localized esophageal cancer. *N Engl J Med* 1998;339:1979–1984.
10. Molloy RG, McCourtney JS, Anderson JR. Laparoscopy in management of patients with cancer of the gastric cardia and oesophagus. *Br J Surg* 1995; 82:352–354.
11. Rosch T. Endosonographic staging of esophageal cancer: a review of literature results. *Gastrointest Endosc Clin North Am* 1995;5:537–547.
12. Roth JA, Putman JB, Rich TA, et al. Cancer of the esophagus. In: De Vita VT Jr, Hellman S, Rosenberg SA, eds. *Cancer: principles and practice of oncology.* 5th ed. Philadelphia: Lippincott-Raven, 1997:980–1021.
13. Teniere P, Hay JM, Fingerhut A, et al. Postoperative radiation therapy does not increase survival after curative resection for squamous cell carcinoma of the middle and lower esophagus as shown by a multicenter controlled trial: French University Association for Surgical Research. *Surg Gynecol Obstet* 1991;173:123–130.
14. Tummala R, Williams SR. Esophageal cancer. In: Djulbegovic B, Sullivan DM, eds. *Decision making in oncology: evidence based management.* Philadelphia: Churchill Livingstone, 1997:169–178.
15. Urba S, Orringer MB, Turrisi A, et al. A randomized trial comparing surgery(s) to preoperative concurrent chemoradiation plus surgery in patients (pts) with resectable esophagus cancer (CA): updated analysis. *Proc Am Soc Clin Oncol* 1997;16:277(abst).
16. Walsh TN, Noonan N, Hollywood D, et al. A comparison of multimodal therapy and surgery for esophageal adenocarcinoma. *N Engl J Med* 1996;335:462–467.
17. Zieren HU, Muller JM, Jacobi CA, et al. Adjuvant postoperative radiation therapy after curative resection of squamous cell carcinoma of the thoracic esophagus: a prospective randomized study. *World J Surg* 1995;19:444–449.

5

Gastric Cancer

George P. Kim and Chris H. Takimoto

Medicine Branch, DCS, National Cancer Institute, National Naval Medical Center, National Institutes of Health, Bethesda, Maryland

EPIDEMIOLOGY

- Gastric cancer represented the leading cause of cancer mortality in the United States in the 1930s and worldwide until the late 1980s, when it was surpassed by lung malignancies.
- Approximately 21,900 new cases of gastric cancer will have been diagnosed in 1999 in the U.S., with 13,500 deaths attributed to the disease.
- In Japan, which has the highest worldwide incidence, stomach cancer continues as the leading cause of cancer-related mortality.
- A worldwide increase in proximal gastric and gastroesophageal (GE) cancers has been reported, and in the U.S., the 4.3% annual rate of GE cancer increase is higher than the rate of lung cancer increase.
- High gastric cancer incidence is observed in Asia, South America (Chile and Costa Rica), Eastern Europe, and the Middle East.

RISK FACTORS

- Age at onset, fifth decade.
- Sex: male (1.67:1.0).
- Race: African-American (1.5:1).
- *Helicobacter pylori* infection, especially childhood exposure, three- to fivefold increase.
- Family history: first degree (two- to threefold); familial clusterings, Napoleon Bonaparte family.
- Alcohol.
- Tobacco use (1.5- to threefold).
- Food preparations: fermenting, smoking result in high salt and nitrosamines content.
- Nutritional deficiencies: vitamins A, C, E, β-carotene, selenium, fiber.
- Previous gastric resection.
- Ménétrier's disease.
- Pernicious anemia (10–20% incidence).
- Blood type A.

SCREENING

- In most countries, screening general populations is not practical because of low incidence. However, screening is worthwhile in Japan where gastric cancer incidence is high.

• Japanese screening guidelines include initial upper endoscopy at age 50 years, with follow-up endoscopy for abnormalities.

PATHOPHYSIOLOGY

The majority of gastric cancers are adenocarcinomas (more than 90%) of two distinct histologic types: intestinal and diffuse.

Intestinal

The "epidemic" form is more differentiated with gland formation and is associated with precancerous lesions, gastric atrophy, and intestinal metaplasia. The intestinal form accounts for the majority of distal cancers and is stable or declining in incidence. These cancers in particular are associated with *Helicobacter pylori* infection, as proposed by Correa. In this carcinogenesis model, the interplay of environmental factors leads to glandular atrophy, relative achlorhydria, and increases in gastric pH. This results in bacterial overgrowth as *H. pylori* and subsequent bacterial production of nitrites and nitroso compounds results in further development of gastric atrophy and intestinal metaplasia, increasing cancer risk.

Diffuse

The "endemic" form is more common in younger patients and exhibits undifferentiated signet-ring histology. There is a predilection for submucosal spread because of lack of cell cohesion, leading to linitis plastica. Contiguous spread to the peritoneum is common. Precancerous lesions have not been identified and, although also associated with *H. pylori* infection, a carcinogenesis model has not been proposed. Genetic predispositions have been reported, as have associations with people with type A blood. These cancers occur in the proximal stomach where worldwide increased incidence has been observed; stage for stage, they have a worse prognosis than do distal cancers.

Molecular analysis

Loss of heterozygosity: chromosomes *5q* or APC gene (deleted in 34% of gastric cancers), *17p*, and *18q* (DCC gene).

• Microsatellite instability: particularly transforming growth factor-β (TGFβ) type II receptor with subsequent growth-inhibition deregulation.
• *p53*: mutated in approximately 40% to 60% by allelic loss and base transition mutations.
• E-cadherin: reduced E-cadherin expression, cell adhesion mediator, observed in diffuse-type undifferentiated cancers.
• Her2/neu and erbB-2/erbB-3 (epidermal growth factors), especially in intestinal forms.
• Epstein–Barr viral genomes detected.
• *ras* mutations: rarely reported, in contrast to other gastrointestinal cancers.

DIAGNOSIS

The most common presenting symptoms are abdominal/epigastric pain and weight loss. Other nonspecific symptoms:

• Gastrointestinal bleeding.
• Dysphagia.
• Early satiety.
• Nausea with emesis.

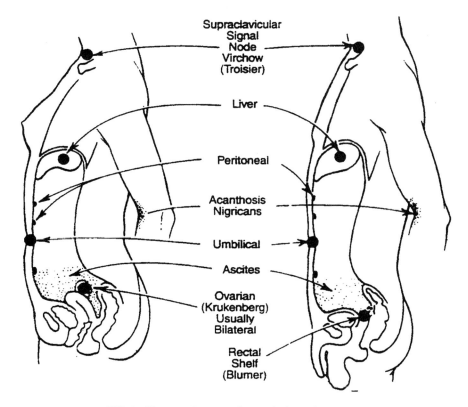

FIG. 1. Diagram of routes of spread of gastric cancer.

- Abdominal wall masses or subcutaneous nodules.
- Lymphadenopathy.
- Excessive belching, reflux.
- Fatigue.

Clinical findings include anemia, weight loss, electrolyte abnormalities, and liver enzyme elevations. Classic physical examination findings (Fig. 1):

- Sister Mary Joseph's nodes or periumbilical lymph nodes, named after Mayo Clinic operating room nurse, which form as tumor spreads along the falciform ligament to subcutaneous sites.
- Virchow's node: left supraclavicular lymph node.
- Irish's node: left anterior axillary lymph node resulting from proximal primary cancer spread to lower esophageal and then intrathoracic lymphatics.
- Blummer's shelf: palpable on rectal examination.
- Krukenberg tumor: ovarian metastases.

Tumor Markers

- Carcinoembryonic antigen (CEA) elevated in 40% to 50% of cases, useful in follow-up but not for screening.

TABLE 1. *Endoscopic findings*

Malignant ulcer	Benign ulcer	Suggestive of a malignant ulcer
Centrifugal radiation of rugal folds Heaped-up borders Diameter >1 cm Rigid stomach wall	Outward radiation of rugal folds	Only diminished distensibility useful

- α-Fetoprotein and CA 19-9 elevated in 30% of gastric cancer patients.
- Medically refractory persistent peptic ulcer disease may prompt barium or endoscopic evaluation.

Endoscopic Findings

- Initial upper gastrointestinal endoscopy or double-contrast barium swallow identify suggestive lesions and have diagnostic accuracy of 95% and 75%, respectively (Table 1).
- Computerized tomography scanning is then useful for assessing local extension, lymph node involvement, and presence of metastasis, although understaging occurs in the majority of cases.
- Endoscopic ultrasonography assesses depth of tumor invasion and lymph node status with 80% accuracy, supplementing preoperative evaluations.

Paraneoplastic Syndromes

Skin syndromes

- Acanthosis nigracans.
- Dermatomyositis.
- Circinate erythemas.
- Pemphigoid.
- Seborrheic keratoses: sign of Leser–Trélat, acute onset.

Central nervous system (CNS) syndromes

- Dementia.
- Cerebellar ataxia.

Miscellaneous syndromes

- Thrombophlebitis.
- Microangiopathic hemolytic anemia.
- Membranous nephropathy.

STAGING

The American Joint Committee on Cancer (AJCC) has designated staging by TNM classification (Table 2). Primary tumor (T) is based on depth of invasion and remains a T2 lesion with penetration of the muscularis propria and extension into gastric ligaments or omentum if visceral peritoneum remains intact. With perforation of peritoneum covering the gastric ligaments or omentum, the tumor becomes T3. A T4 tumor invades adjacent structures including the spleen, transverse colon, liver, diaphragm, pancreas, abdominal wall, adrenal gland, kidney, small intestine, and retroperitoneum. Direct extension to the duodenum or esophagus is

TABLE 2. *TNM/AJCC/UICC staging classification (1997)*

Primary tumor
    TX: Primary tumor cannot be assessed
    T0:   No evidence of tumor in resected specimen
    Tis: Carcinoma in situ
    T1:   Invades lamina propria or submucosa
    T2:   Invades muscularis propria or subserosa with no
            penetration of the visceral peritoneum
    T3:   Invades through the serosa (visceral peritoneum)
    T4:   Invades adjacent structures
Regional lymph nodes
    NX: Nodes cannot be assessed
    N0:   No regional node metastases
    N1:   Involvement of one to six regional lymph nodes
    N2:   Involvement of seven to 15 regional lymph nodes
    N3:   Involvement of >15 regional lymph nodes
Distant metastases
    MX: Presence of distant metastases cannot be assessed
    M0:   No distant metastases
    M1:   Distant metastases present
Staging system
    Stage 0
      Tis N0 M0
    Stage IA
      T1 N0 M0
    Stage IB
      T1 N1 M0
      T2 N0 M0
    Stage II
      T1 N2 M0
      T2 N1 M0
      T3 N0 M0
    Stage IIIA
      T2 N2 M0
      T3 N1 M0
      T4 N0 M0
    Stage IIIB
      T3 N2 M0
    Stage IV
      T4 N1–2 M0
      T any N3 M0
      T any N any M1

classified by the depth of greatest invasion identified. Intraabdominal lymph node groups such as hepatoduodenal, retropancreatic, mesenteric, and paraaortic, previously designated N3 and N4, are presently considered metastatic or advanced-stage disease.

- Two thirds of patients are first seen with stage III or IV disease.
- Lymphadenectomy should contain at least 15 lymph nodes for proper staging.

PROGNOSIS

Factors associated with unfavorable prognosis (Table 3):

- Age: older.

TABLE 3. *Prognosis by stage*

Stage 0	>90%
Stage I	50%
Stage II	29%
Stage III	13%
Stage IV	3%

- Proximal location.
- Weight loss: greater than 10%.
- Linnitus plastica.
- Grade: high or undifferentiated tumors.
- Four or fewer lymph node involvement.
- Aneuploid tumors.
- Elevations in epidermal growth factor/P-glycoprotein.

MANAGEMENT ALGORITHM

Standard of Care

Surgery

Although highly curable if detected early by surgery alone, up to 80% of gastric cancer in the U.S. is advanced at diagnosis. Surgical extirpation of gastric cancer is indicated in patients with stages I, II, and III disease with minimal lymph node involvement (Fig. 2). Tumor size and location dictate the type of surgical procedure. With proximal cardia or distal lesions, subtotal gastrectomy may be performed, provided the fundus or cardioesophageal junction is not involved. Proximal gastrectomy is associated with increased postoperative complications, mortality, and quality-of-life decrement, necessitating thorough consideration of complete gastric resection. Total gastrectomy is more appropriate if tumor involvement is diffuse, and arises in the body of the stomach, with extension to within 6 cm of the cardia.

The regional lymph nodes include N1 and N2 lymph node groups (lesser and greater curvature perigastric, left gastric, common hepatic, splenic, celiac axis nodes). D2 lymphadenectomy involves more extensive N2 lymph node group resection and is reported to improve survival in patients with T1, T2, and some serosa-involved T3 lesions. Factors such as operative time, hospitalization length, and transfusion requirements and thus morbidity are all increased. The greatest benefit may occur in early gastric cancer lesions with small tumors with superficial mucosal involvement, as up to 20% have occult lymph node involvement.

Despite favorable Japanese experience with extended D2 lymph node dissection, a recent randomized trial involving 80 Dutch hospitals compared D1 with D2 lymph node dissection and reported higher morbidity and postoperative mortality but similar cumulative risks of relapse and 5-year survival rates (D1 group, 45%; D2 group, 47%). The routine use of D2 lymphadenectomy continues to be studied.

Postsurgical follow-up should include clinic visits with liver function tests and CEA measurements. A chest radiograph is also warranted. Intervals of every 3 months for the first 2 years, then every 6 months for 3 years, and then every year have been suggested. If total gastrectomy is not performed, yearly upper endoscopy is dictated by a 1% to 2% incidence of second primary tumors. Vitamin B_{12} deficiency develops in most total gastrectomy patients and 20% of subtotal gastrectomy patients, typically within 4 to 10 years. Vitamin B_{12} supplementation is administered at 1,000 µg intramuscularly every month.

Palliative surgery is considered in patients with obstruction, bleeding, or pain and, despite operative mortalities of 25% to 50%, mean survival is increased twofold from gastrojejunos-

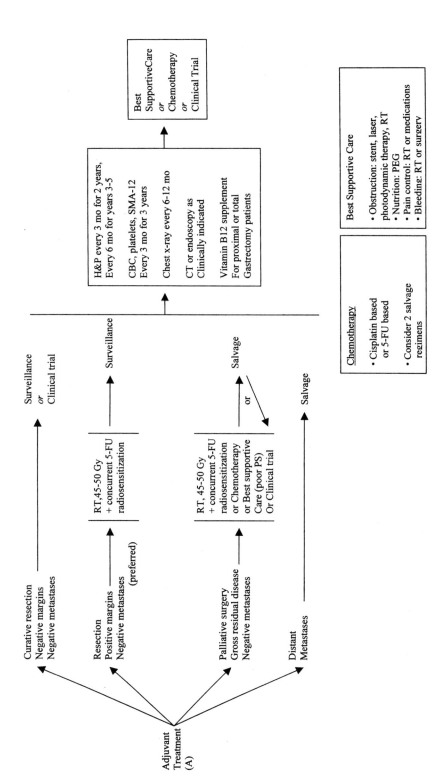

FIG. 2. Adjuvant treatment.

tomy bypass surgery results alone. The selection of patients most likely to benefit from this palliative effort requires further evaluation.

Radiation Therapy

Local Control

Because postsurgical recurrence occurs locally in 40% of patients, radiotherapy is useful in improving local control, but few reports have observed increased survival. This modality is limited by the technical challenges inherent in abdominal irradiation, optimal definition of fields, and the generally diminished performance status, in particular, nutritional state, of potential candidates.

Combined Chemoradiation

Combined chemoradiation is useful in up to 40% of patients, typically in combination with 5-fluorouracil (5-FU) chemotherapy in the neoadjuvant or adjuvant setting. The adjuvant combination of radiotherapy with bolus 5-FU with or without leucovorin leads to 25% 5-year survivals in particular patients with T3 or T4 disease. Combined-modality therapy for unresectable disease leads to 14-month median survival versus 5.9 months for radiation alone.

Palliative Radiation

Palliative radiation is important in managing pain, obstructions, and bleeding.

Treatment Regimens

Adjuvant Therapy for Local and Locally Advanced Disease

The use of adjuvant chemotherapy is dictated by the high rate of recurrence in optimally resected patients. Despite the absence of lymph node involvement, 50% 5-year survival is typical. The risk of recurrence is higher in patients with serosal extension, positive nodes, or positive surgical margins. One of two meta-analyses suggested a small treatment benefit of borderline significance in 1,990 patients from 13 trials who were treated with adjuvant chemotherapy after curative resection. An odds of death ratio of 0.80 (95% CI, 0.66–0.97) was reported in contrast to an odds of death ratio of 0.88 (95% CI, 0.78–1.08) in another meta-analysis of 2,096 adjuvantly treated patients from 11 trials. An Intergroup randomized phase III trial of adjuvant postoperative chemotherapy and radiation therapy in resected gastric cancer is in progress, as well as other investigations in the U.S. and abroad.

Adjuvant chemotherapy regimens have included 5-FU and cisplatin or 5-FU, doxorubicin (Adriamycin), and methotrexate (FAMTX) or etoposide, doxorubicin (Adriamycin), and cisplatin (EAP). Combined-modality 5-FU with and without leucovorin and 4,000 to 5,000 cGy radiotherapy has generally been used with local control improvement (patients with T3 or T4 disease) and prolonged survival trends. Median survivals of 6 to 10 months and 25% 5-year survivals are reported in most studies.

Advanced Disease

The most commonly administered chemotherapeutic agents with objective response rates in gastric cancer include mitomycin C, doxorubicin, 5-FU, and cisplatin. Monotherapy with these agents results in 15% to 20% response rates, and responses with combination chemotherapy regimens increase to 30% to 60%.

5-FU/Leucovorin

Despite the higher responses and toxicity, no clinical or survival benefit for any combination regimens over those of 5-FU alone have been observed. In a study of 252 patients randomized to either 5-FU alone, or 5-FU, doxorubicin, and cisplatin, or 5-FU, doxorubicin, and methyl CCNU (semustine) with triazinate, no survival advantage over the 5-FU alone arm was observed.

The following regimens exhibit variable response rates in phase II studies, but prospective, randomized phase III trials have failed to demonstrate a superior regimen.

- FAM regimen: Initial efforts combined 5-FU, doxorubicin, and mitomycin, and reported a response of 42% with a median survival of 12.5 months.
- FAP regimen: The substitution of mitomycin with cisplatin yielded a response rate of 34% and median survival of 30 weeks but with significant toxicity.
- EAP regimen: The synergy between etoposide and cisplatin resulted in 20% response rates, and addition of doxorubicin increased responses to 50% in patients with metastatic disease. Responses in patients with locoregional tumors were as high as 70%, with median survival of 10 to 17 months. EAP may benefit patients with more locally advanced disease but is less beneficial in patients with peritoneal carcinomatosis and other M1 disease. Significant toxicity was observed; treatment-related deaths approached 10%.
- ELF regimen: The addition of etoposide to leucovorin-modulated 5-FU leads to favorable responses of 48%, with 12% complete responses. A 10-month median survival is observed in this regimen, which is particularly useful in elderly and renal-impaired patients. High-dose leucovorin is suggested to further enhance responses. FAM with leucovorin leads to 50% responses and 11% complete responses.
- FAMTX regimen: The addition of methotrexate to 5-FU and doxorubicin results in response rates of 40%, with up to 12% complete responders, and median survivals of 7 to 10 months. Biochemical modulation of 5-FU with resultant increased incorporation requires sequential administration of methotrexate, typically 1 hour before 5-FU. More moderate doses of methotrexate, 400 mg/m^2 instead of 1,500 mg/m^2, may lead to diminished responses.
- MLP-F regimen: Combined 5-FU modulation with cisplatin, methotrexate, and leucovorin results in 82% responses, 33% complete responders, and median survival of 16 months. This regimen improved outcomes in local and metastatic disease but at the cost of toxicity; 25% of patients required hospitalization. The percentage of complete responders was influenced by supplemental local therapies (i.e., radiation to 50%).

INVESTIGATIONAL APPROACHES

- In the neoadjuvant setting, combined chemoradiation may improve resectability rates to 70% (typically 30–50% of patients), with evidence of downstaging. Clear demonstration of significant pathologic complete responses and resultant overall survival benefit is still unproven. Proximal tumors may benefit most from this approach.
- Intraoperative radiation may benefit up to 20% of patients with locally advanced, marginally resected disease and patients with unresectable tumors. A single dose of 2,000 to 4,000 cGy is typically administered. Local control and survival are improved, especially with the addition of 5-FU chemotherapy.
- Electron-beam radiotherapy delivered intraoperatively may provide a more favorable therapeutic index, as focused high-energy electron delivery to tumor tissue lessens potential normal tissue damage.
- Perioperative intraperitoneal therapy is typically administered, as peritoneal carcinomatosis is the most common site of recurrence, up to 80% in some reports, although rarely the only site of advanced disease. Intraperitoneal therapy typically consists of either 5-FU (FUDR better tolerated), cisplatin, mitomycin C, or the three agents in combination. The use of mit-

omycin C absorbed to activated charcoal resulted in a 67% 2-year survival. Patients at higher risk, with serosal involvement or contiguous structure invasion, also can receive prophylaxis with continuous hyperthermic peritoneal perfusion (CHPP) perioperatively.

• CHPP may benefit some patients with small-volume peritoneal recurrence, as this intraperitoneal therapy has exhibited some complete responses and survival benefit trends.

SUGGESTED READINGS

1. Fuchs CS, Mayer RJ. Gastric carcinoma. *N Engl J Med* 1995;333:32–41.
2. Alexander HR, Kelsen DG, Tepper JC. Cancer of the stomach. In: Devita VT, Hellman S, Rosenberg SA, eds. *Cancer: principles and practices of oncology.* Philadelphia: Lippincott, 1997:1021–1054.
3. Powell SM. *Stomach cancer.* In: Vogelstein B, Kinzler KW, eds. *The genetic basis of human cancer.* New York: McGraw-Hill, 1998:647–652.
4. Bonenkamp JJ, Hermans J, et al. Extended lymph-node dissection for gastric cancer: Dutch Gastric Cancer Group. *N Engl J Med* 1999;340:908–914.
5. Cullinan SA, Moertel CG, Wieard HS, et al. Controlled evaluation of three drug combination regimens versus fluorouracil alone for the therapy of advanced gastric cancer: North Central Cancer Treatment Group. *J Clin Oncol* 1994;12:412–416.
6. Gastrointestinal Tumor Study Group. A comparison of combination chemotherapy and combined modality therapy for locally advanced gastric carcinoma. *Cancer* 1982;49:1771–1777.
7. Hermans J, Bonenkamp JJ, Boon MC, et al. Adjuvant therapy after curative resection for gastric cancer: meta-analysis of randomized trials. *J Clin Oncol* 1993;11:1441–1447.
8. Earle CC and Maroun JA. Adjuvant chemotherapy after curative resection for gastric cancer in non-Asian patients: revisiting a meta-analysis of randomised trials. *Eur J Cancer* 1999;35:1059–1064.

6

Biliary Tract Cancer

Upendra Hegde and Jean Grem

Medicine Branch, DCS, National Cancer Institute, National Institutes of Health, Bethesda, Maryland

Carcinomas of the biliary tract include those cancers arising either in the gallbladder or the bile duct. The term cholangiocarcinoma was initially used to designate tumors of the intrahepatic bile ducts, but more recently refers to the entire spectrum of tumors arising in the intrahepatic, perihilar, and distal bile ducts. The clinical features, staging, and surgical treatment are distinct for carcinomas arising in the gallbladder and bile duct, and these are described separately. The palliative treatment options are similar and are discussed together at the end of the chapter.

EPIDEMIOLOGY

The demographic features are outlined in Table 1.

CARCINOMA OF THE GALLBLADDER

Clinical Features

The most common presenting symptoms and signs include:

- Right upper quarter (RUQ) pain.
- Nausea/vomiting.
- Fatty food intolerance.
- Anorexia.
- Weight loss.
- Jaundice.
- Tenderness.
- Abdominal mass.
- Fever.
- Hepatomegaly.
- Ascites.

A number of radiographic studies are helpful in evaluating the extent of disease. Ultrasound is very sensitive in detecting gallbladder stones. In gallbladder cancer, ultrasound typically shows a thickened gallbladder wall and may demonstrate tumor extension into the liver. Computed tomography (CT) scan is useful in identifying adenopathy and spread of disease into adjacent structures. Endoscopic retrograde cholangiopancreatography (ERCP) and transhepatic cholangiography (THC) can pinpoint the location of biliary obstruction.

TABLE 1. *Demographic features of biliary tract cancer*

Features	Gallbladder cancer	Cancers of the bile duct
Projected cases in U.S.A. (1999)	5,000	3,000
Gender predominance	More common in women (2.5- to 3-fold)	No gender difference
Median age	60–70 yr	60–70 yr
Higher-risk populations	Native Americans Israel Mexico Bolivia Chile Northern Japan	Native Americans Israel Japan

Predisposing factors	Cholelithiasis
	Calcified gallbladder wall
	Typhoid carriers
	Polyps
	Anomalous pancreaticobiliary ductal junction (Asians)
	Obesity
	Chemical carinogens
	  Rubber plant workers
	  Nitrosamines
	  Drugs
	  Estrogens
		Autoimmune diseases
		Ulcerative colitis
		Sclerosing cholangitis
		Hepatolithiasis
		Biliary cystic disease
		
		Cystic dilatation of the intrahepatic bile ducts
		Choledochal cysts
		Bile duct adenomas
		Multiple biliary papillomatosis
		Environmental exposure
		  Parasitosis (liver flukes, Southeast Asia)
		  Radiocontrast agents (Thoratrast)
		  Radionuclides
		  Chemical carcinogens
		    Nitrosamines, dioxin
		  Drugs
		    Isoniazid, methyldopa, oral contraceptives

Pathologic Features and Staging

About 85% of gallbladder cancers are adenocarcinomas, whereas the balance are composed of squamous or mixed tumors (Table 2). Locoregional involvement is common, including lymphatic spread and direct extension into the liver.

Surgical Treatment

The tumor stage influences whether the patient can undergo curative surgical resection. The best prognosis is seen in those patients in whom incidental cancer is found after cholecystectomy for symptomatic cholelithiasis (1–2% of cholecystectomy specimens). For T1 tumors, cholecystectomy alone is adequate, and 5-year survival is approximately 83%. If the tumor invades to or through serosa (T2, T3), resection of the gallbladder and gallbladder bed and porta hepatic lymphadenectomy are recommended; the median survival after "curative" resection is approximately 17 months, and 5-year survival is approximately 33%. The presence of nodal involvement reduces the 5-year survival to less than 15%. In patients who undergo a palliative procedure only, the median survival is 6 months. In patients who have more advanced local or metastatic disease and cannot undergo surgical resection, the median survival is 3 months.

TABLE 2. *AJCC stage groupings for gallbladder cancer*

Stage I	T1, N0, M0	T1a: invades lamina propria
		T1b: invades the muscle layer
Stage II	T2, N0, M0	T2: invades perimuscular connective tissue
Stage III	T3, N0, M0	T3: perforates the serosa and/or directly invades one adjacent organ (<2 cm into liver)
	T1–3, N1, M0	N1: mets in cystic duct, percholedochal, and/or hilar lymph nodes
Stage IVA	T4, N0–1, M0	T4: tumor extends >2 cm into the liver and/or into ≥2 adjacent organs
Stage IVB	Any T, N2, M0	N2: mets in peripancreatic (head only), periduodenal, periportal, celiac, and/or superior mesenteric lymph nodes
	Any T, any N, M1	M1: distant metastases

Mets, metastases.

CARCINOMA OF THE BILE DUCTS

Clinical Features

The most common presenting symptoms and signs include:

- Jaundice.
- Pruritis.
- Nausea/vomiting.
- Anorexia.
- Weight loss.
- Hepatomegaly.

Similar to the case with gallbladder cancer, ultrasound, CT scan, and ERCP are useful. Ultrasound is useful to detect cholelithiasis, mass lesions within the liver, and ductal dilatation throughout the obstructed liver segments. Pancreatic, periampullary, and intrahepatic tumors are more easily detected with conventional CT scanning than are perihilar tumors. The latter are better visualized with intravenous bolu-enhanced spiral CT scanning. CT scan also is useful in identifying regional lymphadenopathy. Cholangiography identifies dilation of bile ducts proximal to obstruction. ERCP is informative for distal primary tumors and simple perihilar tumors, whereas more proximal and sclerotic tumors are best assessed with THC. The invasive procedures permit procurement of bile samples, brush biopsies, and cytologic examination. ERCP is a newer technique with several advantages: it is a noninvasive procedure, does not require administration of exogenous contrast material, and is well tolerated by

TABLE 3. *Radiographic features according to location of the primary tumor*

Intrahepatic tumor involving single lobe with invasion of ipsilateral portal vein	Dilation of intrahepatic ducts in a single "atrophied" hepatic lobe
	Hypertrophy of the contralateral lobe
Perihilar	Dilation of right and left hepatic ducts
	Normal or collapsed gallbladder
Cystic duct	Distended gallbladder
	Normal caliber of intrahepatic or extrahepatic ducts
Distal	Distended gallbladder
	Dilated intra- and extrahepatic ducts

TABLE 4. *AJCC stage groupings for cancers of the bile ducts*

Stage I	T1, N0, M0	T1a: invades subepithelial connective tissue
		T1b: invades the fibromuscular layer
Stage II	T2, N0, M0	T2: invades perimuscular connective tissue
Stage III	T1–2, N1–2, M0	N1: mets to cystic duct, pericholedochal, and/or perihilar nodes
		N2: mets in peripancreatic area (head only), periduodenal, periportal, celiac, superior mesenteric, and/or posterior pancreaticoduodenal nodes
Stage IVA	T3, any N, M0	T3: tumor invades adjacent structures
Stage IVB	any T, any N, M1	M1: distant metastases

Mets, metastases.

patients. Because of the inherent contrast-related properties of fluid in the biliary and pancreatic ducts, ERCP produces images that are similar in appearance to those obtained by invasive radiographic methods. Biliary secretions have high signal intensity (i.e., appear white) on heavily T2-weighted sequences, whereas surrounding tissues have low signals (i.e., appear dark). ERCP offers the potential to reserve invasive procedures for patients in whom a therapeutic or diagnostic procedure is necessary (Table 3).

Pathologic Features and Staging

The vast majority (~95%) of bile duct cancers are adenocarcinomas (Table 4). The location of the primary tumors is distributed as shown in Table 5.

Surgical Treatment

Because of the onset of jaundice earlier in the course of disease than is typical for gallbladder cancer, surgical resection is possible in approximately 20% of proximal cancers and in up to two thirds of distal tumors (Table 6). The surgical management is outlined later. There is no established role for pre- or postoperative radiation therapy or chemotherapy given alone or in combination. The Radiation Therapy Oncology Group plans a randomized trial in biliary tract cancer to evaluate the worth of preoperative chronomodulated infusional 5-fluorouracil (5-FU) chemoradiation. Because the results of orthotopic liver transplantation for patients with intrahepatic cholangiocarcinoma have been poor, most centers are no longer performing transplants in these patients.

Many patients present with unresectable disease, and median survival is less than 1 year. Criteria that exclude a patient from attempts at resection include the following:

- Encasement of the main hepatic artery or portal vein.
- Lymph node involvement outside the hepatic pedicle.
- Distant metastasis.

TABLE 5. *Location of the primary tumors*

Location	Percentage
Intrahepatic	5
Perihilar (Klatskin tumors)	75
Tumors of the bifurcation of the right and left hepatic duct, tumors of the common hepatic duct, distal (common bile duct)	20

TABLE 6. *Surgical treatment with curative intent*

Location of primary	Surgical procedure	5-yr survival
Intrahepatic	Hepatic lobectomy	~35%–45%
Perihilar	En bloc resection of tumor,	~10%–45%
Bismuth types I and II	extrahepatic bile ducts, gallbladder,	
Involvement of common	and regional lymphadenectomy	
hepatic duct	Reconstruction by roux-en-Y	
Tumor at or just below	hepaticojejunostomy to right and	
bifurcation	left hepatic ducts	
	Resect involved lobe if cannot	
	achieve adequate margins	
Perihilar	Right or left hepatic lobectomy alone	~10%–20%
Bismuth type IIIa or IIIb	Lobectomy of involved lobe plus	~20%–35%
Involvement of right hepatic	caudate lobectomy	
duct		
Involvment of left hepatic duct		
Distal	Pancreatic oduodenectomy	Extrahepatic:
	Establish biliary–enteric continuity	~15%–25%
	Roux-en-Y choledochojejunostomy	Ampulla of vater:
	Jejunal loop	~50%–60%

- Bilateral tumor extension into secondary hepatic ducts.
- Bilateral extension of tumor into hepatic parenchyma.
- Ductal involvement of one side with contralateral vascular involvement.

Palliative Treatment for Carcinoma Arising in the Gallbladder and Bile Ducts

Patients with unresectable tumors may still benefit from palliative procedures, as outlined.

Palliative surgery
- Cholecystectomy.
- Roux-en-Y choledochojejunostomy with placement of transhepatic stents.
- Bypass of site of obstruction to left or right hepatic duct.
- Endoscopic or percutaneously placed stents for biliary drainage.
- Advantages of metal versus plastic stents.
  Metal stents have a larger diameter (less prone to become occluded).
  Rarely migrate.
- Local radiation therapy.
- Chemotherapy.
- Pain control.
- Oral analgesics and narcotics.
- Celiac plexus block (chemical splanchiectomy).

External-beam radiotherapy can be given with palliative intent or with a more aggressive approach. In patients with locally advanced and unresectable disease, total doses of 45 to 60 Gy have been given with standard fractions (1.8–2.0 Gy/day). Multishaped ports with three or four fields are typically used; customized blocking is needed to limit the dose of radiation to the liver, duodenum, distal small intestine, spinal cord, and right kidney. Chemotherapy plus radiation therapy has been used, but the data supporting a benefit come from nonrandomized, single-institution studies with relatively small numbers of patients. A phase I trial conducted by the Eastern Cooperative Oncology Group combined external-beam radiation therapy [59.4 Gy in 33 fractions (1.8 Gy) over 6–7 weeks] with concurrent protracted infusional 5-FU given starting on day 1 and continuing until the end of radiation. A 5-FU dose of 250 mg/m^2 was recommended, and the median survival was 11.9 months; 19% of patients were alive at 2 years.

Chemotherapy drugs with phase II single-agent activity include:

- 5-FU.
- Doxorubicin.
- Mitomycin C.
- Gemcitabine.

A number of phase II studies evaluating 5-FU in combination with other agents have reported higher response rates than might be expected with 5-FU alone. One phase II trial using the combination of epirubicin (50 mg/m^2 i.v., day 1), cisplatin (60 mg/m^2 i.v., day 1), and protracted infusional 5-FU (200 mg/m^2, days 1–21) once every 3 weeks was associated with objective responses in eight of 20 evaluable patients with bile duct cancer. These results must be confirmed in a larger study. Randomized trials will be required to establish the relative benefits of combination versus single-agent chemotherapy. Outside of a clinical trial setting, treatment with 5-FU alone or modulated by leucovorin seems reasonable.

CONCLUSIONS

Data from Eurocare II, a European Union project, indicate that the overall 1-year and 5-year survival rates over the period of 1985 through 1989 for 11,589 patients with biliary tract cancer were 26% and 12%, respectively. When the trends in 1-year survival rate for patients over time were considered, there appeared to be an improvement for patients registered between 1987 and 1989 (29%) versus 1978 through 1980 (20%) (relative risk, 0.77). However, there was less improvement in 5-year survival over time: 14% versus 11%. These data suggest that improvements in conventional therapies such as surgery, radiation, and chemotherapy over the decade of the 1990s are unlikely to improve these results dramatically. However, progress for the future may be realized from strategies aimed at prevention and prophylaxis or early detection in high-risk patients.

SUGGESTED READINGS

1. de Groen PC, Gores GJ, LaRusso NF, et al. Biliary tract cancers. *N Engl J Med* 1999;341:1368–1378.
2. Faivre J, Forman D, Esteve J, et al, Survival of patients with primary liver cancer, pancreatic cancer and biliary tract cancer in Europe: EUROCARE Working Group. *Eur J Cancer* 1998;34:2184–2190.
3. Whittington R, Neuberg D, Tester W, et al. Protracted intravenous fluorouracil infusion with radiation therapy in the management of localized pancreaticobiliary carcinoma: a phase I Eastern Cooperative Oncology Group Trial. *J Clin Oncol* 1995;13:227–232.
4. Hejna M, Pruckmayer M, Raderer M. The role of chemotherapy and radiation in the management of biliary cancer: a review of literature. *Eur J Cancer* 1998;34:977–986.
5. Barish MA, Kent Yucel E, Ferrucci JT. Magnetic resonance cholangiopancreatography. *N Engl J Med* 1999;341:258–264.
6. Saini S. Imaging of the hepatobiliary tract. *N Engl J Med* 1997;336:1889–1894.

7

Primary Cancers of the Liver

Upendra Hegde and Jean Grem

*Medicine Branch, DCS, National Cancer Institute, National Institutes of Health,
Bethesda, Maryland*

The incidence of primary cancers of the liver shows striking geographic variation, ranging from approximately five per 100,000 in North and South America, the United Kingdom, and Scandinavia, to 20 to 150 per 100,000 in China, Southeast Asia, and Western/Southern Africa. About 14,000 cases per year were expected in the United States in 1999. The incidence in male subjects is three- to fivefold higher than in female subjects in all regions. Within regions, the incidence varies by race: Asian > blacks > whites. Most primary liver cancers arise from the parenchymal liver cells or hepatocytes, and are called hepatocellular carcinoma (HCC). Tumors arising from the intrahepatic bile ducts are called cholangiocarcinomas; although the etiology is different from that of HCC, the clinical manifestations and surgical management in resectable patients are similar.

ETIOLOGY

Chronic infection with hepatitis B virus and hepatitis C virus is associated with the development of HCC. The majority of patients with HCC have underlying cirrhosis, but cirrhosis due to ethanol abuse and autoimmune chronic active hepatitis also is associated with an increased risk of HCC. Environmental factors may contribute to the development of HCC. The best-studied agent is a product of the *Aspergillus* fungus, aflatoxin B, which is found in regions in which grains are stored unrefrigerated. Chronic ingestion of various plants including *Senecio,* bush trees, and cycad, which contain pyrrolizidine alkaloids, tannic acid, sassafras oil, and cycasin, also is considered a risk factor for HCC. Other risk factors include ingestion of nitrites and nitrate-treated foods, androgenic steroids, exposure to pesticides and insecticides, and exposure to industrial solvents (dioxane, chloroform, carbon tetrachloride, vinyl chloride, polychorinated biphenyls, and trichloroethylene). Those with two metabolic diseases have a high risk of developing HCC: hemochromatosis and hereditary tyrosinemia. Patients with other metabolic diseases including Wilson's disease, α_1-antitrypsin deficiency, porphyria cutanea tarda, glycogen-storage diseases 1 and 3, citrullinemia, and orotic aciduria also are at increased risk of developing HCC.

HISTOLOGY

The vast majority of primary liver cancers arise from epithelial cells and are primarily adenocarcinomas. The spectrum includes typical HCC, the fibrolamellar variant of HCC, cholangiocarcinoma, mixed HCC/cholangiocarcinoma, and undifferentiated cancers. HCC may be manifest in nodular, diffuse, or massive form; the latter two account for the majority of cases.

The nodular form often has multiple lesions in both lobes. In general, the malignant cells are larger than normal hepatocytes, have a polygonal shape, and appear finely granular with eosinophilic cytoplasm. Distinctive histologic patterns include trabecular, compact, acinar, clear cell, and fibrolamellar variants. Fewer than 3% of primary liver tumors arise from mesenchymal cells; these include sarcoma, angiosarcoma, epithelioid tumors, and hemangioendothelioma. Hepatoblastoma is a very rare cancer that occurs in children with an incidence of one per 100,000.

Invasion of the hepatic vein is common with HCC, and the incidence is higher with larger tumors: in resected specimens, the incidence is approximately 20% with primary tumors less than 2 cm in diameter, but ranges from 70% to 90% with tumors more than 5 cm in diameter. HCC may be complicated by thrombosis of the hepatic vein, vena cava, and/or portal veins.

Among the primary tumors of epithelial origin, the fibrolamellar variant is the only one with a more favorable prognosis. This tumor tends to occur in young female subjects, is not associated with cirrhosis, and is often solitary. The histology is distinctive: eosinophilic, polygonal cells separated by lamellar fibrosis.

CLINICAL FEATURES

Abdominal pain is the most common symptom; other symptoms include increasing abdominal girth, weight loss, fullness, anorexia, vomiting, and jaundice. The most common physical signs are hepatomegaly and stigmata of cirrhosis, but may include abdominal bruits (reflecting increased vascularity), ascites, splenomegaly, Budd–Chiari syndrome, Virchow's node, and cutaneous metastasis. HCC may be associated with a variety of paraneoplastic features including hypoglycemia, erythrocytosis, hypercalcemia, hypercholesterolemia, dysfibrinogenemia, carcinoid syndrome, increased thyroxine-binding globulin, sexual changes, and porphyria cutanea tarda. Common chemistry abnormalities include elevations in alkaline phosphatase, liver transaminases, bilirubin, and α_1-globulin. Very high serum bilirubin levels suggest intrahepatic or extrahepatic obstruction of major bile ducts. Poor synthetic function of the liver usually reflects severe underlying cirrhosis. α-Fetoprotein is elevated in about two thirds of patients with HCC in Western countries. The des-γ-carboxy prothrombin protein

TABLE 1. *Imaging modalities for hepatocellular carcinoma*

Imaging study	Diagnostic features and advantages
Abdominal ultrasound	Inexpensive & widely available; useful for screening high-risk populations
Computed tomography, triphasic spiral CT evaluation	Delineates the extent of hepatic involvement, invasion or thrombosis of the portal and hepatic veins, regional lymph node involvement, splenomegaly, and ascites
CT portography: contrast injected in superior mesenteric artery	Contrast enters portal vein and permits good contrast between normal and tumor tissue
Ethiodol (Lipiodol) CT scanning: ethiodized oil emulsion retained by liver tumors	Can be delivered by hepatic artery injection with delayed CT imaging 1–3 weeks later; can detect tumors <5 mm in size
Hepatic angiography	Reveals multiple, tortuous tumor vessels, and a characteristic early venous tumor blush; provides important details about the vascular anatomy in planning hepatic intraarterial therapy
MRI with intravenous gadolinium	T2-weighted spin-echo sequence can detect small hepatic tumors; T2 signal is less intense than seen with hemangiomas

MRI, magnetic resonance imaging.

TABLE 2. *AJCC stage groupings*

Stage I	T1, N0, M0	T1: solitary tumor ≤ 2 cm, no vascular invasion
Stage II	T2, N0, M0	T2: solitary tumor ≤ 2 cm, with vascular invasion; multiple tumors (one lobe only), none >2 cm, no vascular invasion; solitary tumor >2 cm, no vascular invasion
Stage IIIA	T3, N0, M0	T3: solitary tumor >2 cm, with vascular invasion; multiple tumors (one lobe only) with no tumor >2 cm with vascular invasion; multiple tumors (one lobe only) with any tumor >2 cm vascular invasion
Stage IIIB	T1–3, N1, M0	N1: regional lymph node involvement including nodes in hepatoduodenal ligament, hepatic and periportal nodes, and nodes along inferior vena cava, portal vein, and hepatic artery
Stage IVA	T4, any N, M0	T4: multiple tumors in more than one lobe; tumor(s) involving a major branch or portal or hepatic vein
Stage IVB	Any T, any N, M1	M1: distant metastases

induced by vitamin K abnormality is elevated in more than 90% of patients wtih HCC, but is not specific for this disease. Hepatitis A, B, C, and D serology should be measured, and if the hepatitis B serology is positive, hepatitis B DNA or RNA should be quantitated.

A variety of imaging studies are available to assist in staging and evaluation of the disease (Table 1).

For nonsurgical candidates, percutaneous biopsy or fine-needle aspirate for cytology provides the tumor diagnosis. If surgery is planned, an open biopsy at laparotomy is usually preferred to decrease the risk of tumor seeding.

AJCC STAGE GROUPINGS

The TNM staging system (Table 2) has been criticized because it does not evaluate the underlying liver disease, which is clearly a major prognostic factor in patients regardless of tumor stage.

TREATMENT OPTIONS

Surgery

Surgical resection offers the potential for cure, but only a minority of patients are candidates. The best results are seen in patients with clinical stage I and II disease in whom a 2-cm surgical margin of normal liver is achieved. Patients must have adequate hepatic reserve (Child's class A), defined as bilirubin less than 2.0 mg/dL, serum albumin approximately 3.5 g/dL, no ascites, no neurologic dysfunction, and excellent nutritional status. Long-term survival is achieved in 25% to 50% of patients who undergo a potentially curative resection. Long-term survival is unusual if more than one lobe is involved. Although operative mortality varies from center to center, the average is about 15%.

Because many patients with moderate cirrhosis are not good surgical candidates even if they have early-stage HCC, transplantation has become a potential therapeutic option. Liver transplantation offers the potential advantages of curing the HCC as well as the underlying cirrhosis. Results are most favorable for patients with small primary tumors. In contrast, factors that portend a poor outcome after transplantation include tumors larger than 5 cm, multiple tumors, involvement of more than one lobe, vascular invasion, and diffuse tumor infiltration. In selected patients, 5-year survival rates for stages I, II, and III disease are 75%, 60%, and 40%, respectively, whereas fewer than 10% of stage IV patients who have received a transplant are alive at 5 years. The recurrence rate appears to be lower than that expected with surgical resection alone for patients with stage II and III tumors. With additional experience, most transplant centers now exclude patients with macroscopic evidence of vascular invasion by tumor, bilobar HCC (TNM stage IVa), and patients with any stage of HCC displaying hepatitis B virus antigen in plasma or viral DNA in blood. Disadvantages of transplantation include the expense, the availability at only a few selected centers, the limited supply of donor livers, and the potential for tumor progression before a suitable donor liver is available. Preoperative chemoembolization is often used as a temporizing modality and to downstage patients, but the worth of this approach is not yet proven. Because the outcome for patients with cholangiocarcinoma undergoing transplantation has been extremely poor, patients with this diagnosis are not currently considered to be transplant candidates.

Locoregional Approaches for HCC

A variety of regional approaches for the palliation of HCC are available (Table 3). In general, the data supporting benefit of these approaches are derived from single-institution or phase II studies. Transhepatic arterial (chemo)embolization and hepatic arterial infusion of chemotherapy are contraindicated in patients with portal vein thrombosis or advanced cirrhosis. In contrast, regional administration of Lipiodal can be given administered safely to patients with portal vein thrombosis. Three randomized trials comparing different methods of chemoembolization for patients with unresectable disease have failed to show survival benefit over more conservative therapy.

Systemic Therapy

The median survival for HCC patients who are not surgical candidates and who receive no treatment is only a few months. A variety of single chemotherapy agents have been reported to have some activity in HCC (including doxorubicin, 5-FU, epirubicin, cisplatin) in small trials, but more recent phase II trials have generally failed to confirm single-agent response rates higher than 10% to 15% in untreated patients. Combination chemotherapy regimens have not demonstrated a survival benefit. Response rates are usually higher with hepatic arterial administration of chemotherapy, but no survival advantage has been found in randomized trials comparing intravenous with intraarterial therapy.

Factors suggesting potential androgen dependence of hepatocellular carcinoma have led to evaluation of hormonal therapy:

- Male predominance of HCC.
- HCC can be induced by androgen therapy.
- Androgen receptors are physiologically expressed in normal livers but are expressed at high concentration in HCC.
- Some HCC cell lines have receptors for gonadotropin-releasing hormone.

A phase III double-blind trial randomized 244 patients to one of four arms: nilutamide (Anandron) plus placebo; luteinizing hormone–releasing hormone (LHRH) agonist plus placebo; nilutamide plus LHRH agonist; or placebo plus placebo. No significant difference in survival was evident for any of the four arms. The results of 2×2 factorial analysis (Table 4) also failed to demonstrate any benefit for antiandrogen therapy.

Similarly, the observations that estrogens may produce liver adenomas, and that estrogens may be elevated in patients with cirrhosis, have led to the evaluation of tamoxifen in the treatment of HCC. Several small randomized trials suggested an improvement in survival in HCC patients who received tamoxifen, whereas a larger 120-patient trial failed to confirm this. Therefore a large multicenter phase III trial was conducted in which 496 patients with HCC (any stage) were randomized to receive either tamoxifen, 40 mg p.o. qd until death, or best

TABLE 3. *Methods of palliation in hepatocellular carcinoma*

Modality	Rationale	Advantages and disadvantages
Cryosurgery	Freeze the tumor: in situ destruction of tumor by application of subzero temperatures by specially designed probes that contain circulating liquid nitrogen	Can be performed in patients with multifocal lesions and limited hepatic reserve; complications include cracking of the liver, bile leakage, hemorrhage, infection, myoglobinuria, and renal failure
Percutaneous ethanol injections	Alcohol precipitates macromolecules Results in death of HCC cells Alcohol diffuses more readily in tumor tissue than in surrounding cirrhotic tissue	Effective in the control of small tumors in patients not fit for other treatment modalities; involves no loss of cirrhotic tissue; is relatively safe and can be repeated; relatively low cost; best results in single or a few tumors <5 cm in diameter
Transhepatic arterial embolization (a) Lipiodal (iodized poppyseed oil), (b) Gelfoam (gelatin sponge particles)	Devascularize tumor Primary blood supply Tumors: hepatic artery Normal liver: portal vein Lipiodol used as a delivery agent because it is retained in tumor vessels for weeks Use of degradable vasoocclusive particles minimizes collateralization of blood flow by creating more distal vascular blockade (Gelfoam absorbed in 48–72 h)	May be repeated and used before hepatic resection or hepatic transplantation. Chemotherapy drugs can be added to increase the local tumor kill (doxorubicin, cisplatin, mitomycin C); has significant acute morbidity (fever, abdominal pain, acute hepatic failure)
Hepatic arterial infusion of chemotherapy	Use of drugs with high hepatic extraction permits delivery of high local concentrations of drug to the tumor while minimizing systemic exposure. Drugs include 5-FU, FUDR, anthracyclines, and cisplatin	Requires placement of hepatic arterial catheter with risk of bleeding, thrombosis, and infection
External beam radiation	To achieve symptomatic palliation of painful hepatomegaly	Dose limited to 30–35 Gy over 3–4 weeks; conformal radiation techniques may permit higher doses to be delivered safely
Intrahepatic radioisotopes: (a) ^{131}I-Lipiodal or (b) yttrium 90	[127]I in lipiodal can be replaced by ^{131}I, which produces both and irradiation. Yttrium 90 is a pure emitter; delivered via glass microspheres	Lipiodal accumulates in tumor tissue and becomes trapped in the microvasculature; yttrium 90 may allow delivery of higher doses with less potential for systemic toxicity

HCC, hepatocellular carcinoma; 5-FU, 5-fluorouracil; FUDR, fluorodeoxyuridine

TABLE 4. *Antiandrogen treatment in hepatocellular carcinoma*

Hormonal agent?	No	Yes
Antiandrogen		
Male/female	101/18	118/17
Median survival	4.7 mo	3.7 mo
LHRH agonist		
Male/female	99/17	103/18
Median survival	4.8 mo	3.4 mo

LHRH, luteinizing hormone–releasing hormone.

supportive care. No difference was noted in median survival: 16 months versus 15 mont[s] (supportive care). The results of this trial refute any benefit of tamoxifen for the treatment [of] HCC when used in doses expected to exhibit an anti–estrogen receptor effect. Because mo[st] HCCs are not estrogen-receptor positive, others have argued that any potential effect [of] tamoxifen would be exerted through estrogen receptor–independent mechanisms. Therefo[re] an ongoing double-blind, placebo-controlled study in Singapore is comparing placebo wi[th] one of two doses of tamoxifen (80 or 120 mg daily) for 1 year in patients with HCC.

Although initial results with systemic administration of ^{131}I-labeled antiferritin antibo[dy] seemed promising, a randomized trial comparing systemic chemotherapy with doxorubic[in] and 5-FU alone or with [^{131}I]antiferritin antibody showed equivalent response rates a[nd] median survival (6 months). Other primary liver tumors are shown in Table 5.

TABLE 5. *Other primary liver tumors*

Tumor	Characteristics
Hepatoblastoma	Most common primary malignant tumor of the liver in children
	Affects young children (< age 3)
	Abdominal distention
	Sexual precocity due to ectopic sex hormone production
	AFP levels are markedly increased in > 75%
	CT scan: solitary enhancing mass in 80%; speckled calcificatio[n] in 50%
	Angiography: hypervascular
	Surgical resection possible in ½–⅔ of patients; 30–70% are cur[ed]
	More chemosensitive than HCC: active agents include doxorubicin, vincristine, cyclophosphamide, 5-FU
	Preop chemotherapy may increase resectability rate
	Postop adjuvant chemotherapy may improve survival
Angiosarcoma	Highly aggressive tumor (median survival, <6 mo)
	50% develop distant metastases
	85% patients are male
	Peak incidence in 6th and 7th decades
	Abdominal pain most common symptom
	Related to vinyl chloride, arsenic solutions, and Thorotrast
	Surgical resection is treatment of choice
	Insensitive to chemotherapy and radiation therapy
Epithelioid Hemangioendothelioma	Slight female excess
	Median age is 50 yr
	Tumor is generally low grade but can metastasize in 30%
	Tumor stains for factor VIII
	Vinyl chloride exposure is risk factor
	Surgical resection is treatment of choice

AFP, α-fetoprotein; HCC, hepatocellular carcinoma; CT, computed tomography.

PREVENTION

Given the dismal prognosis for most patients with HCC, strategies focusing on primary prevention offer the promise of reducing mortality. It is hoped that more widespread use of the hepatitis B vaccine will decrease the incidence of patients with chronic hepatitis B, although the cost of such vaccination in developing nations may be prohibitive. Transmission of the hepatitis B virus at birth though the vaginal canal is a major source of viral infection, and infants and children exposed to hepatitis B virus have a greater chance of becoming chronic carriers than do newly infected adult patients. These observations form the rationale for a large intervention study, sponsored by the World Health Organization, that is currently under way in Asia involving vaccination of newborns. However, it will take many years of follow-up to ascertain whether this strategy indeed reduces the incidence of HCC.

The use of interferon-α in patients with chronic hepatitis C reduces the onset of liver damage and progression to cirrhosis in about 10% to 30% of the patients. One randomized trial demonstrated that a 12- to 24-week treatment with interferon-α reduced the incidence of HCC in patients with chronic active hepatitis C with cirrhosis. Unanswered questions include the optimal timing, dose, and length of interferon-α therapy. Refrigerated storage of food grains and transportation of grains in refrigerated vehicles should help reduce the risk of ingesting aflatoxin.

Screening of high-risk populations with α-fetoprotein at 4-month intervals and ultrasound at yearly intervals has been shown to identify patients with earlier stages of HCC. Unfortunately, it is not yet clear if screening influences mortality, and if it is a cost-effective strategy.

One randomized trial suggested that the acyclic retinoid polyprenoic acid reduced the incidence of second primaries of HCC after initial resection. If this finding is confirmed in larger trials, this may ultimately improve results in surgically resected patients and provide a strategy for chemoprevention in patients at risk for HCC.

REFERENCES

1. Carr BI, Flickinger JC, Lotze MT. *Hepatobiliary cancers.* In: DeVita VT Jr, Hellman S, Rosenberg SA, eds. *Cancer: principles and practice of oncology.* 5th ed. Lippincott-Raven, 1997:1087–1114.
2. Schafer DF, Sorrell MF. Hepatocellular carcinoma. *Lancet* 1999;353:1253–1257.
3. Soni P, Dusheiko GM, Harrison TJ. Genetic diversity of hepatitis C virus: implications for pathogenesis, treatment, and prevention. *Lancet* 1995;345:562–566.
4. Bottelli R, Tibballs J, Hochhauser D, et al. Ultrasound screening for hepatocellular carcinoma (HCC) in cirrhosis: the evidence for an established clinical practice. *Clin Radiol* 1998;53:713–716.
5. Venook AP. Treatment of hepatocellular carcinoma: too many options? *J Clin Oncol* 1994;12: 1323–1334.
6. Mor E, Kaspa RT, Sheiner P, et al. Treatment of hepatocellular carcinoma associated with cirrhosis in the era of liver transplantation. *Ann Intern Med* 1998;129:643–653.
7. Finch MD, Crosbie JL, Currie E, et al. An 8 year experience of hepatic resection: indications and outcome. *Br J Surg* 1988;85:315–319.
8. Ahmed A, Keeffe EB. Treatment strategies for chronic hepatitis C: update since the 1997 National Institutes of Health consensus development conference. *J Gastroenterol Hepatol* 1999;14(suppl): S12—18.
9. Yoshida H, Shiratori Y, Moriyama M. Interferon therapy reduces the risk for hepatocellular carcinoma: national surveillance program of cirrhotic and noncirrhotic patients with chronic hepatitis C in Japan. *Ann Intern Med* 1999;131:174–181.
10. McGinn CJ, Ten Haken RK, Ensminger WD, et al. Treatment of intrahepatic cancers with radiation doses based on a normal tissue complication probability model. *J Clin Oncol* 1998;16:2246–2252.
11. Grimaldi C, Bleiberg H, Gay F, et al. Evaluation of antiandrogen therapy in unresectable hepatocellular carcinoma: results of a European organization for research and treatment of cancer multicentric double-blind trial. *J Clin Oncol* 1998;16:411–417.

8

Colorectal Cancer

George P. Kim, Chris H. Takimoto, and Carmen J. Allegra

Medicine Branch, National Cancer Institute, National Institute of Health, Bethesda, Maryland

EPIDEMIOLOGY

- Colorectal cancer is the second leading cause of cancer death in the United States after lung cancer.
- Approximately 129,400 new cases will be diagnosed in 1999, and 56,600 Americans will die of this disease.
- Colon cancer comprises more 13% of all cancers in the U.S., with the vast majority of cases occurring in patients after the fifth decade of life.
- Surgery will cure almost half of these patients, although almost 60,000 people each year develop metastatic colorectal cancer.
- The incidence of colon cancer is higher in more economically developed regions such as the U.S. or in Western Europe than in Asia, Africa, or South America. Between 1973 and 1995, the U.S. incidence of colorectal cancer declined by 7.4% and mortality by 20.8%.

RISK FACTORS

Although certain conditions predispose patients to colon cancer development, up to 70% of patients have no identifiable risk factors.

- Age: More than 90% of cases occur in patients older than 50 years.
- Gender: Colon cancer is higher in women (1.20:1.0), whereas rectal cancer is more common in men (1.27:1.0).
- Ethnicity: More common in African-Americans than in whites (1.16:1).
- History of colorectal cancer or adenomas:
    Tubular adenomas (lowest risk).
    Tubulovillous adenomas (intermediate risk).
    Villous adenomas (highest risk).
- Tobacco use: About 2.5-fold increased risk of adenomas.
- Dietary factors: high-fiber, low-caloric-intake, and low-animal-fat diets may reduce risk.
- Calcium deficiency: Daily intake of 1.25–2.0 g of calcium is associated with a reduced risk of recurrent adenomas in a randomized placebo-controlled trial.
- Micronutrient deficiency of folate and vitamins E and D may increase risk.
- Inflammatory bowel disease: Ulcerative colitis increases risk by sevenfold to 11-fold, and Crohn's colitis is associated with a twofold increased risk of colorectal cancer.
- Nonsteroidal antiinflammatory drugs (NSAIDs): An American Cancer Society study reported 40% lower mortality in regular aspirin users, and similar reductions were seen in

prolonged NSAID use in patients with rheumatologic disorders. The new cyclooxygenase-2 (COX-2) inhibitor celecoxib was recently approved by the U.S. Food and Drug Administration (FDA) for adjunctive treatment of patients with familial adenomatous polyposis (FAP).

- Family history: In the general population, one first-degree relative with cancer results in an increased relative risk of 1.72, and if two relatives are affected, relative risk increases to 2.75; also increased risk if first-degree relative develops an adenomatous polyp before age 60 years. True hereditary forms of cancer account for only 6% of colorectal cancers.

Familial Adenomatous Polyposis Syndrome

FAP is an autosomal dominant inherited syndrome with more than 90% penetrance, manifested by hundreds of polyps developing by late adolescence. The risk of invasive cancer over time is virtually 100%. Germline mutations in the adenomatous polyposis coli (APC) gene have been identified.

Hereditary Nonpolyposis Colorectal Cancer

The Lynch syndromes, named after Henry T. Lynch, include Lynch I or the colonic syndrome, which is an autosomal dominant trait characterized by distinct clinical features including proximal colon involvement, mucinous or poorly differentiated histology, pseudodiploidy, and the presence of synchronous or metachronous tumors. Increased survival has been observed despite colon cancer developing before age 50 years, with a lifetime risk of cancer approximating 75%. The Lynch II or extracolonic individuals are susceptible to endometrial, ovary, stomach, hepatobiliary, small intestine, and genitourinary malignancies.

The "Amsterdam Criteria" were established to identify potential kindreds and include:

- Histologically verified colorectal cancer in at least three family members, one a first-degree relative of the other two.
- Colorectal cancer involving at least two successive generations.
- At least one family member diagnosed by age 50 years.

Inclusion of extracolonic tumors as well as clinicopathologic and age modifications were introduced by the "Bethesda Criteria" in 1997. Germline defects in DNA mismatch repair genes (*hMSH2*, *hMLH1*, *hPMS1*, *hPMS2*) have been detected, and resultant microsatellite instability can be identified in virtually all hereditary nonpolyposis colorectal cancer (HNPCC) kindreds and in 15% to 20% of sporadic colon cancers.

SCREENING

Digital Rectal Examination

Digital rectal examination (DRE) has a low rate of risk reduction with limited impact on survival but remains a simple, inexpensive test.

Fecal Occult Blood Testing

Yearly fecal occult blood testing (FOBT) is recommended by the U.S. Preventive Services Task Force for patients older than 50 years. Minnesota researchers reported a 46,551-patient study in which yearly FOBT reduced the cumulative 13-year mortality by 33% (5.88 patients vs. control, 8.83/1,000). In addition, cancers were detected at an earlier stage, with stage A disease increased from 5.5 to 6.9 per 1,000, whereas patients with stage D decreased from 4.4 to 2.3 per 1,000. Conversely, the low positive predictive value of FOBT (less than 20%) can result in unnecessary patient inconvenience and health care expenditure, whereas two thirds of colon cancer patients could die with a negative test.

Flexible Sigmoidoscopy

The detection of precancerous lesions and adenomatous polyps and their removal reduces the risk of colorectal cancer. The National Polyp Study showed a greater than 75% reduction in the subsequent incidence of colorectal cancer after colonoscopic polypectomy. The finding of an adenoma on flexible sigmoidoscopy, which reaches to 60 cm, may warrant colonoscopy to evaluate the more proximal colon for synchronous lesions. The U.S. Preventive Services Task Force recommends performing flexible sigmoidoscopies on all patients after the age of 50 years.

The American Cancer Society has developed screening guidelines:

- Average risk (roughly 70–80% of individuals): Initial screening instituted at age 50 years, with annual FOBT and sigmoidoscopy every 3 to 5 years.
- Moderate risk: Total colonic examination every 3 years, especially if polyps are initially detected. If a patient has a positive FOBT or an abnormal flexible sigmoidoscopy, then the entire colon should be examined with either a barium enema or colonoscopy.
- High-risk patients with strong family history: FAP (screening as early as age 10 years) or HNPCC (screening in early twenties), and colonoscopy annually after age 35 years.

Carcinoembryonic Antigen

Carcinoembryonic antigen (CEA) is not useful for general colorectal cancer screening purposes. CEA has a low positive predictive value whereby approximately 60% of cancers are missed.

K-ras Detection

The k-*ras* gene is mutated in 50% of colorectal cancers, and its detection in stool represents a potential powerful screening strategy. This is currently an active area of clinical investigation.

PATHOPHYSIOLOGY

Colon carcinogenesis involves progression from hyperproliferative mucosa, to polyp formation with dysplastic involvement, to transformation to noninvasive lesions and subsequent tumor cells with invasive and metastatic capabilities. Colorectal cancer is a unique model of multistep carcinogenesis resulting from the accumulation of multiple genetic alterations. Stage-by-stage molecular analysis has revealed this progression to involve several types of genetic instability, including loss of heterozygosity, with chromosomes *8p*, *17p*, and *18q* representing the most common chromosomal losses. The *17p* deletion accounts for loss of *p53* function, and *18q* contains the tumor-suppressor genes deleted in colon cancer (DCC) and deleted in pancreatic cancer 4 (DPC4). The loss of heterozygosity of chromosome *18q* has prognostic significance.

Colon carcinogenesis also is a consequence of defects in the DNA mismatch-repair system. The loss of predominantly hMLH1 and hMSH2 in sporadic cancers leads to accelerated accumulation of additions or deletions in repeating DNA nucleotide units. This microsatellite instability (MSI) contributes to loss of growth inhibition mediated by transforming growth factor-β (TGFβ) due to a mutation in the type II receptor. Mutations in the adenomatous polyposis coli (APC) gene on chromosome *5q21* are responsible for FAP and are involved in cell signaling and cellular adhesion with binding of β-catenin. Alterations in the APC gene occur early in tumor progression. Mutations in the protooncogene *ras* family, including K-*ras* and N-*ras*, are important for transformation and also are common in early tumor development.

More than 90% of colorectal cancers are adenocarcinomas, with proximal tumors becoming increasingly more common. Left-sided cancers tend to be annular, leading to obstruction, whereas right-sided cancers are more commonly polypoid and clinically silent. One third of patients will initially be seen with metastatic disease, whereas 50% will eventually develop metastases.

DIAGNOSIS

Signs and Symptoms

- Abdominal pain, typically intermittent and vague.
- Weight loss.
- Bowel changes, such as pencil-caliber stools.
- Early satiety.
- Gastrointestinal bleeding.
- Fatigue.
- Obstruction, perforation, acute or chronic bleeding, or liver metastasis all contribute to symptom development.
- Unusual presentations include patients with deep venous thrombosis, *Streptococcus bovis* bacteremia, and nephrotic range proteinuria.
- Clinical findings include anemia, weight loss, electrolyte abnormalities, and liver enzyme elevations.

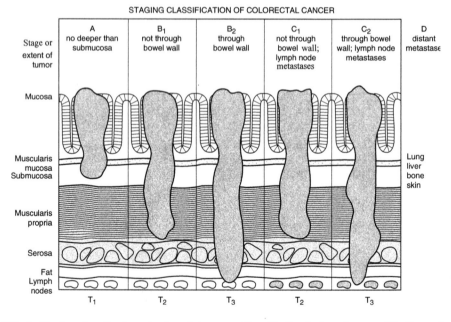

FIG. 1. Staging classification of colorectal cancer. Classification is based on modifications of Dukes' system. Stages B3 and C3 (not shown) signify invasion of contiguous organs or structures (T4). Prognosis also is determined by the number of positive lymph nodes: More than four (N2) predicts a worse outcome than one to three (N1), poor histopathologic differentiation, vascular or lymphatic invasion, and a positive preoperative. CEA >5 ng/mL implies a worse outcome. According to the revised TNM classification system, stage I equals T1 or T2 N0 (Dukes' stage A and B2); stage II equals T3 or T4 N0 (Dukes' stage B2 and B3); stage III equals any T plus N1, N2, or N3 (Dukes' stage C1, C2 and C3); and IV equals any T, any N, plus M2 (Dukes' stage D).

Diagnostic Evaluation

- As an initial evaluation, a double-contrast barium enema may be more cost-effective, but endoscopic studies provide histologic information, potential therapeutic intervention, and overall greater sensitivity and specificity.
- Basic laboratory studies including complete blood count, electrolytes, and liver and renal function tests, chest radiograph, and computerized tomography of the abdomen and pelvis are useful in initial cancer diagnosis, although the relative contributions of these various modalities are undefined.
- CEA elevations occur in non–cancer-related conditions, reducing the specificity of CEA measurements in initial detection of colon cancer.

STAGING

The American Joint Committee on Cancer (AJCC; 1) staging of colon cancer (Fig. 1) by TNM classification was updated in 1997 (Table 1). The tumor designation, or T, is unique in defining extent of bowel wall penetration, as opposed to tumor size. The AJCC staging system accounts for two significant predictors of survival: number of lymph nodes involved, and extent of bowel wall penetration. Four or more positive lymph nodes or gross versus micro-

TABLE 1. *AJCC/UICC staging classification (1997)*

Primary tumor: T
TX: Primary tumor cannot be assessed
T0: No evidence of primary tumor
Tis: Carcinoma in situ: confined within the glandular basement membrane (intraepithelial) or lamina propria (intramucosal) with no extension through the muscularis mucosae into the submucosa
T1: Invades submucosa
T2: Invades into muscularis propria
T3: Invades through muscularis propria into subserosa, or into nonperitonealized pericolic or perirectal tissues
T4: Invades other organs or structures, and/or perforates visceral peritoneum. Direct extension through to the serosal surface is considered T4. A tumor nodule >3 mm in diameter in the perirectal or pericolic fat without histologic evidence of a residual node in the nodule is classified as regional perirectal or pericolic lymph node metastasis. However, a tumor nodule ≤3 mm in diameter is classified in the T category as a discontinuous extension, that is, T3.
Regional lymph nodes: N
NX: Nodes cannot be assessed
N0: No regional node metastases
N1: One to three positive nodes. Metastatic nodules or foci found in the pericolic or perirectal fat or in adjacent mesentery (mesocolic fat) without evidence of residual lymph node tissue are equivalent to regional lymph node metastasis. Multiple metastatic foci seen microscopically only in the pericolic fat should be considered metastasis in a single lymph node for classification. A tumor nodule >3 mm in diameter in the perirectal or pericolic fat without histologic evidence of a residual node is classified as regional perirectal or pericolic lymph node metastasis.
N2: Four or more positive nodes
Distant metastases: M
MX: Presence of distant metastases cannot be assessed
M0: No distant metastases
M1: Distant metastases present. Metastasis in the external iliac or common iliac lymph node is classified as M1
Stage grouping
Stage 0:   Tis N0 M0
Stage I: T1–2 N0 M0
Stage II: T3–4 N0 M0
Stage III: Any T N1–2 M0
Stage IV: Any T any N M1
Stage at initial diagnosis:
Stage I   39.2%
Stage II/III 39.9%
Stage IV   20.9%

TABLE 2. *Five-year survival prognosis by stage*

Stage 0	>90%
Stage I	>75%
Stage II	70–85%
Stage III	55–70%
Stage IV	25%

scopic bowel wall penetration lead to diminished survival. Some stage II patients exhibit a heterogeneous outcome and are at high risk of relapse, with outcomes similar to those of node-positive patients.

PROGNOSIS

Adverse Prognostic Factors

- Advanced stage.
- Serosal penetration.
- Advanced age of patient.
- High tumor grade.
- More than four lymph nodes involved.
- Bowel obstruction or perforation at presentation.
- Tumor thymidylate synthase expression may correlate with decreased survival in rectal cancer (2).
- Biochemical and molecular markers such as p53 mutations or loss of heterozygosity of chromosome 18q also may be predictive of a poor prognosis (Table 2).

MANAGEMENT ALGORITHM

Surgery

- The primary curative intervention requires en bloc extirpation of the involved bowel segment with mesentery by laparotomy with pericolic and intermediate lymphadenectomy for both staging and therapeutic intent. Negative proximal, distal, and lateral surgical margins are of paramount importance.
- Surgical intervention is indicated if polypectomy pathology reveals muscularis mucosal involvement or penetration.
- Surgical palliation may include colostomy or even resection of metastatic disease for symptoms of acute obstruction or persistent bleeding.

Radiation Therapy

- Administration of radiotherapy is limited by bowel-segment mobility. Small bowel toxicity, in particular, limits abdominal radiation, and patients with co-morbidities such as diabetes, previous surgery with adhesion formaton and previous 5-FU exposure are at higher risk. Bowel toxicity ranging from 4 to 8% is expected.
- Local control and improved disease-free survival (DFS) have been reported in patients with T4 lesions or perforations, nodal disease, and subtotal resections treated with 5,000 to 5,400 cGy directed at the primary tumor bed and draining lymph nodes.

Adjuvant Chemotherapy for Colon Cancer

Early clinical trials of adjuvant 5-FU–based chemotherapy in colorectal cancer showed trends favoring DFS, but overall survival (OS) benefit was generally not significant. The first study to demonstrate a significant DFS and overall survival benefit for chemotherapy was the NSABP C-01 study.

NSABP C01

- 1,166 patients were treated with surgery alone versus methyl-CCNU, vincristine, and 5-FU (MOF) chemotherapy or bacille Calmette-Guérin (BCG) immunotherapy, with DFS and OS improved only in initial analysis (3).
- A 1.31 cancer-related death risk reduction was observed despite methyl-CCNU–induced myelodysplasia and leukemia in long-term survivors.

In 1990, a large intergroup trial demonstrated the efficacy of 5-FU and levamisole chemotherapy in stage III colon cancer, leading to a National Institutes of Health (NIH) consensus panel recommendation of 5-FU and levamisole adjuvant therapy for all patients with resected stage III colon cancer.

Intergroup 035

- This trial of 5-FU/levamisole was initiated to validate an earlier pilot NCCTG 784852 study in which 401 patients received either surgery alone versus levamisole alone, or 5-FU and levamisole in combination (4).
- A total of 929 patients with stage III colon cancer was randomized to these same three treatment arms. The 5-FU and levamisole combination reduced the relapse rate by 41% and the overall cancer mortality by 33%.
- Levamisole alone was not significantly different from the surgery alone control arm.

Because of increased response rates in metastatic colorectal cancer for 5-FU and calcium leucovorin (LV) regimens, several more recent studies have examined the value of biochemical modulation of 5-FU in the adjuvant setting.

NSABP C03

- Trial of stage II and III patients randomized to weekly 5-FU and LV (500 mg/m^2 weekly for 6 of 8 weeks for 48 weeks) or MOF chemotherapy.
- A statistically significant increased 3-year DFS (73% vs. 64%; $p = 0.0004$) and overall survival (84% vs. 77%; $p = 0.003$) for the 5-FU and LV arm over the MOF-treated cohort was observed.
- At 3 years of follow-up, patients treated with postoperative 5-FU/LV had a 30% reduction in the risk of developing a treatment failure and a 32% reduction in mortality risk compared with similar patients treated with MOF (5) .

International Multicentre Pooled Analysis of Colon Cancer Trials (IMPACT)

- The International Multicentre Pooled Analysis of Colon Cancer Trials (6) pooled analyses of three trials conducted in Canada, France, and Italy that included 1,493 eligible patients with Dukes' B and C colon cancer randomized to 5-FU and LV or surgery alone.
- Data revealed 3-year recurrence-free and OS rates with statistically significant improvment with adjuvant chemotherapy versus surgery alone, with reduction in failure events by 35% ($p < 0.0001$) and overall mortality reduction of 22% ($p = 0.029$).

Currently a growing number of trials suggest that 5-FU and LV is equivalent to or possibly better than 5-FU and levamisole in combination. Treatment with adjuvant chemotherapy with 5-FU and LV for longer than six cycles does not appear to be necessary.

NSABP-C-04

- A 2,151-patient trial demonstrated that weekly 5-FU/LV is superior or equal to 5-FU plus levamisole–containing arm.
- Increased benefit with six cycles of weekly 5-FU/LV for 6 consecutive weeks of every 8 weeks versus 5-FU and levamisole or 5-FU, LV, and levamisole combination.
- Significantly prolonged DFS, 65% versus 60% ($p = 0.04$) and prolonged OS trend, 74% versus 70% ($p = 0.07$) for the LV-containing arms. No difference was observed when levamisole was added to 5-FU and LV (7).

Adjuvant Chemotherapy Regimens for Colon Cancer

Based on these recent clinical studies of adjuvant chemotherapy, use of one of the following three regimens is recommended for patients with stage III colon cancer.

5-Fluorouracil and calcium leucovorin

- 5-FU, 425 mg/m^2 daily for 5 days, preceded by LV, 20 mg/m^2/day every 4 weeks for six cycles, *OR*
- 5-FU, 500 mg/m^2 with LV, 500 mg/m^2 weekly for 6 weeks, repeated every 8 weeks for 8 months, *OR*

5-FU and levamisole

- 5-FU, 450 mg/m^2 daily times 5 days, and then weekly for 48 weeks, with oral levamisole, 50 mg 3 times a day for 3 days every other week for 12 months.

Adjuvant Chemotherapy for Stage II Colon Cancer

Despite 75% 5-year survival with surgery alone, some stage II patients have a higher risk of relapse, with outcomes similar to those of node-positive patients. Adjuvant chemotherapy provides up to a 33% overall survival advantage, resulting in an overall treatment benefit of roughly 8%. Two retrospective analyses have reported opposite outcomes with adjuvant treatment. The NSABP summary of protocols using various treatments reported a 30% risk reduction (8), whereas a Canadian–European consortium noted no significant benefit. Studies evaluating numerous prognostic factors are ongoing.

Other Approaches to Adjuvant Therapy

5-FU Portal Vein Infusion

A reduction in hepatic metastasis recurrence by treating micrometastatic disease is the rationale for perioperative portal circulation administration of adjuvant chemotherapy. Trials with 7-day perioperative continuous 5-FU followed by standard adjuvant therapy are ongoing.

Immunotherapy

Reithmuller et al. (9) treated 189 patients postoperatively with monoclonal antibody 17-1A, resulting in a 27% decrease in recurrence rate and 30% mortality rate reduction. Studies attempting to eradicate micrometastases with this relatively nontoxic approach are ongoing.

Vaccine trials using irradiated autologous tumor cells combined with BCG have yielded varying results. Vaccines targeting *ras* and the *p53* are currently being studied.

Adjuvant Treatment for Rectal Cancer

In contrast to colon cancer, treatment failures after potentially curative resections tend to occur more locally. Combined-modality adjuvant chemotherapy and radiation therapy is now standard for stage II and III rectal cancer patients.

NCCTG Trial (1991)

- Trial of 204 patients with resected rectal cancer randomized to postoperative 5-FU with oral semustine (methyl-CCNU) plus radiation or radiation alone (10).
- Significant 34% reduction in disease recurrence at 5 years associated with combined modality therapy ($p = 0.0016$) and a significant reduction in cancer-related death by 36% ($p = 0.0071$).

NCCTG Trial (1994)

- Randomized trial of 660 stage II and III rectal cancer patients into four treatment arms (11):
  1. 5-FU plus methyl-CCNU followed by radiation with bolus intravenous 5-FU and then 5-FU plus methyl-CCNU.
  2. 5-FU plus methyl-CCNU followed by radiation with continuous-infusion 5-FU and then 5-FU plus methyl-CCNU.
  3. 5-FU alone followed by radiation with bolus intravenous 5-FU and then 5-FU alone.
  4. 5-FU alone followed by radiation with continuous-infusion 5-FU and then 5-FU alone.
- Continuous infusion of 5-FU was associated with decreased overall tumor relapse, compared with bolus 5-FU when given with radiation: 37% versus 47%, $p = 0.01$. This difference was largely due to a reduction in recurrence at distant metastatic sites; the local recurrence rates were unchanged.
- Methyl-CCNU did not add to the effectiveness of 5-FU therapy and increased toxicity.

Adjuvant Combined-Modality Regimens for Rectal Cancer

- 5-FU by intravenous bolus injection at 500 mg/m^2/day on days 1–5 and 36–40, followed by
- Radiation therapy in 180-cGy fractions given over 5 weeks starting day 64, to a total dose of 4,500–5,400 cGy in association with 5-FU, 225 mg/m^2/day by ambulatory infusion pump during the entire 5-week period of radiation therapy, followed by
- Intravenous bolus of 5-FU, 450 mg/m^2/day given daily for 5 days on days 134–138 and days 169–173, for a total treatment period of 6 months.

FOLLOW-UP AFTER ADJUVANT TREATMENT

Eighty percent of recurrences are seen within 2 years after initial therapy. The American Cancer Society recommends total colonic evaluation with either colonoscopy or double-contrast barium enema within 1 year of resection, followed every 3 to 5 years if findings remain normal. Synchronous cancers must be excluded during initial surgical extirpation, and metachronous malignancies in the form of polyps continue to require detection and excision before more malignant behavior develops.

TREATMENT FOR ADVANCED DISEASE

5-Fluorouracil–Based Chemotherapy

Single-arm phase II studies of 5-FU–based chemotherapy regimens in advanced colorectal cancer have reported response rates ranging from 0 to 70%, but most larger studies have observed objective response rates of 20% to 25%. Median survival times of 8 to 12 months are quite common. Biochemical modulation of 5-FU with calcium LV enhances the intracellular reduced folate pool and prolongs the inhibition of thymidylate synthase by 5-FU metabolites. Leucovorin with 5-FU is the most frequently used regimen for metastatic colorectal cancer and has been associated with higher response rates and a trend toward improved survival compared with single-agent bolus 5-FU regimens. A variety of 5-FU schedules and LV doses have been used, but two common regimens are listed.

Bolus 5-FU and Leucovorin

- Daily for five days: 5-FU at 425 mg/m^2 preceded by 20 mg/m^2 LV daily × 5 days every 4–5 weeks (12).
- Weekly: LV, 500 mg/m^2 infused over 2 hours with 5-FU, 600 mg/m^2 as an intravenous bolus 1 hour after the start of the LV infusion weekly for 6 weeks, repeated every 8 weeks (13).

The toxicity profile of these two regimens differs. Myelosuppression is more common with the daily regimen. Diarrhea and mucositis may be seen with either schedule. Cryotherapy with ice held in the mouth during the 5-FU infusion may help to lessen the mucositis associated with therapy.

The combination of 5-FU with a variety of other agents including methotrexate, methyl-CCNU, vincristine, and mitomycin C has been studied in the past, but none of these combinations shows any particular advantage over 5-FU and LV. 5-FU with levamisole has no role in metastatic disease.

Continuous Infusion of 5-FU

Continuous infusion of 5-FU may have efficacy equivalent to that of bolus 5-FU and LV (14) and is generally well tolerated, despite the inconvenience of a prolonged intravenous infusion apparatus. 5-FU at 300 mg/m^2/day is infused continuously by ambulatory infusion pump. Toxicities include mucositis; however, myelosuppression is less common. Palmar–plantar erythrodysesthesia (hand–foot syndrome) is very common and may respond to pyridoxine, 50–150 mg/m^2/day. Continuous infusions of 5-FU may have modest activity in patients who have progressed on a bolus 5-FU regimen (15).

Irinotecan/CPT-11

Irinotecan is a topoisomerase I–targeting agent with activity in patients with advanced colorectal cancer who have previously been treated with 5-FU. Response rates range from 15% to 25%. Irinotecan can be given at 125 mg/m^2 infused over 90 minutes weekly for 4 weeks followed by a 2-week rest, or at 350 mg/m^2 over 90 minutes every 3 weeks. Delayed-onset diarrhea must be managed by administering high-dose loperamide, 4 mg initially and then 2 mg every 2 hours during the day and 4 mg every 4 hours at night, until all bowel movements stop for at least 12 hours. Neutropenia and mild nausea and vomiting also are common. Significant survival advantages have been shown for using irinotecan as second-line therapy after 5-FU compared with supportive care or with continuous-infusion 5-FU regimens.

In preliminary studies, the combination of irinotecan and 5-FU and LV in untreated patients with colorectal cancer is highly promising. A three-arm randomized phase III study has compared 5-FU and LV (425 mg/m^2 and 20 mg/m^2 daily × 5) with irinotecan alone (125 mg/m^2 weekly) and with the combination of irinotecan, 125 mg/m^2, and weekly 5-FU, 500 mg/m^2, and LV, 20 mg/m^2 (16). A significantly improved overall response rate was noted for the irinotecan and 5-FU combination (33%) compared with 5-FU and LV alone (18%; $p < 0.001$) or with irinotecan alone (17%). Toxicity was not substantially worse with the combination arm. Another preliminary randomized study comparing the same regimen of 5-FU, LV, and irinotecan with 5-FU and LV alone also found a significantly better response rate for the combination (17). If confirmed, these data would support the use of irinotecan and 5-FU combination therapy as initial therapy in newly diagnosed patients with advanced disease who can tolerate these combination regimens.

OTHER CHEMOTHERAPEUTIC AGENTS IN DEVELOPMENT

Capecitabine: 5-FU prodrug with preferential tumor tissue activation by thymidine phosphorylase. Side-effect profile and efficacy similar to those of continuous 5-FU infusion.

Uracil-ftorafur (UFT): oral combination of fluorinated pyrimidine and dihydropyrimidine dihydrogenase (DPD) inhibitor.

Eniluracil (776C85): an irreversible oral inactivator of DPD, which blocks 5-FU catabolism and may enhance the therapeutic index of oral 5-FU.

Raltitrexed (Tomudex): antifolate-specific thymidylate synthase inhibitor.

Oxaliplatin: European data suggest enhanced 5-FU response when given in combination with the platinum analogue oxaliplatin, with response rates ranging from 26% to 57%. Toxicity profile includes peripheral neuropathy, acute dysesthesias, and nausea and vomiting. Renal dysfunction and myelosuppression are uncommon.

CONTROVERSIES

CEA

Carcinoembryonic antigen is an acid glycoprotein localized to the cell membrane, facilitating release into blood and surrounding body fluids. CEA is elevated in nonneoplastic processes such as smoking and inflammatory bowel disease and in cancers involving the breast, lungs, or pancreas. The degree of tumor differentiation correlates with CEA expression, and up to 30% of colon cancers, in particular poorly differentiated tumors, exhibit no CEA elevation. Elevation is typically defined as greater than 5 ng/mL and is associated with increased recurrence rate and decreased survival. A measurement of greater than 25 ng/mL is highly suggestive of metastatic disease. In patients preoperatively evaluated with CEA measurements, sensitivity of 43% and specificity of 90% were reported.

Persistent elevation of CEA postoperatively may suggest residual tumor or early metastasis. The routine use of CEA alone for evaluating treatment response is not recommended, as up to 20% of patients have conflicting declines in CEA levels despite disease progression. Patients with initially negative levels can become positive. Serial postinitial therapy determinations may identify patients benefiting from curative resections, in particular involving solitary liver or lung metastases, but this is rare. Data from studies such as the Ohio State study report a 31% 5-year survival in very selected populations with aggressive CEA surveillance and second-look laparotomy to detect early recurrences. A joint NIH and United Kingdom trial failed to demonstrate survival differences with serial CEA measurements. The American Society of Clinical Oncology recommends CEA testing in patients with previous colorectal cancer diagnoses who would be eligible or considered for surgical resection.

Hepatic Metastasis

The liver is the most common site for metastasis, with one third involving the liver only, and median survival less than 1 year with 13% 3-year survival; two thirds of patients dying of colon cancer have liver involvement. Approximately 25% are resectable, with 30% 5-year survival after resection possible in certain patient subsets and 3-5% operative morbidity/mortality. Intraoperative ultrasound is the most sensitive test for initial detection, followed by computed tomography (CT) or magnetic resonance imaging (MRI).

Nonresectable high-risk patients are treated with locoregional (via hepatic artery infusion; HAI) or systemic chemotherapy, typically an LV-modulated 5-FU approach, with 33% to 40%

2-year survival rates comparable to resected patient survival. Postoperative chemotherapy trials have exhibited little survival benefit and were actually closed because of low accrual. Focus on oral agents with postulated increased portal vein delivery and preoperative chemotherapy with newer agents is ongoing.

REFERENCES

1. American Joint Committee on Cancer. *AJCC cancer staging manual.* 5th ed. Philadelphia: Lippincott-Raven, 1997.
2. Johnston PG, Fisher ER, et al. The role of thymidylate synthase expression in prognosis and outcome of adjuvant chemotherapy in patients with rectal cancer. *J Clin Oncol* 1994;12:2640–2647.
3. Wolmark N, Fisher B, Rockette H, et al. Postoperative adjuvant chemotherapy or BCG for colon cancer: results from NSABP protocol C01. *J Natl Cancer Inst* 1988;80:30–36.
4. Moertel CG, Fleming TR, Macdonald JS, et al. Levamisole and fluorouracil for adjuvant therapy of resected colon carcinoma [see comments]. *N Engl J Med* 1990;322:352–358.
5. Wolmark N, Rockette H, Fisher B, et al. The benefit of leucovorin-modulated fluorouracil as postoperative adjuvant therapy for primary colon cancer: results from National Surgical Adjuvant Breast and Bowel B, Project protocol C03. *J Clin Oncol* 1993;11:1879–1887.
6. IMPACT. Efficacy of adjuvant fluorouracil and folinic acid in colon cancer: International Multicentre Pooled Analysis of Colon Cancer Trials (IMPACT) investigators [see comments]. *Lancet* 1995;345:939–944.
7. Wolmark N, Rockette H, Mamounas E, et al. Clinical trial to assess the relative efficacy of fluorouracil and leucovorin, fluorouracil and levamisole, and fluorouracil, leucovorin, and levamisole in patients with Dukes' B and C carcinoma of the colon: results from National Surgical Adjuvant Breast and Bowel Project C04. *J Clin Oncol* 1999;17:3553–3559.
8. Mamounas E, Wieand S, Wolmark N, et al. Comparative efficacy of adjuvant chemotherapy in patients with Dukes' B versus Dukes' C colon cancer: results from four National Surgical Adjuvant Breast and Bowel Project adjuvant studies (C01, C02, C03, and C04) [see comments]. *J Clin Oncol* 1999;17:1349–1355.
9. Riethmuller G, Schneider-Gadicke E, Schlimok G, et al. Randomised trial of monoclonal antibody for adjuvant therapy of resected Dukes' C colorectal carcinoma: German Cancer Aid 171A Study Group [see comments]. *Lancet* 343:1177–1183.
10. Krook JE, Moertel CG, Gunderson LL, et al. Effective surgical adjuvant therapy for high-risk rectal carcinoma [see comments]. *N Engl J Med* 1991;324:709–715.
11. O'Connell MJ, Martenson JA, Wieand HS, et al. Improving adjuvant therapy for rectal cancer by combining protracted infusion fluorouracil with radiation therapy after curative surgery. *N Engl J Med* 1994;331:502–507.
12. Poon MA, O'Connell MJ, Wieand HS, et al. Biochemical modulation of fluorouracil with leucovorin: confirmatory evidence of improved therapeutic efficacy in advanced colorectal cancer [see comments]. *J Clin Oncol* 1991;9:1967–1972.
13. Petrelli N, Herrera L, Rustum Y, et al. A prospective randomized trial of 5-fluorouracil versus 5-fluorouracil and high-dose leucovorin versus 5-fluorouracil and methotrexate in previously untreated patients with advanced colorectal carcinoma. *J Clin Oncol* 1987;5:1559–1565.
14. Leichman CG, Fleming TR, Mussia FM, et al. Phase II study of fluorouracil and its modulation in advanced colorectal cancer: a Southwest Oncology Group study [see comments]. *J Clin Oncol* 1995;13:1303–1311.
15. Falcone A, Allegrini G, Lenconi M, et al. Protracted continuous infusion of 5-fluorouracil and low-dose leucovorin in patients with metastatic colorectal cancer resistant to 5-fluorouracil bolus-based chemotherapy: a Phase II study. *Cancer Chemother Pharmacol* 1999;44:159–163.
16. Saltz LB, Locker PK, Pirotta N, et al. Weekly irinotecan (CPT11), leucovorin (LV), and fluorouracil (FU) is superior to daily × 5 LV/FU in patients (PTS) with previously untreated metastatic colorectal cancer (CRC). *Proc Am Soc Clin Oncol* 1999;18:233a.
17. Douillard JY, Cunningham D, Roth AD, et al. A randomized phase III trial comparing irinotecan (IRI) + 5-FU/folinic acid (FA) to the same schedule of 5-FU/FA in patients with metastatic colorectal cancer as front line chemotherapy. *Proc Am Soc Clin Oncol* 1999;18:233a.

9

Pancreatic Cancer

James Gulley and *Chris H. Takimoto

*Laboratory of Tumor Immunology and Biology, Experimental Oncology Section, Division of Basic Sciences, National Cancer Institute, Bethesda, Maryland 20892; and *Medicine Branch, National Cancer Institute, National Naval Medical Center, Bethesda, Maryland 20889-5105*

EPIDEMIOLOGY

- In 1999, an estimated 29,900 new cases will have been diagnosed.
- Fifth leading cause of death from cancer in the United States.
- Responsible for 5% of all cancer-related deaths.
- 28,900 will die of this disease.
- The 5-year survival rates range from 1% to 4%.
- African-Americans have a higher mortality rate than any other ethnic group.

RISK FACTORS

Pathophysiology

The pancreas is involved with both endocrine and exocrine functions; however, about 80% of the cells in the pancreas are acinar cells, and 10% to 15% are ductal cells. Approximately 95% of malignant pancreatic cancer arises in the exocrine pancreas, with about two thirds in the head of the pancreas (Table 1). The sites where the cancer arises determine the symptoms, with lesions arising in the head of the pancreas causing duct obstruction, jaundice, and pain, whereas tumors arising in the body or tail are less likely to cause symptoms before metastasis.

- Pain from localized disease is usually described as mid to upper back pain, from tumor invasion of the celiac and mesenteric plexi.
- Most patients develop glucose intolerance to some degree.
- K-*ras* mutations are reportedly associated with a majority of cases of pancreatic cancer.

STAGING

Staging classification is reviewed in Table 2.

PROGNOSIS

Tumor size, presence of lymph node metastasis, and histologic differentiation each have independent prognostic values, with larger tumors, lymph node metastasis, and poor differentiation having worse prognoses. The 36-month survival for node-negative patients is between

107

TABLE 1. *Risk factors*

Environmental	
Cigarette smoking	*N*-nitrosoamines, may increase risk by 1.5- to 2.0-fold. Up to 30% of pancreatic cancer associated with this.
Dietary factors	Increased risk with fat and meat, decreased with vegetables. Caffeine and alcohol link is controversial.
Disease states	
Diabetes mellitus	Long-standing NIDDM.
Chronic pancreatitis	Associated with 5% of cases.
PUD surgery	Associated with increased serum gastrin levels.
Genetic	
MEN I	
Hereditary pancreatitis	
Lynch syndrome II	
von Hippel–Lindau	
Ataxia–telangiectasia	
Occupational	
Chemicals	Petrochemical products, benzidine, β-naphthylamine.

PUD, peptic ulcer disease; NIDDM, non–insulin-dependent diabetes mellitus; MEN, multiple endocrine neoplasia.

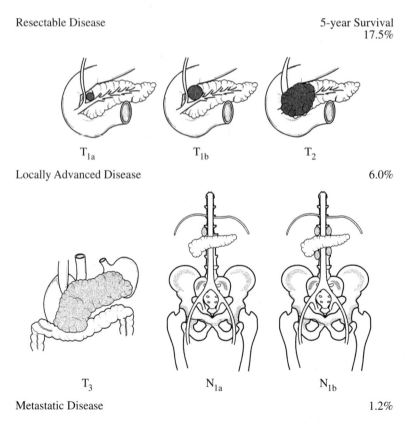

Fig. 1. Resectable Disease/Locally Advanced Disease/Metastatic Disease

TABLE 2. *AJCC/UICC staging classification (1997)*

Primary tumor
TX	Primary tumor cannot be assessed
T0	No evidence of primary tumor
Tis	*In situ* carcinoma
T1	Tumor limited to the pancreas ≤2 cm
T2	Tumor limited to the pancreas >2 cm
T3	Tumor extends directly to any of the following: duodenum, bile duct, or peripancreatic tissue
T4	Tumor extends directly to any of the following: stomach, spleen, colon, adjacent large vessels

Regional lymph nodes
NX	Regional lymph nodes cannot be assessed
N0	No regional lymph node metastasis
N1	Regional lymph node metastasis
	pN1a Metastasis in a single regional lymph node
	pN1b Metastasis in multiple regional lymph nodes

Distant metastasis
MX	Distant metastasis cannot be assessed
M0	No distant metastasis
M1	Distant metastasis

Stage grouping
Stage 0	Tis	N0	M0
Stage I	T1–2	N0	M0
Stage II	T3	N0	M0
Stage III	T1–3	N1	M0
Stage IVA	T4	Any N	M0
Stage IVB	Any T	Any N	M1

25% and 30%, whereas there is only a 6- to 8-month median survival for node-positive patients. In patients who successfully undergo a potentially curative surgical resection, long-term survival is seen in about 20%.

DIAGNOSIS

- Screening tests: There are no good screening tests for pancreatic cancer.
  CA19-9, a sialated Lewis antigen, is elevated in 70% to 90% of patients with pancreatic cancer; however, because of low specificity, it is not useful as a screening test.
  The CA19-9 may have greater utility in monitoring recurrent or advanced disease.
- Imaging techniques: chest radiographs, abdominal computed tomography (CT; with spiral CT showing more precise details), ultrasound, endoscopic retrograde cholepancreatography (ERCP), and endoscopic ultrasound
- Pathologic diagnosis may be achieved with ERCP, laparoscopy, peritoneal cytology, or CT-guided biopsy.

MANAGEMENT

For management considerations, pancreatic cancer can be divided into resectable disease (potentially curable), locally advanced disease, and metastatic disease (see Fig. 2).

Management alorithm

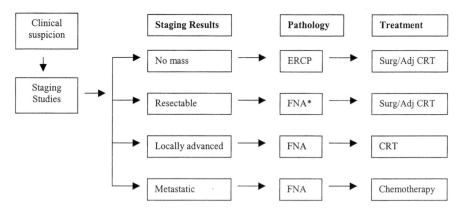

Fig. 2. Staging studies should include CT (spiral CT with contrast preferred) as well as laparoscopy for potentially resectable cancers. *For FNA there remains some controversy regarding seeding of the needle tract for potentially curable (i.e., resectable) disease and in some centers surgeons will take patients to a planned Whipple procedure and obtain tissue at the time of surgery. Adj CRT, adjuvant chemoradiation; FNA, fine needle aspiration; ERCP, endoscopic retrograde cholangiopancreatography.

Resectable Disease

Fewer than 10% of patients with pancreatic cancer have resectable disease at diagnosis. Resectable disease is confined to the pancreas without lymph node evolvement, encasement of the celiac axis or superior mesenteric artery, and with a patent superior mesenteric–portal vein confluence. Patients may have isolated involvement of the superior mesenteric vein, portal vein, or hepatic artery, however. A Whipple or modified (pylorus-sparing) Whipple procedure is the surgical procedure of choice. Even after complete resection, there is a greater than 70% risk of locoregional recurrence. This has led to numerous studies of adjuvant chemotherapy and radiation therapy after surgical resection. The original GITSG trial (4) had 21 chemoradiation patients versus 22 controls but showed a significantly prolonged median survival of 20 months versus 11 months for controls with 43% 2-year actuarial survival (vs. 18% for the control arm) and 25% 5-year survival. Based on this relatively small trial, the standard of care is to give a split course of 4,000 cGy in 200-cGy fractions with bolus 5-fluorouracil (5-FU; 500 mg/m^2/day for the first 3 days of each 200-cGy segment of radiotherapy) followed by weekly 5-FU (500 mg/m^2/week) for up to 2 years. Some investigators have elected to give this same overall dose of radiation as a continuous-course regimen, avoiding the split-course schedule in combination with daily 5-FU, 500 mg/m^2/day for the first 3 days and last 3 days of radiation therapy (10). The postradiation treatment of weekly 5-FU also has been shortened from 2 years to 4 to 6 months (10). Several large randomized ongoing trials should give more information regarding effectiveness of conventional adjuvant therapy.

Locally Advanced Disease

Another 25% of patients have regional involvement at diagnosis. Chemoradiation has been shown to improve survival significantly over that with radiation alone and chemotherapy

TABLE 3. *Gemcitabine versus 5-FU therapy*

	Clinical benefit response[a]	Response rate	Median survival	1-yr surv.
Gemcitabine	23.8%	5.4%	5.7 mo	18%
5-FU	4.8%	0	4.4 mo	2%

[a]Clinical benefit responders showed improvement in at least one of the following without decrease in any other: pain, performance status, and weight.

alone in locally advanced, unresectable disease for patients with good performance status. One commonly used regimen is 4,500 to 5,400 cGy in divided doses with 5-FU, 500 mg/m^2/day daily on the first and last 3 days of radiation (9). The treatment schema is identical to those used for adjuvant treatment of resectable disease as described earlier. Median survival is approximately 10 months with treatment. Use of gemcitabine in locally advanced disease is under investigation (see later).

Metastatic Disease

Approximately half of new diagnoses of pancreatic cancer have metastasis, with common sites including the liver and lungs. Treatment of metastatic disease is purely palliative and should be offered to patients with a good performance status (ECOG, 0–2). Historically, 5-FU has been the most extensively evaluated agent for metastatic pancreatic cancer. However, gemcitabine has recently become the treatment of choice for first-line therapy for metastatic pancreatic cancer, despite having an objective response rate of less than 10%. In a study of 126 untreated pancreatic cancer patients randomized to receive gemcitabine, 1,000 mg/m^2 i.v. weekly for 3 of 4 weeks or single-agent 5-FU, 600 mg/m^2 i.v. bolus weekly, a benefit in quality-of-life scores and median survival was seen for the gemcitabine therapy (see Table 3). Gemcitabine has even been advocated for palliation for poor-performance status patients. For single-agent 5-FU, response rates of 0 to 35% have been reported, with median survival from 2 to 6 months. 5-FU combination regimens including streptozotocin, mitomycin, and 5-FU (SMF), and 5-FU, doxorubicin, and mitomycin (FAM) also have been studied, but none has been shown to be superior to 5-FU alone. Many clinicians give leucovorin in conjunction wityh 5-FU.

Palliation

Pain remains a significant problem with pancreatic cancer and can be palliated with narcotics, external beam radiation, and, if indicated, a nerve block to an involved plexus. Obstruction also is a common local issue and can be relieved with stents or surgical procedures.

TREATMENT OPTIONS

Localized Disease

Whipple procedure followed by adjuvant chemoradiation with a standard split course of 40-Gy external beam radiation in 2-Gy fractions with

- Fluorouracil, 500 mg/m^2/day by i.v. bolus for the first 3 days of each 20-Gy segment of radiotherapy (total dose/3-day course of fluorouracil, 1,500 mg/m^2), followed by
- Fluorouracil, 500 mg/m^2/week by i.v. bolus injection, weekly for up to 2 years.

This adjuvant treatment can increase long-term survival as well as prolong disease-free survival.

Locally Advanced Disease

For those patients with good performance status (PS, 0–2), clinical trials are the preferred treatment, with chemoradiation or gemcitabine available as standard treatments. The chemoradiation is given as described earlier, and chemotherapy consists of

- Gemcitabine, 1,000 mg/m^2/week i.v. weekly for 3 weeks (days 1, 8, and 15) followed by 1 week without gemcitabine (total dose/cycle, 3,000 mg/m^2).
- Treatment cycles are repeated every 28 days.

For those patients with poor performance status, supportive care is recommended. The goal of treatment for locally advanced disease is to prolong survival.

Metastatic Disease

For patients with good performance status, clinical trials are the preferred treatment, with 5-FU–based chemotherapy, gemcitabine, or supportive care available as standard treatments. The latter two treatments may be considered for those patients with poor performance status.

- Gemcitabine, 1,000 mg/m^2/week i.v. weekly for 3 weeks (days 1, 8, and 15), followed by 1 week without gemcitabine (total dose/cycle, 3,000 mg/m^2). Treatment cycles are repeated every 28 days.
- Fluorouracil, 600 mg/m^2/day by i.v. bolus injection once a week.

The goal of treatment for metastatic disease remains to decrease symptoms.

REFERENCES

1. *AJCC cancer staging manual.* 5th ed. 1997:121–126.
2. Burris HA III, Moore MJ, Andersen J, et al. Improvements in clinical survival and clinical benefit with gemcitabine as first line therapy for patients with advanced pancreas cancer: a randomized trial. *J Clin Oncol* 1997;15:2403–2413.
3. Evans DB, Abbruzzese JL, Rich TA. In: DeVita VT Jr, Hellman S, Rosenberg SA, eds. *Cancer: principles and practice of oncology.* 5th ed. Philadelphia: Lippincott-Raven, 1997:1054–1087.
4. Gastrointestinal Study Group. Further evidence of effective adjuvant combined radiation and chemotherapy following curative resection of pancreatic cancer. *Cancer* 1987;59:2006–2010.
5. Ghaneh P, Kawesha A, Howes N, et al. Adjuvant therapy for pancreatic cancer. *World J Surg* 1999;23:937–945.
6. Moertel CG, Frytak S, Hahn RG, et al. Therapy of locally unresectable pancreatic carcinoma: a randomised comparison of high dose (6000 rads) radiation alone, moderate dose radiation (4000 rads) + 5-fluorouracil, and high dose radiation + 5-fluorouracil. *Cancer* 1981;48:1705–1710.
7. National Cancer Institute. SEER cancer statistics review 1973-1996. http://www-seer.ims.nci.nih.gov/
8. National Comprehensive Cancer Network. NCCN practice guidelines for pancreatic cancer. *Oncology* 1997;11:41–55.
9. Sporn JR. Practical recommendations for the management of adenocarcinoma of the pancreas. *Drugs* 1999;57:69–79.
10. Yeo CJ, Abrams RA, Grochow LB, et al. Pancreaticoduodenectomy for pancreatic adenocarcinoma: postoperative adjuvant chemoradiation improves survival. *Ann Surg* 1997;225:621–636.

10

Anal Cancer

Muhammad Wasif Saif and J. Michael Hamilton

National Cancer Institute, National Institutes of Health, Bethesda, Maryland

Anal cancer is a relatively rare malignancy constituting only 1% to 2% of all large bowel cancers, and it can sometimes affect young adults. Three significant prognostic factors include size, site, and differentiation.

EPIDEMIOLOGY

In the United States, annual incidence of anal cancer is six per 1,000,000 population in whites and is more frequent in female than male subjects, showing an incidence of nine of 1,000,000 in nonwhite women versus five per 1,000,000 in white and Hispanic men (F/M ratio, 2:1). However, cancer of the anal margin is more frequent in men. More than 80% of anal cancer develops in patients age 50 to 60 years. Epidemiologic studies during the last decade suggest that the incidence of anal cancer in men younger than 35 years has increased, reversing the gender ratio in this age group; it also is related to receptive anal intercourse.

ETIOLOGY AND RISK FACTORS

In most cases of anal cancer, no etiologic factor has been recognized. Environmental factors are predominantly implicated in the carcinogenesis of anal cancer.

- **Infections.**
  Viral infections: The human papillomavirus is a prime suspect in the genesis of anal cancer. Human immunodeficiency virus (HIV) also has been implicated, with an enhanced risk, but this may be limited to men who engage in anal-receptive intercourse. Anal tumors are very rare in intravenous drug abusers. Other associated viral infections include herpes simplex virus type 2.
  Bacterial infections: Gonorrhea in men and *Chlamydia trachomatis* in women have been reported to be associated with a mild increase in risk of anal cancer.
- **Immunosuppression:** Renal transplant patients have been noted to have a 100 times increased incidence of anal and anogenital malignancies.
- **Smoking:** Cigarette smoking is associated with an 8 times increase in the risk of anal cancer.
- **Radiation exposure:** Previous radiation exposure also has been reported to be linked with the development of anal cancer.
- **Associated diseases:** Diseases associated with anal cancer include anal fissures, anal fistulae, hemorrhoids, chronic local inflammation, Crohn's disease, lymphogranuloma venereum, condylomata acuminata, carcinoma of the cervix, and carcinoma of the vulva.

• Anal-receptive intercourse: Anal-receptive intercourse in men (but not in women) has been found to be implicated in an increased risk of anal cancer at a risk ratio of 33. Studies showed that the incidence rate of anal cancer for single men is 6 times higher than that for married men.

No racial, dietary, or genetic factors are known as risk factors in predisposition to anal cancer.

PATHOLOGY

Anatomy

The anal canal is a 3- to 4-cm-long tubular structure. The junction between the anal canal and the perineal skin is called Hilton's line/anal verge (Figure 1). Cancer of the anal area may be divided into

• carcinoma of the anal canal, and
• carcinoma of anal the margin (Tables 1 and 2).

The World Health Organization (WHO) defines carcinoma of the anal canal as lesions arising from the anorectal ring proximally to the dentate line distally, whereas carcinoma of the anal margin is defined as lesions arising distal to the dentate line to the junction of perineal skin with the hair-bearing skin of the buttocks.

Presentation

Symptoms

Signs

Physical examination should include digital anorectal examination, anoscopy, proctoscopy, and palpation of inguinal lymph nodes (Table 3).

TABLE 1. *Pathology of anal cancer*

Histologic type	%
Squamous cell carcinoma	63
Transitional cell carcinoma (cloacogenic)	23
Mucinous adenocarcinoma	7

TABLE 2. *Other pathologies of anal cancer*

Pathology	%	Site
Malignant melanoma of anus	1–2	Pectinate line
Paget's disease	1–2	Intraepidermal portion of apocrine glands

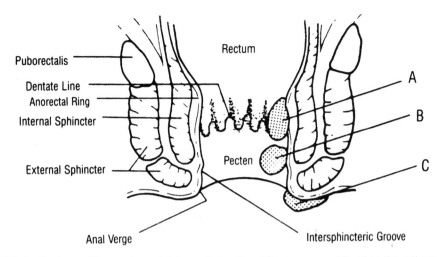

FIG. 1. Anatomy of the anal canal. A tumor in location A is always considered anal canal cancer; in location C, it is anal margin cancer. A tumor in location B has been called canal or margin cancer, depending on institutional preference, but now should be called anal canal cancer by the AJCC/UICC definition.

Biopsy

An incisional biopsy is preferred to confirm diagnosis. Suggestive inguinal lymph nodes should be examined to rule out metastatic disease.

Staging and Prognostic Factors

Staging workup should include physical examination, with special attention to digital rectal/pelvic examination and inguinal nodes, chest radiograph, and liver function tests. Pelvic computed tomography (CT) scan and endoscopic ultrasound of the anal canal may be beneficial.

The UICC (Union Internationale Contre le Cancer) and AJCC (American Joint Committee on Cancer) have proposed a practical staging system for anal cancer. Cancer of the anal margin is staged identically to squamous cell cancer of skin. The staging system for both types of tumors is outlined in Tables 4 and 5.

TABLE 3. *Symptoms of anal cancer*

Symptom	Occurrence
Bleeding	50%
Pain	40%
Sensation of a mass	25%
Pruritus	15%
Asymptomatic	25%

TABLE 4. *AJCC classification of anal canal tumors*

Primary tumor (T)
TX	Primary tumor cannot be assessed
T0	No evidence of primary tumor
Tis	Carcinoma in situ
T1	Tumor ≤2 cm in greatest dimension
T2	Tumor >2 cm but <5 cm in greatest dimension
T3	Tumor >5 cm in greatest dimension
T4	Tumor of any size that invades adjacent organs [e.g., vagina, bladder, urethra; involvement of sphincter muscle(s) *alone* is not classified as T4]

Regional lymph nodes (N)
NX	Regional lymph nodes cannot be assessed
N0	No regional lymph node metastasis
N1	Metastasis in perirectal lymph node(s)
N2	Metastasis in unilateral internal iliac and/or inguinal lymph node(s)
N3	Metastasis in perirectal and inguinal lymph node(s) and/or bilateral internal iliac and/or inguinal lymph nodes

Distant metastasis (M)
MX	Distant metastasis cannot be assessed
M0	No distant metastasis
M1	Distant metastasis

Grade (G)
GX	Grade of differentiation cannot be assessed
G1	Well differentiated
G2	Moderately differentiated
G3	Poorly differentiated
G4	Undifferentiated

Stage groupings
Stage 0	Tis	N0	M0
Stage I	T1	N0	M0
Stage II	T2	N0	M0
	T3	N0	M0
Stage IIIA	T1–3	N1	M0
	T4	N0	M0
Stage IIIB	T4	N1	M0
	Any T	N2–3	M0
Stage IV	Any T	Any N	MI

TABLE 5. *TNM classification of anal margin tumors*

Primary tumor (T)[a]
T4	Tumor invades deep extradermal structures

Regional lymph nodes (N)
N1	Ipsilaterial inguinal nodes

Metastases (M)
M1	Distant metastases

Stage groupings[b]
Stage III	T4	N0	M0
	Any T	N1	M0

[a]Designation as for anal canal tumors, except T4.
[b]Stage groupings as for anal canal tumors, except stage III (no stage IIA or IIIB).
Adapted from Sobin LH, Wittekind C (eds). *UICC International Union Against Cancer: TNM classification of malignant tumors.* 5th ed. New York: John Wiley & Sons, 1997, with permission.

Major Prognostic Factors

There are three major prognostic factors:

- Site: anal canal versus perianal skin.
- Size: primary tumors less than 2 cm in size have a better prognosis.
- Differentiation: well-differentiated tumors are more favorable than are poorly differentiated tumors.

TREATMENT

Because anal cancer is a rare tumor, most studies include a small number of patients accrued over several years. The absence of data from randomized trials makes treatment difficult in certain circumstances. A major determinant of appropriate treatment is the location of the primary tumor.

Traditionally the treatment of the anal canal has been surgical, often involving an antero-posterior (AP) resection. However, small localized tumors may be treated with wide excisions alone. Tumors that involve (a) the dentate line, (b) are greater than 2 cm, or (c) involve greater than half the bowel circumference are probably best managed with combined-modality treatment. This integrated approach improves overall survival and may allow radical surgery to be avoided. In the last several years, several studies have used combined-modality treatments with radiation and chemotherapy after local resection. Therefore, the primary therapeutic modalities for anal cancer are a combination of chemotherapy and radiation therapy. Combined chemoradiation is aimed at cure and preservation of anal function. AP resection is used as salvage therapy in patients with chemoradiation-resistant disease. Table 6 shows results of a few of these trials.

Preliminary results of a phase II study of high-dose radiation therapy and neoadjuvant plus concomitant 5-fluorouracil with cis-diaminedichloroplatinum (CDDP) chemotherapy for patients with anal canal cancer: a French cooperative study (Peiffert D et al) showed tumor response defined as the complete response (CR) and partial response (PR) rates of 11% and 61%, respectively, after induction chemotherapy, 59% and 31% after concomitant radiochemotherapy, and 96% and none 2 months after completion of the treatment.

Primary chemoradiation therapy with fluorouracil and cisplatin for cancer of the anus (Doci R et al) revealed CR in 33 (94%) patients; nine patients with metastatic lymph nodes also had CR. Two patients had a PR; both underwent abdominoperineal resection, which was not curative.

Treatment of anal canal carcinoma with high-dose radiation therapy and concomitant fluorouracil–cisplatin (Gerard JP et al) produced an overall survival of 84% and 77%, cancer-specific survival of 90% and 86%, and colostomy-free survival of 71% and 67% at 5 and 8 years, respectively.

The 5-year survival derived from the comparison of phase II studies involving radiation therapy combined with fluorouracil and CDDP and those involving fluorouracil and mitomycin is 65% to 80% and 84% to 96%, respectively. Radiation with continuous infusion of 5-FU with cisplatin are also under evaluation.

Treatment options according to the stage are shown in Table 7.

Stage 0

Surgical resection is the treatment of choice for the lesions of the perianal area that do not involve the anal sphincter.

Stage I

- Tumors of the perianal skin or anal margin not involving the anal sphincter. Wide local excision (for small tumors).

TABLE 6. *Selected results of concurrent radiation and fluorouracil and mitomycin chemotherapy*

Chemotherapy regimens	Radiation (dose/fractions/time)	Primary tumor control	Regional node control	5-yr survival	Reference
Fluorouracil, 1,000 mg/m² per day, CIVI for 8 days, days 1–4, 29–32 (total dose/course, 8,000 mg/m²) Mitomycin, 15 mg/m² i.v. bolus day 1 (total dose/course, 15 mg/m²)	30 Gy/15/days 1–21	31/34 (91%) (≤5 cm) 7/10 (70%) (>5 cm)	NS	80% crude	Leichman et al.
Fluorouracil, 1,000 mg/m² per day, CIVI for 8 days, days 2–5, 28–31 (total dose/course, 8,000 mg/m²) Mitomycin, 10 mg/m² i.v. bolus day 1 X (total dose/course, 10 mg/m²)	40.8 Gy/24/days 1–35	22/26 (85%) (>3 cm) 32/50 (64%) (≥3 cm)	NA	73%, 3 yr actuarial	Sischy et al.
Fluorouracil, 1,000 mg/m² per day, CIVI for 8 days, days 1–4, 43–46 (total dose/course, 8,000 mg/m²) Mitomycin, 10 mg/m² per dose i.v. bolus for 2 doses, days 1 and 43 (total dose/course, 20 mg/m²)	48–50 Gy/24–20/days 1–58 (split course)	25/27 (93%) (≤5 cm) 16/20 (80%) (>5 cm or T)	4/5	65%, actuarial	Cummings et al.
Fluorouracil, 1,000 mg/m² per day, CIVI for 8 days, days 1–4, 29–32 (total dose/course, 8,000 mg/m²) Mitomycin, 10 mg/m² per dose i.v. bolus for 2 doses, days 1 and 29 (total dose/course, 20 mg/m²)	50 Gy/25–28/days 1–35 ± boost	21/22 (95%) (≤X cm) 14/19 (74%) (>5 cm or T4)	3/4	77%, actuarial	Schneider et al.
Fluorouracil, 600 mg/m² per day, CIVI for 5 days, days 1–5 (total dose/course, 3,000 mg/m²) Mitomycin, 12 mg/m² i.v. bolus day 1 (total dose/course, 12 mg/m²)	42 Gy/10/days 1–19 plus interstitial boost	No data in original publication 57/70 (81%) (≥4 cm)	NS	NS	Papillon and Montbarbon, 1987
Fluorouracil, 1,000 mg/m² per day, CIVI for 4 days, days 1–4 (total dose/course, 4,000 mg/m²) Mitomycin, 10–15 mg/m² i.v. bolus day 1 (total dose/course, 10–15 mg/m²)	50–54 Gy/25–27/days 1–35 (≤5 cm)	28/30 (93%) (>5 cm or T4) 42/56 (75%)	NS	72%, actuarial	Tanum et al., 1991
Fluorouracil, 1,000 mg/m² per day, CIVI for 4 days, days 1–4 (total dose/course, 4,000 mg/m²) Mitomycin, 10 mg/m² i.v. bolus day 1 (total dose/course, 10 mg/m²)	50 Gy/20/days 1–28 (≤5 cm)	3/3 (>5 cm or T4) 11/13 (85%)	3/3	75%, actuarial	Cummings et al., 1984
Fluorouracil, 750 mg/m² per day, CIVI for 8 days, days 1–5, 43–47 (total dose/course, 8,000 mg/m²) Mitomycin, 15 mg/m² per dose i.v. bolus for 3 doses, days 1, 43, and 85 (total dose/course, 45 mg/m²)	54–60 Gy/30–33/days 1–53 (split course)	28/38 (74%) (≤5 cm) 9/17 (53%) (>5 cm)	8/8	81%, actuarial	Doci et al., 1992

CIVI, continuous intravenous infusion; NS, not stated; NA, not applicable; T, tumor invading adjacent organs; T4, tumor invading deep extradermal structures.
From Cohen AM, Winawer SJ, eds. *Cancer of the colon, rectum and anus.* New York: McGraw Hill, 1995, with permission.

TABLE 7. *Treatment options for anal cancer*

Stage	Treatment options
0	Surgery
I	Radiation
	Chemoradiation
	Surgery
	Interstitial iridium 192 after external beam radiation
II	Chemoradiation
	Surgery
IIIa	Treatment as for I and II
IIIb	Chemoradiation with surgical resection of residual disease
IV	Palliative surgery
	Palliative irradiation
	Palliative chemoradiation
	Clinical trials

• Anal canal cancer.
Stage I involving the anal sphincter and those that are too large for complete local resection are treated with external beam radiation therapy with or without chemotherapy. Results from the UKCCCR randomized trial of radiotherapy alone versus radiotherapy, 5-fluorouracil, and mitomycin revealed that combined chemoradiation is more effective than radiation therapy alone (see Table 6).
Radical resection is reserved for residual cancer in the anal canal after chemoradiation therapy.
Interstitial iridium 192 implantation after external beam radiotherapy may aid some patients with residual disease to have CR.
The optimal dose of external beam radiation with concurrent chemotherapy still must be determined.

Stage II

• Tumors of the perianal skin or anal margin not involving the anal sphincter: wide local resection (of small tumors).
• Cancers of the anal canal (involving the anal sphincter and those that are too large to be completely excised locally).
Chemoradiation therapy (see Table 6).
Salvage chemotherapy with fluorouracil and cisplatin combined with a radiation boost may avoid a permanent colostomy in patients with residual tumor after initial nonoperative therapy, as suggested by a phase III randomized intergroup study (Flam M et al.)
Radical resection for residual disease in the anal canal after the initial nonoperative treatment.

Stage IIIA

Stage IIIA anal cancer presents clinically as stage II anal cancer in most patients but is upstaged to IIIA by presence of perirectal nodal disease or adjacent organ involvement. Endoscopic ultrasound (endoanal or endorectal) may help in staging.

• Treatment is similar to stage I/II disease involving chemoradiation.
• Salvage chemotherapy combined with a radiation boost as shown by Flam et al.
• Postoperative radiation therapy.

Stage IIIB

Though the cure of this stage is possible, the presence of metastatic disease secondary to the involvement of inguinal lymph nodes (unilateral or bilateral) constitutes a poor prognostic sign.

- Chemoradiation (as described for stage II) with surgical resection of residual disease at the primary site plus unilateral or bilateral superficial and deep inguinal lymph node dissection.
- Because of the poor prognosis of these patients, they should be recruited for clinical trials whenever possible.

Stage IV

There is no standard chemotherapy for stage IV disease. Palliation of symptoms constitutes the backbone of management. Patients with stage IV anal cancer should be included in clinical trials.

- Palliative surgery.
- Palliative radiation therapy.
- Palliative combined chemotherapy and radiation therapy.
- Clinical trials.

RECURRENT ANAL CANCER

Local recurrences after initial treatment with either chemoradiation or surgical resection can be effectively controlled by alternate treatment options (Table 8) including:

- Surgical resection after radiation (salvage APR).
- Postoperative radiation.

FOLLOW-UP

Patients with anal cancer should be monitored

- Every 3 months for the first 3 years.
- Every 6 months for an additional 2 years.

TABLE 8. *Dosage of chemoradiation in anal cancer*

Treatment modality	Dose
External beam radiation	4,500–5,000 cGY
RTOG	170 cGY/day for 27 days, days 2–28 (total dose, 4,500–5,000 cGY)
Milan	180 cGY/day for 4 weeks followed by a 2-week rest (total dose, 5,400 cGY)
Chemotherapy	
Mitomycin	
RTOG	Mitomycin, 10 mg/m^2 i.v. bolus on day 2
Milan	Mitomycin, 15 mg/m^2 i.v. bolus on day 1
Fluorouracil	
RTOG	Fluorouracil, 1,000 mg/m^2 per day CIVI for days 2–4 and 28–32 (total dose/course, 8,000 mg/m^2)
Milan	Fluorouracil, 750 mg/m^2 per day CIVI for 5 days, days 1–5 (total dose/course, 3,750 mg/m^2)

TABLE 9. *5-year disease-free survival rates*

Stage	%
Primary disease	65–80
Persistent or recurrent disease	40–50

- And then annually.

The following specific recommendations should be undertaken:

- Medical history.
- Physical examination.
- Complete blood counts.
- Liver function tests.
- Chest radiograph.
- CT scan every 6 to 12 months for the first 3 years.
  Prognosis: 5-year disease-free survival (Table 9).

Prevention

Awareness of the disease by the physician and the recognition of a high-risk group (homosexual men, patients with cervical or vulvar cancer) may aid patients by early detection. Yearly anoscopy may be indicated in such a group. Role of the Papanicolaou smear still must be studied.

ANAL CARCINOMA IN HIV-INFECTED PATIENTS

The incidence of anal cancer is increasing in patients with HIV infection, especially with the advent of new antiretroviral medications.

Epidemiology

The San Francisco Study revealed an incidence of anal carcinoma in homosexual men at between 25 and 87 cases per 100,000, as compared with 0.7 cases per 100,000 in the entire male population.

Etiology

- Human papillomavirus (HPV), especially oncogenetic serotypes 16 and 18, which are found to be associated with anal intraepithelial neoplasia (AIN), which designates a precursor lesion. The same subtypes of HPV are implicated in malignant transformation in anal cancer as in cervical cancer.
- Perianal herpes simplex.
- Anal condylomas.
- Anal-receptive behavior in homosexual or bisexual men, especially with multiple sexual partners.

Clinical Presentation

- Rectal pain.
- Rectal bleeding.
- Rectal discharge.
- Symptoms secondary to obstruction.

Diagnosis

Diagnosis workup is similar to determination of local disease extent and staging for dissemination in immunocompetent patients.

Pathology

• Squamous cell carcinoma.
• Grading for AIN is similar to that for cervical intraepithelial neoplasia (CIN).

Staging

The staging of anal cancer in HIV-infected patients is similar to that in HIV-negative patients.

Prognosis

HIV-infected patients with severe immunosuppression, as evidenced by CD4 counts less than $50/mm^3$, may result in more aggressive and advanced disease.

Treatment

• The treatment of choice for squamous cell carcinoma of the anus is combined modality therapy with:
• Mitomycin, 10 mg/m^2 , day 1; (total dose/course, 10 mg/m^2) IV bolus
• Fluorouracil, 1,000 mg/m^2/day continuous intravenous infusion for 4 days, days 1–4 (total dose/course, 4,000 mg/m^2), *PLUS*
• External beam radiation therapy
• Appropriate radiation dosage still must be investigated in HIV infection. Anecdotal experience indicates that HIV-infected patients have a decreased tolerance to full pelvic radiotherapy, resulting in myelotoxicity and mucositis, thereby limiting the size of treatment fields. Surgical excision with or without local radiotherapy may be considered for small localized cancer with minimal depth of invasion.
• Treatment of AIN:
• Treatment of AIN in HIV-infected patients is similar to CIN in women and may include electrocautery, cryoablation, or laser ablation.

Screening

Anal Pap smears have a reported sensitivity of approximately 70% (equal to that associated with uterine cervix Pap testing). There are currently no standard recommendations for screening for anal cancer in this population. Anoscopy with anal cytology should be undertaken in patients with abnormal discharge, bleeding, pruritis, bowel irregularity, rectal or pelvic pain, and those with a history of previous preinvasive lesions or abnormal Pap smears. Other patients who should be screened include HIV-negative men with a history of anal-receptive intercourse, HIV-positive men and women with CD4 cell counts less than $500/mm^3$, and HIV-positive and -negative women with a history of high-grade CIN.

SUGGESTED READINGS

Staging of Anal Cancer

American Joint Committee on Cancer. *AJCC cancer staging manual*. 5th ed. Philadelphia: Lippincott-Raven, 1997:91–95.

Anal Canal. In: Hrmanek P, Sobin LH, eds. *TNM classification of malignant tumors.* 4th ed. Berlin: Springer-Verlag, 1987:50–52.

Treatment of anal cancer

UKCCCR Anal Canal Trial Working Party. Epidermoid anal cancer: results from the UKCCCR randomized trial of radiotherapy alone versus radiotherapy, 5-fluorouracil, and mitomycin. *Lancet* 1996;348:1049–1054.

Peiffert D, Seitz JF, Rougier P, et al. Preliminary results of a phase II study of high-dose radiation therapy and neoadjuvant concomitant 5-fluorouracil with CDDP chemotherapy for patients with anal canal cancer: a French cooperative study. *Ann Oncol* 1997;8(6):575–581.

Flam M, John J, Pajak TF, et al. Role of mitomycin in combination with fluorouracil and radiotherapy, and of salvage chemoradiation in the definitive nonsurgical treatment of epidermoid cancer of the anal canal: results of a phase III randomized intergroup study. *J Clin Oncol* 1996;14:2527–2539.

Doci R, Zucali R, La Monica G, et al. Primary chemoradiation therapy with fluorouracil and cisplatin for cancer of the anus: results in 35 consecutive patients *J Clin Oncol* 1996;14(12):3121–3125.

Sandhu AP, Symonds RP, Robertson AG, et al. Interstitial iridium-192 implantation combined with external radiotherapy in anal cancer: ten years experience. *Int J Radiat Oncol Biol Phys* 1998;40:575–581.

Longo WE, Vernava AM, Wade TP, et al. Recurrent squamous cell carcinoma of the anal canal: predictors of initial treatment failure and results of salvage therapy. *Ann Surg* 1994;220:40–49.

Nigro ND, Seydel HG, Considine B, et al. Combined preoperative radiation and chemotherapy for squamous cell carcinoma of the anal canal. *Cancer* 1983;51:1826–1829.

Sischy B, Doggett RL, Krall JM, et al. Definitive irradiation and chemotherapy for radiosensitization in management of anal carcinoma: interim report on Radiation Therapy Oncology Group study no. 8314. *J Natl Cancer Inst* 1989;81:850–856.

Grabenbauer GG, Schneider IH, Gall FP, et al. Epidermoid carcinoma of the anal canal: treatment by combined radiation and chemotherapy. *Radiother Oncol* 1993;27:59–62.

Gerard JP, Ayzac L, Hun D, et al. Treatment of anal canal carcinoma with high dose radiation therapy and concomitant fluorouracil-cisplatinum. Long-term results in 95 patients. *Radiother Oncol* 1998;46(3):249–256.

Tanum G, Tveit K, Karlsen KO, et al. Chemotherapy and radiation therapy for anal carcinoma: survival and late morbidity. *Cancer* 1991;67:2462–2466.

Doci R, Zucali R, Bombelli L, et al. Combined chemoradiation therapy for anal cancer: a report of 56 cases. *Ann Surg* 1992;215:150–156.

Anal Cancer in HIV-Infected Patients

Peddada AV, Smith DE, Rao AR, et al. Chemotherapy and low-dose radiotherapy in the treatment of HIV-infected patients with carcinoma of the anal canal. *Int J Radiat Oncol Biol Phys* 1997;37:1101–1105.

Palefsky JM, Holly EA, Hogoboom CJ, et al. Anal cytology as a screening tool for anal squamous intraepithelial lesion. *J Acquir Immun Defic Syndr Hum Retrovirol* 1997;14:415–422.

Palefsky JM, Holly EA, Ralston ML, et al. High incidence of anal high grade squamous intraepithelial lesions among HIV-positive and HIV-negative homosexual and bisexual men. *AIDS* 1998;12:495–503.

SECTION 4

Breast

11

Breast Cancer

Jame Abraham and Jo Anne Zujewski

Medicine Branch, DCS, National Cancer Institute, National Institutes of Health, Bethesda, Maryland

Breast cancer is the most common cancer diagnosis in women in North America, and it is second only to lung cancer as a cause of cancer death in women. When diagnosed early, breast cancer is highly treatable with surgery, radiation, and systemic therapy (chemotherapy or hormonal therapy). At the time of diagnosis, more than 90% of patients will have only localized disease. Of women with metastatic disease, 20% are alive at 5 years. Since 1994 there has been a 1% to 2% reduction in mortality in the United States, Canada, Sweden, and the United Kingdom. This decrease in mortality has been attributed to the use of screening mammography and systemic adjuvant therapy.

EPIDEMIOLOGY

- In the U.S., 184,200 new cases of invasive breast cancer were diagnosed in 2000.
- About 27,000 new cases of noninvasive breast cancer (DCIS) were diagnosed in the U.S. in 1999.
- In 2000, 41,200 women were expected to die of breast cancer in the U.S.
- About 1,400 cases of breast cancer were diagnosed in men in 2000.
- Lifetime risk of developing breast cancer in North American women (who live up to 85 years) is one in eight.
- The incidence of breast cancer increases with age, but the rate of increase slows after menopause.
- The 5-year survival rate of all patients with breast cancer is 85%.

RISK FACTORS *(Table 1)*

Hereditary breast cancer syndromes

- **BRCA1 or BRCA2:** Individuals with a mutation of BRCA1 (chromosome 17q21) or BRCA2 (chromosome 13q12-13) have a 50% to 85% lifetime risk of developing breast cancer.
- **Li–Fraumeni syndrome:** Mutations in one p53 suppressor allele lead to this syndrome (other malignancies associated are soft tissue sarcomas, brain tumors, leukemias, lung cancer, and adrenocortical cancer).
- **Cowden's syndrome:** Rare syndrome associated with hamartomatous lesions of skin and oral cavity; in 50% of patients, breast cancer develops.

TABLE 1. *Risk factors for breast cancer in females*

History of breast cancer
Increasing age
Family history of breast cancer
Early menarche
Late menopause
Nulliparity
Atypical lobular hyperplasia or atypical ductal hyperplasia
Early exposure to ionizing radiation
BRCA1 or BRCA2 mutations
Prior breast biopsies
Long-term postmenopausal estrogen replacement
Alcohol consumption

PATHOPHYSIOLOGY

- In sporadic cases, abnormalities of HER-2/neu (overexpressed in 20% to 30% of breast cancers), p53, cyclin D, or bcl-2 genes are seen.
- Many factors stimulate or inhibit the growth and proliferation of breast cancer cells.
- Gonadal steroid hormones: Estrogens, progestins, and androgens
- Growth factors: Epidermal growth factors (EGFs), transforming growth factors (TGF-α and -β), and insulin-like growth factors I and II.

PATHOLOGY

- **High-risk lesions**
    Atypical ductal hyperplasia (ADH)
    Lobular carcinoma in situ (LCIS) or lobular neoplasia
- **Carcinoma in situ: Ductal carcinoma in situ (DCIS)**
- **Infiltrating carcinoma**
    Infiltrating ductal carcinoma (NOS): Medullary, tubular, papillary
    Infiltrating lobular
- **Unusual histologies**
    Inflammatory breast cancer (tumor invasion of the dermal lymphatics)
    Spindle cell (pseudosarcomatous sarcoma)
    Adenoid cystic carcinoma
    Apocrine carcinoma
    Signet-ring cell carcinoma
    Carcinoid tumor
- **Paget's disease of the nipple**

PREVENTION

Chemoprevention

Tamoxifen

A large randomized trial (NSABP P-1) showed a 49% reduction in the incidence of invasive breast cancer in high-risk subjects who took tamoxifen, 20 mg daily.

- Women eligible for this trial were at least 35 years old and had an absolute risk of ≥1.66% over 5 years using Gail Model or a pathologic diagnosis of LCIS.

- Gail model is a statistical model that calculates a woman's absolute risk of breast cancer by using the following criteria: Age, age at menarche, age at first live birth, number of previous biopsies, and number of first-degree relatives with breast cancer. For a free computer disk of this model, call 1-800-4-cancer or visit the NCI web site (http://www.nci.nih.gov).
- This reduction in breast cancer incidence is associated with an increase in endometrial cancer (risk ratio of 2.53) and thrombotic events (pulmonary embolism, with a risk ratio of 3.01) in patients who are older than 50 years.
- Use of tamoxifen in patients should be individualized.

Raloxifene

There is an ongoing clinical trial, Study of Tamoxifen And Raloxifene (STAR), in which tamoxifen is compared with raloxifene in postmenopausal women for prevention of breast cancer.

Prophylactic Surgery

Prophylactic Mastectomy

- Indications for prophylactic mastectomy are controversial.
- Recent data show that in women with high risk of breast cancer, prophylactic mastectomy can reduce the incidence of breast cancer by 90–95%.

Oophorectomy

- Oophorectomy before age 40 years has been shown to decrease the risk of breast cancer by 45%, even in women who subsequently receive hormone replacement therapy (HRT).

Screening

- Regular mammographic screening results in early diagnosis of breast cancer and a 25% to 30% decrease in mortality in women older than 50 years.
- A 17% reduction in mortality is seen in women aged between 40 and 49 years.
- The National Cancer Institute recommends annual mammography every one to two years for women age 40 years and older.

High-Risk Family

Women with high-risk families, especially with BRCA1 and BRCA2 mutations, are often advised to start mammographic screening at the age of 25 years, or 5 years earlier than the earliest age at which the family member was diagnosed with breast cancer.

Clinical Features

Clinical features are listed in Table 2.

DIAGNOSIS

1. History and physical examination.
2. Bilateral mammogram (has 80% to 90% accuracy).

TABLE 2. *Clinical features of breast cancer*

Local effects
Breast lump
Skin thickening or alteration
Peau d'orange
Dimpling of the skin
Nipple inversion or crusting (Paget's disease)
Unilateral nipple discharge
Lymph nodes
Axillary and supraclavicular lymph node enlargement
Distant effects
Pleural effusion
Pericardial effusion
Bone tenderness or fracture
Abdomen
  Hepatomegaly
  Ascites
  Other masses
CNS involvement
  Metastatic lesions of the brain
  Cord compression
  Carcinomatous meningitis
Systemic features
Fatigue
Weight loss
Bone pain
Headache
Paresthesia

CNS, central nervous system.

3. Biopsy: Any distinct mass should be considered for a biopsy, even if the mammograms are negative.
   The standard methods of diagnosis are:
   • Fine-needle aspiration.
   • Core-needle biopsy.
   • Incisional or excisional biopsy.
   In nonpalpable breast lesions, the options are:
   • Ultrasound-guided core-needle biopsy.
   • Stereotactic core-needle biopsy under mammographic localization.
   • Needle localization under mammography followed by surgical excision.
   • Magnetic resonance imaging (MRI)-guided biopsy is under development.
4. Laboratory studies
   • Complete blood count, liver function tests, and alkaline phosphatase.
   • The use of tumor markers is not recommended.
5. Pathology review to determine:
   • Histology and diagnosis (invasive versus *in situ*).
   • Pathologic grade of the tumor.
   • Tumor involvement of the margin.
   • Special studies: ER/PR status, HER2/neu status, indices of proliferation (e.g., mitotic index, Ki-67, or S phase).
6. Radiographic studies are done as per the history and physical examination and screening blood tests.

- Computed tomography (CT) scan of the chest and abdomen.
- Imaging of the brain with CT or MRI.
- Bone scan.
- Chest radiograph.

Staging of Breast Cancer (AJCC) (Tables 3–5)

Prognostic Factors
1. Number of positive axillary lymph nodes.
   - Most powerful prognostic indicator.
   - Axillary lymph node dissection should have at least 10 lymph nodes available for evaluation to be considered adequate.
2. Tumor size.
   - Tumors less than 1 cm in size have good prognosis in patients without lymph node involvement.
3. Histologic or nuclear grade.
   - Poorly differentiated histology and higher nuclear grade have worse prognosis.
   - Commonly used system is Scarff–Bloom–Richardson (SBR) classification and Fisher's nuclear grade.

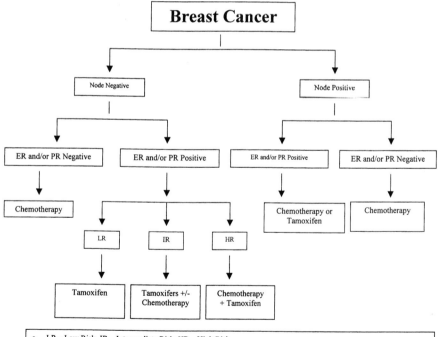

Fig. 1. Treatment algorithm for breast cancer.

TABLE 3. *Staging of breast cancer (AJCC)*

Primary tumor (T)
TX: Primary tumor cannot be assessed
T0: No evidence of primary tumor
Tis: Carcinoma in situ; intraductal carcinoma, lobular carcinoma in situ, or Paget's disease of the nipple with no associated tumor. Note: Paget's disease associated with a tumor is classified according to the size of the tumor.
T1: Tumor ≤2.0 cm in greatest dimension
    T1mic: Microinvasion ≤0.1 cm in greatest dimension
    T1a: Tumor >0.1 but ≤0.5 cm in greatest dimension
    T1b: Tumor >0.5 cm but ≤1.0 cm in greatest dimension
    T1c: Tumor >1.0 cm but ≤2.0 cm in greatest dimension
T2: Tumor >2.0 cm but ≤5.0 cm in greatest dimension
T3: Tumor >5.0 cm in greatest dimension
T4: Tumor of any size with direct extension to (a) chest wall or (b) skin
    T4a: Extension to chest wall
    T4b: Edema (including peau d'orange) or ulceration of the skin of the breast or satellite skin nodules confined to the same breast
    T4c: Both of the above (T4a and T4b)
    T4d: Inflammatory carcinoma
Regional lymph nodes (N)
NX: Regional lymph nodes cannot be assessed (e.g., previously removed)
N0: No regional lymph node metastasis
N1: Metastasis to movable ipsilateral axillary lymph node(s)
N2: Metastasis to ipsilateral axillary lymph node(s) fixed to each other or to other structures
N3: Metastasis to ipsilateral internal mammary lymph node(s)

TABLE 4. *Pathologic classification (pN)*

pNX: Regional lymph nodes cannot be assessed (not removed for pathologic study or previously removed)
pN0: No regional lymph node metastasis
pN1: Metastasis to movable ipsilateral axillary lymph node(s)
    pN1a: Only micrometastasis (none >0.2 cm)
    pN1b: Metastasis to lymph node(s), any >0.2 cm
        pN1bi: Metastasis in one to three lymph nodes, any >0.2 cm, and all <2.0 cm in greatest dimension
        pN1bii: Metastasis to four or more lymph nodes, any >0.2 cm and all <2.0 cm in greatest dimension
        pN1biii: Extension of tumor beyond the capsule of a lymph node metastasis <2.0 cm in greatest dimension
        pN1biv: Metastasis to a lymph node ≥2.0 cm in greatest dimension
pN2: Metastasis to ipsilateral axillary lymph node(s) fixed to each other or to other structures
pN3: Metastasis to ipsilateral internal mammary lymph node(s)
Distant metastasis (M)
MX: Presence of distant metastasis cannot be assessed
M0: No distant metastasis
M1: Distant metastasis present (includes metastasis to ipsilateral supraclavicular lymph nodes)

Adapted from AJCE Manual 1997.

TABLE 5. *AJCC stage groupings*

Stage 0	Tis	N0	M0
Stage I	T1	N0	M0
Stage IIA	T0	N1	M0
	T1	N1	M0
	T2	N0	M0
Stage IIB	T2	N1	M0
	T3	N0	M0
Stage IIIA	T0	N2	M0
	T1	N2	M0
	T2	N2	M0
	T3	N1	M0
	T3	N2	M0
Stage IIIB	T4	Any N	M0
	Any T	N3	M0
Stage IV	Any T	Any N	M1

Adapted from AJCE Manual 1997.

4. ER/PR status.
   - ER positive has better prognosis.
5. Histologic tumor type.
   - Prognoses of infiltrating ductal and lobular carcinoma are similar.
   - Medullary and tubular cancers have good prognosis if the size is less than 3 cm.
   - Inflammatory breast cancer has poor prognosis.

MANAGEMENT OF BREAST CANCER

High-Risk Lesions

Atypical ductal hyperplasia (ADH)

- Fourfold to fivefold increase in risk of breast cancer in patients with ADH.
- There is wide variation in the diagnostic criteria used in the diagnosis of ADH.
- Managed by close follow-up.
- Clinical breast examination and mammogram.
- NSABP-P1 study: 86% risk reduction was seen in patients who received tamoxifen.

Lobular carcinoma in situ (LCIS)

- LCIS is not considered a cancer, but a marker of increased risk for developing invasive breast cancer.
- Also known as lobular neoplasia or atypical lobular hyperplasia.
- It is usually multicentric and bilateral.
- There is a 21% chance of developing breast cancer in 15 years for patients with LCIS.
- Managed by close follow-up.
- Clinical breast examination every 4 to 12 months and annual mammogram.
- Tamoxifen may be used for prevention of breast cancer (56% reduction in risk as per the NSABP-P1 study).
- Bilateral prophylactic mastectomy may be considered in selected patients.

Noninvasive Breast Cancer

Ductal carcinoma in situ

- With the extensive use of mammograms, the diagnosis of DCIS has increased over the past few years.
- Microcalcification or soft-tissue abnormality is seen in mammogram.

Different histologic types of DCIS

- Comedocarcinoma.
- Noncomedo carcinoma: micropapillary, papillary, solid, cribriform.

Treatment

- Lumpectomy plus radiation treatment is the recommended treatment option.
- In patients who had lumpectomy and radiation, tamoxifen reduced the risk of breast cancer recurrence (ipsilateral and contralateral).
- Simple mastectomy is an alternative to lumpectomy with radiation.

Invasive Breast Cancer

Early-stage breast cancer

1. **Surgery.** No survival difference is seen in patients who are treated with modified radical mastectomy versus lumpectomy plus radiation treatment. Breast preservation with lumpectomy with radiation therapy is the preferred treatment.
   Contraindications for lumpectomy.
   - Two or more gross tumors in separate quadrants of the breast.
   - Diffuse, indeterminate, or malignant-appearing microcalcifications.
   - Central location of the tumor mass.
   Contraindications for radiation.
   - History of therapeutic irradiation to the breast region.
   - Connective tissue disorders (scleroderma).
   - Pregnancy.
   Axillary lymph node dissection (ALND)
   - This procedure primarily provides prognostic information. It has minimal therapeutic benefit, especially in clinically negative axillae.
   - Histologically positive axillary lymph nodes are the most important prognostic factor.
   - Of patients with clinically negative axillary lymph nodes, 30% will have positive histology after dissection.
   - Associated with approximately 10% to 25% risk of lymphedema, which can be mild to severe.
   Sentinel node biopsy
   - A minimally invasive procedure for staging.
   - A radioactive substance or blue dye is injected into the area around the tumor.
   - The ipsilateral axilla is explored, and the node that has taken up the dye or radioactive material is excised, and very carefully examined pathologically.
   - In expert hands, this procedure identifies a node in more than 85% of patients.
   - Many clinical trials are ongoing to validate this approach in clinical practice.
2. **Radiotherapy**
   - It is part of the breast-conserving treatment (lumpectomy).

- Breast radiation up to 4,500 to 5,000 cGy ± 1,000 to 1,500 cGy boost to tumor-excision site.
- Usually it is given after chemotherapy in patients who need chemotherapy, or after lumpectomy in those who are not receiving chemotherapy.
- Postmastectomy radiation treatment to the chest wall and supraclavicular lymph nodes decreases the risk of locoregional recurrence in patients with four or more positive lymph nodes.
- Whether postmastectomy radiation is beneficial in patients with one to three positive lymph nodes and whether it improves overall survival in patients is a subject of recent controversy.

3. **Systemic treatment for early breast cancer**
   For risk stratification of patients with lymph node–negative breast cancer, see the St. Gallen recommendations (Table 6). The algorithm for systemic treatment of breast cancer is shown in Fig. 1.
   Chemotherapy
   - Combination chemotherapy can reduce the annual risk of death by 20%, and in 10 years produces an absolute improvement in survival of 7% to 11% in women younger than 50 years (Table 7).
   - Effect of chemotherapy is less pronounced in older women.
   Hormonal therapy: Tamoxifen.
   - Tamoxifen is a selective estrogen-receptor modulator (SERM).
   - In early-stage breast cancer, tamoxifen decreases the risk of recurrence by 42% and the absolute risk of death by 22% in both pre- and postmenopausal women with ER-positive tumors.
   - In hormone receptor–positive patients, when tamoxifen was added to chemotherapy, it caused a 25–30% reduction in recurrence, compared with chemotherapy alone.

TABLE 6. *Risk categories for patients with node-negative breast cancer*

Factors[a]	Minimal/low risk (has all listed factors)	Intermediate risk (risk classified between the other two categories)	High risk (has at least one listed factor)
Tumor size[b]	≤1 cm	>1–2 cm	>2 cm
Estrogen receptor (ER) and/or progesterone receptor (PgR) status[c]	Positive	Positive	Negative
Grade[d]	Grade 1 (uncertain relevance for tumors ≤1 cm)	Grade 1–2	Grade 2–3
Age (y)[e]	≥35		<35

[a]Some panel members also recognize lymphatic and/or vascular invasion as important features that include an increased risk.

[b]It was generally agreed by the panel members that pathology tumor size (i.e., size of the invasive component) was the most important prognostic factor for defining the additional risk of relapse.

[c]ER status and PgR status are important biologic characteristics that identify responsiveness to endocrine therapies.

[d]Histologic and/or nuclear grade.

[e]Patients who develop breast cancer at a young age are considered to be at high risk of relapse, although an exact age threshold for this increased risk has not been defined.

Adapted from Ref. 5.

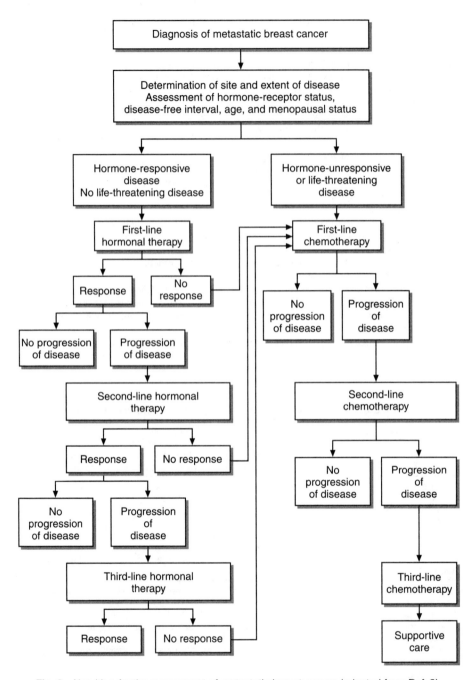

Fig. 2. Algorithm for the mangement of metastatic breast cancer (adapted from Ref. 3).

- Tamoxifen decreases the incidence of breast cancer in the contralateral breast by approximately 50%.
- Recommended treatment is tamoxifen, 20 mg/day p.o. for 5 years.

Locally Advanced Breast Cancer and Inflammatory Breast Cancer

- Tumor ≥5 cm.
- Tumors of any size with direct invasion of the skin of the breast or chest wall (T4).
- Any tumors with fixed or matted axillary lymphadenopathy (NZ).

Treatment

1. Initial surgery is limited to biopsy to confirm the diagnosis and to identify the receptor status.
2. Neoadjuvant (primary) chemotherapy.
   - In more than 65% of the women treated with neoadjuvant chemotherapy, the tumor shrinks by 50% and allows surgical resection with clear margins.
3. Surgery is done after the best response to preoperative chemotherapy.
4. Radiation therapy to the chest wall and supraclavicular area is done after the surgery.

Metastatic Breast Cancer

- Treatment goal is palliation.
- All patients should be considered for ongoing clinical trials.
- In 5% to 15% of patients, durable complete remission can be achieved with systemic therapy.
- Local control may be achieved by surgery and/or radiation treatment.
- In hormone receptor–positive patients with soft-tissue, bone, or asymptomatic visceral disease, consider hormonal agents as the first-line therapy (Table 8).
- Chemotherapy regimens can be used as the initial treatment in hormone receptor–negative disease or patients with symptomatic visceral disease.
- Patients with progressive disease after anthracycline treatment can be considered for paclitaxel or docetaxel.
- Capecitabine has been approved for use in metastatic breast cancer patients whose cancer has progressed after anthracycline and paclitaxel.
- Patients with HER2/neu-positive tumors have an increased response and survival with paclitaxel and trastuzumab (Herceptin) than with paclitaxel alone.
- Bisphosphonates should be used in patients with bony metastatic disease, as they decrease pain and fractures.

Algorithm for the treatment of metastatic breast cancer is shown in Fig. 2. Commonly used chemotherapy agents in metastatic breast cancer are:

About 30% to 50% response rate:
- Docetaxel.
- Doxorubicin.
- Epirubicin.
- Paclitaxel.
- Vinorelbine.
- Capecitabine.

About 10% to 30% response rate:
- Cisplatin.
- Cyclophosphamide.
- 5-Fluorouracil.
- Ifosamide.
- Methotrexate.
- Mitomycin C.
- Mitoxantrone.
- Thiotepa.
- Vinblastine.
- Vincristine.

TABLE 7. *Commonly used chemotherapy regimens*

Regimens	Treatment description	References
AC	Doxorubicin, 60 mg/m^2 i.v. on day 1 (total dose/cycle, 60 mg/m^2) Cyclophosphamide, 600 mg/m^2 i.v. on day 1 　(total dose/cycle, 600 mg/m^2) Treatment cycles are repeated every 21–28 days depending 　on hematologic recovery	1
CMF	Cyclophosphamide, 100 mg/m^2 per day p.o. for 14 days, 　days 1–14 (total dose/cycle, 1,400 mg/m^2) Methotrexate, 40 mg/m^2 per dose i.v. for two doses, days 1 　and 8 (total dose/cycle, 80 mg/m^2) Fluorouracil, 600 mg/m^2 per dose i.v. for 2 doses, days 1 and 8 　(total dose/cycle, 1,200 mg/m^2) Treatment cycles are repeated every 28 days	2
AC → P	Doxorubicin, 60 mg/m^2 i.v. on day 1 (total dose/cycle, 60 mg/m^2) Cyclophosphamide, 600 mg/m^2 i.v. on day 1 × four cycles 　(total dose/cycle, 600 mg/m^2) **Followed by** Paclitaxel 175 mg/m^2 per dose i.v. over 3 h every 3 weeks × 　four cycles (total dose/cycle, 175 mg/m^2) Treatment cycles are repeated every 21 days Doxorubicin and cyclophosphamide followed by Paclitaxel 　has demonstrated a survival advantage in women with +LN	3
CAF	Cyclophosphamide, 100 mg/m^2 p.o. for 14 days, days 1–14 　(total dose/cycle, 1,400 mg/m^2) Doxorubicin, 30 mg/m^2 i.v. for two doses on days 1 and 8 　(total dose/cycle, 60 mg/m^2) Fluorouracil, 500 mg/m^2 i.v. for two doses on days 1 and 8 　(total dose/cycle, 1,000 mg/m^2) Treatment cycles are repeated every 28 days	4

From the following references:

1. Fisher B, Brown AM, Dimitrov NV, et al. Two months of doxorubicin-cyclophosphamide with and without interval reinduction therapy compared with 6 months of cyclophosphamide, methotrexate, and fluorouracil in positive-node breast cancer patients with tamoxifen-nonresponsive tumors: results from the National Surgical Adjuvant Breast and Bowel Project B-15. *Clin Oncol* 1990;8(9):1483–1496, with permission.

2. Bonadonna G, Brusamolino E, Valagussa P, et al. Combination chemotherapy as an adjuvant treatment in operable breast cancer. *N Engl J Med* 1976;294(8):405–410, with permission.

3. Henderson IC, Berry D, Demetri G, et al. Improved disease free (DFS) and overall survival (OS) from the addition of sequential paclitaxel but not from the escalation of doxorubicin dose level in the adjuvant chemotherapy of patients with node positive primary breast cancer. *Proc ASCO* 1998;17:390A, with permission.

4. Falkson G, Gelman RS, Tormey DC, et al. The Eastern Cooperative Oncology Group experience with cyclophosphamide, adriamycin, and 5-fluorouracil (CAF) in patients with metastatic breast cancer. *Cancer* 1985;56(2):219–224, with permission.

Trastuzumab (Herceptin™)

- Indicated in patients with metastatic disease whose tumor overexpresses HER2/neu protein (3+ by immunohistochemistry).
- About 30% of the patients overexpress HER2/neu.
   1. As a single agent in patients who have received one or more chemotherapy regimens for metastatic disease (the response rate is about 13% as a single agent).

2. As a combination with paclitaxel in patients who have not received chemotherapy for metastatic disease.

Treatment dosage and schedule of trastuzumab

- Initial dosage is trastuzumab, 4 mg/kg i.v. over 90 minutes, followed at weekly intervals by
- Maintenance with trastuzumab, 2 mg/kg i.v. over 30 minutes if the initial infusion rate was well tolerated.
- Common adverse effects during administration include fever and chills in up to 40% of patients.
- Mild to moderate symptoms may be successfully treated with acetaminophen, diphenhydramine, and meperidine (12.5–25 mg/dose i.v. or i.m.) with or without interrupting or slowing trastuzumab administration.
- Preexisting cardiac disease and cardiomyopathies associated with prior treatments (e.g., anthracycline drugs and radiation to the chest) may be exacerbated by trastuzumab.
- The probability of cardiac dysfunction is greatest in patients who receive it concurrent with anthracycline drugs (e.g., doxorubicin).

High-dose chemotherapy (HDCT)

- Rationale
  1. High dose of chemotherapy can overcome drug resistance and eradicate micrometastatic disease.
  2. Breast cancer is a moderately chemosensitive tumor, and there is a dose–response correlation.
- Many single-institution phase II studies showed promising results with HDCT.
- Recently reported phase III studies failed to show a survival advantage with HDCT, in either the adjuvant or the metastatic treatment of breast cancer.
- HDCT should be used only in the context of a well-designed clinical trial.

Oophorectomy

- Can be considered in premenopausal patients.
- It can be done with surgical, radiation, or chemical methods.

Recurrent Breast Cancer

Local recurrence

1. After mastectomy
   - 80% of local recurrences occur within 5 years.
   - The treatment of choice is surgical excision and radiotherapy (RT).
   - May consider systemic therapy, although the survival advantage is not clear.
2. After lumpectomy
   - Mastectomy is the treatment of choice for patients who have only isolated breast cancer recurrence.
   - The 5-year relapse-free survival is 60% to 75%, if treated only with mastectomy.

Breast Cancer in Pregnancy

- Breast cancer diagnosis may be delayed in pregnant women.
- Breast cancer during pregnancy was thought to be more aggressive, but the overall poor outcome is likely related to advanced stage at the time of diagnosis.
- Breast biopsy is safe in all stages of pregnancy and should be done for any suggestive mass.

TABLE 8. *Hormonal agents used in metastatic breast cancer*

SERM with combined estrogen agonist and estrogen antagonist activity
Tamoxifen (Nolvadex, others), 20 mg/day p.o.
Toremifene (Fareston), 60 mg/day p.o.
Progestins
Megestrol acetate (Megace, others), 40 mg/dose p.o. 4 times daily
Aromatase inhibitors
Anastrozole (Arimidex), 1 mg/day p.o.
Letrozole (Femara), 2.5 mg/day p.o.
Aminoglutethimide, 250 mg/dose p.o. 4 times daily; hydrocortisone replacement to offset
cortisol suppression associated with aminoglutethimide
LHRH agonist analogue in premenopausal women
Leuprolide (Lupron Depot), 7.5 mg/dose i.m. monthly, *OR*
Leuprolide (Lupron Depot), 22.5 mg/dose i.m. every 3 mo, *OR*
Leuprolide (Lupron Depot), 30 mg/dose i.m. every 4 mo
GnRH agonist analogue
Goserelin (Zoladex), 3.6 mg/dose s.c. implant into the abdominal wall every 28 days *OR*
Goserelin (Zoladex), 10.8 mg/dose s.c. implant into the abdominal wall every 12 weeks
Used in patients who have tumors that express either ER or PR receptors or both receptors.

Treatment

- Lumpectomy and axillary dissection can be performed in the third trimester, and RT can be safely delayed until after delivery.
- Modified radical mastectomy is the treatment of choice in the first and second trimesters, as radiation treatment is contraindicated during pregnancy.

Chemotherapy

- Should not be administered during the first trimester.
- No chemotherapeutic agent has been found to be completely safe during pregnancy.
- An anthracycline combined with cyclophosphamide (e.g., AC given every 3 weeks for four cycles) has been used in the adjuvant setting during the second or third trimesters.
- Chemotherapy should be scheduled to avoid neutropenia and thrombocytopenia at the time of delivery.
- Paclitaxel is teratogenic and should not be used during pregnancy.
- Tamoxifen is teratogenic and should not be used in pregnant women.
- Therapeutic abortion does not change the survival rate.

MALE BREAST CANCER

- Uncommon.
- Risk factors are family history, BRCA2 germline mutation, Kleinfelter syndrome, and radiation.
- Presence of gynecomastia is not a risk factor for breast cancer.
- First seen with a mass beneath the nipple or ulceration.
- Mean age is 60 to 70 years.
- Of male breast cancer, 80% are hormone receptor positive.

Treatment

- Modified radical mastectomy.
- Lumpectomy is rarely done, as it does not offer any cosmetic benefit.
- Systemic treatment with chemotherapy and tamoxifen should follow the general guidelines for female patients.
- None of the adjuvant treatment modalities has been tested in a randomized clinical trial setting in men.

FOLLOW-UP FOR PATIENTS WITH OPERABLE BREAST CANCER

1. History and physical examination every 3 to 6 months for the first 3 years, every 6 to 12 months for the next 2 years, and then annually.
2. Monthly breast self-examination.
3. Annual mammogram of the contralateral and ipsilateral (remaining breast after lumpectomy) breast.
4. Annual Pap smear and pelvic examinations in women who are taking, or have taken, tamoxifen.
5. Complete blood count, liver function tests, and alkaline phosphatase with physical examination.
   - Serum tumor markers (CA 27, 29, CA 15-3) are not recommended.
   - Bone scan, imaging of the chest, abdomen, pelvis, and brain are not recommended routinely, but they are done if symptoms or laboratory abnormalities are present.
6. Annually or every 2 years: rectal examination, occult blood testing, and skin examination.

(Adapted from recommendations by American Society of Clinical Oncology)

REFERENCES

1. Overgaard M, Hansen PS, Overgaard J, et al. Postoperative radiotherapy in high-risk premenopausal women with breast cancer who receive adjuvant chemotherapy. *N Engl J Med* 1997;337:949–955.
2. Karg D, Weaver D, Ashikaga T, et al. The sentinel node in breast cancer. *N Engl J Med* 1998;339: 941–946.
3. Hortobagyi GN. Treatment of breast cancer. *N Engl J Med* 1998;339:974–984.
4. Early Breast Cancer Trialists' Collaborative Group. Tamoxifen for early breast cancer: an overview of the randomised trials. *Lancet* 1998;351:1451–1465.
5. Goldhirsch A, Glick JH, Gelber RD, et al. Meeting highlights: International Consensus Panel on the Treatment of Primary Breast Cancer. *J Natl Cancer Inst* 1998;90:1601–1608.
6. Struewing JP, Hartge P, Wacholder S, et al. The risk of cancer associated with specific mutations of BRCA1 and BRCA2 among Ashkenazi Jews. *N Engl J Med* 1997;336:1401–1408.
7. Hartmann LC, Schaid DJ, Woods JE, et al. Efficacy of bilateral prophylactic mastectomy in women with a family history of breast cancer. *N Engl J Med* 1999;340:77–84.
8. Fisher B, Dignam J, Wolmark N, et al. Tamoxifen in the treatment of intraductal breast cancer: NSABP B-24 randomized controlled trial. *Lancet* 1999;353:1993–2000.
9. Goldenberg MM. Trastuzumab, a recombinant DNA-derived humanized monoclonal antibody: a novel agent for the treatment of metastatic breast cancer. *Clin Ther* 1999;21:309–318.
10. Fisher B, Constatino JP, Wickerham DL, et al. Tamoxifen for prevention of breast cancer; report of NSABP P-1 study. *J Natl Cancer Inst* 1998;90:1371–1388.
11. Gradishar WJ, Jordan VC. Hormonal therapy for breast cancer. *Hematol Oncol Clin North Am* 1999; 13:435–455.
12. Hoskins KF, Stopfer JE, Calzone KA, et al. Assessment and counseling for women with a family history of breast cancer: a guide for clinicians. *JAMA* 1995;273:577–585.

SECTION 5

Genitourinary

12

Renal Cancer

Hung T. Khong and Susan Bates

Medicine Branch, National Cancer Institute, Bethesda, Maryland

EPIDEMIOLOGY

- Of adult malignancies, 3%, with 30,000 new cases and 12,000 deaths estimated each year.
- Male/female ratio is 2:1.
- In the United States, the incidence rates for renal cell carcinoma (RCC) are higher among blacks than whites (Table 1).
- Age at diagnosis is usually older than 40 years, with median age in the mid-60s.
- Cancer of the renal tubular epithelium, RCC, accounts for 90% of all malignancies arising in the kidney. Most of the remaining cases are transitional cell carcinoma of the renal pelvis.
- The incidence and mortality rates for RCC increased steadily in all race and sex groups from 1975 through 1995 (SEER, 1975–1995) (Figs. 1 and 2; Table 1).

ETIOLOGY AND RISK FACTORS

- Tobacco use contributes to one third of all cases of RCC in the U.S.: 40% higher risk in current smokers than nonsmokers; risk increased per pack-year history.
- High consumption of fried or sauteed meat.
- Obesity: particularly in women
- Exposure to asbestos and petroleum products
- End-stage renal disease with development of acquired cystic disease of the kidney; 30 times higher risk in dialysis patients with cystic changes in the kidney than in the general population.
- Hereditary disease:
  1. von Hippel–Lindau (VHL) disease: a familial syndrome with an autosomal dominant inheritance pattern, associated with retinal hemangiomas, central nervous system (CNS) hemangioblastomas, renal cysts and RCC, pheochromocytoma, and epididymal cysts.

TABLE 1. *Age-adjusted incidence rates per 100,000 person-years*

Race/Sex	Incidence rate	% Increase per year
White men	9.6	2.3
White women	4.4	3.1
Black men	11.1	3.9
Black women	4.9	4.3

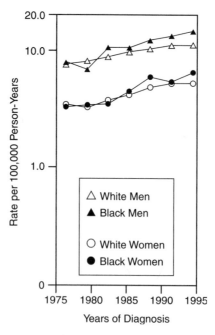

FIG. 1. Age-adjusted incidence rates for renal cell carcinoma.

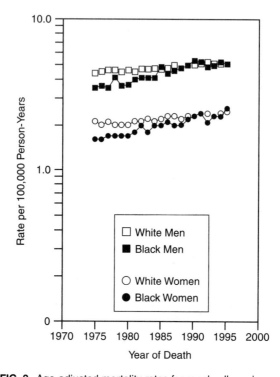

FIG. 2. Age-adjusted mortality rates for renal cell carcinoma.

RCC developed in 25% of VHL patients (data collected from literature reviews: total VHL patients, 706; total RCC cases reported, 176). The mean age at onset was 44 years.

2. Hereditary nonpapillary RCC: translocation between short arm of chromosome 3 (3p) and chromosome 6, 8, or 11 seen in some familial RCC kindreds.
3. Hereditary papillary RCC (HPRCC): not associated with abnormality of chromosome 3p or mutation of VHL gene; gene(s) associated with HPRCC currently unknown.

PATHOLOGIC CLASSIFICATION

For pathologic classification, see Table 2.

CLINICAL PRESENTATION

The classic triad of hematuria, abdominal pain, and abdominal mass occurs in only 10% of patients (Tables 3–7).

DIAGNOSIS

For diagnosis, see Table 8.

TABLE 2. *Pathologic classification of renal cell carcinoma*

Type	Frequency (%)	Genetic changes	5-yr survival (%)
Clear cell	70–80	−3p (81–98%), Von Hippel–Lindau (VHL) gene mutation (57%)[a]	55–60
Papillary	10–15	Trisomies (3q, 7, 12, 16, 17, and 20), −Y, and c-met gene mutation	80–90
Chromophobe	5	Monosomy of multiple chromosomes (1, 2, 6, 10, 13, 17, and 21) and hypodiploidy	90
Collecting duct	<1	−18, −Y	<5
Unclassified	4–5		

Sarcomatoid variant is not a histologic type of renal cancer, but a high-grade change that has been found to arise in all types.

[a]VHL gene, a tumor-suppressor gene, is located on chromosome 3p, which is deleted in 81–98% of sporadic clear cell RCC. Therefore, −3p implies loss of one allele of the VHL gene. The remaining allele is mutated in 57% of cases.

TABLE 3. *AJCC stage (1987 version: T1, ≤2.5 cm; T2, >2.5 cm) at diagnosis*

Stage	Frequency (%)
I	9.3
II	39.5
III	16
IV	24.6
Unknown	10.6

There is a shift from stage II to stage I under the 1997 version of the AJCC stage, which defines T1 as ≤7 cm and T2 as >7 cm. From one recent study, stage I is reported to be 45%, and stage II 13%, with the 1997 version.

TABLE 4. *Common presenting symptoms or laboratory abnormality*

Symptom/lab finding	% of patients
Hematuria	56–59
Pain	38–41
Abdominal mass	36–45
Weight loss	28
Anemia	21
Fever	11
Nonmetastatic hepatic dysfunction	7
Polycythemia	<5
Hypercalcemia	<5 (up to 25% in metastatic disease)
Acute varicocele	2

TABLE 5. *Common sites of metastatic involvement*

Site	%
Lung	75
Lymph node/Soft tissue	36
Bone	20
Liver	18
Skin	8
CNS	8

CNS, central nervous system.

TABLE 6. *Adverse prognostic factors in patients with metastatic RCC*

Karnofsky performance status <80%
LDH >1.5 × upper limit of normal
Hemoglobin <lower limit of normal
Corrected serum calcium >10 mg/dL
Absence of prior nephrectomy

LDH, lactate dehydrogenase.

TABLE 7. *Risk groups based on prognostic factors in Table 6*

Risk group	Risk factors	Median survival time (mo)	Survival rate (%)		
			1-yr	2-yr	3-yr
Favorable	0	20	71	45	31
Intermediate	1 or 2	10	42	17	7
Poor	3 or more	4	12	3	0

TABLE 8. *Initial evaluation*

H & P
CBC/Chemistry profiles (including PT/PTT)
Urinalysis
CT abdomen and pelvis with contrast
CXR
CT chest if
    1. Abnormal CXR, or
    2. Large primary tumor, or
    3. IVC involvement
Bone scan not done routinely unless
    1. Presence of bone pain or
    2. Elevation of serum alkaline phosphatase

A recent study found pelvic CT to have a negligible yield in the staging of 119 patients with RCC (no malignancy found).

STAGING AND PROGNOSIS

Two commonly used staging systems for RCC are the modified Robson system and the TNM system (AJCC) (Tables 9 and 10). The TNM system is preferred because it more accurately describes the extent of tumor involvement (Fig. 3, Table 11).

TREATMENT

Surgery

- Radical nephrectomy is the only curative treatment for localized RCC.
- Radical nephrectomy is defined as resection of the kidney, ipsilateral adrenal gland, regional lymph nodes, and perirenal fat.
- Lymph node dissection is not therapeutic but allows more accurate staging.
- Ipsilateral adrenalectomy may be reserved for patients with large upper-pole disease, and/or with tumor involvement of the adrenal gland, as suggested by CT.
- Partial nephrectomy may be performed in patients in whom standard nephrectomy would significantly impair renal function. Recent studies have shown that in patients with localized tumors 4 cm or less (including those with unilateral disease and a normal contralateral kidney), nephron-sparing surgery offered long-term disease survival comparable to that obtained after radical nephrectomy.
- In selected stage IV patients who have (or relapse) with a solitary metastasis, nephrectomy and resection of the metastasis may be the primary treatment of choice.
- Adjuvant therapies (radiation or systemic therapy) have not been shown to prevent or decrease relapse rates.

TABLE 9. *Robson staging system for renal cell carcinoma*

Extent of disease	Stage
Tumor limited to kidney	I
Tumor extending through renal capsule and confined to Gerota's fascia	II
Tumor invading renal vein or vena cava	IIIA
Tumor involving lymph nodes	IIIB
Combination of two preceding stages	IIIC
Invasion of surrounding organs or distant metastases	IV

TABLE 10. *TNM staging of renal cell carcinoma*

Primary tumor (T)
TX	Primary tumor cannot be assessed
T0	No evidence of primary tumor
T1	Tumor ≤7 cm in greatest dimension, limited to the kidney
T2	Tumor >7 cm in greatest dimension, limited to the kidney
T3	Tumor extends into major veins or invades adrenal gland or perinephric tissues but not beyond Gerota's fascia
T3a	Tumor invades adrenal gland or perinephric tissues but not beyond Gerota's fascia
T3b	Tumor grossly extends into renal vein(s) or vena cava below diaphragm
T3c	Tumor grossly extends into vena cava above diaphragm
T4	Tumor invades beyond Gerota's fascia

Regional lymph nodes (N)[a]
NX	Regional lymph nodes cannot be assessed
N0	No regional lymph node metastasis
N1	Metastasis in a single regional lymph node
N2	Metastasis in more than one regional lymph node

Distant metastasis (M)
MX	Distant metastasis cannot be assessed
M0	No distant metastasis
M1	Distant metastasis

Stage grouping
Stage I	T1	N0	M0
Stage II	T2	N0	M0
Stage III	T1	N1	M0
	T2	N1	M0
	T3a	N0–N1	M0
	T3b	N0–N1	M0
	T3c	N0–N1	M0
Stage IV	T4	Any N	M0
	Any T	N2	M0
	Any T	Any N	M1

From Fleming ID, Cooper JS, Henson DE, et al., eds. *AJCC cancer staging manual.* 5th ed. Philadelphia: Lippincott-Raven, 1997:231–234, with permission.

Data from recent studies indicate that a subdivision of T1 into T1a (<4 cm) and T1b (≥4 cm) would be more prognostically useful. Tumors ≥5 cm have a recurrence rate of 55.8% compared with 4% for those <5 cm. In addition, partial nephrectomy in patients with localized tumor ≤4 cm results in long-term survival comparable to that of radical nephrectomy.

[a]Laterality does not affect the N classification

Systemic Treatment

Hormone Therapy and Chemotherapy

- Little effect in the treatment of metastatic RCC
- A review of 155 trials that studied 80 single chemotherapeutic agents showed a median overall response rate of 4%. The overall response rates for vinblastine, and 5-fluorouracil (5-FU) or FUDR were 6% to 9%, and 5% to 8%, respectively. A recent trial combining gemcitabine with infusional 5-FU reported a 17% response rate (Rini BI et al).
- Patients should be encouraged to enroll in clinical trials.

Interleukin-2

- High-dose interleukin-2 (IL-2) is the only drug approved by the Food and Drug Administration (FDA) for the treatment of metastatic RCC (Table 12).

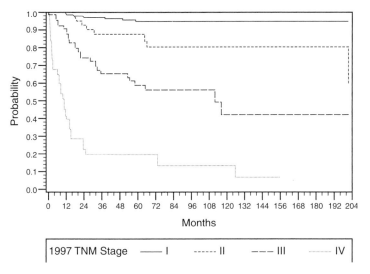

FIG. 3. Survival rates in RCC by AJCC/ICC stage (1997 version) at diagnosis.

• Durable response was seen in a small number of patients treated with high-dose IL-2 (7% complete responses, 8% partial responses, with a median response duration of 54 months for all responses. Median duration for all complete responses has not been reached). These results have been confirmed in other clinical studies.

High dose: 600,000 to 720,000 U/kg i.v. infused over 15 minutes every 8 hours until toxicity or 14 doses for 5 days. Repeat the cycle once after a 7- to 10-day rest, with one or two additional courses repeated every 6 to 12 weeks if there is evidence of tumor stabilization or regression (Fyfe G, Fisher RI, Rosenberg SA, et al: J Clin Oncol 13: 688-696, 1995).

Low dose (i.v.): 72,000 U/kg i.v. bolus every 8 hours to a maximum of 15 doses every 7 to 10 days for two cycles (one course), with an additional course if there is evidence of tumor stabilization or regression. One or two additional courses may be given if further regression is observed. (Yang JC, Topalian SL, Parkinson D, et al: J Clin Oncol 12: 1572-1576, 1998).

Low dose (SQ): First 5-day cycle: 18 million units/day s.c., for 5 days (week 1). Subsequent 5-day cycles: 9 million units/day s.c., for 2 days, and then 18 million units/day s.c., 3 days/week (weeks 2 through 6).

Interferon-α

• Response rates around 12% to 15%; complete responses (2% to 5%) are generally seen in patients with pulmonary metastases.

TABLE 11. *Five-year survival rates (%) in renal cell carcinoma based on sex and race[a]*

Stage	White men	White women	Black men	Black women
Localized	89	86	75	84
Regional	62	59	52	44
Distant	9	7	7	8
Unstaged	31	21	21	35

[a]SEER, 1975–1995; Time period from 1986 to 1995.

TABLE 12. *Treatment regimens with recombinant interleukin-2 (rIL-2) and/or recombinant interferon-α (rIFN-α)*

Regimen	Treatment	Comment	Reference
High-dose rIL-2	600,000–720,000 U/kg i.v. over 15 min q8h until toxicity or 14 doses for 5 days	Repeat once after a 7- to 10-day rest	Fyfe G, Fisher RI, Rosenberg SA, et al., 1995
Low-dose rIL-2 (i.v.)	72,000 U/kg i.v. bolus q8h to a maximum of 15 doses q7–10 days for 2 cycles (1 course)	One more course if tumor stabilization or regression occurred; one or two more courses if there is further tumor regression	Yang JC, Topalian SL, Parkinson D, et al., 1998
Low-dose rIL-2 (s.c.)	18 MU/d s.c. for 5 days, then 9 MU/d s.c. for 2 days, then 18 MU/d s.c. 3 days a week, for 6 weeks		Sleijfer DTh, Janssen RAJ, Buter J, et al., 1992
rIFN-α2	5 to 10 MIU/m² s.c., 3 to 5 times a week, or daily		Horoszewicz JS, Murphy GP, 1989
rIL-2 +	20 MU/m² s.c., days 3–5, weeks 1 and 4; 5 MU/m² s.c., days 1, 3, 5, weeks 2, 3, 5, and 6	Repeat cycle every 8 weeks	Atzopodien J, Kirchner H, Hannien EL, et al., 1993
rIFN-α2	6 MU/m² s.c., day 1, weeks 1 and 4; 6 MU/m² s.c., days 1, 3, and 5, weeks 2, 3, 5, and 6		

- Usual regimens: 5 to 10 MU/m² s.c., three to five times a week, or daily. (Horoszewicz JS, Murphy GP).

Combination of Interleukin-2 and Interferon-α

- Interleukin-2 (rIL-2): 20 million units/m² s.c., days 3 to 5, weeks 1 and 4; 5 million units/m² s.c., days 1, 3, and 5, weeks 2, 3, 5, and 6.
- Interferon-α (rIFNα2): 6 million units/m² s.c., day 1, weeks 1 and 4; 6 million units/m² s.c., days 1, 3, and 5, weeks 2, 3, 5, and 6. Repeat cycle every 8 weeks.

Note: Several trials reported response rates and overall survival of combination regimens (IL-2 and IFN-α, with or without 5-FU) similar to that of high-dose IL-2 alone.

REFERENCES

1. Motzer RJ, Russo P. Systemic therapy for renal cell carcinoma. *J Urol* 2000;163:408–417.
2. Hartmann JT, Bokemeyer C. Chemotherapy for renal cell carcinoma. *Anticancer Res* 1999; 19:1541–1544.
3. Minasian LM, Motzer RJ, Gluck L, et al. Interferon alfa-2a in advanced renal cell carcinoma: treatment results and survival in 159 patients with long-term follow-up. *J Clin Oncol* 1993;11:1368–1375.
4. Motzer RJ, Mazumdar M, Bacik J, et al. Survival and prognostic stratification of 670 patients with advanced renal cell carcinoma. *J Clin Oncol* 1999;17:2530–2540.
5. Negrier S, Escudier B, Lasset C, et al. Recombinant human interleukin-2, recombinant human interferon alfa-2a, or both in metastatic renal-cell carcinoma. *N Engl J Med* 1998;338:1273–1278.
6. Parkinson DR, Sznol M. High-dose interleukin-2 in the therapy of metastatic renal cell carcinoma. *Semin Oncol* 1995;22:61–66.

7. Motzer RJ, Mazumdor M, Bacik J, et al. Effect of cytokine therapy on survival for patients with advanced renal cell carcinoma. *J Clin Oncol* 2000;18:1928–1935.
8. Fyfe G, Fisher RI, Rosenberg SA, et al. Results of treatment of 255 patients with metastatic renal cell carcinoma who received high-dose recombinant interleukin-2 therapy. *J Clin Oncol* 1995;13: 688–696.
9. Yang JC, Topalian SL, Parkinson D, et al. Randomized comparison of high-dose and low-dose intravenous interleukin-2 for the therapy of metastatic renal cell carcinoma: an interim report. *J Clin Oncol* 1998;12:1572–1576.
10. Sleijfer DT, Janssen RAJ, Buter J, et al. Phase II study of subcutaneous interleukin-2 in unselected patients with advanced renal cell cancer on an outpatient basis. *J Clin Oncol* 1992;10:1119–1123.
11. Horoszewicz JS, Murphy GP. An assessment of the current use of human interferons in therapy of urological cancers. *J Urol* 1989;142:1173–1180.
12. NCI-PDQ Web-Page at http://cancernet.nci.nih.gov/clinp_a/Renal_cell_cancer_Physician.html
13. Atzopodiem J, Kirchner H, Hannien EL, et al. European studies of interleukin-2 in metastatic renal cell carcinoma. *Semin Oncol* 1993;20:23.
14. Rini BI, Vogelzang NJ, Dumas MC, et al. Phase II trial of weekly intravenous gemcitabine with continuous fluoroucil in patients with metastatic renal cell cancer. *J Clin Oncol* 2000;18:2419–2426.
15. Chow WH, Devesa SS, Warren JL, et al. Rising incidence of renal cell cancer in the United States. *JAMA* 1999;281:1628–1631.
16. Javidan J, Stricker HJ, Tamboli P, et al. Prognastic significance of the 1997 TNM classification of renal cell carcinoma. *J Urol* 1999;162:1277–1281.

13

Prostate Cancer

Kevin Knopf and William Dahut

Medicine Branch, DCS, National Cancer Institute, National Institutes of Health, Bethesda, Maryland

EPIDEMIOLOGY

Prostate cancer (CaP) is the most common noncutaneous malignancy in American men, and the second greatest cause of cancer-related mortality (1,2). Risk increases progressively with age, and the median age at diagnosis is 72 years, although there is no "peak" age. Black men have a lower age at diagnosis than do white men.

Incidence rates peaked in 1992/1993 after widespread screening and have been declining since then. Mortality rates have increased over the past 20 years but have declined in recent years. Incidence and mortality rates are higher in blacks than in whites.

Frequency of clinically aggressive disease varies by geography, although frequency of occult tumors does not; this suggests a role of environmental factors in the etiology of CaP. Studies of Japanese immigrants to the United States show that incidence increases after migration.

RISK FACTORS FOR PROSTATE CANCER

- Age (incidence increases with age).
- Family history (risk increased 2 times with a first-degree relative).
- Race (in the U.S.: black > white > Asian).
- Geographic location (lowest in Asia, high in Scandinavia and U.S.).
- Dietary fat: putative but not definitive.

SCREENING

Screening for prostate cancer is performed with prostate specific antigen (PSA) and/or digital rectal examination (DRE). There is much debate with regard to screening asymptomatic men for prostate cancer; this debate centers on whether biologically and clinically significant cancers are actually being detected at an early enough stage to reduce mortality. Screening is associated with high false-positive rates. Autopsy series have shown approximately a 50% rate of occult prostate cancer in men in their 80s, and more men die with, rather than of, prostate cancer. Many of the cancers detected by PSA have already metastasized at the time of diagnosis, and many of the tumors detected are indolent and probably would not have affected the patient's life expectancy. In addition, treatment is associated with significant morbidity, and no randomized controlled trial has convincingly shown a decrease in mortality from screening.

Incidence greatly exceeds mortality, and the fact that mortality does not vary between geographic regions with different incidence or screening patterns argues against the benefits of screening.

Despite the controversy, use of PSA for CaP screening is widespread in the U.S. Advocates of screening recommend commencement of annual screening for average-risk men at 50 years and for African-Americans and men with a family history of CaP at age 40 years.

CHEMOPREVENTION

Chemoprevention trials examining treatment of asymptomatic men with compounds that may be capable of preventing CaP are under way. The Prostate Cancer Prevention Trial is a large-scale study examining finasteride, a 5-α reductase inhibitor, versus placebo in the prevention of CaP in men older than 50 years.

A large-scale 2×2 factorial study compared dietary supplementation with vitamin E and/or β-carotene and/or placebo in male Finnish smokers, with a 2×2 factorial design. Although the Finnish trial showed an increase in lung cancer in the β-carotene arm, a secondary analysis showed that there were fewer prostate cancers in those men who received vitamin E. Another separate, multiinstitutional trial tested supplementation with selenium versus placebo to prevent skin cancer. In a secondary analysis, men who received selenium experienced only 33% as many prostate cancers as did men who received placebo, a statistically significant difference. A retrospective study of selenium levels in men with and without CaP also showed a protective effect in men with the highest amount of selenium.

These interesting retrospective data led to the development of a prospective placebo-controlled, 2×2 factorial study to examine selenium and vitamin E in the prevention of CaP.

PATHOLOGY

Of prostate cancers, 95% are adenocarcinomas; rarely other histologies (sarcoma, lymphoma, small cell carcinoma, transitional carcinoma) are found. Although visceral metastases or osteolytic bone metastases are found in a minority of patients with metastatic adenocarcinoma of the prostate, a careful examination of pathology should be performed to determine if a nonadenocarcinoma variant is present in this setting, as treatment regimens are different for these other histologies.

Adenocarcinoma typically arises in the peripheral zone of the prostate (approximately 70%).

The Gleason Score (GS) (Table 1) is obtained by examining the histologic architecture of the biopsy. Two ratings are given for the two most predominant areas of cancer on a scale from 1 to 5 (most to least differentiated) in the form X + Y. For example, a GS score of 5+4 is a total score of 9, whereas a GS of 3+3 is a total score of 6. Total GS of 2 to 4, 5 to 6, 7, and 8 to 10 represent well-, moderately, moderately poorly, and poorly differentiated tumors, respectively. However, there is a growing belief that the highest, most predominant score is most predictive of clinical outcome.

There is often a change in GS at the time of radical prostatectomy, with 20% of men being upgraded to a higher score.

TABLE 1. *Risk of metastatic disease*

Gleason score	Risk of developing metastatic disease
2–4	20%
5–7	40%
8–10	75%

SIGNS AND SYMPTOMS

Men with local or regional disease can be asymptomatic or have symptoms similar to benign prostatic hypertrophy (BPH) (i.e., symptoms of urinary outflow obstruction). Occasionally men with regional disease have hematuria. The presence of metastatic disease can be seen as bone pain or weight loss, rarely with symptoms of spinal cord compression. With the advent of widespread screening by PSA, the vast majority of men are asymptomatic at the time of diagnosis.

WORKUP AND STAGING

CaP is usually detected by an abnormal PSA and/or DRE followed by a transrectal ultrasound with core biopsy (sextant, three from each side of the prostate). Biopsy is typically obtained for a PSA >4, although available normograms suggest a higher threshold in older men (with BPH) and a lower threshold in younger men or African-Americans. A negative biopsy should prompt reassessment in 6 months with PSA/DRE and repeated biopsy as needed.

Age enters into the decision-making process; older men with major comorbid illnesses and limited life expectancy are less likely to benefit from definitive treatment than are younger, otherwise healthy men. For men with a life expectancy of less than 5 years who are asymptomatic in whom CaP is detected, one option is deferral of further workup and treatment until symptoms present; however, many patients prefer a more aggressive course.

For men in whom treatment is planned, a bone scan is indicated for symptomatic bone pain, T3/T4, GS >7, or PSA >10 ng/mL; otherwise the positive yield is very low. Obtaining a "baseline" bone scan in other patients has not been shown by clinical evidence to improve survival.

TABLE 2. *Staging of prostate cancer: TNM system*

T1	Tumor not palpable or visible by imaging			
T1a	Tumor incidental finding in ≤5% of tissue resected (TURP)			
T1b	Tumor incidental finding in >5% of tissue resected (TURP)			
T1c	Tumor identified by needle biopsy alone (after PSA found to be elevated)			
T2	Tumor confined to the prostate			
T2a	Tumor involves one lobe			
T2b	Tumor involves both lobes			
T3	Tumor extends through the prostatic capsule			
T3a	Extracapsular extension (unilateral or bilateral)			
T3b	Tumor invades the seminal vesicle(s)			
T4	Tumor is fixed or invades adjacent structures other than seminal vesicles: bladder neck, external sphincter, rectum, levator muscles, and/or pelvic wall			
N0	No regional lymph node metastasis			
N1	Metastases in regional lymph node(s)			
M0	No distant metastases			
M1	Distant metastases (M1a, nonregional LN; M1b, bone(s); M1c, other).			
Stage grouping				
I	T1a	N0	M0	Any GS
II	T1a	N0	M0	GS 2,3, or 4
	T1b,c	N0	M0	Any GS
	T1/2	N0	M0	Any GS
III	T3	N0	M0	Any GS
IV	T4	N0	M0	Any GS
	Any T	N1	M0	Any GS
	Any T	Any N	M1	Any GS

TURP, transurethral resection of the prostate; PSA, prostate specific antigen.

TABLE 3. *Modified Jewett system*	
A:	Clinically undetectable tumor confined to the prostate gland/incidental at prostate surgery
A1:	Well differentiated, focal involvement
A2:	Moderately or poorly differentiated, involves multiple foci of the gland
B:	Tumor confined to the prostate gland
B0:	Nonpalpable, PSA detected
B1:	Single nodule in one lobe of the prostate
B2:	More extensive involvement of one lobe or both lobes
C:	Tumor localized to the periprostatic area but extending through the prostatic capsule or involving the seminal vesicles
C1:	Clinical extracapsular extension
C2:	Extracapsular tumor producing bladder outlet or ureteral obstruction
D:	Metastatic disease
D0:	Clinically localized disease with persistently elevated acid phosphatase
D1:	Regional lymph nodes only
D2:	Distant lymph nodes, metastases to bone or visceral organs
D3:	D2 patients who relapse after adequate endocrine therapy

Computed tomography (CT) or magnetic resonance imaging (MRI) is obtained for T3, T4 lesions to detect the presence of enlarged lymph nodes for men in whom surgery is considered. If lymph nodes appear enlarged, a fine-needle aspiration (FNA) can be performed, potentially sparing surgery. CT scans are often needed for treatment planning for radiation therapy, especially 3-D conformational approaches.

Baseline laboratory tests include complete blood count (CBC), creatinine, PSA (if not yet done), and alkaline phosphatase, and preoperative studies if surgery is being considered (Tables 2 and 3).

PROGNOSTIC FACTORS AT THE TIME OF DIAGNOSIS

- Stage.
- Grade (Gleason score).
- PSA level.
- DNA ploidy in stage C/D1 patients: diploid is better.
- Age.
- Serum acid phosphatase level.

TREATMENT

Surgery

Radical prostatectomy (RP) is performed via the perineal or retropubic approach. Pelvic lymph node dissection may be performed at the time of RP, although it may not be necessary in patients with T1c disease whose PSA is less than 10 and GS is less than 7, in which the results will alter therapeutic decision less than 1% of the time. For patients at high risk of having positive lymph nodes, pelvic laparoscopic lymph node dissection can be performed initially.

Formula for predicting percentage chance of positive pelvic lymph nodes:

$$\% \text{ Positive pelvic LN} = 2/3 \times PSA + (GS-6) \times 10 \ (1)$$

Nerve-Sparing Surgery

This procedure is appropriate for men with small-volume disease in an attempt to spare potency. However, much higher impotence rates after nerve-sparing RP have been reported in the community than in the original reports from certain tertiary referral centers. Talcott et al. (3) reported data on 94 patients who underwent RP and were queried before surgery and for up to 12 months afterward. At 12 months after surgery, 79% of the men who had bilateral nerve-sparing surgery reported erections inadequate for sexual intercourse, compared with 33% before surgery. No benefit in potency was provided by unilateral nerve-sparing surgery. These numbers are significantly lower than those published previously in several retrospective studies. Studies have shown that a younger age at diagnosis and the absence of capsular penetration or seminal vesicle invasion correlate with a greater likelihood of potency after surgery.

Incontinence rates vary from single-institution experiences, and various definitions of incontinence make interpretation of studies difficult. In one prospective study evaluating urinary control at 3, 12, and 24 months after RP, it was reported that 58%, 35%, and 42% of patients, respectively, wore pads in their underwear, and 24%, 11%, and 15% of patients, respectively, reported "a lot" of urine leakage or worse symptoms.

Much work is ongoing in evaluating quality of life in CaP treated with surgery, radiation therapy, and hormones. The Prostate Cancer Outcomes Study, with a community sample of more than 3,000 men from the SEER sites, is evaluating patterns of care and quality of life; the latter uses an instrument that includes many specific questions about urinary, sexual, and rectal functioning.

Neoadjuvant Therapy

The role of neoadjuvant hormonal therapy before RP is still under investigation. A recent randomized trial comparing neoadjuvant treatment with 3 versus 8 months (leuprolide plus flutamide) for clinically confined CaP was reported (4). The proportion of men with negative margins and organ-confined disease was significantly higher in the group receiving 8 months of neoadjuvant hormonal therapy, suggesting that 3 months is not the optimal duration. It is too early in this study to determine survival.

Extracapsular extension or positive margins in the surgical specimen portends a high incidence of disease recurrence, and such patients can be considered for clinical trials involving postoperative radiation, chemotherapy, or hormonal treatment.

After surgery a detectable PSA indicates a relapse, either local or systemic, although PSA increase may be slow and not necessarily indicate immediate treatment. In a study of nearly 2,000 men whose PSA was measured every 3 months after surgery, the median time for the development of metastases after an elevated PSA was detected (>0.2 ng/mL) was 8 years. PSA doubling time, Gleason score, and time from surgery to biochemical failure were predictive of time to metastases after an elevated PSA (5).

Surgical Complications

Complications include immediate morbidity/mortality (2%) from surgery, impotence (35% to 60%), urinary incontinence (>30%), urinary stricture, fecal incontinence (approximately 10% to 20%).

Radiation Therapy

External Beam

The traditional four-field box arrangement is used, with approximately 70 Gy given over 7 to 8 weeks. Prophylactic radiation of pelvic LNs has not been shown to improve survival.

Ten-year cause-specific survival rates with RT:

- T1, 79%.
- T2, 66%.
- T3, 55%.
- T4, 22%.

Adjuvant Treatment with GnRH agonists and RT

Adjuvant treatment with a gonadotropin-releasing hormone (GnRH) agonist starting 1 month before radiotherapy and continuing for 3 years has been shown to improve overall survival at 5 years in patients with "high risk" locally advanced tumors. An RTOG study (85-31) (6) randomized men with clinical stage T3 CaP, or patients with stages T1 or T2 if there was evidence of spread to regional lymph nodes, to RT with goserelin administered during the last week of radiotherapy (3.6 mg subcutaneously q month) continuing indefinitely or at the time of progression versus goserelin given at the time of relapse. A statistically significant survival advantage in the group given adjuvant hormonal treatment was found for patients with GS of 8 to 10, with an absolute survival difference of 11%. However, all patients achieved a higher relapse-free and disease-free survival.

A European study (7) examined the same question, although they included patients with stage T1 and T2 high-grade histologies, and T3/T4 without lymph node or metastatic involvement. This trial randomized patients to RT alone, with an option of goserelin on relapse, versus RT with goserelin started on day 1 of RT (3.6 mg subcutaneously q month) and continuing for 3 years. This study again found a statistically significant improvement in overall survival at 5 years in favor of the group receiving RT + immediate goserelin (79% vs. 62%). The percentage of patients with stage T1/T2 tumors was less than 20%, and randomization was stratified by stage. The groups were well balanced by initial PSA. However, 19% of patients receiving goserelin reported adverse reactions, and 4% stopped goserelin before 3 years because of toxicity. A major criticism of this study has been that the decision to start hormonal therapy was left up to the individual practitioner in the arm that received RT alone as initial treatment, and thus may have been delayed compared with patterns of care in the U.S.

Investigations are being initiated to test the addition of adjuvant chemotherapy in this setting.

3-D Conformational/High-dose Radiation Therapy

With careful treatment planning using 3-D conformational techniques, higher doses of radiation (up to 80 Gy over 7–8 weeks) can be delivered to the prostate while sparing normal tissue. This approach appears promising in that it may offer higher dosages to the tumor and thus greater efficacy and less toxicity to the surrounding structures.

Brachytherapy

Interstitial brachytherapy with radioactive palladium or iodine (I 125) seeds has been used for patients with T1/T2 tumors. Initially this approach required retropubic implantation (which required laparotomy), but within the last 10 years, CT and/or transrectal ultrasound have been used to guide seed placement, and the procedure is performed on an outpatient basis. Better definition of tumor volume and radiation dosimetry have made this technique more accurate. Initial results have been very promising, but no randomized trials have compared brachytherapy with external beam RT, 3D RT, or surgery.

External Beam and Brachytherapy

The use of combined external beam and brachytherapy has come into increasing use (8,9). A 10-year review of experience with this combination showed a biochemical (i.e., normal

PSA) relapse-free survival of 79% in T3 tumors, suggesting a strong role for the combination in these lesions (10). However, there are no randomized trials comparing this combination with external beam or brachytherapy alone, and thus this treatment approach remains investigational at this point.

Complications of RT

- Acute (during treatment): cystitis, proctitis, enteritis, fatigue.
- Long term: impotence (less than with RP), incontinence (7%), frequent bowel movements (10%, more than with RP), urethral stricture [delay RT by 4 weeks after transurethral resection of the prostate (TURP)].

Cryosurgery

Cryosurgery involves destruction of prostate cancer cells through probes that subject the prostate tissue to freezing followed by thawing. Some believe that cryosurgery is a good option for men with high-grade tumors (Gleason 8 to 10), high PSA levels (20 to 40 ng/mL), or stage C tumors, who potentially do not respond well to RT or surgery. This technique is still early in development, and long-term efficacy is not fully established. Side effects include incontinence, impotence, and injury to the bladder outlet and rectal tissues.

Observation

In several European countries, observation of patients with prostate cancer, particularly of low stage/low or moderate grade, is commonplace. Particularly with elderly patients, survival equivalent to aggressive treatment has been reported.

Hormonal Therapy

Hormonal therapy is used most commonly for metastatic prostate cancer, although it has been used in treatment of localized disease and also in the neoadjuvant, and adjuvant, settings with RT.

Androgen blockade is achieved through bilateral surgical castration or depot injections of GnRH agonists (leuprolide, goserelin, buserelin), which offer equivalent efficacy. Maximal androgen blockade can be achieved by adding an oral antiandrogenic agent (nilutamide, flutamide, bicalutamide); however, this is controversial, and if a benefit exists, it is small.

Tumor flare is possible with the use of GnRH agonists, which initially cause an increase in luteinizing hormone (LH) and follicle-stimulating hormone (FSH) before decreasing these levels to a therapeutic value. Because the prostate cancer cells are androgen sensitive, this increase in testosterone-inducing hormones can exacerbate symptoms of prostate cancer and elevate PSA. Tumor flare can be prevented by the use of oral antiandrogens, which compete with androgens at the androgen-receptor site, at low dose for several weeks before beginning therapy. There is a reduced risk of tumor flare with a lower volume of disease. The use of estrogen [as diethylstilbestrol (DES)] has fallen into disfavor because of its side-effect profile. Therapeutic doses were shown to induce a high frequency of cardiovascular complications and mortality in a population predisposed to cardiovascular disease. DES is no longer available in the U.S.

Intermittent androgen ablation (IAA) is a newer approach to treating patients with hormone-sensitive prostate cancer. This is treatment with hormonal therapy for 2 to 3 months beyond the "best response" followed by a discontinuation of hormonal therapy, restarting the hormones at some predetermined point (e.g., a PSA value). IAA has the potential advantage of improved quality of life during the time the patient is not receiving hormonal therapy. It is unknown, however, what effect these manipulations have on the time that a tumor remains hormonally sensitive. A large randomized trial by SWOG is under way to evaluate this.

The rationale for continued androgen blockade, antiandrogen withdrawal, and additional hormonal therapy (e.g., ketoconazole and aminoglutethimide) are discussed later under second-line hormonal therapy.

Dosages and Side Effects of Hormonal Therapy

- **Bilateral orchiectomy.**
  Side effects: tumor flare (see later), impotence, loss of libido, gynecomastia, hot flashes, osteoporosis.
- **GnRH agonists.**
  1. Goserelin acetate (Zoladex), 3.6 mg s.c. every month;
     Side effects: same as with orchiectomy.
  2. Leuprolide acetate (Lupron), 7.5 mg s.c. every month or 22.5 mg s.c. every 3 months, or 30 mg s.c. every 4 months. Comparable efficacy with long-acting formulations.
     Side effects: same as with orchiectomy.
- **Oral antiandrogens.**
  1. Flutamide (Eulexin), 250 mg p.o. t.i.d.
     Side effects: diarrhea, nausea, breast tenderness, hepatotoxicity [liver function tests (LFTs) must be monitored], loss of libido, impotence.
  2. Bicalutamide (Casodex), 50 mg daily.
     Side effects: nausea, breast tenderness, hepatotoxicity
     (LFTs must be monitored), hot flashes, loss of libido, impotence.
  3. Nilutamide (Nilandron), 150 mg p.o. daily.
     Side effects: pulmonary fibrosis (rare), visual field changes (i.e., night blindness/abnormal adaptation to darkness), hepatotoxicity (LFTs must be monitored), impotence, loss of libido, hot flashes, nausea.

Hot flashes from hormonal therapy can be treated with clonidine (0.1 mg/day), low-dose estrogens, or possibly antidepressants. Painful gynecomastia can be treated with external beam radiation therapy to the breasts.

Osteoporosis is an increasingly noted side effect of orchiectomy or therapy with GnRH agonists (11) because of the lack of the beneficial effects of androgens on bone density. This side effect is most likely to occur with long duration of hormone therapy use and in men who had baseline osteoporosis before starting antiandrogen therapy. Bone densitometry can be performed to assess presence and/or severity of osteoporosis. Treatment that does not interfere with the benefits of antiandrogen is occasionally used (e.g., oral bisphosphonates).

COMPARISON OF PRIMARY TREATMENT MODALITIES

Comparison of treatment modalities with respect to primary outcomes (overall survival, disease-free survival) is difficult because of variability in study design, patient selection, and technique of each therapy.

No satisfactory randomized trials comparing RT with RP have been conducted. The major study conducted by the Veterans Affairs group is considered to have many flaws, including higher-staged patients in the radiation arm. Another multiinstitutional randomized trial failed to accrue a sufficient number of patients, and it is unlikely that another randomized trial will be done in the U.S. at this time.

In general, comparing single-modality studies is difficult because of disparities in treatment groups; men receiving RT tend to be older and to have more comorbid illnesses. A major problem is that men receiving RT will have had clinical staging of their cancer only, whereas many patients receiving surgery will have had pathologic staging that upstages their tumor, including the discovery of positive pelvic lymph nodes (metastatic disease). One way to compare the two modalities is by PSA and PSA-free survival (also called biochemical relapse-free survival), provided that the patients have reproducible PSA values on repeated measurement before their definitive, primary therapy.

In the "PSA era," RT and RP appear to have equivalent survival in appropriately matched patients at 5 years, but differ in side effect type and frequency.

Brachytherapy appears to be promising, although most studies have been conducted in patients with early-stage, low-grade disease only, who are thought to be the most appropriate men for this treatment modality. One comparison of 3-D conformational RT with ^{125}I implants in comparable patients concluded equivalent efficacy, with some higher urinary complications in the brachytherapy group.

Continuing research in quality of life may allow more informed choices among the various treatment modalities.

INITIAL TREATMENT, BY STAGE

Treatment decisions should be made with regard to the patient's age and comorbid conditions (i.e., life expectancy) and preferences, as well as tumor-related factors (stage, grade, PSA). Enrollment in clinical trials is appropriate at each stage of disease.

T1a

Observation is often appropriate for elderly patients with low-grade disease. Consider definitive treatment for high PSA/GS if life expectancy is long with (a) RT (external beam, 3-D, brachytherapy) and (b) RP.

Localized Disease (T1b through T2c)

Two factors in particular are important in deciding whether to treat. These are (a) the probability of having organ-confined disease: normograms are available based on PSA and GS[12], and (b) the patient's overall life expectancy. Observation can be considered in selected patients.

For a long life expectancy and a reasonable chance of having organ-defined disease, RT (including 3-D/high dose or brachytherapy) or RP remains the standard of care. Surgery is usually reserved for patients younger than 70 years. For a short life expectancy, RT (external beam, 3-D, brachytherapy), hormonal therapy, or deferring treatment until the presentation of symptoms is recommended.

Patients in whom surgery would pose a great risk (e.g., cardiovascular or pulmonary disease) should have RT (external beam, 3-D, brachytherapy). Otherwise, patient preference should play a major role in deciding primary treatment choice, after informed discussions have occurred.

Certain patients should be considered for neoadjuvant hormonal therapy in combination with RT (see earlier discussion). The role of neoadjuvant hormonal therapy in surgical patients remains investigational (see earlier).

If pelvic lymph nodes are found to be grossly positive at the time of surgery, prostatectomy should not be performed. A recently presented randomized trial (13) compared men with T1 or T2 lesions and microscopically positive lymph nodes. Men were randomized to immediate hormonal therapy (orchiectomy or goserelin) versus observation (with hormonal therapy started at the time of metastases or symptomatic local recurrences). Prostate cancer–specific mortality rate was 4.3% in the arm receiving immediate hormonal therapy versus 30.8% in the observation arm ($p < 0.01$). In the immediate hormonal therapy arm, 18.8% of men recurred by any parameter versus 75% in the observation arm ($p < 0.001$).

If the tumor is found to have extracapsular extension on the pathologic specimen, consideration can be given to enrolling in clinical trials using adjuvant radiation therapy, hormonal therapy, or a combination of the two. As yet these strategies have unproven mortality benefits.

There are insufficient data to claim a mortality benefit for surgery versus radiation as a primary treatment modality.

Stage III (T3, N0, M0)

RP can be considered for well-differentiated tumors. Other patients should probably receive RT (external beam) with or without neoadjuvant hormonal therapy. Hormonal therapy alone (surgical castration or GnRH agonist) is another option.

Some patients are treated with brachytherapy followed by external beam RT, but results are preliminary at this point.

T3b, T3c, T4N0

These patients are unlikely to have a significant chance of cure by surgery. Viable treatment options include hormonal therapy, RT alone, or RT with hormonal therapy. With node-positive disease, patients are considered metastatic at the time of diagnosis, and local therapy should be used primarily for symptom management. Observation is a viable option for this group of patients, given the side effects of hormonal therapy and RT and their primarily palliative role.

N+ or M1

There are no firm data that RT or RP improves survival in patients who are node positive. Hormonal therapy remains the standard of care. Surgical castration or medical orchiectomy with GnRH agonists offer equivalent efficacy. There is no proven survival benefit in comparing maximal androgen blockade (surgical castration + oral antiandrogen) with surgical castration alone. A randomized study of leuprolide with or without flutamide alone showed a slight survival advantage (14); however, a similar study design that used orchiectomy in lieu of GnRH agonists showed equivalent survival (15). In the trial with orchiectomy + flutamide versus flutamide alone, quality of life was shown to be reduced in the group receiving antiandrogen therapy in addition to castration (16). The reason for the discrepancy between these two trials is not completely known. A meta-analysis found an overall survival advantage for combined blockade at 5, but not 2, years; however, the magnitude of the difference is of questionable clinical significance (17).

Another area of controversy is the use of delayed or immediate hormonal therapy in patients who are initially metastatic or whose tumors later recur. The Medical Research Council Trial (18) randomized patients with locally advanced or asymptomatic metastatic CaP to immediate versus deferred orchiectomy/GnRH agonist. They showed a significant difference in deaths of prostate cancer, especially in M0 patients. However, this study has often been criticized. In the comprehensive, evidence-based review conducted by the Agency for Health Care Policy and Research (AHCPR), they concluded that there is no evidence favoring immediate compared with deferred androgen suppression; however, many practitioners tend toward treating earlier, and newer evidence is beginning to mount favoring early antiandrogen therapy. Again, quality-of-life issues should play a role in decision analysis.

ADJUVANT TREATMENT AFTER RP WITH POSITIVE MARGINS OR LOCAL RELAPSE

The use of RT after RP for patients with margin-positive disease has been used, either soon after surgery or delayed until PSA progression occurs. For men with T3 lesions who have PSA progression and a negative metastatic workup, the use of RT has shown a return of PSA to normal in at least 50% of men. No long-term follow-up suggests a survival advantage, because of the newness of this approach. A combination of RT and hormonal therapy after local relapse is also being examined. Additionally, some patients with a negative metastatic workup and local recurrence after RT can be considered for salvage surgery; the evidence for this is even less well defined.

FOLLOW-UP OF DEFINITIVELY TREATED PATIENTS

Patients treated with curative intent should have PSA ascertained at least every 6 months for 5 years and then annually. Annual DRE is appropriate to detect annual recurrences.

After treatment with RP, any reproducible, detectable PSA indicates a relapse. PSA failure after RT is defined as three consecutive PSA increases. Treatment of patients who relapse after radiation is not standardized; participation in clinical trials should be encouraged. Hormonal treatment and salvage surgery (if a metastatic workup is negative and patient is in good health) are options.

For patients with a short life expectancy treated with observation alone, some would consider surveillance and PSA measurement as optional. Treatment should be guided by symptoms. For patients with a longer life expectancy, annual DRE and PSA are appropriate measures of disease progression if watchful waiting is selected as the primary treatment.

For patients with metastatic disease, intensity and type of follow-up is determined by the degree of clinical progression; for patients responding well to hormonal therapy, follow-up at 3 months (with PSA) is reasonable. Bone scans are ordered depending on clinical symptoms, but should not be routinely ordered. Patients with bony metastases are at risk for spinal cord compression, and MRI should be ordered when signs or symptoms are suggestive of this complication, because early identification and treatment are vital.

It is important to note that there is interlaboratory variation in PSA levels.

RESPONSE CRITERION IN PROSTATE CANCER

Response rates (RRs) in this chapter are shown as percentage of patients with a PSA decline greater than 50%, which is a generally agreed-on criterion (19). Ranges of RRs are given when available. Confidence intervals are not shown around the RR, but in most trials, they were fairly wide. Because of differences in patient selection, it is difficult to compare clinical trials by RRs alone. Quality of life is an extremely important consideration in treating patients with prostate cancer, and may be a primary consideration in the choice of chemotherapy agents for metastatic AIPC. An important caveat, however, is that some agents (particularly cytostatic agents) may upregulate or downregulate PSA expression independent of their effect on cell growth.

HORMONAL THERAPY FOR METASTATIC DISEASE

Metastatic prostate cancer tends to present at the spine/axial skeleton. Visceral metastases are uncommon, and brain metastases are even rarer.

Prostate cancer cells usually respond to hormonal manipulations that block the production of androgen (20), with durable remissions and significant palliation. Duration of response ranges from 12 to 18 months, with 20% of patients having a complete biochemical response at 5 years. However, ultimately androgen-independent CaP cells emerge and lead to progression of disease.

The use of maximal androgen blockade is not currently considered standard of care in the initial treatment of metastatic disease. For patients who progress on GnRH agonists or surgical castration, the addition of an antiandrogen agent may result in responses in up to 10% of men.

Antiandrogen Withdrawal

Once GnRH agonists are started, they should be continued for life. It has been shown that metastatic CaP can reactivate if testosterone levels are allowed to increase or exogenous testosterone is administered, and anecdotal evidence has shown a worsening of disease in patients who have had discontinuation of GnRH agonists. However, for patients progressing on maximal androgen blockade, discontinuation of the oral antiandrogen has resulted in responses in up to 20% of patients (range, 15–33% RR), although they are relatively short-lived (median duration, 3–5 months). Decreased cancer-related anemia and decreased pain were also reported. Antiandrogen withdrawal response occurs within 4 to 6 weeks, depending on the half-life of the agent.

Second-line Hormonal Therapy

Even after androgen withdrawal has failed, some patients will benefit from switching classes of antiandrogens or initiating treatment with aminoglutethimide, ketoconazole, or glucocorticoids. One month should be allowed to assess for a response.

Bicalutamide at 200 mg can be used in patients who have not received it before; this agent exhibits a dose response, and thus the rationale for the higher dose (RR = 23%). Similarly, flutamide can be given in patients who previously received bicalutamide. A minority of patients will respond, and responses are usually not long in duration, but these agents offer much less toxicity than chemotherapy.

Adrenal Androgen Inhibitors

Adrenal androgen inhibitors work by achieving a "medical adrenalectomy," which further decreases androgen production. Responses have been seen in patients after antiandrogen withdrawal. It is important to use steroid replacements in patients receiving adrenal androgen inhibitors; often this is started at 20 mg qa.m. and 10 mg qp.m., but is increased to 20 mg p.o. b.i.d if patients show symptoms of glucocorticoid insufficiency (e.g., fatigue).

Adrenal Androgen Inhibitors: Regimens and Toxicities

Aminoglutethimide + hydrocortisone (21,22) (RR = 49%).
- Aminoglutethimide (Cytadren), 125 p.o. q.i.d., increasing to 250 mg q.i.d. + hydrocortisone, 20 mg p.o. b.i.d.
- Side effects: sedation, skin rashes, fever
- Rarer side effects: ataxia, hypothyroidism, abnormal LFTs, peripheral edema
Ketoconazole + hydrocortisone (RR = 78–80%) (21).
- Ketaconazole (Nizoral), 200 mg p.o. t.i.d., increasing to 400 mg p.o. t.i.d. + hydrocortisone, 20 mg p.o. b.i.d.
- Side effects: impotence, pruritis, nail changes, adrenal insufficiency, nausea, emesis, hepatotoxicity. LFTs need to be monitored. (Ketoconazole is absorbed at an acidic pH; therefore the concomitant use of H_2 blockers, antacids, or omeprazole should be avoided.)

Corticosteroids (RR = 18–22%)
- Corticosteroids (23) alone have been shown to improve pain in patients with symptomatic bone metastases.
- Prednisone, 5 mg p.o. qa.m. and 2.5 mg p.o. qp.m., increasing to 5 mg p.o. b.i.d. Side effects as for any medical use of Prednisone.

CHEMOTHERAPY FOR ANDROGEN-INDEPENDENT PROSTATE CANCER

Patients have a median survival of 6 to 9 months after developing androgen-independent prostate cancer. Chemotherapy has not been shown to prolong survival, although it has achieved palliation in androgen-independent prostate cancer patients (20). Participation in clinical trials of novel agents or combinations should be encouraged. Antiangiogenic agents in particular are undergoing studies in AIPC, and there is growing accrual to trials of immunotherapy/tumor vaccines.

Estramustine phosphate (EMP, Emcyte) is a compound that combines estradiol and nitrogen mustard. It works by binding to microtubule-associated proteins. Many phase II trials of single-agent estramustine have been conducted. However, there appears to be synergy when estramustine is combined with other agents that have activity against the microtubule proteins (e.g., vinblastine, the taxanes), and thus estramustine is usually given in combination.

Estramustine (Emcyte)/vinblastine (24) (RR = 31–50%).
- 4 mg/m^2 vinblastine i.v. per week for 6 weeks, with 2 weeks off + 600 mg/m^2 estramustine p.o. daily for 7 weeks with 1 week off.
- Side effects: nausea (40%), granulocytopenia (10%), grade II nausea (26%), extremity edema (22%).

Estramustine (Emcyte)/paclitaxel (Taxol) (25) (RR = 65%).
- Estramustine, 600 mg/m^2 p.o. qD beginning on D1, 24 hours before paclitaxel + paclitaxel, 120 mg/m^2 over 96 hours starting D2. Premeds for paclitaxel: cimetidine, 300 mg, and diphenhydramine, 60 mg, 30 min before starting paclitaxel.
- Cycle is repeated every 21 days for patients without progressive disease or unacceptable toxicity.
- Side effects: leukopenia (38%), thrombocytopenia (13%), anemia (54%), nausea (50%), edema (38%), increase in LFTs (approximately 30%), diarrhea (29%), and fatigue (33%).

Estramustine (Emcyte)/docetaxel (Taxotere) (26) (RR = 62%).
- Estramustine, 280 mg p.o. t.i.d., administered 1 hour before or 2 hours after meals, D1-5 +
  1. Minimally pretreated patients: docetaxel, 70 mg/m^2 i.v. D2.
  2. Extensively pretreated patients: docetaxel, 60 mg/m^2 D2.
- Cycle repeated every 21 days.
  1. Minimally pretreated: Two or fewer prior chemotherapy treatments, two or fewer prior RT treatments, no history of radioisotope therapy, no history of whole pelvic RT, no evidence of "superscan" on bone scan.
  2. Extensively pretreated: all other patients.
- Side effects: granulocytopenia (68%), neutropenic fevers (3%), thrombocytopenia (24%), elevated LFTs (approximately 47%), esophagitis (3%), edema (65%), hypocalcemia (59%), alopecia (18%), nausea (29%), vomiting (12%).
- Estramustine (Emcyte)/etoposide (VP-16R) (27) (RR = 52%).
- This regimen has the advantage of being completely p.o.

Estramustine, 15/mg/kg/day p.o. q.i.d., days 1–21.
- VP-16, 50 mg/m^2/day p.o. b.i.d., D 1–21.
- Repeat cycle on D28, if no progressive disease and AGC more than 1,000/μL and Plts more than 50,00/μL.
- VP-16R was lowered by 25% for AGC less than 1,000/μL or Plts less than 100,000/μL (i.e., 50 mg/m^2/day, alternating with 25 mg/m^2/day).
- Side effects: alopecia (100%), leukopenia (57%), anemia (55%), edema (48%), thrombocytopenia (36%), fatigue (31%), nausea (29%), diarrhea (12%); 10% or less for anorexia, stomatitis, vomiting, venous thrombosis, allergic reaction, constipation, or cardiac toxicity in one patient [congestive heart failure (CHF) and possible myocardial infarction (MI) within 3 weeks of initiating therapy]. Neutropenic fever: five episodes in 236 cycles of therapy.

Mitoxantrone (Novantrone) + Prednisone (RR = 33%) (28).
- This regimen has been shown to improve quality of life, but not DFS or OS, in an RCT versus Prednisone alone, and is a regimen in much current use.
- Prednisone, 5 mg p.o. b.i.d, D1, + mitoxantrone, 12 mg/m^2 i.v., D21; delayed if not recovered hematologically.

- Mitoxantrone was stopped at a cumulative dose of 140 mg/m². Prochlorperazine was used as an antiemetic.
- Side effects: cardiac abnormalities in 6% of patients in the mitoxantrone arm only (2% with CHF), neutropenic fever (1.1%), neutropenia (45%), thrombocytopenia (5%), nausea/vomiting (29%), alopecia (26%); exacerbation of diabetes in 1 patient.

SELECTED MANAGEMENT ISSUES

CNS metastases are relatively rare, but not unheard of, in prostate cancer. Visceral metastases occur in about 20% of patients; the majority of patients have symptoms related to bone metastases.

Bone Metastases

The use of radiation therapy to localized painful bone metastases has been shown to provide palliation. Usually the painful vertebra and the two vertebrae superior and inferior to the lesion are treated with 3,000 cGy in 10 fractions. Pain relief occurs in approximately 80% of patients; side effects generally are limited to fatigue and an anemia that is usually reversible. The tolerance of the spinal cord is approximately 5,000 cGy, so retreating areas with 2,000 cGy can sometimes be attempted, albeit with caution.

For widespread disease, hemibody irradiation has been used, as has the radioisotope strontium-89 (Metastron), a calcium analogue that preferentially localizes to tumor. Palliation of pain with strontium has been reported in up to 75% of cases, and typically occurs after 1 to 3 weeks of treatment and may continue for several months. Toxicities of strontium include the potential for flare (15%) that is often associated with a later response and a reversible thrombocytopenia in 25% of patients that is usually resolves by 3 months. Strontium can often be readministered.

Samarium-153 phosphonic acid is a newer radioisotope with treatment indications similar to those of strontium, and a shorter half-life.

Bisphosphonates, agents that inhibit osteoclastic bone resorption, are under investigation in prostate cancer, but appear very promising for pain control and preservation of bone mass.

Careful attention to pain control with narcotics and adjuncts should be maintained in patients with bone metastases.

Spinal Cord Compression

Spinal cord compression, an oncologic emergency, is not uncommon in patients with metastatic prostate cancer who have widespread bony metastases. This largely consists of vertebral column metastases impinging on the spinal cord.

More than 90% of patients have pain as an early sign; pain that is worsening is particularly worrisome. There may be pain present over the involved spine, muscle weakness, or abnormalities in the neurologic examination. Later signs, often indicative of irreversible damage, include weakness and/or sensory corresponding to the level of the spinal cord compression. Signs such as genitourinary or gastrointestinal dysfunction (e.g., urinary retention or constipation) or autonomic dysfunction are late signs, and spinal cord compression usually progresses rapidly at this point.

One should have a high index of suspicion for spinal cord compression in patients known to have osseous metastases in prostate cancer, particularly with new signs or any symptoms related to spinal cord compression. Diagnosis requires a thorough history and physical, with special attention to the musculoskeletal and neurologic examinations. The standard for diagnosing and localizing epidural cord compression is an MRI, usually with gadolinium. A myelogram is still used in patients with contraindications to MRI (e.g., a pacemaker).

Steroids should be started (dexamethasone, 100 mg i.v., followed by 4 mg i.v. or p.o., every 6 hours) as soon as history or neurologic examination suggests spinal cord compression. Radiation therapy, given as 3,000 cGy in 10 fractions to the involved vertebra and to the two superior and two inferior vertebrae, is the usual treatment modality, and early consultation with radiation oncology is warranted. Surgical resection of the vertebral body is generally used in patients who have had previous RT to the involved area, if patients require procedures for spinal stability, experience progression despite treatment with steroids and RT, or if RT facilities are not locally available. It should also be considered in patients with a rapidly progressive neurologic deficit, as the relief from RT is slower (by days) compared with a surgical decompressive procedure. Neurologic or orthopedic surgeons should be consulted early in the diagnosis of spinal cord compression as well.

REFERENCES

1. Brawley OW, Knopf K, Merrill R. The epidemiology of prostate cancer. I: Descriptive epidemiology. *Semin Urol Oncol* 1998;16:187–192.
2. Brawley OW, Knopf K, Thompson I. The epidemiology of prostate cancer. II: The risk factors. *Semin Urol Oncol* 1998;16:193–201.
3. Talcott JA, Rieker P, Propert KJ, et al. Patient reported impotence and incontinence after nerve-sparing radical prostatectomy. *J Natl Cancer Inst* 1997;88:1117–1123.
4. Gleave M, Goldenberg LS, et al. Randomized comparative study of 3 vs. 8 months of neoadjuvant hormonal therapy prior to radical prostatectomy: biochemical and pathological effects. Abstract, *1999 American Urological Association Annual Meeting.*
5. Pound CR, Partin AW, Eisenberger MA, et al. Natural history of progression after PSA elevation following radical prostatectomy. *JAMA* 1999;281:1591–1597.
6. Pilepich MV, Caplan R, Byhart RW, et al. Phase III trial of androgen suppression using goserelin in unfavorable-prognosis carcinoma of the prostate treated with definitive radiotherapy: report of Radiation Therapy Oncology Group protocol 85-31. *J Clin Oncol* 1997;15:1013–1021.
7. Bolla M, Gonzalez D, Warde P, et al. Improved survival in patients with locally advanced prostate cancer treated with radiotherapy and goserelin. *N Engl J Med* 1997;337:295–300.
8. Dattoli M, Wallner K, Sorace R, et al. [103]Pd brachytherapy and external beam irradiation for clinically localized, high-risk prostatic carcinoma. *Int J Radiat Oncol Biol Phys* 1996;35:875–879.
9. Ragde H, Elgamal AA, Snow PB, et al. Ten-year disease free survival after transperineal sonography-guided iodine-125 brachytherapy with or without 45-Gray external beam irradiation in the treatment of patients with clinically localized, low to high Gleason grade prostate carcinoma. *Cancer* 1998;83:989–1001.
10. Kovacs G, Galalae R, Loch T, et al. Prostate preservation by combined external beam and HDR brachytherapy in nodal negative prostate cancer. *Strahlenther Onckol* 1999;175S:87–88.
11. Daniell HW. Osteoporosis after orchiectomy for prostate cancer. *J Urol* 1997;157:439–444.
12. Partin AW, Kattan MW, Subong EN, et al. Combination of prostate-specific antigen, clinical stage, and Gleason score to predict pathological stage of localized prostate cancer: a multi-institutional update. *JAMA* 1997;277:1445–1451.
13. Messing E, Manola J, Sarosdy M, et al. Immediate hormonal therapy compared with observation after radical prostatectomy and pelvic lymphadenectomy in pen with node-positive prostate cancer. *N Engl J Med* 1999;341:1781–1788.
14. Crawford ED, Eisenberger MA, McLeod DG, et al. A controlled trial of leuprolide with and without flutamide in prostatic carcinoma. *N Engl J Med* 1989;321:419–424.
15. Eisenberger MA, Blumenstein BA, Crawford ED, et al. Bilateral orchiectomy with or without flutamide for metastatic prostate cancer. *N Engl J Med* 1998;339:1036–1042.
16. Moinpour CM, Savage MJ, Troxel A, et al. Quality of life in advanced prostate cancer: results of a randomized therapeutic trial. *J Natl Cancer Inst* 1998;90:1537–1544.
17. Agency for Health Care Policy and Research. *Relative effectiveness and cost-effectiveness of methods of androgen suppression in the treatment of advanced prostatic cancer* (AHCPR Publication No. 99-E012) www.ahcpr.gov
18. The Medical Research Council Prostate Cancer Working Party Investigators Group. Immediate versus deferred treatment for advanced prostatic cancer: initial results of the Medical Research Council trial. *Br J Urol* 1997;79:235–246.

19. Bubley GJ, Carducci M, Dahut W, et al. Eligibility and response guidelines for phase II clinical trials in androgen-independent prostate cancer: recommendations from the prostate-specific antigen working group. *J Clin Oncol* 1999;17:3461–3467.
20. Oh WK, Kantoff PW. Management of hormone refractory prostate cancer: current standards and future prospects. *J Urol* 1998;160:1220–1229.
21. Dawson NA. Treatment of progressive metastatic prostate cancer. *Oncology* 1993;7:17–27.
22. Sartor O, Cooper M, Weinberger M, et al. Surprising activity of flutamide withdrawal, when combined with aminoglutethimide, in treatment of "hormone-refractory" prostate cancer. *J Natl Cancer Inst* 1994;86:222–227. [Erratum appears in *J Natl Cancer Intst* in 1994;86:463].
23. Tannock I, Gospodarowicz M, Meakin W, et al. Treatment of metastatic prostatic cancer with low-dose prednisone: evaluation of pain and quality of life as pragmatic indices of response. *J Clin Oncol* 1989;7:590–597.
24. Amato RJ, Ellerhorst J, Bui C, et al. Estramustine and vinblastine for patients with progressive androgen-independent adenocarcinoma of the prostate. *Urol Oncol* 1995;1:168.
25. Hudes GR, Nathan FE, Khater C, et al. Paclitaxel plus estramustine in metastatic hormone-refractory prostate cancer. *Semin Oncol* 1995;22:41.
26. Petrylac DP, Macarthur RB, O'Connor J, et al. Phase I trial of docetaxel with estramustine in androgen-independent prostate cancer. *J Clin Oncol* 1999;17:958–967.
27. Pienta KJ, Redman B, Hussein M, et al. Phase II evaluation of oral estramustine and oral etoposide in hormone-refractory adenocarcinoma of the prostate *J Clin Oncol* 1994;12:2005.
28. Tannock IF, Osaba D, Stockler MR, et al. Chemotherapy with mitoxantrone plus prednisone or prednisone alone for symptomatic hormone-resistant prostate cancer: a Canadian randomized trial with palliative end points. *J Clin Oncol* 1996;14:1756–1764.

14

Bladder Cancer

Sattva S. Neelapu and William Dahut

*Medicine Branch, DCS, National Cancer Institute, National Institutes of Health,
Bethesda, Maryland*

EPIDEMIOLOGY

In 1999, bladder cancer had an estimated incidence of approximately 54,200 cases and was estimated to cause 12,100 deaths. Bladder cancer is the fourth leading site of cancer in men and the eighth leading site of cancer in women. Bladder cancer is 2.6 times more common in men than in women and two times more common among whites than among African-Americans. Most bladder cancers occur in patients between the ages of 50 and 80 years.

ETIOLOGY

Cigarette smoking is the single most common cause of bladder cancer in developed countries. Smokers have twice the risk of nonsmokers. Workers in dye, rubber, and leather industries also are at an increased risk for bladder cancer. The risk of transitional cell bladder cancer (TCC) is increased 6.5-fold by phenacetin and ninefold by cyclophosphamide. Chronic infection due to *Schistosoma hematobium* causes squamous metaplasia and increases the risk of squamous cell carcinoma (SCC) in endemic areas such as Egypt.

PATHOLOGY

TCC accounts for 90% to 95% of all tumors of the bladder in the United States. Five percent to 10% are SCC, and 1% to 2% are adenocarcinomas. Pathologically, bladder cancers are divided into superficial tumors and invasive tumors. Superficial bladder tumors are tumors that have not invaded the muscularis propria and account for 75% of bladder cancers. Tumors that have invaded the muscularis propria, perivesical tissues, or adjacent structures are invasive bladder carcinomas. Patients with muscle-invasive disease have a 50% likelihood of having occult distant metastases at the time of diagnosis. The usual sites of metastases are pelvic lymph nodes, liver, lung, bone, adrenal glands, and intestine. Carcinoma in situ (CIS) usually presents as diffuse urothelial involvement in patients with superficial bladder tumors. When present in association with superficial bladder tumors, CIS increases the risk of subsequent invasive disease and recurrence.

CLINICAL FEATURES

Painless gross or microscopic hematuria is seen in 85% of patients. Symptoms of bladder irritability are seen in 20% of patients. Patients with invasive disease may have flank pain due to ureteral obstruction, bladder mass, or lower extremity edema. Weight loss, abdominal pain, or bone pain may be present in patients with advanced disease.

DIAGNOSIS

- The diagnostic workup of a patient with suspected bladder cancer includes intravenous pyelography or ultrasonography or both, urinary cytologic studies, and cystoscopy with full evaluation of bladder mucosa and urethra.
- Tumor markers such as bladder tumor antigen (BTA) and nuclear matrix protein (NMP) 22 have low sensitivity and specificity. More recently, assessment of urinary telomerase level has been shown to have an overall sensitivity of 80% and specificity of 70%. This may be useful both for diagnosing TCC and in monitoring for recurrence.

STAGING

The clinical staging of carcinoma of the bladder (Fig. 1 and Table 1) requires a cystoscopic examination that includes a biopsy, bladder and urethral mapping, and examination under anesthesia. Preoperative staging should include serum creatinine, liver function tests, chest radiograph, and excretory urography. A bone scan is recommended for muscle-invasive bladder cancer. A computed tomography (CT) scan of the abdomen and pelvis is useful in assessing the extent of the primary tumor, pelvic and paraaortic lymphadenopathy, and liver and adrenal metastases.

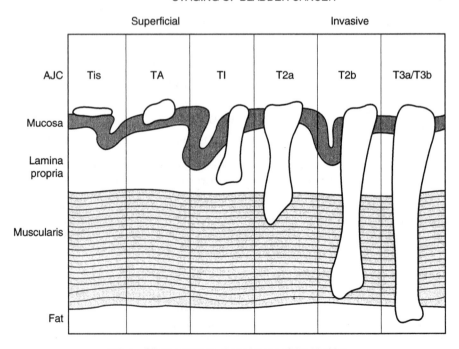

FIG. 1. Clinical staging of carcinoma of the bladder.

TABLE 1. *TNM staging of bladder cancer*

Primary tumor (T)
  The suffix "m" should be added to the appropriate T category to indicate multiple lesions.
    The suffix "is" may be added to any T to indicate the presence of associated carcinoma in
    situ
  TX: Primary tumor cannot be assessed
  T0: No evidence of primary tumor
  Ta: Noninvasive papillary carcinoma
  Tis: Carcinoma in situ: "flat tumor"
  T1: Tumor invades subepithelial connective tissue
  T2: Tumor invades muscle
    T2a: Tumor invades superficial muscle (inner half)
    T2b: Tumor invades deep muscle (outer half)
  T3: Tumor invades perivesical tissue
    T3a: microscopically
    T3b: macroscopically (extravesical mass)
  T4: Tumor invades any of the following: prostate, uterus, vagina, pelvic wall, or abdominal
    wall
    T4a: Tumor invades the prostate, uterus, vagina
    T4b: Tumor invades the pelvic wall, abdominal wall
Regional lymph nodes (N)
  Regional lymph nodes are those within the true pelvis; all others are distant lymph nodes
  NX: Regional lymph nodes cannot be assessed
  N0: No regional lymph node metastasis
  N1: Metastasis in a single lymph node, $\leq$2 cm in greatest dimension
  N2: Metastasis in a single lymph node, >2 cm but $\leq$5 cm in greatest dimension; or
    multiple lymph nodes, none >5 cm in greatest dimension
  N3: Metastasis in a single lymph node >5 cm in greatest dimension
Distant metastasis (M)
  MX: Distant metastasis cannot be assessed
  M0: No distant metastasis
  M1: Distant metastasis
Stage grouping
  Stage 0a: Ta, N0, M0
  Stage 0is: Tis, N0, M0
  Stage I: T1, N0, M0
  Stage II: T2a, N0, M0 or T2b, N0, M0
  Stage III: T3a, N0, M0 or T3b, N0, M0 or T4a, N0, M0
  Stage IV: T4b, N0, M0 or any T, N1–N3, M0 or any T, Any N, M1

PROGNOSIS

- The major prognostic factors are tumor stage at the time of diagnosis, especially the depth of invasion of the bladder wall and degree of differentiation of the tumor.
- Five-year relative survival rates for patients with superficial tumors, regional, and metastatic disease are 95%, 50%, and 6%, respectively.
- Older age, expression of p53, aneuploidy, tumor multifocality, and palpable mass are other adverse prognostic factors.

Treatment

Carcinoma In Situ

Transurethral resection (TUR) followed by intravesical bacillus Calmette–Guérin (BCG) therapy is the most common treatment of choice for CIS of the bladder (Fig. 2). It produces

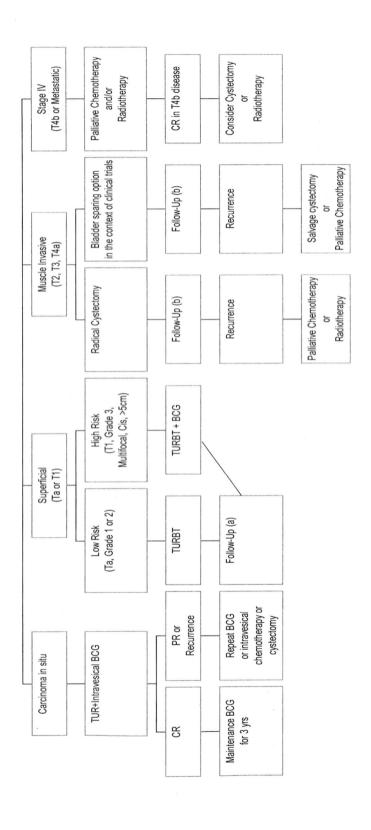

a) Cystoscopy and urine cytology q 3 mo x 2 yrs, and then q 6 mo x 2 yrs, and then yearly for life.
b) CT scan q 6 mo, IVP or U/S q 12 mo, cystoscopy and urine cytology q 3 mo x 1 yr and then q 6 mo, serum creatinine, LFT and Vit B12 q 3-6 mo.

FIG. 2. Treatment of bladder cancer.

70% to 80% complete response rate and a 5-year disease-free survival of more than 75%. Intravesical chemotherapy agents like thiotepa, doxorubicin, and mitomycin produce complete response rates in 30% to 50% of patients and 5-year disease-free survival in 20% to 40%.

Superficial Bladder Cancer

- TUR is the primary therapy for superficial bladder cancer. Approximately 80% of these patients survive for 5 years if treated with TUR alone, but in 71% of these patients, tumor recurrence develops.
- In high-risk patients, the tumor recurrence rate is decreased to about 20% with adjuvant intravesical BCG therapy.

Muscle-Invasive Bladder Cancer

- Radical cystectomy with bilateral pelvic lymph node dissection remains the standard of therapy for muscle-invasive bladder cancer. In men, the surgery involves radical cystoprostatectomy. A total urethrectomy is indicated if there is involvement of the prostatic urethra. In women, radical cystectomy involves wide excision of the bladder, urethra, uterus, adnexa, and anterior vaginal wall.
- Recent studies have shown that bladder-sparing options, which include aggressive TUR in combination with radiotherapy and/or chemotherapy, can be considered in selected patients with T2/T3a disease without compromising survival; however, this approach remains investigational.
- External beam radiotherapy with or without radiation-sensitizing agents such as cisplatin or 5-fluorouracil is an option for poor surgical candidates. Randomized trials have not shown any benefit for preoperative radiotherapy followed by radical cystectomy over radical cystectomy alone.
- Preliminary studies with adjuvant chemotherapy have shown benefit in disease-free and overall survival, but these studies were of small sample size and had several statistical and methodologic problems. Adjuvant therapy is currently not the standard of care; however, it may be considered for high-risk muscle-invasive bladder cancer.
- Randomized prospective phase III trials comprising 100 to 300 patients could not distinguish a difference in survival between definitive local treatment alone and neoadjuvant chemotherapy followed by definitive local treatment. However, a large prospective randomized study (Medical Research Council/European Organization for Research and Treatment of Cancer Trial) comprising 975 patients is currently under way to assess the role of neoadjuvant chemotherapy before definitive local treatment.

Stage IV Bladder Cancer

- Cisplatin, methotrexate, paclitaxel, and gemcitabine are some of the most active single agents in bladder cancer, with response rates of 30% to 45%.
- M-VAC is the only combination chemotherapy regimen that has been shown in randomized trials to be superior to single-agent cisplatin (4) and the three-drug regimen CISCA (6) (Tables 2 and 3). M-VAC has a response rate of 40% to 72% but is associated with significant toxicity including neutropenia, sepsis, mucositis, and renal failure.
- More recently, several phase II trials, which included docetaxel (9), gemcitabine (10), and paclitaxel (12) as first-line agents, had response rates of 40% to 70% with potentially less toxicity (Table 4).

TABLE 2. *Combination chemotherapy regimens in advanced urothelial carcinoma*

Regimen	Treatment description	Cycle duration	Comments	Reference
CISCA	Cyclophosphamide, 650 mg/m² i.v. day 1 (total dose/cycle, 650 mg/m²) Doxorubicin, 50 mg/m² i.v. day 2 (total dose/cycle, 50 mg/m²) Cisplatin, 100 mg/m² i.v. day 2 (total dose/cycle, 100 mg/m²)	21–28 days		6, 7
CMV	Methotrexate, 30 mg/m² i.v. days 1 and 8 (total dose/cycle, 60 mg/m²) Vinblastine, 4 mg/m² i.v. days 1 and 8 (total dose/cycle, 8 mg/m²) Cisplatin, 100 mg/m² i.v. infusion over 4 h on day 2, ≥12 h after methotrexate and vinblastine (total dose/cycle, 100 mg/m²)	21 days		8
Docetaxel + cisplatin[a]	Docetaxel, 75 mg/m² slow i.v. infusion over 1 h, day 1 (total dose/cycle, 75 mg/m²) Cisplatin, 75 mg/m² i.v. day 1 (total dose/cycle, 75 mg/m²)	21 days		9
Gemcitabine + cisplatin	Gemcitabine, 1,000 mg/m² i.v. days 1, 8, and 15 (total dose/cycle, 3,000 mg/m²) Cisplatin, 75 mg/m² i.v. day 1 (total dose/cycle, 75 mg/m²)	28 days		10
ITP[a]	Ifosfamide, 1,500 mg/m² per day i.v. for days 1–3 (total dose/cycle, 4,500 mg/m²) Mesna, 300 mg/m² i.v., 30 min before ifosfamide, and then Mesna, 300 mg/m² i.v. 4 and 8 h after ifosfamide, *or* Mesna, 600 mg/m² p.o. 4 and 8 h after ifosfamide Paclitaxel, 200 mg/m² i.v. infusion over 3 h, day 1 (total dose/cycle, 200 mg/m²) Cisplatin, 70 mg/m² i.v. day 1 (total dose/cycle, 70 mg/m²)	28 days	Regimen included primary hematopoietic growth factor support with filgrastim, 5 μg/kg per day, s.c.	11
M-VAC	Methotrexate, 30 mg/m² i.v. days 1, 15, and 22 (total dose/cycle, 90 mg/m²) Vinblastine, 3 mg/m² i.v. days 2, 15, and 22 (total dose/cycle, 9 mg/m²) Doxorubicin, 30 mg/m² i.v. day 2 (total dose/cycle, 30 mg/m²) Cisplatin, 70 mg/m² i.v. day 2 (total dose/cycle, 70 mg/m²)	28 days	Withhold methotrexate and vinblastine on d 15 and 22 if WBC count is <2.5 × 10³/μL and platelets <100 × 10⁹/μL	4, 5
Paclitaxel + carboplatin[a]	Paclitaxel, 200 mg/m² i.v. infusion over 3 h, day 1 (total dose/cycle, 200 mg/m²) Carboplatin i.v. after paclitaxel; dosage is calculated by the Calvert formula to achieve a target AUC of 5 mg/mL per min (Calvert reference)[b]	21 days		12

[a]Antineoplastic regimen included primary prophylaxis with antihistamines and corticosteroids against hypersensitivity reactions before taxoid (paclitaxel or docetaxel) administration.

[b]Calvert formula: Total dose (mg) = [Target AUC (mg/mL/min) × [GFR (mL/min) + 25]. From Calvert AH, Newell DR, Gumbrell LA, et al. Carboplatin dosage: prospective evaluation of a simple formula based on renal function. *J Clin Oncol* 1989;7:1748–1756, with permission.

AUC, graphically represented area under the plasma concentration versus time curve for carboplatin; GFR, glomerular filtration rate. In clinical application, urinary creatinine clearance during 24 h approximates the GFR; i.v., intravenously; p.o., orally; s.c., subcutaneously; WBC, white blood cell.

TABLE 3. *Randomized trials in patients with advanced urothelial carcinoma*

Randomized trial	Overall response rate	Median survival
M-VAC vs. cisplatin[4]	39% vs. 12%	12.5 mo vs. 8.2 mo
M-VAC vs. CISCA[6]	65% vs. 46%	48 wk vs. 36 wk

TABLE 4. *Newer agents in untreated advanced urothelial carcinoma patients*

Phase II trials	No. of evaluable pts.	Overall response rate
Docetaxel + cisplatin[9]	25	60%
Gemcitabine + cisplatin[10]	47	66%
Ifosfamide + paclitaxel + cisplatin[11]	29	79%
Paclitaxel + carboplatin[12]	35	51.5%

REFERENCES

1. Levin RM, Crawford DE. Bladder, renal pelvis, and ureters. In: Haskell CM, ed. *Cancer treatment.* 4th ed. Philadelphia: WB Saunders, 1995:567–588.
2. Sher HI, Shipley WU, Herr HW. Cancer of the bladder. In: DeVita VT Jr, Hellman S, Rosenberg SA, eds. *Cancer: principles and practice of oncology.* 5th ed. New York: Lippincott-Raven, 1997: 1300–1322.
3. NCCN. Urothelial cancer practice guidelines. *Oncology* 1998;3:225–271.
4. Loehrer PJ Sr, Einhorn LH, Elson PJ, et al. A randomized comparison of cisplatin alone or in combination with methotrexate, vinblastine, and doxorubicin in patients with metastatic urothelial carcinoma: a cooperative group study [published erratum appears in *J Clin Oncol* 1993;11:384. *J Clin Oncol* 1992;10:1066–1073.
5. Sternberg CN, Yagoda A, Scher HI, et al. Preliminary results of M-VAC (methotrexate, vinblastine, doxorubicin and cisplatin) for transitional cell carcinoma of the urothelium. *J Urol* 1985;133: 403–407.
6. Logothetis CJ, Dexeus FH, Finn L, et al. A prospective randomized trial comparing MVAC and CISCA chemotherapy for patients with metastatic urothelial tumors. *J Clin Oncol* 1990;8: 1050–1055.
7. Logothetis CJ, Dexeus FH, Chong C, et al. Cisplatin, cyclophosphamide and doxorubicin chemotherapy for unresectable urothelial tumors: the MD Anderson experience. *J Urol* 1989;141:33–37.
8. Harker WG, Meyers FJ, Freiha FS, et al. Cisplatin, methotrexate, and vinblastine (CMV): an effective chemotherapy regimen for metastatic transitional cell carcinoma of the urinary tract: a Northern California Oncology Group study. *J Clin Oncol* 1985;3:1463–1470.
9. Sengelov L, Kamby C, Lund B, et al. Docetaxel and cisplatin in metastatic urothelial cancer: a phase II study. *J Clin Oncol* 1998;16:3392–3397.
10. Kaufman D, Stadler W, Carducci M, et al. Gemcitabine plus cisplatin in metastatic transitional cell carcinoma: final results of a phase II study. *Proc Am Soc Clin Oncol* 1998;7:320(Abst)1235.
11. Bajorin DF, McCaffrey JA, Hilton S, et al. Treatment of patients with transitional-cell carcinoma of the urothelial tract with ifosfamide, paclitaxel, and cisplatin: a phase II trial. *J Clin Oncol* 1998; 16:2722–2727.
12. Redman BG, Smith DC, Flaherty L, et al. Phase II trial of paclitaxel and carboplatin in the treatment of advanced urothelial carcinoma. *J Clin Oncol* 1998;16:1844–1848.

15

Testicular Carcinoma

Philippe C. Bishop and *Barnett S. Kramer

*Division of Clinical Trial Design and Analysis, Food and Drug Administration,
Center for Biologics Evaluation and Research, Rockville, Maryland 20852-1448;
and *Division of Cancer Prevention and Control, National Cancer Institute,
Bethesda, Maryland 20892*

Testicular cancer is rare (less than 1% of all tumors), but represents one of the most frequently occurring malignancies in young men. For most tumors, the reproductive organs are the sites of the primary tumors; they usually arise from the malignant transformation of primordial germ cells. It is highly curable, and life expectancy for affected individuals is long. Consequently, careful long-term follow-up of survivors is required. Not only oncologists but also primary care providers are likely to observe an increasing number of successfully treated patients in their practice. For these patients, careful monitoring for recurrent disease and therapy-related long-term sequelae is imperative.

CLINICAL FEATURES

Epidemiology

- For 2000, 6,900 new cases and 300 deaths were estimated (1).
- It includes 1% of all malignancies in men.
- Incidence in whites is greater than that in African-Americans.
- Peak frequency is in early adulthood (greatest incidence between age 20 and 35 years).
- Uncommon after age 40 years.

Risk Factors

- Cryptorchid testes (intraabdominal testes more than inguinal testes).
- Testicular cancer in contralateral testis.
- Klinefelter's syndrome (increased risk of mediastinal germ cell tumors).

History/Signs/Physical Examination

- Asymptomatic nodule or swelling.
- Testicular mass, feeling of heaviness, pain, and/or hardness.
- Patients with advanced disease may have back or abdominal pain (due to retroperitoneal adenopathy), weight loss, gynecomastia [due to elevated β-human chorionic gonadotropin (HCG)], supraclavicular lymphadenopathy, superior vena cava syndrome (from mediastinal disease), urinary obstruction, dyspnea and hemoptysis (secondary to extensive pulmonary metastases), and headaches or seizures (due to brain metastases).

DIFFERENTIAL DIAGNOSIS

- Epididymitis (may coexist with germ cell tumors).
- Hydrocele/varicocele/spermatocele/orchitis.
- Lymphoma.
- Leukemia.
- Metastasis from prostate cancer, melanoma, lung cancer.
- Tuberculosis/gumma/other infectious causes.

DIAGNOSTIC

Goals

- Any testicular mass in a man requires prompt evaluation to exclude testicular carcinoma.
- Testicular cancer is highly curable (85% of cases).
- Histologic determination of tumor type has prognostic and therapeutic significance.

Evaluation

The diagnostic workup is outlined in Fig. 1.

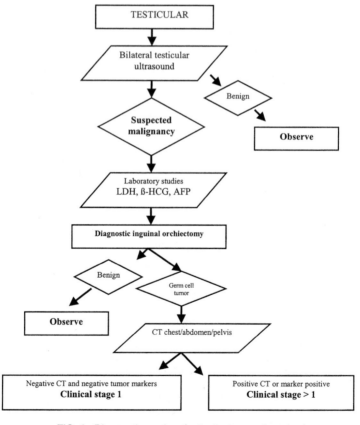

FIG. 1. Diagnostic workup for testicular carcinoma.

Imaging

- **Ultrasound:** to detect the presence of testicular parenchymal abnormality.
- **Radiographic studies:** standard two-view chest radiograph to rule out pulmonary metastases.
- **Computed tomography (CT)** scans of chest, abdomen, and pelvis: to establish extent of disease dissemination.
- **Magnetic resonance imaging (MRI):** especially when results of the physical examination and testicular ultrasound are equivocal.

Laboratory

Serum α-fetoprotein (AFP)

- Biologic half-life is approximately 5 to 7 days.
- Commonly excreted by embryonal cell cancers.
- Not produced by pure seminoma, and its detection implies the presence of nonseminomatous elements (primary or metastatic site).

Serum β-HCG

- Half-life is approximately 24 hours.
- May be biologically active, leading to enhanced estrogen production by the testes and consequent gynecomastia.
- Secreted by syncytiotrophoblastic giant cells.
- Present in choriocarcinomas.

Serum LDH

- Independently useful as a prognostic factor.
- Can reflect tumor burden and growth rate.

PATHOLOGIC EVALUATION

Inguinal orchiectomy with complete removal of the testis and spermatic cord through the inguinal ring is the procedure of choice for pathologic evaluation of suspected testicular tumors. Transcrotal testicular biopsy is not recommended for fear of local and nodal dissemination of tumor, although scientific evidence supporting this notion is weak.

- Germ cell tumors display an array of histopathology (Table 1).

TABLE 1. *Histopathologic characteristics of germ cell tumors*

Tumor type	Pathologic feature
Germinal cell tumors (95%)	**Seminomas** (40–50%)
Single cell tumors (60%)	Primordial germ cell
Combination tumors (40%)	**Nonseminomas** (50–60%)
	Embryonal cell tumors
	Yolk sac tumors
	Teratomas
	Choriocarcinomas
Tumors of gonadal stroma (1–2%)	Leydig cell
	Sertoli cell
	Primitive gonadal structures
Gonadoblastoma	Germinal cell + stromal cell

TABLE 2. *American Joint Committee TNM Classification and Staging*

Primary tumor (pT) (The extent of primary tumor is classified after radical orchiectomy)

pTX	Primary tumor cannot be assessed (if no radical orchiectomy has been performed)
pT0	No evidence of primary tumor (e.g., histologic scar in testis)
pTis	Intratubular germ cell neoplasia (carcinoma in situ)
pT1	Tumor limited to testis and epididymis without lymphatic/vascular invasion
pT2	Tumor limited to testis and epididymis with vascular/lymphatic invasion, or tumor extending through the tunica albuginea with involvement of the tunica vaginalis
pT3	Tumor invades the spermatic cord with or without vascular/lymphatic invasion
pT4	Tumor invades the scrotum with or without vascular/lymphatic invasion

Regional lymph nodes (N)

NX	Regional lymph nodes cannot be assessed
N0	No regional lymph node metastasis
N1	Metastasis in a single lymph node, ≤2 cm in greatest dimension
N2	Metastasis in a single lymph node, >2 cm but ≤5 cm in greatest dimension; or multiple lymph nodes, none >5 cm in greatest dimension
N3	Metastasis in a lymph node >5 cm in greatest dimension

Distant metastasis (M)

MX	Presence of distant metastasis cannot be assessed
M0	No distant metastasis
M1	Distant metastasis
M1a	Nonregional nodal or pulmonary metastasis
M1b	Distant metastasis other than to nonregional nodes and lungs

Serum tumor markers (S)

	LDH		β-HCG (mIU/mL)		AFP (ng/mL)
SX	Marker studies not available or not performed				
S0	NL		NL		NL
S1	<1.5 × ULN	and	<5,000	and	<1,000
S2	1.5–10 × ULN	or	5,000–50,000	or	1,000–10,000
S3	>10 × ULN	or	>50,000	or	>10,000

TABLE 3. *AJCC Stage Groupings*

Stage 0	pTis, N0, M0, S0
Stage I	pT1–4, N0, M0, SX
Stage IA	pT1, N0, M0, S0
Stage IB	pT2–4, N0, M0, S0
Stage IS	any pT/Tx, N0, M0, S1–3
Stage II	any pT/Tx, N1–3, M0, SX
Stage IIA	any pT/Tx, N1, M0, S0–1
Stage IIB	any pT/Tx, N2, M0, S0–1
Stage IIC	any pT/Tx, N3, M0, S0–1
Stage III	any pT/Tx, any N, M1, SX
Stage IIIA	any pT/Tx, any N, M1a, S0–1
Stage IIIB	any pT/Tx, N1–3, M0, S2
	any pT/Tx, any N, M1a, S2
Stage IIIC	any pT/Tx, N1–3, M0, S3
	any pT/Tx, any N, M1a, S3
	any pT/Tx, any N, M1b, any S

HCG, human chorionic gonadotropin; AFP, α-fetoprotein.

- Placental alkaline phosphatase (PLAP)-positive midline tumors of uncertain histogenesis, negative for low-molecular-weight keratins by immunohistochemistries, are suggestive of seminomas. Those that express low-molecular-weight keratins are usually embryonal carcinomas.
- Germ cell tumors usually are hyperdiploid.
- Loss of heterozygosity is often demonstrated in early-stage disease and is not associated with progression of disease.
- 80% of cases have an isochromosome of the short arm of chromosome 12[i(12p)], implicating one or more genes on 12p in the malignant transformation of primordial germ cells.

STAGING

Tables 2 and 3 contain the American Joint Committee TNM Classification and Staging criteria.

PROGNOSIS

Table 4 outlines the International Consensus Risk Classification for Germ Cell Tumors, and Table 5, expected survival.

THERAPY

Treatment Modalities According to Histology and Stage

Testicular cancer is highly treatable, and can be broadly divided into seminoma and nonseminoma types (Figs. 2–4). Seminomas are more sensitive to radiation therapy. For patients

TABLE 4. *International Consensus Risk Classification for germ cell tumors*

Prognosis	Nonseminoma	Seminoma
Good	Testis/retroperitoneal primary and no nonpulmonary visceral metastases and AFP <1,000 µg/mL HCG <5,000 IU/L (1000 µg/ml) LDH <1.5 × upper limit of normal	Any primary site and no nonpulmonary visceral metastases and AFP <1,000 µg/mL any HCG any LDH
Intermediate	Testis/retroperitoneal primary and no nonpulmonary visceral metastases and AFP ≥1,000 and ≤10,000 µg/ml or HCG ≥5,000 IU/L and ≤50,000 IU/L or LDH ≥1.5 × N1 and ≤10 × N1	Any primary site and nonpulmonary visceral metastases and AFP <1,000 µg/mL Any HCG Any LDH
Poor	Mediastinal primary *or* nonpulmonary visceral metastases or AFP >10,000 µg/mL *or* HCG >50,000 IU/L (10,000 µg/ml) or >10 × upper limit of normal	No patients classified as poor prognosis

TABLE 5. *Expected survival*

	5-year progression-free survival (%)		5-year overall survival (%)	
Prognosis	Seminoma	Nonseminoma	Seminoma	Nonseminoma
Good	82	89	86	92
Intermediate	67	75	72	80
Poor	—	41	—	48

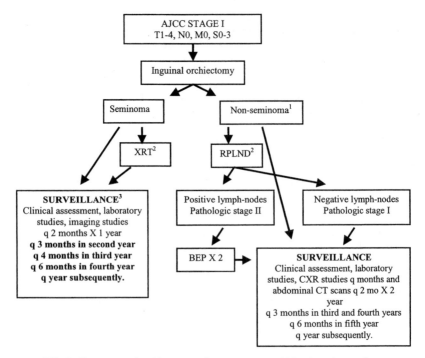

FIG. 2. Treatment algorithm according to stage and histology (stage I).

[1] With normal post-orchiectomy tumor marker levels.
[2] Salvage therapy in the surveillance group yields equivalent testicular carcinoma cure rates. XRT is associated with an increased rate of secondary solid tumors. RPLND is associated with an increased morbidity.
[3] Suggested surveillance intervals are arbitrary.

with seminoma (all stages combined), the cure rate exceeds 90%. For those with low-stage disease, the cure rate approaches 100%. Tumors that have a mixture of seminoma and non-seminoma components should be managed as nonseminomas. Tumors that appear to have a seminoma histology with elevated serum levels of α-fetoprotein (AFP) should be treated as nonseminomas. Elevation of the β subunit of human chorionic gonadotropin (β-HCG) alone is found in approximately 10% of patients with pure seminoma. Patients with brain metastasis should receive whole brain radiotherapy in addition to chemotherapy (Table 6).

- A randomized study has shown similar overall survival and time to treatment failure results for BEP and PVB regimens. Another randomized study has shown similar results for BEP and VIP.
- BEP causes fewer paresthesias, abdominal cramps, and myalgias than does PVB.
- VIP is more toxic and myelosuppressive than BEP.
- Four cycles of EP were equivalent to three cycles of BEP in a randomized study.

Salvage therapy

- Usually given to patients who fail to achieve an initial complete response.
- VIP is commonly used as a first-line salvage therapy.
- High-dose chemotherapy with autologous bone marrow/peripheral stem cell support is experimental and may represent a therapeutic option for selected patients.

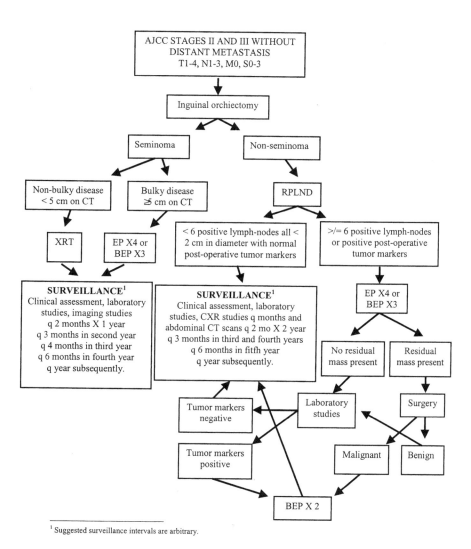

FIG. 3. Treatment algorithm according to stage and histology: stage II and stage III without distant metastases.

Therapy-Related Toxicity

Fertility

- Many patients have oligospermia or sperm abnormalities before therapy.
- Virtually all become oligospermic during chemotherapy.
- Sperm banking should be recommended for all patients desiring to father children after therapy; however, many recover sperm production after completion of therapy and can father children.
- Children of treated patients do not appear to have an increased risk of congenital malformations.

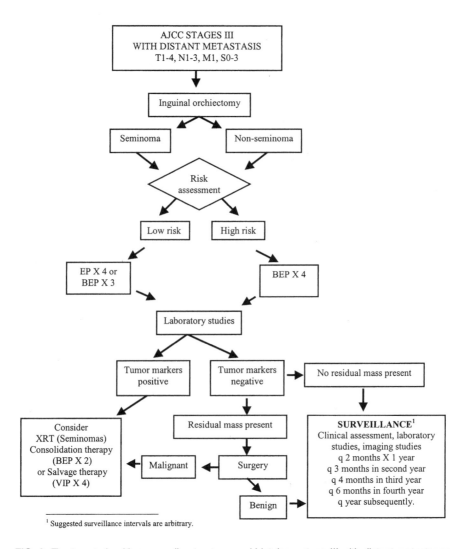

FIG. 4. Treatment algorithm according to stage and histology: stage III with distant metastases.

Pulmonary Toxicity

- Associated with bleomycin.
- Rarely fatal at total cumulative doses of bleomycin less than 400 units.
- Bleomycin should be discontinued if early signs of pulmonary toxicity develop.
- Asymptomatic decreases in pulmonary function are frequent and are reversible after the completion of chemotherapy.
- Routine use of pulmonary function tests (e.g., PFTs, DLCO) is rarely indicated and should be reserved for patients with signs and symptoms of pulmonary toxicity (e.g., dry rales on physical examination, SOB, DOE).

TABLE 6. *Commonly used chemotherapy regimens*

Regimen		
EP	Etoposide, 100 mg/m² i.v. daily × 5 days Cisplatin, 20 mg/m² i.v. daily × 5 days	Four cycles administered at 21-day intervals
BEP	Bleomycin, 30 units i.v. weekly on days 2, 9, 16 Etoposide, 100 mg/m² i.v. daily × 5 days Cisplatin, 20 mg/m² i.v. daily × 5 days	Two to four cycles administered at 21-day intervals
VIP	Vinblastine, 0.11 mg/kg weeks 1 and 2 Ifosfamide, 1.2 g/m² i.v. daily × 5 days Mesna, 400 mg/m² i.v. q8h × 5 days Cisplatin, 20 mg/m² i.v. daily × 5 days	Three to four cycles administered at 21-day intervals
PVB	Cisplatin, 20 mg/m² i.v. daily × 5 days Vinblastine, 0.11 mg/kg weeks 1 and 2 Bleomycin, 30 units i.v. weekly on days 2, 9, 16	Three cycles administered at 21-day intervals

- Patients should be encouraged to stop smoking.
- If deemed medically necessary, supplemental oxygen should be used with caution, minimizing exposure and using low F_iO_2 settings.
- If fluids are indicated, i.v. colloids rather than crystalloids are preferred.

Nephrotoxicity

- Minor decreases in creatinine clearance can occur with platinum-based regimens, but these appear to remain stable in the long term without clinically significant deterioration.

Neurologic

- Hearing deficits occur with cisplatin-based regimen, but they generally occur at sound frequencies outside the range of conversational tones; for most patients, routine monitoring for deficit is not indicated, and use of hearing aids after therapy is rarely needed.

Cardiovascular

- Hypertension.
- Raynaud's phenomenon.
- Hypercholesterolemia.

Secondary Malignancies

- Associated with the prolonged use of alkylating agents, etoposide, and the use of radiation.
- Secondary leukemias: primarily of myeloid lineage and associated with etoposide-containing regimens; often characterized by an 11q23 translocation; and usually occurs within several years after therapy.
- Cancers of the stomach, the bladder, and possibly the pancreas: associated with radiation therapy, which is often used in the management of pure seminomatous germ cell cancers; often limited to the radiation portal; may have a latency period of a decade or more.

ANNOTATED BIBLIOGRAPHY

1. American Cancer Society. *Cancer facts and figures 1999.* Atlanta, GA: American Cancer Society, 1999.
2. Baniel J, Foster RS, Gonin R, et al. Late relapse of testicular cancer. *J Clin Oncol* 1995;13: 1170–1176.
3. Bosl GJ, Chaganti RSK. The use of tumor-markers in germ-cell malignancies. *Hematol Oncol Clin North Am* 1994;8:573–587.
4. Bosl GJ, Motzer RJ. Testicular germ-cell cancer. *N Engl J Med* 1997;337:242–253.
5. Bosl GJ, Steinfeld J, Barjorin DF, et al. Cancer of the testis. In: DeVita VT, Hellman S, Rosenberg SA, eds. *Cancer: principles and practice of oncology.* 5th ed. Philadelphia: Lippincott-Raven, 1997: 1397–1425.
6. Einhorn LH. Testicular cancer: an oncological success story. *Clin Cancer Res* 1997;3:2630–2632.
7. Einhorn LH, Donohue JP. Advanced testicular cancer: update for urologists. *J Urol* 1998; 160:1964–1969.
8. Fox EP, Loehrer PJ. Chemotherapy for advanced testicular cancer. *Hematol Oncol Clin North Am* 1991;5:1173–1187.
9. Harland SJ, Cook PA, Fossa SD, et al. Intratubular germ cell neoplasia of the contralateral testis in testicular cancer: defining a high risk group. *J Urol* 1998;160:1353–1357.
10. Lehne G, Johansen B, Fossa SD. Long-term follow-up of pulmonary function in patients cured from testicular cancer with combination chemotherapy including bleomycin. *Br J Cancer* 1993;68: 555–558.
11. Mead GM. Testicular cancer: staging, treatment and outcome. *Eur J Cancer* 1997;33:6.
12. Mead GM, Stenning SP, Cook P, et al. International germ cell consensus classification: a prognostic factor-erased staging system for metastatic germ cell cancers. *J Clin Oncol* 1997;15:594–603.
13. Miller KD, Loehrer PJ, Gonin R, et al. Chemotherapy with vinblastine, ifosfamide, and cisplatin in recurrent seminoma. *J Clin Oncol* 1997;15:1427–1431.
14. Murty VS, Bosl GJ, Houldsworth J, et al. Allelic loss and somatic differentiation in human male germ-cell tumors. *Oncogene* 1994;9:2245–2251.
15. Osanto S, Bukman A, Vanhoek F, et al. Long-term effects of chemotherapy in patients with testicular cancer. *J Clin Oncol* 1992;10:574–579.
16. Stephenson WT, Poirier SM, Rubin L, et al. Evaluation of reproductive capacity in germ-cell tumor patients following treatment with cisplatin, etoposide, and bleomycin. *J Clin Oncol* 1995;13: 2278–2280.
17. Travis LB, Curtis RE, Storm H, et al. Risk of second malignant neoplasms among long-term survivors of testicular cancer. *J Natl Cancer Inst* 1997;89:1429–1439.
18. Vanbasten JP, Koops HS, Sleijfer DT, et al. Current concepts about testicular cancer. *Eur J Surg Oncol* 1997;23:354–360.

SECTION 6

Gynecologic

16

Ovarian Cancer

Kevin Knopf and Elise Kohn

Medicine Branch, DCS, National Cancer Institute, National Institutes of Health, Bethesda, Maryland

EPIDEMIOLOGY

Epithelial ovarian cancer is the fifth leading cause of cancer death among women in the United States and the most common cause of death in women in whom gynecologic cancer develops.

For 1999, 25,200 cases and 14,500 deaths were predicted (1). Ovarian cancer represents 25% of the malignancies of the female genital tract, yet has the highest mortality rate because 75% of ovarian cancer patients have advanced-stage disease at the time of diagnosis. However, the overall 5-year survival rate has improved from 36% in the 1970s to 47% in the early 1990s.

Median age for epithelial ovarian cancer is between 60 and 65 years, and fewer than 1% of cases occur in women younger than 30 years. Incidence increases with age, peaking in the mid to late 70s. A woman's lifetime risk of developing ovarian cancer is approximately one in 70, or 1.4%. Ovarian cancer is more common in whites than in blacks, and occurs most frequently in industrialized countries.

CA125: A TUMOR MARKER IN OVARIAN CANCER

CA125 is an antigenic epitope expressed on a glycoprotein, and testing for this antigen can reveal elevated CA125 levels, which are present in 60% of epithelial ovarian cancers. Unfortunately, CA125 levels can be elevated in a variety of benign conditions as well, and its low specificity limits its use in screening (see later). Preoperatively, a serum CA125 level of more than 95 U/mL has a positive predictive value of 96% in postmenopausal women. In premenopausal women, however, benign conditions (e.g., endometriosis, benign tumors, fibroids) often raise CA125, so it has a low positive predictive value preoperatively. CA125 has its greatest utility in monitoring patients treated for ovarian cancer, as elevations may indicate a relapse, depending on the relative value and trend; additionally it can serve as a marker of response during treatment. Changes in CA125 levels are occasionally used as a response criterion if they are clearly abnormal and changing; for example, the Gynecologic Oncology Group uses serial doubling or a value over 100 U/mL to constitute a relapse without a biopsy. Patients who did not express CA125 preoperatively may not benefit from having their CA125 levels monitored.

SCREENING

There is no currently accepted screening modality for ovarian cancer. Several trials are under way, including the Prostate, Lung, Colon, and Ovarian screening trial (PLCO), conducted by the National Cancer Institute, although this trial may be underpowered to show any benefit. A recently completed randomized trial involving 20,000 women was reported (2). These investigators used a combination of CA125, followed by ultrasound, for patients with elevated CA125 values. They did not find a significant difference in early-stage disease between the screened and unscreened groups. Although median survival of women with screen-detected ovarian cancer was longer than those with ovarian cancer in the control group, the number of deaths from ovarian cancer did not differ significantly. The real objective in developing a screening method for ovarian cancer is to identify early-stage, and thus more curable, disease.

The National Institutes of Health (NIH) recommends screening for women with one of the known genetic syndromes (familial breast/ovarian cancer syndrome or hereditary nonpolyposis colorectal cancer) consisting of semiannual rectovaginal pelvic examinations, CA-125 determination every 6 months, and transvaginal ultrasound with color Doppler flow annually. There are additional recommendations of oral contraceptive use for prevention in high-risk families until after childbearing (see later) and consideration of prophylactic TAH/BSO after age 40 years.

PATHOGENESIS OF OVARIAN CANCER

Although risk factors have been defined for ovarian cancer, the etiology and even the cell of origin remain unknown.

The most plausible explanation relates to ovulatory activity. Constant, uninterrupted ovulation may lead to an increased risk of ovarian cancer because each ovulatory cycle involves proliferation of the ovarian surface epithelium, with the possibility of transformation.

Other, less convincing biologic mechanisms posited are (a) increased pituitary gonadotropin levels and (b) alterations in blood flow to the ovaries. Transtubal transportation of carcinogens is a risk factor but is not thought to be etiologic.

RISK FACTORS

Most cases of ovarian cancer are sporadic, occurring in women without any known risk factors (Table 1). Ovarian cancer risk does increase with age.

GENETIC SYNDROMES

Genetic syndromes are responsible for 5% to 10% of ovarian cancers.

TABLE 1. *Risk factors*

Risk factors for ovarian cancer	Relative risks
First- or second-degree relative with ovarian cancer	RR 2–3
BRCA1 or BRCA2 mutation carrier	RR 5–35
Nulliparity	RR 1.5–2.0
Infertility and/or use of fertility drugs	RR 1.5–2.0
Northern European/North American descent	RR 1.5
White	RR 1.5
Postmenopausal hormone replacement therapy use	RR 1.15
Talc use in the perineal area before first live birth	RR 0.9–1.8
Early menarche/late menopause	

Hereditary Breast and Ovarian Cancer Syndrome: BRCA1 and BRCA2

- These patients have a younger age at presentation, on average 10 years younger than patients without mutations in BRCA1 and/or BRCA2.
- Estimated risk by age 80 is 27.8% (3).
- BRCA1 may account for 4.4% of ovarian cancer diagnoses.
- BRCA2 is associated with approximately 4.5% of ovarian cancers.
- Patients in families with ovarian cancer alone probably represent a subset of women with BRCA1/BRCA2 mutations or variable phenotypic expression.

Lynch II Syndrome (Hereditary Nonpolyposis Colorectal Cancer)

- Ovarian, endometrial, breast, colon, pancreatic [other gastrointestinal (GI), genitourinary (GU) possible].
- Associated with DNA mismatch repair enzyme mutations (hMSH-2, hMLH1, hPMS1, hPMS2, and GTBP) (4).

However, in a small case series of 116 ovarian cancer patients, there were 13 germline mutations present in 12 patients: 10 in BRCA1, one each in hMSH2 and hMLH1, and one in BRCA2. Interestingly, more than 50% of patients with BRCA1 mutations had "unremarkable" family histories, and the majority of patients with a maternal history of ovarian or breast cancer tested negative for germline mutations (5). This work is preliminary but is suggestive of variable penetrance and discordance between family history and presence of a germline mutation.

Protective Factors for Ovarian Cancer

1. Oral contraceptive use (combination estrogen/progesterone).
   - Protection increases with duration of use.
   - Shown to be protective for patients with known family history or a genetic syndrome.
   - The benefits with newer low-estrogen formulations, with or without progestin 2nd of pair are not yet established.
2. Prophylactic oophorectomy can be considered for women with a family history or known genetic syndrome. There will still be a risk of developing peritoneal cancer at remaining sites.
3. Pregnancy of any duration.
4. Lactation with nursing.

PATHOLOGY

Epithelial adenocarcinoma (90% of ovarian cancers).

- Serous.
- Mucinous.
- Endometrioid.
- Transitional (Brenner).
- Clear cell.

Malignant mixed mullerian tumor.
"Borderline" tumors for each of the five histologies.
Stromal and germ-cell tumors (10% of ovarian cancers).

Stromal tumors.

- Granulosa tumor.
- Sertoli–Leydig tumor.

Germ cell tumors.

- Dysgerminoma.
- Endodermal sinus tumor.
- Malignant teratoma.
- Embryonal carcinoma.
- Primary choriocarcinoma.

DIAGNOSIS AND WORKUP

Signs and Symptoms

Ovarian cancer has an insidious onset, and the signs and symptoms are nonspecific, which accounts in part for the preponderance of late stages at diagnosis. A pelvic mass is sometimes detected on routine pelvic examination, prompting further workup. Advanced-stage disease can present with abdominal discomfort, swelling from ascites, and occasionally bladder or rectal symptoms. Pleural effusions can be symptomatic.

The workup of an undiagnosed pelvic mass should include a complete history and physical examination, laboratory work including CA125, and an ultrasound or computed tomography (CT) scan of the abdomen/pelvis (if clinically warranted). If the woman is younger than 30 years, an α-fetoprotein and β-human chorionic gonadotropin (β-HCG) should be performed to rule out germ cell tumors. A pelvic radiograph can be used to look for the presence of a mature teratoma, which can appear as a calcified mass. Preoperative endometrial sampling should be performed in women with abnormal vaginal bleeding. A chest radiograph is warranted before surgical intervention.

The majority of advanced-stage cases of ovarian cancer can be identified preoperatively. However, an exploratory laparotomy is warranted for all suggestive masses. Laparoscopy has some proponents but is still considered investigational.

TABLE 2. *FIGO staging of ovarian cancer*

Stage I	**Growth limited to the ovaries.**
IA	Growth limited to one ovary; no ascites; no tumor on the external surfaces; capsule intact
IB	Growth limited to both ovaries; no ascites; no tumor on the external surfaces; capsule intact
IC	Tumor either stage IA or IB but with tumor on the surface of one or both ovaries; capsule ruptured; ascites present containing malignant cells; or positive peritoneal washings
Stage II	**Growth involving one or both ovaries with pelvic extension**
IIA	Extension and/or metastases to the uterus and/or fallopian tubes
IIB	Extension to other pelvic organs
IIC	Tumor either stage IIA or IIB but with tumor on the surface of one or both ovaries; capsule(s) ruptured; ascites present containing malignant cells; or positive peritoneal washings
Stage III	**Tumor involving one or both ovaries** with peritoneal implants outside the pelvis and/or positive retroperitoneal or inguinal nodes; metastases to the surface of the liver equals stage III; tumor is limited to the true pelvis but with histologically verified malignant extension to the small bowel or omentum
IIIA	Tumor grossly limited to the true pelvis with negative nodes but with histologically confirmed microscopic seeding of abdominal peritoneal surfaces
IIIB	Tumor of one or both ovaries; histologically confirmed implants of abdominal peritoneal surfaces, none >2 cm in diameter; node negative
IIIC	Abdominal implants >2 cm in diameter and/or positive retroperitoneal or inguinal nodes
Stage IV	**Growth involving one or both ovaries** with distant metastases; if pleural effusion is present, there must be positive cytologic test results to allot a case to stage IV; parenchymal liver metastasis equals stage IV

STAGING

Ovarian cancer spreads by local shedding into the peritoneal cavity with implantation into the peritoneum and omentum and by local invasion of the bladder and bowel. Spread across the diaphragm to the pleural cavity is common. Tumor cells may also spread via pelvic and periaortic nodes, and may block diaphragmatic lymphatics, possibly contributing to ascites.

Staging (Table 2) is based on a properly performed staging laparotomy.

PROGNOSTIC FACTORS

Favorable Prognostic Factors

- Younger age (e.g., younger than 50 years) at the time of diagnosis.
- Good performance status.
- Cell type other than clear cell.
- Early stage.
- Well-differentiated tumor.
- Diploid tumors.
- No overexpression of HER2/neu.
- No overexpression of vascular endothelial growth factor (VEGF) in early ovarian cancer.
- Smaller disease volume before any surgical debulking.
- Absence of ascites.
- Optimal residual disease after primary cytoreductive surgery (<1–2 cm) (6).
- Patients with germline BRCA1 mutations.
- Surgery performed by a gynecologic oncologist.

Unfavorable Prognostic Factors for Stage I Ovarian Cancer

- High grade.
- Dense adherence.
- Large-volume ascites.
- Increased angiogenesis.
- Clear cell histology.

What Constitutes a Proper Operation?

- Performed by a gynecologic oncologist.
- Midline vertical incision, at least supraumbilical, preferred to xiphoid process.
- TAH/BSO[1]: noting characteristics of primary tumor (i.e., adhesions, extracapsular extension, rupture).
- Omentectomy.
- Debulking of as much gross tumor as possible, ideally to less than 1 cm ("optimal debulking") (6).
- Random sampling of all four quadrants/gutters of the abdominal peritoneum.
- Ascites and/or pleural fluid, if present, submitted for cytologic evaluation.
- In patients without ascites, peritoneal washings from the pelvis and pericolic gutters should be obtained. The diaphragm should be sampled, and washings from the undersurface of the diaphragm should be obtained. If there are no suggestive areas, random peritoneal biopsies should be performed.
- Pelvic and paraaortic node sampling should be performed.

Occult metastases were detected in 30% of initially staged patients at stage I or II who had incomplete staging but were subsequently restaged.

---

[1] With early-stage, low-grade ovarian cancers, a unilateral salpingo-oophorectomy can be performed in a young wonan who desires to preserve reproductive poential, if she has stage 1, grade 1 or 2 disease.

TABLE 3. *Five-year survival rate by stage*

Stage	Survival rate
IA/IB, grade 1	90–98%
I, "poor prognosis"	60–80%
III, minimal or no residual tumor	30–50%
III, bulky residual tumor	10%
IV	<10%

Incidence of Positive Lymph Nodes at Primary Surgery

Frequency of pelvic node involvement is equal to paraaortic node involvement.

- Clinical stage I (24%).
- Clinical stage II (50%).
- Clinical stage III (74%).
- Clinical stage IV (73%; Table 3).

TREATMENT OF OVARIAN CANCER

Clinical Trials

With the possible exception of favorable stage I disease (defined later) not requiring postoperative chemotherapy, enrollment in clinical trials is appropriate for women with ovarian cancer at every stage of disease and should be encouraged (7).

Primary Disease

Primary treatment modalities include surgery and postoperative chemotherapy in all but selected patients with early stage at diagnosis. Radiation therapy is considered to be of limited use in the U.S. in newly diagnosed patients, although it is more commonly used in Canada and Europe.

Treatment of Borderline Tumors/Tumors of Low Malignant Potential

The primary treatment of borderline tumors is surgical resection. There is no apparent benefit from postoperative chemotherapy or radiation therapy. Occasionally a unilateral salpingo-oophorectomy is possible in early-stage tumors for women who desire to preserve fertility. Treatment (Table 4) is to be considered for patients with microinvasive implants, aneuploidy, residual disease, or advanced stage.

Treatment of Early-Stage Disease (I and II)

If the workup of a pelvic mass is suggestive of cancer, patients should undergo a laparotomy with TAH/BSO and comprehensive staging (see Table 3). If a patient has a stage 1, grade 1 tumor and desires to preserve fertility, a unilateral salpingo-oophorectomy can be performed, when technically feasible (8).

Patients with stage IA or IB, grade 1 disease do not benefit from chemotherapy. Current recommendations for patients with stage IC disease, stage IA or IB with grade 2 or 3 or clear cell histology, or stage II disease is three to six cycles of paclitaxel with either cisplatin or carboplatin (see Table 4).

TABLE 4. *Standard chemotherapy regimens for initial treatment of ovarian cancer*

Paclitaxel, 135 mg/m^2 i.v. continuous infusion over 24 h on day 1
  (total dose/cycle, 135 mg/m^2) *followed by*
Cisplatin, 75 mg/m^2 i.v. over 60 min on day 2, after completion of paclitaxel
  (total dose/cycle, 75 mg/m^2)[13]
Cycle is repeated every 21 days
or
Paclitaxel, 175 mg/m^2 i.v. over 3 h on day 1
  (total dose/cycle, 175 mg/m^2) *followed by*
Carboplatin i.v. over 60 min on day 1. Dosage is calculated by the Calvert formula to achieve a
  target AUC of 5–7.5 mg/mL per min (see Table 4)[7]
Cycle is repeated every 21 days

Calvert formula[14]: Total dose (mg) = [Target AUC (mg/mL/min)] × [GFR (mL/min) + 25].

Patients with incompletely staged IA or IB grade 1 tumors, who may be referred to you for treatment, present a dilemma. Options in this scenario are (a) chemotherapy followed by observation; if CA125 becomes persistently elevated or a recurrent mass is detected, surgical reexploration is warranted; or (b) observation alone. Recent data from Europe support option b.

All stage II ovarian cancer patients should receive postoperative chemotherapy (Table 4).

Debulking: Optimal Versus Suboptimal

The size of residual masses of tumor after debulking correlates with prognosis. Optimal debulking is defined as no residual tumor mass larger than 1 to 2 cm, and suboptimal debulking as residual tumor masses greater than 1 to 2 cm. It is not clear whether it is the act of debulking or the biologic nature of the tumor that permits optimal debulking that is responsible for the prognosis; nevertheless, all patients should be debulked to the smallest amount of residual tumor that is technically feasible.

Treatment of Advanced Stage Disease (III and IV)

Optimally Debulked Patients

After optimal debulking, the standard of care for patients with advanced-stage disease is to receive paclitaxel and either cisplatin or carboplatin for six cycles (Table 4). In patients who achieve a complete response (CR) after six cycles of chemotherapy, clinical trials are evaluating the possible benefit of (a) several additional cycles of chemotherapy beyond the sixth cycle, and (b) prolonged maintenance chemotherapy.

Suboptimally Debulked Patients

Patients with bulky stage III/IV who are not candidates for surgery at the time of diagnosis, or who are unable to be debulked initially because of medical or surgical reasons, may be considered for neoadjuvant chemotherapy, if pathologic diagnosis has been confirmed.

INTERVAL CYTOREDUCTION FOR SUBOPTIMAL ADVANCED OVARIAN CANCER

A European Organization for Research and Treatment of Cancer randomized trial showed a survival advantage for patients who underwent interval surgical cytoreduction after three cycles of cisplatin plus cyclophosphamide. This trial, after several additional years of follow-up, is still showing a survival advantage for interval cytoreduction. Results of a current trial performed by the Gynecologic Oncology Group with cisplatin/paclitaxel are awaited.

Failure to normalize CA125 by three cycles of chemotherapy is a poor prognostic sign.

Is Reoperation Needed for Referred Patients Diagnosed by Previous Surgery?

It is important to review a patient's medical record to determine if their prior surgery was complete and adequate. If staging is inadequate, then a reoperation is recommended, followed by stage-appropriate standard care as explained earlier. Some would consider initial chemotherapy with the possibility of a second-look laparotomy a viable option for stage III or IV patients if there was a low level of suspicion of residual disease from the previous surgery.

Second-Look Laparotomy

The role of second-look laparotomy is still being debated. The current standard of care is that it is acceptable and appropriate in a clinical trial; otherwise second-look laparotomy is not mandated. Second-look laparotomy has not been shown in a randomized trial to prolong survival. If it is performed and residual disease is found, patients should continue on their prior chemotherapy if they were responding; otherwise they should be treated with salvage therapy. Residual disease, including microscopic residual disease, will be found in approximately 50% of patients who have had a CR to chemotherapy, as documented by physical examination, CT scan, and CA125 level.

Debulking of residual disease at the time of second-look laparotomy is also controversial. Because some trials have reported a survival advantage for patients who achieved optimal secondary debulking, it would seem reasonable to perform debulking surgery in patients undergoing second-look laparotomy.

FOLLOW-UP OF OVARIAN CANCER PATIENTS

The standard of community care is:

- Visits every 3 months for 2 years, and then every 6 months for 3 years with H&P.
- CA125 levels should be measured each visit if they were initially elevated.
- Complete blood count (CBC) annually.
- Chest radiograph may be obtained for patients with initial disease of stage III/IV.

It is important to ensure that breast cancer screening is being performed. Women who are suspected of having a BRCA mutation should have mammographies starting at age 35 years. Those who are not suspected of having a BRCA mutation should begin mammography at age 40 to 50 years.

Other tests are to be ordered as indicated by signs/symptoms, including abdominal/pelvic CT scans.

TREATMENT OF RECURRENT, REFRACTORY, AND PROGRESSIVE OVARIAN CANCER

Primary Progressive Disease

Patients whose tumors progress on primary chemotherapy have an extremely poor prognosis.

These patients can be offered participation in a clinical trial or second-line therapy, as in Table 5. Supportive care is an acceptable option for patients with a very poor performance status, depending on patient preference (9,10).

TABLE 5. *Second-line agents for recurrent ovarian cancer*

Drugs	Treatment description	Cycle duration	Response rates (CR + PR)
Altretamine (Hexalen®, Hexamethyl-melamine)[15,16]	Altretamine, 65 mg/m² per dose p.o. 4 times daily (not to exceed 400 mg/day), after meals and at bedtime, for 14 days (d 1–14; total dose/cycle, 3,640 mg/m²)[15] *OR* Altretamine, 1.5 mg/kg per dose p.o. 4 times daily, after meals and at bedtime, for 21 days (d 1–21; total dose/cycle, 126 mg/kg)	28 days 28 days	14% in platinum-refractory patients 18% in platinum-refractory patients
Oral etoposide (VePesid®)[17,18]	Etoposide, 100 mg/day p.o. for 14 days (d 1–14; total dose/cycle, 1,400 mg/m²) A "low-toxicity" regimen *OR* Etoposide, 50 mg p.o. twice daily for 7 days (cycle 1, d 1–7; total dose/cycle, 700 mg/m²) (cycle 2, d 1–10; total dose/cycle, 1,000 mg/m²) (cycle 3–6, d 1–14; total dose/cycle, 1,400 mg/m²) If tolerated, treatment duration may be increased from 7 to 10 d, and then 14 d during repeated cycles	21 days 21 days, for six cycles	26% in platinum-resistant patients
Fluorouracil + leucovorin[19]	Leucovorin, 500 mg/m² per day i.v. daily over 30 min for 5 days (d 1–5; total dose/cycle, 2,500 mg/m²), followed by Fluorouracil, 375 mg/m² per day i.v. bolus daily for 5 days (d 1–5; total dose/cycle, 1,875 mg/m²) 5-FU started 1 h after completing leucovorin	21 days	10–17%
Gemcitabine (Gemzar®)[20]	Gemcitabine, 1,000 mg/m² per week i.v. over 30 min, weekly for 3 wk (d 1, 8, & 15; total dose/cycle, 3,000 mg/m²)	28 days	19%
Ifosfamide (Ifex)[21]	Ifosfamide, 1,000 mg/m² per day i.v., daily for 5 days (d 1–5; total dose/cycle, 5,000 mg/m²), *PLUS* Mesna, 200 mg/m² i.v. for three doses each day for 5 days (d 1–5; total dose/cycle, 3,000 mg/m²) Immediately before ifosfamide and at 4 h and 8 h after ifosfamide *OR* Ifosfamide, 1,200 mg/m² per day i.v., daily for 5 days (d 1–5; total dose/cycle, 6,000 mg/m²), *PLUS* Mesna, 240 mg/m² i.v. for three doses each day for 5 days (d 1–5; total dose/cycle, 3,600 mg/m²) Immediately before ifosfamide and at 4 h and 8 h after ifosfamide	28 days, for six cycles	12% in platinum-refractory patients
Liposomal Doxorubicin (Doxil)[22]	Liposomal doxorubicin, 50 mg/m² i.v. (d 1; total dose/cycle, 50 mg/m² For ADRs ≥grade 3 severity, decrease dose to 40 mg/m² For ADRs ≥grade 1 severity that persist until the start of a subsequent cycle, increase cycle duration by 1 wk (up to 5 wk)	21 days	26% in 35 evaluable platinum-refractory patients
Tamoxifen[23]	Tamoxifen, 20 mg p.o. twice daily (total dose/day, 40 mg)	Continuously	13% in platinum-refractory patients
Topotecan[24] (Hycamtin®)	Topotecan, 1.5 mg/m² per day i.v. over 30 min daily for 5 days (d 1–5; total dose cycle, 7.5 mg/m²)	21 days	5.9–13.3% in platinum-refractory patients
Vinorelbine[25] (Navelbine®)	Vinorelbine, 25 mg/m² i.v. weekly (total dose/week, 25 mg/m²)	Weekly	15% in platinum-refractory patients

5-FU, 5-fluorouracil; ADR, adverse drug reaction; CR, complete response; PR, partial response.

Persistent Disease

Patients who have persistently elevated CA125 and/or clinically evident disease after primary surgery and chemotherapy but have a reduced tumor burden compared with their immediate postoperative level are said to have "persistent disease" and a poor prognosis. Patients who have microscopic disease discovered at second-look laparotomy are a subset of this group; however, they have a better prognosis. Options include prolonged chemotherapy with the initial agents (i.e., paclitaxel with either carboplatin or cisplatin), participation in a clinical trial, or use of one of the second-line agents in Table 6.

Recurrent Disease

Although up to half of patients will achieve a complete clinical response with surgery and taxane/platinum-containing chemotherapy, most of these patients will relapse within the first 3 years after therapy. Patients who relapse less than 6 months after the completion of therapy are considered platinum and taxane resistant (if treated with the standard taxane/platinum-based regimen); they should be treated with a second-line agent (Table 6) alone or be considered for a clinical protocol.

Patients who relapse more than 6 months after their initial chemotherapy are considered "potentially platinum (and taxane) sensitive" (11). They may still respond to platinum-based agents or paclitaxel and preferably should be treated with these agents as monotherapy or in combination, reserving second-line therapy for patients whose tumors progress. Response rates to platinum retreatment range from 25% to 56%. For patients whose tumors progress with cisplatin or carboplatin, paclitaxel treatment can be considered. Regimens for potentially platinum/taxane-sensitive patients are listed in Table 5.

Potentially platinum/taxane-sensitive patients whose tumors progress with platinum and/or paclitaxel can be enrolled in clinical trials (including intraperitoneal chemotherapy) or treated with one of the second-line agents (Table 6). There is no definitive evidence for superiority of one second-line agent over another; although the response rates are different, this cannot be used to compare regimens because of variation in patient selection. Toxicity profile, performance status, and quality of life should all be considered in the decision about which agent to recommend. There is no proven benefit for combinations of second-line agents versus monotherapy in platinum-resistant patients.

TABLE 6. *Treatment of relapsed patients with potentially platinum-sensitive ovarian cancer*[7,9]

Carboplatin i.v. over 60 min on day 1; dosage is calculated by the Calvert formula to achieve a target AUC of 5–7.5 mg/mL per min[8]
Treatment cycle repeats every 3–4 wk
OR
Paclitaxel, 175 mg/m^2 i.v. over 3 h; treatment cycle repeats every 3 wk
(total dose/cycle, 175 mg/m^2)
OR
Paclitaxel, 75–80 mg/m^2 i.v. over 1 h weekly
(total dose/cycle, 75–80 mg/m^2 per wk)
OR
Paclitaxel, 175 mg/m^2 i.v. over 3 h on day 1
(total dose/cycle, 175 mg/m^2) *PLUS*
Carboplatin i.v. over 60 min on day 1; dosage is calculated by the Calvert formula to achieve a target AUC of 5–7.5 mg/mL per min[a]
Treatment cycle repeats every 3–4 wk

[a]Calvert formula[14]: Total dose (mg) = [Target AUC (mg/mL/min)] × [GFR (mL/min) + 25].

Median overall survival is less than 12 months in platinum-refractory patients treated with second-line chemotherapy. There is no consistent correlation between response rate and progression-free survival.

Recurrent Disease Manifest by Increasing CA125 Alone

For patients found to have elevated CA125 during follow-up, with a normal abdominal/pelvic CT and physical examination, there is no evidence that immediate cytotoxic chemotherapy achieves an improvement in survival. Patients can continue to be monitored for clinical relapse before initiating therapy for recurrent disease, although many oncologists feel strongly about initiating therapy in a minimal disease state. In the interim, tamoxifen, an agent with a demonstrated response rate in platinum-refractory disease and relatively low toxicity, is a reasonable nonprotocol treatment option.

NEWER METHODS OF ADMINISTERING CHEMOTHERAPY

Intraperitoneal Chemotherapy

A randomized trial demonstrated a survival advantage with the use of intraperitoneal (i.p.) cisplatin + i.v. cyclophosphamide versus i.v. cisplatin + cyclophosphamide (12). Not all patients are appropriate candidates for i.p. chemotherapy, and optimal benefit was observed in women whose maximal diameter of tumor after debulking was less than 0.5 cm. If i.p. chemotherapy is desired, it is best at this time to enroll patients in ongoing clinical trials.

High-Dose Chemotherapy with Stem Cell Transplant

There is no convincing evidence that high-dose chemotherapy with stem cell (or bone marrow) transplantation is superior to conventional chemotherapy in relapsed ovarian cancer; no randomized controlled trials have been completed. Further clinical trials are ongoing.

SPECIAL TOPICS

Supportive Care

The terminal phase of ovarian cancer involves caring for patients with various cancer-related complications, the most common being pain, bowel obstruction, urinary tract obstruction, and anorexia and cachexia.

- Adequate pain control should be maintained in patients; level of pain should be included among the vital signs evaluated during every examination.
- Bowel obstruction: Supportive. If not resolving, laparotomy with lysis of adhesions or intestinal bypass as needed and safe to perform.
- Urinary tract obstruction: Nephrostomy tubes (usually placed percutaneously; occasionally endoscopically).

REFERENCES

1. Landis SH, Murray T, Bolden S, et al. *Cancer statistics, 1999. CA Cancer Clin J* 1999;49:8–32.
2. Jacobs I, Skates SJ, MacDonald N, et al. Screening for ovarian cancer: a pilot randomised controlled trial. *Lancet* 1999;353:1207–1210.
3. Whitmore AS, Gong G, Intyre J. Prevalence and contribution of BRCA1 mutations in breast cancer and ovarian cancer: results from three U.S. population-based case-control studies of ovarian cancer. *Am J Hum Genet* 1997;60:496–504.
4. Terdiman JP, Conrad PG, Sleisenger MH. Genetic testing in hereditary colorectal cancer: indications and procedures. *Am J Gastroenterol* 1999;94:2344–2356.

5. Rubin SC, Blackwood A, Bandera C, et al. BRCA1, BRCA2, and hereditary nonpolyposis colorectal cancer gene mutations in an unselected ovarian cancer population: relationship to family history and implications for genetic testing. *Am J Obstet Gynecol* 1998;178:670–677.
6. Hoskins WJ, McGuire WP, Brady MF, et al. The effect of diameter of largest residual disease on survival after primary cytoreductive surgery in patients with suboptimal residual epithelial ovarian carcinoma. *Am J Obstet Gynecol* 1994;170:974–979.
7. Ozols RF. Update of the NCCN ovarian cancer practice guidelines. *Oncol Am* 1997;11:95–105.
8. Young RC, Walton LA, Ellenberg SS, et al. Adjuvant therapy in stage I and stage II epithelial ovarian cancer. *N Engl J Med* 1990;332:1021–1027.
9. Sabbatini P, Spriggs D. Salvage therapy for ovarian cancer. *Oncology* 1998;12:833–851.
10. Alberts DS. Treatment of refractory and recurrent ovarian cancer. *Semin Oncol* 1999;26:8–14.
11. Markman M, Rothman R, Hakes T, et al. Second-line cisplatin treatment in patients with ovarian cancer previously treated with cisplatin. *J Clin Oncol* 1991;9:389–393.
12. Alberts DS, Liu PY, Hannigan EV, et al. Intraperitoneal cisplatin plus intravenous cyclophosphamide versus intravenous cisplatin plus intravenous cyclophosphamide for stage III ovarian cancer. *N Engl J Med* 1996;335:1950–1995.
13. McGuire WP, Hoskins WJ, Brady MF, et al. Taxol and cisplatin improve outcome in patients with advanced ovarian cancer as compared to cytoxan/cisplatin. *N Engl J Med* 1996;334:1–6.
14. Calvert AH, Newell DR, Gumbrell LA, et al. Carboplatin dosage; prospect of evaluation of a simple formula based on renal function. *J Clin Oncol* 1989;7:1748–1756.
15. Manetta A, MacNeill C, Lyter JA, et al. Hexamethylmelamine as a single second-line agent in ovarian cancer. *Gynecol Oncol* 1990;36:93–96.
16. Vergote I, Himmelmann A, Frankendal B, et al. Hexamethylmelamine as second-line therapy in platinum-resistant ovarian cancer. *Gynecol Oncol* 1992;47:282–286.
17. Hoskins PJ, Swenerton KD. Oral etoposide is active against platinum-resistant epithelial ovarian cancer. *J Clin Oncol* 1994;12:60–63.
18. Seymour MT, Mansi JL, Gallagher CJ, et al. Protracted oral etoposide in epithelial ovarian cancer: a phase II study in patients with relapsed or platinum-resistant disease. *Br J Cancer* 1994;69:191–195.
19. Reed E, Jacob J, Ozols RF, et al. 5-Fluorouracil (5-FU) and leucovorin in platinum-refractory advanced stage ovarian cancer. *Gynecol Oncol* 1992;46:326–329.
20. Shapiro JD, Millward MJ, Rischin D, et al. Activity of gemcitabine in patients with advanced ovarian cancer: responses seen following platinum and paclitaxel. *Gynecol Oncol* 1996;63:89–93.
21. Markman M, Hakes T, Reichman B, et al. Ifosfamide and mesna in previously treated advanced epithelial ovarian cancer: activity in platinum-resistant disease. *J Clin Oncol* 1992;10:243–248.
22. Muggia F, Hainsworth JD, Jeffers S, et al. Phase II study of liposomal doxorubicin in refractory ovarian cancer: antitumor activity and toxicity modification by liposomal encapsulation. *J Clin Oncol* 1997;15:987–993.
23. Markman M, Iseminger KA, Hatch KD, et al. Tamoxifen in platinum-refractory ovarian cancer: a Gynecologic Oncology Group ancillary report. *Gynecol Oncol* 1996;62:4–6.
24. Creemers GJ, Bolis G, Gore M, et al. Topotecan, an active drug in the second-line treatment of epithelial ovarian cancer: results of a large European phase II study. *J Clin Oncol* 1996;14:3056–3061.
25. Bajetta E, Di Leo A, Biganzoli L, et al. Phase II study of vinorelbine in patients with pretreated advanced ovarian cancer: activity in platinum-resistant disease. *J Clin Oncol* 1996;14:2546–2551.

17

Endometrial Carcinoma

Margaret Wojtowicz[*], Hung T. Khong[**], Samir Khleif[*]

[*]Medicine Branch, DCS, National Cancer Institute, National Institutes of Health, Bethesda, Maryland; [**]Surgery Branch, DCS, National Cancer Institute, National Institutes of Health, Bethesda, Maryland

EPIDEMIOLOGY

- The most common pelvic gynecologic malignancy (13% of all cancers in women).
- 37,400 new cases are diagnosed in 1999 (the incidence has been constant since the 1980s of 22/100,000).
- An estimated 6,400 deaths due to this malignancy are predicted yearly (the mortality rate has been constant since 1989 at 3/100,000).
- Mortality is around 2 times higher in African-American (AA) than in white women. However, the incidence is 1.4 times higher in white women than in AA.
- Peak incidence is in the sixth and seventh decades of life (5% of cases are diagnosed before age 40 years; 20% to 25% will be diagnosed before menopause).

RISK FACTORS

Unopposed estrogens, which include:
1. Endogenous source secondary to:
   - Polycystic ovary disease.
   - Anovulatory menstrual cycles.
   - Obesity: overweight by 21 to 50 lb increases the risk threefold, and by more than 50 lb, increases the risk tenfold.
   - Granulosa cell tumor of the ovary (or other estrogen-secreting tumors).
   - Advanced liver disease.
   - Early menarche and late menopause. Menopause at older than 52 years increases the risk 2.4-fold.
2. Exogenous, including tamoxifen (TAM), a weak estrogen that increases the relative risk (RR) of developing endometrial cancer to 2.3.
   - Irregular menses, infertility, and nulliparity: Nulliparous women have twice the risk of developing uterine cancer compared with women with one child, and this risk increases to three times as compared with women with five or more children.
   - Diabetes mellitus (DM).
   - Hypertension.
   - Family history. History of endometrial cancer in a first-degree relative increases risk three times, and history of a colorectal cancer in a first-degree relative increases risk of an endometrial cancer by two times.
   - Patient history of breast, ovarian, or colorectal cancer.

PROTECTIVE FACTORS

- Oral contraceptives: there is a 50% decrease in an RR when used for at least 12 months. This protection lasts for at least 10 years after discontinuation.
- Cigarette smoking: there appears to be a modest protective role of cigarette smoking. However, this is strongly outweighed by the significant increased risk of lung cancer and other major health hazards.

DIAGNOSIS/SCREENING

- There is no role for routine screening for endometrial cancer in asymptomatic women.
- Women taking tamoxifen should have a gynecologic evaluation as per the recommendation for women who are not taking this drug. Endometrial biopsy should be done when the patient is symptomatic (vaginal bleed or spotting).

Signs and Symptoms

- Abnormal vaginal bleeding (most common in ~90% of cases). Premenopausal women with prolonged and/or heavy menses, or intermenstrual spotting require endometrial biopsy. All postmenopausal women with vaginal bleeding should be evaluated for endometrial cancer (20% of these patients will ultimately be diagnosed with the malignancy). Biopsy is also recommended in women taking estrogen therapy for menopausal symptoms who may have withdrawal bleeding.
- Asymptomatic patients with abnormal Pap smear should be evaluated for endometrial cancer if cervical cancer was excluded (~10% of uterine cancer cases are detected by a Pap smear). Pap smear, however, is not an adequate tool for detection of endometrial malignancy.
- Palpable, locally advanced tumor, detected on pelvic examination.
- Signs and symptoms of advanced disease (manifestation in <10% of cases): bowel obstruction, jaundice, ascites, pain, etc.

Procedures

- Endocervical curettage and outpatient endometrial biopsy.
- Pap smear is of limited value (see earlier).
- Fractional curettage under anesthesia: this method involves scraping of the endocervical canal and then walls of the uterus in a set sequence. It is a procedure of choice for the diagnosis of endometrial cancer, used in symptomatic women with negative or inadequate endometrial biopsy.
- Transvaginal ultrasound (U/S): available data suggest a correlation between endometrial stripe, as seen on U/S, with endometrial thickness and subsequent risk of endometrial cancer. Either less than 4 mm or less than 5 mm "cutoff" of endometrial stripe has been used as a diagnostic criterion; however, occasional cases of endometrial cancer could still be missed. Therefore there is no general agreement on a cutoff thickness of endometrial stripe for the recommendation of endometrial biopsy. All patients taking TAM have thicker endometrium than their counterparts with no TAM.

HISTOLOGY

- Endometrioid (75% to 80%).
- Uterine papillary serous (<10%).
- Mucinous (1%).
- Clear cell (4%).
- Squamous cell (<1%).

- Mixed (10%).
- Undifferentiated.

Endometrial carcinoma may also be divided into two types (I and II) according to its dependence on estrogen:

Type I: Estrogen related. It is the more common type, associated with DM and obesity, tends to have better prognosis (more differentiated; higher incidence of superficial invasion, lower grade, and lower stage; higher progesterone receptor levels; and younger patients).

Type II: Unrelated to estrogen stimulation and endometrial hyperplasia, less common, usually has a short duration of symptoms, poor differentiation, deep myometrial invasion, poor prognosis, more aggressive histology (serous, clear cell).

Adenomatous hyperplasia: An estrogen-dependent lesion, which could be seen along with type I but not type II endometrial carcinoma. Other more favorable histologic subtypes such as endometrioid, mucinous, and secretory are also associated solely with type I disease.

PRE-THERAPY EVALUATION

- Physical examination.
- Chest radiograph (CXR).
- Urinary imaging studies (i.v. pyelogram/renal scan), cystoscopy, proctoscopy (very rarely done).
- Routine blood and urine studies.
- Evaluation of specific symptoms or physical examination findings, as indicated.
- Routine use of U/S, computed tomography (CT) scan, magnetic resonance imaging (MRI), and bone scan rarely adds useful information and is not recommended.

STAGING

- Staging for endometrial carcinoma is surgical (Table 1), by using information from hysterectomy, bilateral salpingo-oophorectomy (BSO), peritoneal cytology, pelvic and periaortic lymph node (LN) dissection.

  Endometrial cancer distribution by stage:

  Stage I: 73%.
  Stage II: 12%.
  Stage III: 12%.
  Stage IV: 3%.

PROGNOSTIC FACTORS

Uterine

- Histologic type.
- Histologic differentiation.
- Stage of disease [5-year survival (%) distribution by stage: I- 86%; II- 66%; III- 44%; IV- 16%).
- Myometrial invasion.
- Vascular space invasion (gives ~25% rate of disease recurrence).

  Extrauterine

- Positive peritoneal cytology (rate of disease recurrence seen was ~15%).

TABLE 1. *Staging for endometrial cancer: 1988*

Stage IA G123	Tumor limited to endometrium
Stage IB G123	Invasion to less than one half of the myometrium
Stage IC G123	Invasion to more than one half of the myometrium
Stage IIA G123	Endocervical glandular involvement only
Stage IIB G123	Cervical stromal invasion
Stage IIIA G123	Tumor invades aeorea and/or adroxa, and/or positive peritoneal cytology
Stage IIIB G123	Vaginal metastases
Stage IIIC G123	Metastases to pelvic and/or paraaortic lymph nodes
Stage IVA G123	Tumor invasion of bladder and/or bowel mucosa
Stage IVB	Distant metastases including intraabdominal and/or inguinal lymph nodes

Histopathology: Degree of differentiation

Cases of carcinoma of the corpus should be classified (or graded) according to the degree of histologic differentiation, as follows:

G1, 5% of a nonsquamous or nonmorular solid growth pattern
G2, 6% to 50% of a nonsquamous or nonmorular solid growth pattern
G3, >50% of a nonsquamous or nonmorular solid growth pattern

Notes on pathologic gradings
1. Notable nuclear atypia, inappropriate for the architectural grade, raises the grade of a grade 1 or grade 2 tumor by 1.
2. In serious adenocarcinomas, clear-cell adenocarcinomas, and squamous cell carcinomas, nuclear grading takes precedence.
3. Adenocarcinomas with squamous differentiation are graded according to the nuclear grade of the glandular component.

Rules related to staging
1. Because corpus cancer is now staged surgically, procedures previously used for determination of stages are no longer applicable, such as the findings from fractional dilation and curettage to differentiate between stage I and II.
2. It is appreciated that there may be a small number of patients with corpus cancer who will be treated primarily with radiation therapy. If that is the case, the clinical staging adopted by FIGO in 1971 should still apply, but designation of that staging system would be noted.
3. Ideally, width of the myometrium should be measured along with the width of tumor invasion.

FIGO, Federation Internationale de Gynecogie et d'Obstetrique.
Adopted from DiSaia PJ, Creasman WT. *Clinical gynecologic oncology.* 5th ed. St. Louis: Mosby, 1997:140–141, with permission.

- **LN metastasis:** Involvement of pelvic LN or peritoneal metastases poses ~25% risk for disease recurrence, whereas metastasis to periaortic LN increases this risk to 40%.
- **Adnexal metastasis** (~15% recurrence risk). Also:
- **Tumor hormone-receptor status:** the presence of estrogen receptor (ER)/progesterone receptor (PgR) and their levels were found to be inversely proportional to histologic grade and associated with a longer survival.
- **Tumor size:** Tumors of more than 2 cm have worse prognosis.
- **Molecular factors:** DNA ploidy, p53 overexpression (however, most studies are small, use different techniques and cutoff values; more standardization is needed before conclusions can be drawn).

MANAGEMENT

- **Endometrial hyperplasia:** TAH/BSO is the treatment of choice for patients with persistent endometrial hyperplasia after the failure of adequate therapy with progestin.
- **Endometrial carcinoma:** Therapy should be individualized.

Stage I, IIA

1. **Total abdominal hysterectomy with bilateral salpingo-oophorectomy (TAH/BSO); selected pelvic LN may be removed).** This is considered adequate for patients with well or moderately differentiated tumors, with negative peritoneal cytology (if no peritoneal fluid is found during surgery, peritoneal washing with normal saline should be done); no vascular space invasion; and less than 50% myometrial invasion.
2. **TAH/BSO combined with paraortic and selective pelvic LN sampling/dissection.** If there are no medical or technical contraindications (e.g., morbid obesity), this should be done in: tumors involving more than 50% of outer myometrium, tumor presence in cervical isthmus, or the adnexal and other extrauterine metastases, in cases of serous, clear cell, undifferentiated, or squamous histology, as well as in cases of LN enlargement (visible or palpable).
3. **Followed by postoperative total pelvic irradiation** for tumors with deep myometrial invasion, grade 2 or 3 histology, and vascular space invasion, as well as with cervical involvement. Radiation doses of 45 to 50 Gy of standard fractionation and daily treatments of multiple fields with small-bowel protection are applied.

Special Considerations

- Patients who are not surgical candidates should be treated with radiation therapy alone; however, this may achieve an inferior cure rate as compared with surgery.
- Combined surgery and external radiation carries a higher complication rate than either treatment alone (e.g., bowel complications, 4%). Therefore, special attention should be given to appropriate patient selection, choice of surgical techniques [e.g., with retroperitoneal approach, fewer complications are seen, as well as with LN sampling vs. LN dissection (trials comparing conventional TAH/BSO and pelvic, periaortic LN dissection vs. laparascopic pelvic and periaortic LN dissection, BSO, and vaginal hysterectomy are ongoing)].
- Pelvic surgery carries an increased risk for pelvic and lower extremities thrombophlebitis; hence, low-dose heparin or venodyne boots should be used in these patients.
- In case of papillary serous tumor histology, because of higher rate of vaginal, pelvic, and upper abdomen recurrences seen with this histology, treatment recommendations include whole-abdominal irradiation for up to 30-Gy dose and additional treatments to reach a pelvic dose of 50 Gy. A vaginal cylinder or colpostats can be used to give an additional surface dose of 40 Gy (5-year survival of 50% was documented with this approach).

Stage IIB

1. **Hysterectomy, bilateral salpingo-oophorectomy, and periaortic LN sampling, followed by postoperative radiation.** The radiation therapy is administered as an external beam to a dose of 45 to 50 Gy along with vaginal irradiation with vaginal cylinder or colpostats to bring the vaginal surface dose to 80 to 90 Gy (5-year disease-free survival of 80% and locoregional control of 90% were seen with this treatment).
2. **Combination of preoperative intracavitary radiation** (consisting of uterine tandem and vaginal colpostat insertions with a standard Fletcher applicator delivering 20 to 25 Gy to a point A[1]) and external beam radiation (dose of 40 to 45 Gy with standard fractionation delivered to multiple fields). In patients with extensive cervical involvement precluding initial hysterectomy, the external beam radiation should be followed in 4 to 6 weeks by hysterectomy and bilateral salpingo-oophorectomy with periaortic LN sampling (this approach, can provide 5-year disease-free survival of 70% to 80%).
3. **Radical hysterectomy and pelvic LN dissection** (selected cases).

---

[1]Point A is defined as a point located 2 cm caudal and 2 cm lateral to the cervical os.

Stage III

Surgery and combination of intracavitary and external beam radiation:

- Special considerations.
- Women with isolated ovarian metastasis form a subgroup with a relatively better prognosis. Five-year disease-free survival ranges between 60% and 82% (depending on the histologic grade of tumor and the depth of myometrial invasion). The pelvic radiation doses given are 45 to 50 Gy in standard fractionation and vaginal boost with a cylinder or colpostats adding 30 to 35 Gy to the vaginal surface. However, some believe that this represents double primary tumors rather than true metastasis from primary endometrial cancer.
- If tumor extends to the pelvic wall, patients would be considered inoperable and should be treated with radiation.
- When parametrial extension is present, preoperative radiation (external and intracavitary) is applied.
- If the pelvic and/or paraaortic LNs are involved with tumor, patients should be treated with extended-field radiation (encompassing pelvic and periaortic regions) by using 45- to 50-Gy doses, and they may be candidates for clinical trials including radiation and/or chemotherapy, as they are at higher risk for recurrence (see earlier).
- Patients who are not candidates for either surgery or radiation are treated with progestational agents (see later).
- Whole-abdominal radiation should be considered for patients with positive peritoneal washings or micrometastases in the upper abdomen.
- Stage III patients are at high risk for distant metastases (in the upper abdomen and extraabdominal sites). Therefore these patients are candidates for experimental clinical trials.

Stage IV and Recurrent Disease

- Therapy recommendations depend on the sites of metastasis or recurrent disease and the disease-related symptoms.
- **Pelvic exenteration** can be considered for patients with disease extending only to the bladder or rectum (tumor tissue should be checked for ER and PgR levels) and for isolated central recurrence after irradiation (some long-term survivals have been reported).
- **Radiation** (palliative): applied for localized recurrences, e.g., pelvic (external-beam radiation together with brachytherapy boost), paraaortic LN, or distant metastases.
- In isolated vaginal recurrence (if not previously given), irradiation may be curative.
- **Hormonal therapy** produces responses in 15% to 30% of patients associated with improved survival (two times longer than those seen in nonresponders). On average, responses last 1 year.
- When distant metastases are present (most common sites are abdominal cavity, liver, and lungs), hormonal therapy can be given (hormone-receptor levels and degree of tumor differentiation correlate well with responses).

Drugs and Regimens Most Frequently Used in Uterine Cancer

Hormonal Therapy

- Medroxyprogesterone acetate (Depo-Provera), 400 to 1,000 mg i.m. weekly for 6 weeks, and then monthly, *OR*
- Oral medroxyprogesterone (Provera), approximately 150 mg p.o. daily.
- Megestrol acetate (Megace), 40 to 80 mg p.o. 4 times daily.
- Tamoxifen, 10 mg p.o. twice daily.

Only modest response rates were seen; one report documented responses in nine patients out of 17 treated with the higher doses of 40 mg/day, but it remains unclear whether this will translate into a more favorable outcome.

Chemotherapy for Palliative Purposes Only

- No standard chemotherapy is available.
- Chemotherapy use is restricted mainly to stage IVB or recurrent disease or nonresponders to hormonal therapy.
- On average, duration of responses is around 4 months, and survival is 9 months.
- The most active agents are Doxorubicin (35–40% RR), cisplatin (36% RR), and Paclitaxel (35.7% RR).
- Multiple reported trials tested various combination regimens, but to date there has been no prospective comparison of doxorubicin with combination regimens that show superiority of the combination. However, one phase III trial conducted by GOG (comparing doxorubicin, 60 mg/m² every 3 weeks, with doxorubicin, 60 mg/m² plus cisplatin, 50 mg/m² every 3 weeks) has shown a superior response rate for the combination versus doxorubicin alone (45% vs. 27%). Thus far, progression-free interval and survival were similar. This has been reported only in abstract form.

Combination of Chemotherapy and Hormonal Therapy

Response rates of 17% to 86% were reported, similar to results achieved with chemotherapy alone. Hormonal therapy followed by chemotherapy would be the preferred therapeutic strategy. However, initiation of treatment with chemotherapy or use of progestins/chemotherapy combination may be considered in patients with life-threatening or rapidly progressive metastatic disease.

All patients should be considered for clinical trials.

ESTROGEN-REPLACEMENT THERAPY

In patients with endometrial cancer, this remains controversial.

POST-THERAPY SURVEILLANCE (SUGGESTED)

- No standard schedule is available.
- Most recurrences are seen in the first 3 years after primary therapy.
- Asymptomatic patients with no evidence of disease could be monitored:
  Every 3 months for the first year.
  Every 3 to 4 months during the second year.
  Every 6 months during the third to fifth years.
  Annually after 5 years.

REFERENCES

1. DiSaia PJ, Creasman WT. *Clinical gynecologic oncology.* 5th ed. St. Louis: Mosby, 1997.
2. Ball HG, Elkadry EA. Endometrial cancer: current concepts and management. *Surg Oncol Clin North Am* 1998;7:271–284.
3. Yamada SD, McGonigle KF. Cancer of the endometrium and corpus uteri. *Curr Opin Obstet Gynecol* 1998;10:57–60.
4. Sabbatini P, Aghajanian C. Chemotherapy in gynecologic cancers. *Curr Opin Oncol* 1998;10:429–433.
5. Bergman C, Boente M. Surgery for gynecologic malignancies. *Curr Opin Oncol* 1998;10:434–438.
6. Thigpen T, Blessing J, Homsley H, et al. Phase III trial of doxorubicin +/- cisplatin in advanced or recurrent endometrial carcinoma: a Gynecologic Oncology Group study. *Proc ASCO* 1993;12:261.
7. Barakat RR, Greven K, Muss HB. Endometrial cancer. In: Pazdur R, Coia LR, Hoskins WJ, et al., eds. *Cancer management: a multidisciplinary approach.* 3rd ed. New York: PRR Melville, 1999:269–285.
8. NCI-Pdq Pahe at http://cancernet.nci.nih.gov/clinpdq/soa/Cervical cancer Physician.html

18

Cervical Cancer

Margaret Wojtowicz*, Hung T. Khong**, and Samir Khleif*

*Medicine Branch, DCS, National Cancer Institute, National Institutes of Health,
Bethesda, Maryland; **Surgery Branch, DCS, National Cancer Institute,
National Institutes of Health, Bethesda, Maryland*

EPIDEMIOLOGY

Worldwide

- One of the most common cancers in women (6% of all female malignancies).
- More than 470,000 new cases are diagnosed each year.
- 350,000 women will die each year as a consequence of this disease.
- Only second after breast cancer in incidence of mortality.

United States

- 16,000 new cases of invasive cervical cancer are diagnosed annually.
- 5,000 deaths per year is still higher than expected, even if adequate screening with Pap smear and pelvic examination is done on all eligible women (about one third of eligible women do not have appropriate screening).
- The lifetime risk for developing cervical cancer is 0.88%. The lifetime risk of dying from it is 0.29%.
- Incidence of cervical carcinoma. The incidence is higher among women with a history of sexually transmitted diseases [e.g., human papillomavirus (HPV) infection and herpes simplex virus (HSV) infection].

RISK FACTORS

Human Papilomavirus (HPV)

- 85% to 93% of cervical cancers harbor HPV DNA. A history of genital warts increases the risk of developing cervical cancer by 18-fold.
- HPV types 6, 11, 42, 43, and 44 are some of the viruses of "low oncogenic potential" that are associated with benign cervical lesions.
- HPV types 16, 18, 31, and 45 are viruses of "high oncogenic potential" that are associated with high-grade cervical intraepithelial neoplasia (CIN) and invasive cervical cancer.
- The oncogenic effect appears to be mediated by E6 and E7 proteins of high-risk HPV subtypes. The E6 and E7 proteins have been shown to inactivate tumor-suppressor genes p53

and pRb, respectively, with subsequent loss of the cell-cycle regulatory mechanism leading to malignant transformation.

- Based on current clinical data, there is no evidence that knowing whether a cervical cancer harbors HPV would affect clinical outcome or management. Therefore, routine HPV typing is not recommended except in a clinical trials setting.

Demographic Factors

- Race: Higher among Latin American, African-American, American Indian women.
- Socioeconomic status: More prevalent in lower socioeconomic classes.
- Education: Higher among undereducated.
- Age: More common in older women.

Personal/Sexual Factors

- Sexual partners: History of more than six sexual partners increases the relative risk (RR) to 2.2 times background incidence. Women married to a man whose previous partner developed cervical cancer have threefold increase in the risk of developing the disease. History of genital warts increases the incidence by 18-fold. Penile cancer in a man places a woman at higher risk for cervical cancer.
- Age at first intercourse before 18 years, RR = 1.6.
- Smoking: RR increased to 1.7.
- Oral contraceptive use for more than 10 years, RR = 2.2.
- Nutrition: Higher risk in patients on diets that are deficient in folate, carotene, or vitamin C.

Medical/Gynecologic Factors

- Parity: More common among multiparous women (RR = 1.5–5.0) and early parous women
- PAP (Papanicolaou) smear: Prior abnormal PAP smear or documented dysplasia is associated with an increased risk.
- Immunosuppression: Renal transplant (RR = 5.7), human immunodeficiency virus (HIV) infection [cervical cancer in HIV(+) women defines acquired immunodeficiency syndrome (AIDS) as per the Centers for Disease Control (CDC) criteria] (8).

SCREENING

- As per the American Cancer Society recommendations: asymptomatic, low-risk, 20 years old or older women and women younger than 20 years who are sexually active should have PAP smear annually for 2 consecutive years and at least every 3 years until the age of 65.
- American College of Obstetricians and Gynecologists recommends screening with annual PAP smear for all women who are or who have been sexually active or are 18 years old. After three consecutive normal annual PAP smears, low risk women can be screened at less frequent intervals at the discretion of her physician, e.g., every 2- to 3- years. If they are at high risk, PAP smear should continue to be done on an annual basis.
- Any patient with a history of cervical dysplasia should be screened minimally at yearly intervals.
- Cervical cytology (Table 1).

TABLE 1. *Nomenclature in cervical cytology*

	Classification	
Papanicolaou	World Health Organization	Bethesda system
Class I: Absence of atypical or abnormal cells	Normal	Negative, within normal limits
Class II: Atypical cytology but no evidence of malignancy	Atypical	Reactive or reparative changes Atypical squamous cells of undetermined significance (ASCUS) Atypical glandular cells of undetermined significance (AGCUS)
Class III: Cytology suggestive of but not conclusive for malignancy	Dysplasia Mild dysplasia	Squamous intraepithelial lesion (SIL) Low-grade squamous intraepithelial lesion (LGSIL)
	Moderate dysplasia Severe dysplasia	High-grade squamous intraepithelial lesion (HGSIL)
Class IV: Cytology strongly suggestive of malignancy	Carcinoma in situ	High-grade squamous intraepithelial lesion (HGSIL)
Class V: Cytology conclusive for malignancy	Squamous cell carcinoma Adenocarcinoma	Suggestive of or positive for malignancy Squamous cell carcinoma Adenocarcinoma

Adopted from Wright TC, Richart RM. Pathogenesis and diagnosis of pre-invasive lesions of the lower genital tract. In: Orr JW, Shingleton HM. *Cancer of the cervix.* Philadelphia, JB Lippincott, 1995:40, with permission.

PRECURSOR LESIONS

• Dysplasia and cervical intraepithelial neoplasia (CIN).
• CIN III if left untreated will progress to invasive cancer over the period of 20 years in more than 12% of cases.

SIGNS AND SYMPTOMS

• Abnormal vaginal bleeding (i.e., postcoital, intermenstrual, and menorrhagia) is usually a first manifestation.
• Vaginal discharge (serosanguineous or yellowish, sometimes foul smelling) usually represents a more advanced lesion.
• Fatigue and other anemia-related symptoms are seen in patients with chronic bleeding.
• Pain in lumbosacral or gluteal area, possibility of iliac or periaortic lymph node (LN) involvement with extension to the lumbar roots or hydronephrosis.
• Urinary or rectal symptoms (hematuria, rectal bleeding, etc.) can be seen with bladder or rectal involvement.
• Leg edema (persistent, unilateral or bilateral) results from lymphatic and venous blockage due to extensive pelvic wall disease.

PHYSICAL EXAMINATION

• Can be normal.
• Most frequent findings: visible cervical lesion or abnormal bimanual pelvic examination.

DIAGNOSTIC WORKUP

- History.
- Physical examination (including bimanual pelvic and rectal examinations).

Diagnostic Procedures

- PAP smear, if no gross lesion
- Colposcopy.
- Conization (subclinical tumor).
- Punch biopsies (edge of gross tumor, four quadrants).
- Dilatation and curettage.
- Cystoscopy, rectosigmoidoscopy (stages IIB, III, IVA).

Radiologic Studies

- Chest radiograph (CXR).
- Intravenous pyelography or computed tomography (CT) scan with i.v. contrast.
- Barium enema (stage III, IVA, and earlier stages if there are symptoms referable to colon or rectum).
- Magnetic resonance imaging (MRI) if needed for better disease evaluation.

Laboratory Studies

- Complete blood count.
- Blood chemistries.
- Urinalysis.

HISTOLOGY

Cervical carcinoma originates at the squamous–columnar junction of the cervix (transformation zone). Of cervical cancers, 85% to 90% are of squamous cell histology. The remaining 10% to 15% are mostly adenocarcinomas.

STAGING

- In contrast to other gynecologic malignancies, cervical cancer is a clinically staged disease (Table 2).
- Surgical staging is more accurate than clinical staging; however, there is no evidence that it will lead to improvement in the overall survival. Therefore surgical staging should be done only as part of a clinical trial.

PROGNOSTIC FACTORS

Based on Gynecologic Oncology Group (GOG) experience (where para-aortic LN staging was obligatory), multivariate analysis showed:

TABLE 2. *International Federation of Gynecology and Obstetrics Staging of Carcinoma of the Cervix (1994)*

Stage	Definition
Stage 0	Carcinoma in situ, intraepithelial carcinoma; cases of Stage 0 should not be included in any therapeutic statistics for invasive carcinoma
Stage I	The carcinoma is strictly confined to the cervix (extension to the corpus should be disregarded).
Stage IA	Invasive cancer identified only microscopically. All gross lesions, even with superficial invasion, are stage IB cancers. Invasion is limited to measured stromal invasion with a maximum depth of 5 mm and no wider than 7 mm. (The depth of invasion should not be >5 mm taken from the base of the epithelium, either surface or glandular, from which it originates. Vascular space involvement, either venous or lymphatic, should not alter the staging.)
Stage IA1	Measured invasion of stroma ≤3 mm in depth and no wider than 7 mm
Stage IA2	Measured invasion of stroma >3 mm and no greater than 5 mm in depth and no wider than 7 mm
Stage IB	Clinical lesions confined to the cervix or preclinical lesions greater than IA
Stage IB1	Clinical lesions ≤4 cm
Stage IB2	Clinical lesions >4 cm
Stage II	The carcinoma extends beyond the cervix, but has not extended onto the pelvic wall; the carcinoma involves the vagina, but not as far as the lower third
Stage IIA	No obvious parametrial involvement
Stage IIB	Obvious parametrial involvement
Stage III	The carcinoma has extended onto the pelvic wall; on rectal examination there is no cancer-free space between the tumor and the pelvic wall; the tumor involves the lower third of the vagina; all cases with a hydronephrosis or nonfunctioning kidney should be included, unless they are known to be due to other cause
Stage IIIA	No extension onto the pelvic wall, but involvement of the lower third of the vagina
Stage IIIB	Extension onto the pelvic wall or hydronephrosis or nonfunctioning kidney
Stage IV	The carcinoma has extended beyond the true pelvis or has clinically involved the mucosa of the bladder or rectum
Stage IVA	Spread of the growth to adjacent organs
Stage IVB	Spread to distant organs

(Adapted from International Federation of Gynecology and Obstetrics. Staging announcement: FIGO staging of gynecologic cancers: cervical and vulva. *Int J Gynecol Cancer* 1995;5:319 with permission)

- Para-aortic LN involvement as the most important negative prognostic factor, followed by pelvic LN involvement, larger tumor size, younger age, and advanced stage: 5-year survival (%) is dependent on the stage: 0, 95% to 100%; I, 80%; II, 60; III, 30%; IV, 5%.
- Lymph–vascular invasion and tumor grade.
- It remains controversial whether adenocarcinoma of the cervix carries a worse prognosis than does squamous cell cancer.

MODE OF SPREAD

Cervical cancer is a locally progressive and destructive tumor with the following spread pattern.

- Local: into vaginal mucosa or myometrium, or direct extension into adjacent structures or parametria.
- Lymphatic: most commonly involved LNs are pelvic, paraaortic.
- Hematogenous: most common sites are lung, liver, and bone.

MANAGEMENT

Stage 0 (CIN)

Loop electrosurgical excision procedure (LEEP) allows excision of the entire transformation zone of the cervix with a low-voltage diathermy loop (usually 25–50 watts, but the larger the loop, the higher the wattage needed) (Fig. 1).

In very selected situations, a LEEP may be an acceptable alternative to cold-knife conization because it is a quick, outpatient procedure requiring only local anesthesia. However, current data do not support LEEP as a adequate replacement for conization.

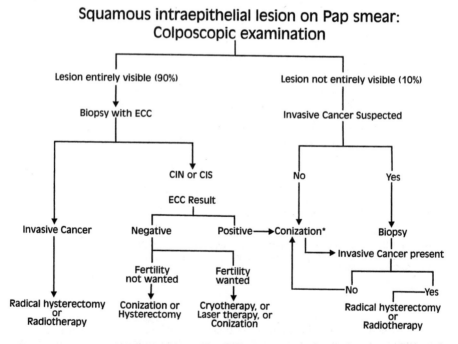

FIG. 1. Management of patients with positive PAP smear cytologies and early cervical carcinoma of the uterine cervix. *CIS*, Carcinoma in situ; *ECC*, endocervical curettage. *If invasion is not found on conization, patients are followed up with Pap smears, biopsies, or repeated conization, depending on the patient and patient's age.

Invasive Cervical Cancer

- Treatment in each stage may vary, depending on the size of the tumor.
- Results from five recently reported randomized phase III trials demonstrated an overall survival advantage for cisplatin-based chemotherapy given concurrent with radiation therapy. These trials have demonstrated an overall reduction in reduction in risk of death by 30% to 50% in patients with FIGO stage IB2 to IVA, and in patients with FIGO I to IIA with poor prognostic factors (pelvic LN involvement, parametrial disease, positive surgical margins). Therefore, strong consideration should be given to concurrent cisplatin-based chemotherapy and radiation treatment in women who require radiation therapy for treatment of cervical cancer.

Cisplatin doses various regimens, doses (cisplatin, 40–75 mg/m^2 i.v.), and schedules (cisplatin daily or weekly) have been used for concurrent cisplatin-based chemotherapy and radiation. The optimal therapy for locally advanced cervical cancer has not yet been established.

Some regimens use cisplatin as a single agent, once weekly, 40 mg/m^2 i.v. for a maximum of six doses given concurrent with radiation.

When chemotherapy is used in combination [e.g., 5-fluorouracil (5-FU)/cisplatin], a cisplatin dose of 50 to 75 mg/m^2 has been given on various schedules concomitant with radiation.

Stage IA1

See Fig. 2.

Stage IA2, IB, IIA

1. Radical hysterectomy with bilateral pelvic LN dissection and para-aortic LN sampling.

or

2. Radiation therapy: external beam pelvic irradiation with intracavitary applications.
   - Radiation dose is defined as the energy absorbed per unit mass (joule per kilogram of tissue: J/kg). The unit of absorbed dose is the Gray (Gy): 1 Gy equals 1 J/kg and is equivalent to 100 centigray (cGy) or 100 rad.
   - Higher central doses of radiation can be delivered with the combination of external beam radiation and intracavitary irradiation as compared with the external radiation therapy alone. This combination method leads to an improved pelvic control and survival.
   - HDR (high dose rate, 200–300 cGy/min) versus LDR (low dose rate, 50–60 cGy/h) brachytherapy is still controversial, and it is being tested.
   - Radioactive isotopes (e.g., cesium 137) are introduced into the uterine cavity and vaginal fornices with special applicators (the most commonly used applicator is the Fletcher–Suit intrauterine tandem and vaginal ovoids).
   - The important issues that must be addressed in delivering radiation for therapy of cervical cancer are the maximum bladder and rectal doses and the dose delivered to the three standard pelvic points: A, B, and P (Fig. 3).
   - **Point A** is located 2 cm caudal and 2 cm lateral to the cervical os. Anatomically it correlates with the medial parametrium/lateral cervix, the point where the ureter and uterine artery cross. **Point B** is located 5 cm lateral to the center of the pelvis at the same level as point A. Anatomically it correlates to the obturator LN or lateral parametrium.
   - **Point P** is located at the most lateral point of the bony pelvic sidewall. Represents the minimal dose to the external iliac LN.

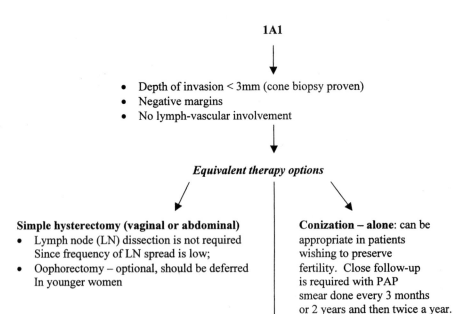

1A1

- Depth of invasion < 3mm (cone biopsy proven)
- Negative margins
- No lymph-vascular involvement

Equivalent therapy options

Simple hysterectomy (vaginal or abdominal)
- Lymph node (LN) dissection is not required
  Since frequency of LN spread is low;
- Oophorectomy – optional, should be deferred
  In younger women

Conization – alone: can be appropriate in patients wishing to preserve fertility. Close follow-up is required with PAP smear done every 3 months or 2 years and then twice a year.

Intracavitary radiation alone (reserved for inoperable patients)
- 1 or 2 insertions with tandem and ovoids for a total dose of approximately 5.500 cGy to point A (see below)
- no external beam radiation is required since frequency of LN(--) is low

FIG. 2. Management of stage 1A cervical cancer.

- Typical doses of external radiation are 40 to 50 Gy followed by 40 to 50 Gy to point A with brachytherapy for a total dose of 80 to 90 Gy to point A. Depending on the extent of disease, a parametrial boost may be applied to point B or P for a total dose of 60 Gy with external beam radiation and brachytherapy.

- Surgery and radiation are equivalent treatment options for stages IB and IIA with identical 5-year overall survival (OS) and disease-free survival (DFS). Expected cure rate is 75% to 80% (85–90% in small-volume disease).
- The choice of surgery versus radiation depends on many factors including tumor size, younger women wishing to preserve their ovaries, other comorbid conditions, and the availability of local expertise.
- For bulky (4 cm or greater) stage IB2 disease, the pelvic control, which is 57%, and survival, which is 40%, are lower than for nonbulky tumors (smaller than 4 cm; total pelvic control and survival rates are 93% and 82%, respectively) if treated with radiation alone. Adjuvant hysterectomy could potentially improve these statistics. Based on current data, both radiation alone and radiation combined with hysterectomy are acceptable local therapy options for bulky IB2 disease. However, recently published data from

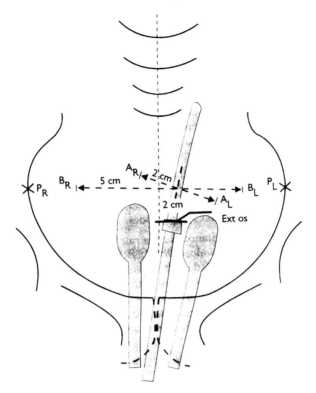

FIG. 3. GOG definitions of points A, B, and P.

the GOG study support addition of (weekly) cisplatin (40 mg/m^2 for up to six doses) to radiotherapy followed by hysterectomy, because it reduces recurrence and death rate in this patient population. The use of adjuvant hysterectomy remains controversial in disease of smaller than 4 cm IB2 disease.

- Postradiation surgery may be a consideration in patients with residual tumor confined to the cervix or in patients with suboptimal brachytherapy due to vaginal anatomy (Table 3).
3. **Postoperative pelvic irradiation (with or without chemotherapy) after radical hysterectomy and bilateral pelvic LN dissection** applied to patients with negative pelvic nodes who are at risk for pelvic failure (primary tumor greater than 4 cm, outer third cervical stromal invasion, lymph–vascular space invasion, close vaginal margins (less than 0.5 cm). This provides reduction in recurrence rate and improved survival.
  - It is also recommended for patients with positive pelvic nodes, as this was shown to reduce pelvic failure rates by 25%. However, radiation therapy alone did not improve survival compared with surgery.

Radiation doses used are 45 to 50 Gy by external pelvic radiation, with boosts given to specific sites (as needed) with external beam, intracavitary, or interstitial radiation.

TABLE 3. *Radiation versus surgery for stages IA₂, IB, and IIA*

Therapy	Advantages	Disadvantages
Radiation	Can be applied to all patients	0–1% operative mortality in the case of intercavitary application 2–6% serious bladder/bowel damage, destruction of ovary function, vaginal stenosis, and sexual dysfunction, especially common in postmenopausal women
Surgery	Possible ovary conservation; documents exact tumor extent; complications appear early and are correctable; more functional vagina	<1% operative mortality, 3–4% long-term bladder dysfunction, 1–2% urinary fistulas/strictures. Postop radiation needed in 10–15% cases; vaginal shortening and sexual dysfunction; cannot be applied in morbidly obese and some elderly patients

Modified from Orr JW. Cervical cancer. *Surg Oncol Clin North Am* 1998;7:299–317, with permission.

Special considerations:

- Patients with suspected or confirmed paraaortic nodal disease should receive extended-field radiation encompassing pelvic and paraaortic areas. Current data confirm survival advantage (in stage IB, larger than 4 cm, IIA, IIB) with addition of external beam paraaortic radiation over external beam pelvic irradiation alone. Some patients with small-volume disease in paraaortic LNs and controllable pelvic disease can potentially be cured. However, in gross paraaortic disease, the role of radiation is limited, as tolerance of surrounding organs (bowel, kidney, spinal cord) precludes delivery of adequately high radiation doses.
- Toxicity from paraaortic LN radiation is somewhat greater than that in pelvic radiation alone, but is seen mostly in patients with prior abdominopelvic surgery.
- Different surgical techniques alter the rate of complications (e.g., extraperitoneal LN sampling led to fewer complications than seen in transperitoneal approach).

Stages IIB, III, IVA

The role of surgery as a curative treatment decreases when tumor spreads beyond the cervix and vaginal fornices. Patients presenting with tumors at these stages are treated with:

- Radiation therapy plus chemotherapy: where brachytherapy is given for central pelvic disease and external beam radiation is for lateral parametrial and pelvic nodal disease. Chemotherapy used is cisplatin-based (see earlier for details). In the GOG, standard therapy is weekly cisplatin chemotherapy combined with radiation.
- For patients without paraaortic LN involvement: external beam pelvic radiation of 45 to 50 Gy followed by brachytherapy with 40 to 50 Gy to point A for a total dose of 80 to 90 Gy (applies to stages IB2–IVA). Patients with paraaortic LNs involved will benefit from extended-field radiation covering the paraaortic area.

- Special considerations:
- Based on multivariate analysis, therapeutic factors associated with improved pelvic tumor control and survival in cervical cancer patients were: use of intracavitary radiation, total

dose of more than 8,500 cGy to point A (stage III only), and overall treatment time less than 8 weeks.

Stage IVB

Radiation is used for palliation of central disease or distant mets.
Chemotherapy

- No standard chemotherapy provides substantial palliation.
- All patients are appropriate candidates for clinical trials.
- The most active single agents include:
  1. Cisplatin, 50 mg/m^2 (usual dose as a single agent or in combination regimens) i.v. once every 3 weeks for a maximum of six cycles. RR of 18% to 31% is documented. Higher doses (e.g., 100 mg/m^2 i.v. once every 3 weeks) produce higher RRs, but toxicity is greater, and response duration, survival, and progression-free survival were similar to those seen with the 50-mg/m^2 dose.
  2. Carboplatin: 15% RR. Less nephrotoxicity and neurotoxicity as compared with cisplatin; thus carboplatin may be considered an alternative to cisplatin in selected patients.
  3. Ifosfamide, lead to 16% to 33% RR in advanced disease, 15% RR in recurrent disease.
  4. Paclitaxel, has 17% to 25% RR.
  5. Irinotecan, provides 13% to 21% RR.

Combination chemotherapy has not been consistently shown to be superior to single agent (e.g., cisplatin).

- Responses are of brief duration.
- Benefit of chemotherapy with or without radiation versus best supportive care in this group of patients has not yet been established.

Recurrent disease

No standard therapy is available for recurrent disease outside previous surgical or radiation field (Table 4).

TABLE 4. *Recurrent disease*

Stage	Site of failure (%)	
	Pelvic	Distant metastases
IB	10	9
IIA	17	17
IIB	23	15
III	42	20
IVA	74	22

Adopted from Perez CA, Grigsby PW, Camel HM, et al. Irradiation alone or combined with surgery in stage IB, IIA and IIB carcinoma of uterine cervix: update of a nonrandomized comparison. *Int J Radiat Oncol Biol Phys.* In Hoskins WJ, Perez CA, Young RC. *Principles and practice of gynecologic oncology.* 2nd ed. Philadelphia: Lippincott, 1997:840, with permission.

1. **Radiation combined with 5-FU ± mitomycin chemotherapy:**
   • Used for recurrence in the pelvis after radical surgery.
   • From 40% to 50% of these patients may be cured.
2. **Pelvic exenteration** (resection of the bladder, rectum, vagina, uterus/cervix).
   • Used for locally recurrent disease.
   • From 32% to 62% 5-year survival can be achieved in selected patients.
   • Reconstruction is possible; continent urinary conduit, rectal anastomosis, myocutaneous neovagina.
3. **Chemotherapy:** palliative, not curative. Agents tested: see list for IVB (provides low response rates, short response duration and overall survival).

TREATMENT OF CERVICAL CANCER IN PREGNANCY

• Preinvasive lesion: No therapy is warranted; colposcopy is recommended to rule out invasive cancer.
• Invasive cancer: Treatment depends on the tumor stage and gestational age. If cancer is diagnosed before fetal maturity, immediate appropriate cancer therapy for the relevant stage is recommended. However, some reports suggest that with stage IA and early IB treatment, delay to allow fetal maturity may still be a reasonable option. If diagnosis is made in the final trimester, treatment may be delayed.

TREATMENT OF CERVICAL CANCER IN HIV-INFECTED WOMEN

• These women have more aggressive and more advanced disease with poorer prognosis than do the HIV-negative cervical cancer patients.
• The same standard therapy is used for preinvasive lesions and invasive cervical cancer in HIV-positive as in HIV-negative patients.
• Response to therapy is usually worse than that in patients with no HIV infection.

FOLLOW-UP AFTER PRIMARY THERAPY

Optimal post-treatment surveillance has not been determined. 80% to 90% of tumor recurrences appear in the first 2 years after therapy. Therefore most oncologists schedule follow-up visits frequently: e.g., every 3 to 4 months for 1 year, every 4 months for 1 year, every 6 months for 3 years and then annually to detect any potentially curable recurrences.

ACKNOWLEDGMENT

We would like to thank Dr. Helen Frederickson for critical review of this chapter.

REFERENCES

1. Hoskins WJ, Perez CA, Young RC. *Principles and practice of gynecologic oncology.* 2nd ed. Philadelphia: Lippincott-Raven, 1997.
2. Orr JW, Shingleton HM. *Cancer of the cervix.* Philadelphia: JB Lippincott, 1995.
3. Orr JW. Cervical cancer. *Surg Oncol Clin North Am* 1998;7:299–317.
4. Elkas J, Farias-Eisner R. Cancer of the uterine cervix. *Curr Opin Obstet Gynecol* 1998;10:47–50.
5. Morris M, Eifel PJ, Lu J. Pelvic radiation with concurrent chemotherapy compared with pelvic and para-aortic radiation for high risk cervical cancer. *N Engl J Med* 1999;340:1137–1143.
6. Rose P, Bundy B, Watkins E. Concurrent cisplatin-based radiotherapy and chemotherapy for locally advanced cervical cancer. *N Engl J Med* 1999;340:1144–1153.

7. Keys H, Bundy B. Cisplatin, radiation, and adjuvant hysterectomy compared with radiation and adjuvant hysterectomy for bulky stage IB cervical cancer. *N Engl J Med* 1999:340:1154–1161.
8. Coleman RL, Miller DS. Topotecan in the treatment of gynecological cancer. *Semin Oncol* 1997; 24(suppl 20):S20–S63.
9. Sabbatini P, Aghajanian C, Spriggs D. Chemotherapy in gynecological cancer. *Curr Opin Oncol* 1998;10:429–433.
10. Bergman C, Boente M. Surgery for gynecologic malignancies. *Curr Opin Oncol* 1998;10:434–438.
11. Pazdur R, Coia LR, Hoskins WJ, et al. Cancer management: a multidisciplinary approach. In: *Medical, surgical and radiation oncology.* 3rd ed. New York: PRR Melville, 1999:xx–xx.
12. NCI-PDQ Page at http://cancernet.nci.nih.gov/clinpdq/soa/Cervical_cancer_Physician.html.
13. National Cancer Institute. Concurrent chemoradiation for cervical cancer: February 1999. NCI Cancer Resource Page available at http://cancertrials.nci.nih.gov/NCI CANCER TRIALS/zones/TrialInfo/News/cervcan/clinann.html.
14. Canavan TP, Doshi NR. Cervical cancer. *Am Fam Physician* 2000;61(5):1369–1376.
15. Koh WJ, Panwala K, Greer B. Adjuvant therapy for high-risk, early stage cervical cancer. *Semin Radiat Oncol* 2000;10(1):51–60.
16. Ostor AG. Natural history of cervical intraepithelial neoplasia: a critical review. *Int J Gynecol Pathol* 1993;12(2):186–192.

19

Vulvar Cancer

Margaret Wojtowicz*, Hung T. Khong**, and Samir Khleif*

*Medicine Branch, DCS, National Cancer Institute, National Institutes of Health, Bethesda, Maryland; **Surgery Branch, DCS, National Cancer Institute, National Institutes of Health, Bethesda, Maryland

EPIDEMIOLOGY

- Accounts for 4% of all female genital malignancies.
- Most frequent in women between 65 and 75 years old, occasionally diagnosed before 40 years.

ETIOLOGY/RISK FACTORS

- Etiology remains unclear.
- Human papillomavirus (HPV) DNA, especially type 16, found in 80% of intraepithelial lesions and 10% to 15% of invasive vulvar cancers (especially squamous cell).
- Association with veneral or granulomatous lesions has been documented.
- Lichen sclerosis was reported to coexist with up to 25% of vulvar cancers.
- Vulvar intraepithelial neoplasia (VIN), especially high grade (VIN III) increases risk for development of vulvar cancer.
- Classic risk factors such as hypertension, diabetes mellitus, and obesity most probably represent conditions associated with aging, and not truly independent risk factors for this malignancy.

HISTOLOGY

Squamous cell carcinomas (SCCs) constitute more than 90% of cases, and melanomas from 5% to 10%. The remainder are adenocarcinoma, basal cell carcinoma, verrucous, sarcoma, and other rare tumors.

VULVAR SQUAMOUS CELL CARCINOMA

Vulvar squamous cell carcinoma is commonly indolent, with slow extension and late metastases. Signs and symptoms in order of decreasing frequency are pruritus, mass, pain, bleeding, ulceration, dysuria, and discharge.

Diagnostic workup

- Biopsy, cystoscopy, proctoscopy, chest radiograph (CXR), and i.v. urography if needed, based on extent of disease.
- Suspected bladder or rectal involvement must be biopsied.

Indications for excisional biopsy of vulvar lesions:

- Any gross lesion
- Red, white, dark brown, or black skin patches.
- Areas firm to palpation.
- Pruritic, tingling, or bleeding lesions.
- Any nevi in the genital tract.
- Enlarged or thickened areas of Bartholin's glands, especially in postmenopausal women.

Location and metastatic spread pattern of vulvar SCC

- Found on labia majora in 50% of cases, and in labia minora in 15% to 20%; the reminder are on the clitoris and perineum.
- Tends to grow locally, with subsequent spread to inguinal, femoral, and pelvic lymph nodes (LNs). Hematogenous spread usually takes place after LN involvement.

Staging (Table 1)

- Vulvar cancer is a surgically staged disease.

Prognostic factors and survival (true for most histologies).

- Depends on stage, LN involvement, depth of invasion, structures involved, and tumor location.
- Survival is most dependent on the pathologic status of the inguinal LNs and the size of the primary lesion (<2-cm lesion, inguinal LN(−): 98% 5-year survival; any size lesion, three or more unilateral LN(+), or two or more bilateral LN(+), 29% 5-year survival.
- Lymph node metastases are related to tumor size, clinical stage, and depth of invasion.

Management

Stage 0

The following are equally effective therapeutic approaches:

1. **Wide local excision**, laser beam therapy, or their combination.
2. Skinning vulvectomy ± grafting.

In some cases, a 5% fluorouracil (FU) cream can be used [Response rate (RR) 50–60%], but it is not a first choice of therapy.

Recurrences are seen regardless of type of procedure used for initial treatment (most common sites: perianal skin, presacral area, clitoral hood).

Stage I

- Less than 1-mm invasion: **wide local excision.**
- From 1- to 5-mm invasion: **modified radical vulvectomy with ipsilateral superficial inguinal lymphadenectomy** for lesions located laterally, and **bilateral node dissection** for centrally placed lesions.

TABLE 1. *Staging*

TNM		Staging (FIGO) 1988	
T Primary tumor			
Tis	Preinvasive carcinoma (carcinoma in situ)	Stage 0 Tis	Carcinoma in situ; intraepithelial carcinoma
		Stage I T1 N0 M0	Tumor confined to the vulva and/or *perineum*—2 cm or less in greatest dimension. *No nodal metastases*
T 1	Tumor confined to the vulva and/or *perineum*—2 cm or less in diameter		
T 2	Tumor confined to the vulva and/or *perineum*—more than 2 cm in diameter	Stage II T2 N0 M0	Tumor confined to the vulva and/or *perineum*—more than 2 cm in greatest dimension. *No nodal metastases*
T 3	Tumor of any size with adjacent spread to the urethra, vagina, anus or all of these	Stage III T3 N0 M0 T3 N1 M0	Tumor of any size with the following: (1) Adjacent spread to the lower urethra, the vagina, the anus, and/or the following: (2) *Unilateral regional lymph node metastases*
T 4	Tumor of any size infiltrating the bladder mucosa or the rectal mucosa or both, including the upper part of the urethral mucosa or fixed to the anus	Stage IVA T1 N1 M0 T1 N2 M0 T2 N2 M0 T3 N2 M0 T4 any N M0	Tumor invades any of the following: Upper urethra, bladder mucosa, rectal mucosa, pelvic bone, and/or *bilateral regional lymph node metastases*
N Regional lymph nodes			
N 0	No nodes palpable		
N 1	*Unilateral regional lymph node metastases*		
N 2	*Bilateral regional lymph node metastases*		
M Distant metastases		Stage IVB any T, any N, M1	*Any distant metastases, including pelvic lymph nodes*
M 0	No distant metastases		
M 1	Distant metastases (*including pelvic lymph node metastases*)		

Italicized words indicate changes from the pre-1988 definitions.
Adopted from Creasman WT. *Obstet Gynecol* 1990;75:287, with permission.

Special considerations:

• Inoperable patients can be treated with radiation therapy, achieving long-term survival.
• Surgical complications: mortality, 2% to 5%; wound breakdown/infection, sepsis, thromboembolism, chronic leg lymphedema (use of separate incision for the groin LN dissection reduces wound breakdown and leg edema), urinary tract infection, stress urinary incontinence, and poor sexual function.

Stage II

Modified radical vulvectomy and bilateral inguinal lymphadenectomy can be used if at least 1 cm of negative margins can be achieved with preservation of midline structures.

Stages III and IV

• See Figure 1. Special considerations:
• Management of positive groin nodes: one LN, no further therapy; two or more LNs, groin and pelvic radiation therapy (based on GOG randomized trial data in which improved survival was documented as compared with pelvic LN dissection).
• Suggested doses of localized adjuvant radiation: 45 to 50 Gy.
• Radiation can be used preoperatively in stage III and IV to shrink the lesion thus improving its resectability. Suggested dose of preoperative radiation: 55 Gy with concomitant 5-FU.

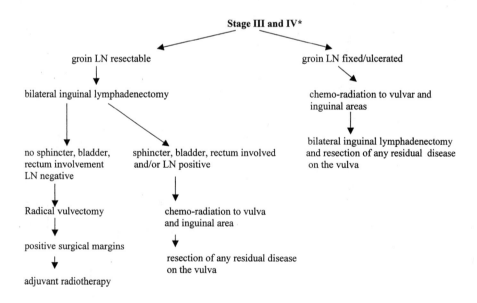

*Adopted from DiSaia PJ and Creasman WT, "Clinical Gynecologic Oncology", 5th ed. Mosby,1997:222.

FIG. 1. Management algorithm for stage III and IV disease.

- Inoperable patients can achieve long-term survival with radical radiation therapy.
- When radiation is given as primary definitive treatment, it is suggested that the addition of 5-FU ± cisplatin be considered [four different phase II clinical trials showed a complete response (CR) rate of 53% to 89% in patients treated for unresectable primary disease or before exenterative surgery. Two reports cited disease-free survival of 47% to 84% at median follow-up of 37 months].
- Radiation fraction size of less than or equal to 180 cGy proved to minimize the radiation complication rate (late fibrosis, atrophy, telangiectasia, necrosis). Total doses of 54 to 65 Gy should be used.

Recurrent/Metastatic Disease

- Treatment and outcome depend on site and extent of recurrence.
- **Local recurrence** can be treated with wide local re-excision ± radiation (5-year survival of 56% if regional LNs are negative). In small localized recurrence, radiation ± 5-FU can be curative in some patients.
- Another option is radical vulvectomy and pelvic exenteration.
- **Groin nodes:** radiation and surgery.
- **Distant recurrence:** no standard systemic chemotherapy is available for metastatic disease. These patients are appropriate candidates for clinical trials. Agents such as cisplatin, methotrexate, cyclophosphamide, bleomycin, and mitomycin C have shown a partial RR of only 10% to 15%, and they are of short duration (few months).

VERRUCOUS CARCINOMA

- Very rare; can be confused with condyloma acuminatum because of exophytic growth pattern.
- Locally destructive, rarely metastasizes.
- Associated with HPV type 6.
- Main treatment is surgery; LN dissection is of questionable value unless LN are obviously involved. Radiation is contraindicated because it is not effective and can potentially lead to more aggressive behavior.

PAGET'S DISEASE

- Preinvasive lesion.
- Most frequent symptoms: pruritus, tenderness, or vulvar lesion (hyperemic, well demarcated, thickened, with areas of induration and excoriation).
- Can be associated with underlying adenocarcinoma of the vulva (1–2%). These patients should be treated the same way as are patients with other vulvar malignancies.

MALIGNANT MELANOMA

- Rare tumor (5% of all melanoma cases).
- Majority are located on the labia minora and clitoris.
- Prognosis depends on size of the lesion and depth of invasion.
- Staging as for skin melanoma.
- Suggested therapy has been radical vulvectomy with inguinal and pelvic lymphadenectomy (lately tendency for a more conservative approach). 2-cm margins for thin (up to 7 mm) lesions and 3 to 4 cm margins for thicker lesions are suggested for most well-demarcated lesions.

BARTHOLIN'S GLAND
Adenocarcinoma

- Very rare tumor (1% of all vulvar malignancies).
- Peak incidence in the mid-60s.
- Enlargement of the Bartholin's gland area in postmenopausal women requires evaluation for malignancy.
- Therapy includes radical vulvectomy with wide excision to achieve adequate margins and inguinal lymphadenectomy.

Adenoid Cystic

- Very rare tumor.
- Frequent local recurrences and very slow progression.
- Recommended therapy: wide local excision with ipsilateral inguinal lymphadenectomy.

Basal Cell Carcinoma

- Natural history and therapeutic approach similar to those for primary tumors seen in other sites (i.e., wide local excision).

ACKNOWLEDGMENT

We would like to thank Dr. Helen Frederickson for critical review of this chapter.

REFERENCES

1. DiSaia PJ, Creasman WT. *Clinical gynecologic oncology.* 5th ed. St. Louis: Mosby, 1997.
2. Nash JD, Curry S. Vulvar cancer. *Surg Oncol Clin North Am* 1998;7:xx–xx.
3. NCI-PDQ Page at: http://cancernet.nci.nih.gov/clinpdq/soa/Cervical_cancer_Physician.html

SECTION 7

Musculoskeletal

20

Sarcomas and Malignancies of the Bone

V. Koneti Rao[*] and Lee Helman[**]

[*]Medicine Branch, DCS, National Cancer Institute, National Institutes of Health,
Bethesda, Maryland; [**]Pediatric Branch, DCS, National Cancer Institute,
National Institutes of Health, Bethesda, Maryland

Malignancies of the soft tissue (6.1%) and bones (4.7%) account for more than 10% of newly diagnosed cancers in children, adolescents, and young adults. Fortunately, benign musculoskeletal neoplasms are 100 times more common than malignant soft-tissue tumors. Median age at diagnosis of rhabdomyosarcoma (RMS) is 5 years, with a male preponderance. Osteosarcomas account for approximately 60% of malignant bone tumors in the first two decades of life. Most of the remaining bone malignancies in children and adolescents are Ewings' sarcomas and the histologically similar and genetically identical peripheral primitive neuroectodermal tumors (PNETs). Together, these tumors are often referred to as the Ewings' family of tumors (EFT). Chondrosarcomas are seen in older adults. Identification of specific, recurrent genetic alterations in RMS and Ewing's sarcoma has improved diagnosis by clarifying pathogenesis. Better supportive care and systematic application of effective multimodality treatment have improved survival dramatically during the past 30 years (Fig. 1, Table 1).

RHABDOMYOSARCOMA

Clinical Presentation

RMS has been encountered in almost all anatomic sites (Table 2). It is associated with development of a mass, and often, the child is not unwell unless there is metastatic disease. Orbital tumors present early with signs of proptosis. Tumors in the nasopharynx have a characteristically long history of nasal discharge and obstruction and may involve local extension into the base of the skull and posterior orbit, with the potential for associated cranial nerve palsies or visual loss and parameningeal extension. Tumors within the genitourinary tract present as a vaginal polyp or discharge (vaginal and uterine tumors), urinary obstruction (bladder and prostate tumors), or as a paratesticular scrotal mass (Fig. 2).

Pathophysiology

These tumors are of mesenchymal origin, characterized by myogenic differentiation. They are histologically distinguished into two main forms, embryonal (80%) and alveolar (15–20%) subtypes. Botryoid RMS and spindle cell sarcoma are both morphologic variants of embryonal RMS. Most alveolar RMSs demonstrate a recurrent chromosomal translocation, t(2,13)(q35;q14), or less frequently, a variant t(1;13)(p36;q14). These involve the *FKHR* gene

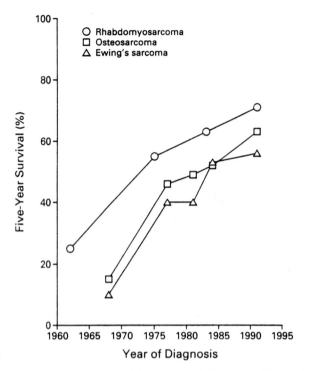

FIG. 1. Five-year survival rates among children and adolescents with rhabdomyosarcoma, those with osteosarcoma, and those with ewing's sarcoma. Data are from Link and Eilber, Horowitz et al., Crist and Kun, and the Surveillance, Epidemiology and End Results Program.

on chromosome 13, the *PAX3* gene on chromosome 2, and the *PAX7* gene on chromosome 1. Embryonal RMS shows consistent loss of heterozygosity (LOH) in the chromosome 11p15.5 locus that also happens to be the location for the *IGH-II* gene. Hyperdiploid DNA content is associated with embryonal histology, whereas tetraploid DNA content is associated with alveolar histology (Fig. 3).

Diagnosis

Diagnostic Radiology

Staging investigations must include adequate imaging of the primary site [computed tomography (CT) and/or magnetic resonance imaging (MRI)] and accurate assessment of sites of potential metastatic spread [lungs, bones, bone marrow, and cerebrospinal fluid (CSF)].

Biopsy and Pathologic Diagnosis

Aside from conventional histology showing morphologic evidence of myogenesis, immunohistochemistry (particularly for desmin and myoD1), and the identification of *PAX-FKHR* fusion genes using reverse transcription–polymerase chain reaction (RT-PCR) are

TABLE 1. *Outcome of therapy for musculoskeletal tumors of childhood and adolescence*

Type of tumor	Commonly used agents	Duration of therapy (mo)	Long-term survival (%)	Additional treatment
Rhabdomyosarcoma				
Low-risk group (those with group I or II embryonal tumors at sites with a favorable outcome or group III orbital tumors)	Vincristine, dactinomycin	8–12	90–95	Resection of primary tumor for all but orbital tumors; irradiation of group II or III tumors
Intermediate-risk group	Vincristine, dactinomycin, cyclophosphamide	8–12	70–80	Irradiation of primary tumor and metastases, if present
High-risk group [all those with metastases (group IV) except patients under 10 years old who have embryonal tumors]	Vincristine, dactinomycin, cyclophosphamide; new agents; high-dose therapy with hematopoietic stem-cell transplantation	8–12	20	Irradiation of primary tumor and all metastatic lesions
Osteosarcoma				
Localized to limb	Doxorubicin, high-dose methotrexate, ifosfamide, cisplatin	8–12	58–76	Surgery for control of tumor
Metastatic	Doxorubicin, methotrexate, ifosfamide, cisplatin	8–12	14–50	Resection of primary tumor and metastases needed for cure
Ewing's sarcoma				
Localized	Vincristine, doxorubicin, cyclophosphamide, dactinomycin, etoposide-ifosfamide	8–12	50–70	Surgery, radiation therapy, or both for local control of tumor
Metastatic	Vincristine, doxorubicin, cyclophosphamide, dactinomycin, etoposide-ifosfamide; high-dose therapy with hematopoietic stem-cell transplantation	8–12	19–30	Surgery, radiation therapy, or both for local control of tumor

The estimated rates of survival at 3–5 years without the need for retreatment (progression-free or relapse-free survival) are shown.

TABLE 2. *Associated risk factors for rhabdomyosarcoma*

Genetic	Familial cancer risk	Li–Fraumeni syndrome
	Germline mutant p53	Risk of breast cancer in female relatives[a]
	Congenital abnormalities	
	Neurofibromatosis type I	
Environmental	Parental habits	Smoking
		Recreational drugs
		Occupational chemical exposure
		Fetal alcohol syndrome

[a]Link between rhabdomyosarcoma and risk of breast cancer in a female relative plays an important role in cancer surveillance in at-risk families.

likely to become increasingly important in clarifying the diagnosis of RMS, in distinguishing it from other soft tissue or small round-cell tumors (e.g., lymphoma, neuroblastoma, and EFT), and in confirming histologic subtypes. Needle biopsy may restrict access to fresh and frozen tissue for cytogenetic and molecular genetic investigations. Open biopsy should preferably be undertaken at an oncology center, where the optimal use of diagnostic material can be achieved and the initial surgical approach determined by a multidisciplinary team responsible for the patient's subsequent treatment.

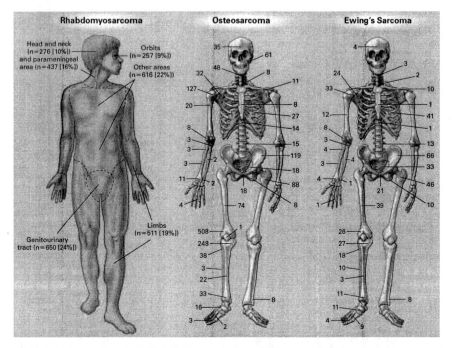

FIG. 2. Primary sites of rhabdomyosarcoma, osteosarcoma, and Ewing's sarcoma. The numbers of patients with primary tumors at specific sites are shown.

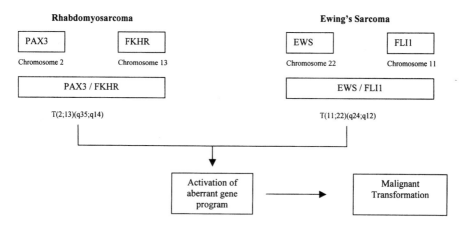

FIG. 3. Molecular pathogenetic mechanisms in rhabdomyosarcoma and Ewing's sarcoma.

Treatment Strategies Overview

The diversity of primary sites, the distinctive surgical and radiation therapy treatments for each primary site, and the subsequent site-specific rehabilitation underscore the importance of treating children and young adults with RMS in the context of a clinical trial at a major medical center with appropriate experience in all therapeutic modalities (Table 3).

Surgery

Local tumor control is the cornerstone of therapy, especially for patients with nonmetastatic disease. Primary tumor resection should be undertaken only if there is no evidence of lymph node or metastatic disease and if the tumor can be excised with good margins without functional impairment or mutilation. Surgery has little or no role in the primary management of orbital tumors, and only a limited role in the local control of head and neck tumors. However, the morbidity of radical surgery necessary to achieve local control may be preferred, to avoid pelvic irradiation in very young children.

Radiation Therapy

Radiation therapy is recommended for patients with microscopic or gross residual disease after initial surgical resection or chemotherapy. Moreover, radiation therapy may also benefit group I (completely resected tumors) patients who have less favorable prognoses (e.g., alveolar histology). In general, patients with microscopic residual disease (group II) receive 4,100 cGy and patients with gross residual disease (group III) in IRS (Intergroup Rhabdomyosarcoma Society)-IV standard treatment arm receive 5,040 cGy. The treated volume should be determined by the extent of tumor at diagnosis before surgical resection and chemotherapy, and includes a 2-cm margin adjacent to the primary tumor. Patients with parameningeal disease with intracranial meningeal extension receive whole-brain radiation (2,340–3,060 cGy) in addition to treatment of the primary tumor.

TABLE 3. *Treatment options, local control, and potential toxicity in rhabdomyosarcoma*

Treatments	Local control	Sequelae			
		Sterility	Kidneys	On growth	Esthetics
Part I. Orbit					
Radical surgery then VA ± C	++	-	-	±	±
Biopsy then radiation + V ± C	++	±	-	++	++
Biopsy then IVA/VAC	±	±	±	-	-
No complete remission:					
Radical surgery				++	++
or Radiotherapy				++	++
Part II. Paratesticular					
Surgery + VA	±	-	-	-	-
Surgery + VAC/IVA	++	±	±	-	-
Part III. Limbs					
Surgery + VA	+	-	-	-	±
Surgery + IVA	++	±	±	-	±
Part IV. Vagina					
IVA/VAC, complete remission then monitoring	+	±	±	-	-
IVA then elective surgery or interstitial radiation	++	±	±	+	+
Part V. Bladder/prostate					
Radical surgery then IVA/VAC ± selective radiotherapy	++	±	±	+	+
IVA/VAC then local surgery	+	±	±	-	±
No complete remission, radiation	±				
Part VI. Thorax, abdomen, pelvis					
IVA/VAC then selective radiation, then IVA/VAC		++	±	±	± ±
IVA/VAC,CR ± surgery then IVA/VAC	±	±	±	±	-
Part VII. Parameningeal					
IVA/VAC then extensively early radiation, then IVA/VAC	++	±	±	++	
IVA/VAC, then delayed limited radiation then IVA/VAC	±	±	±	+	
Part VIII. Nonparameningeal head and neck					
Radical surgery then VA	++	-	-	-	++
Biopsy then IVA/VAC, then either CR	±	±	±	-	-
Or non-CR and radiation				++	+
Or non-CR and surgery				-	±

IVA, ifosfamide–vincristine–actinomycin D; CR, complete remission; VA, vincristine–actinomycin D; VAC, vincristine–actinomycin D–cyclophosphamide.

Chemotherapy

It has long been recognized that neoadjuvant combination, multiagent chemotherapy given for extensive (primarily unresectable) tumors could reduce the extent of subsequent surgery or radiation therapy (Fig. 4).

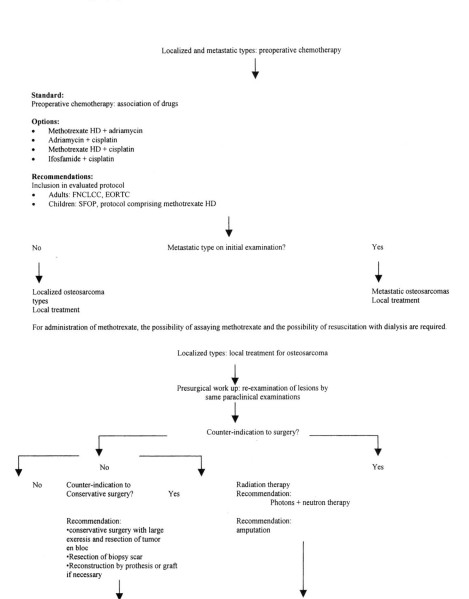

Fig. 4. Treatment options schema in osteosarcoma.

OSTEOSARCOMA

Peak incidence occurs during the pubescent growth spurt (ages 15 to 19 years) in the metaphyses of the most rapidly growing bones. Risk factors are listed in Table 4.

Symptoms

The majority of tumors arise around the knee joint in the metaphysis of the femur or tibia. The commonest mode of presentation is with bone pain and swelling. Typical radiologic features are destruction of bone with a consequent loss of normal trabeculae and the appearance of radiolucent areas. New bone formation is typical, both within the bone itself and in the soft-tissue extension. Some tumors appear completely lytic, whereas others are predominantly sclerotic. The radiologically descriptive "sunburst sign" is due to periosteal elevation caused by the tumor penetrating the cortical bone.

Diagnosis and Staging

Histologic diagnosis depends on the presence of a frankly malignant sarcomatous stroma associated with the production of tumor osteoid. It is highly recommended that if the surgeon suspects a primary malignant bone lesion after a preliminary assessment with a history, physical examination, and plain radiographs, all invasive procedures, especially the placement and technique of biopsy, be done by an experienced orthopedic oncologist.

Laboratory Investigations and Biopsy

Generous amounts of fresh and frozen tissue should be available to perform various prognostic assays including measurement of tumor DNA content, molecular genetic evaluations, and P-glycoprotein estimation. Serum lactic dehydrogenase (LDH) levels are also a powerful prognostic factor and may be elevated in 30% of patients without metastases.

Diagnostic Radiology

MRI accurately estimates tumor boundaries. It assesses the intraosseous extent of tumor and extent with respect to surrounding muscle groups, subcutaneous fat, joints, and major neurovascular structures. This helps in determining the level of amputation or in planning limb-salvage resections. T1-weighted MRI images are appropriate for this purpose and should include the entire involved bone in a longitudinal plane to detect skip metastases. Radionuclide bone scan is also indicated in the initial diagnostic evaluation to screen for metastatic disease and skip lesions. Metastases are most likely to occur in the lungs (90%), whereas regional and distant lymph node metastases are rare. CT scan of the chest is more sensitive than a plain radiograph in detection of and surveillance for pulmonary metastases. Approximately 15% to 20% of patients have clinically detectable metastases at presentation.

TABLE 4. Risk factors for osteosarcoma

Familial cancer	Li–Fraumeni syndrome
Secondary osteosarcoma	Irradiated bones
	Bilateral retinoblastoma (Independent of therapy modality)
Loss of tumor-suppressor genes	p53 and Rb (retinoblastoma)

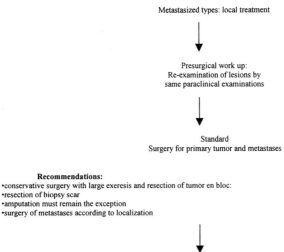

Fig. 5. Treatment options in metastatic osteosarcoma.

Management

Virtually all patients with osteosarcoma have subclinical micrometastatic disease. Thus treatment requires surgical ablation of the primary tumor (amputation or limb-sparing resection) and treatment of micrometastatic disease with chemotherapy (Figs. 4–7)

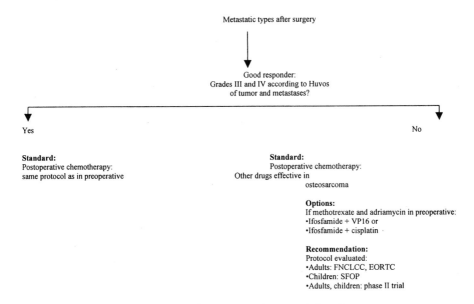

Fig. 6. Treatment options in post-operative metastatic osteosarcoma.

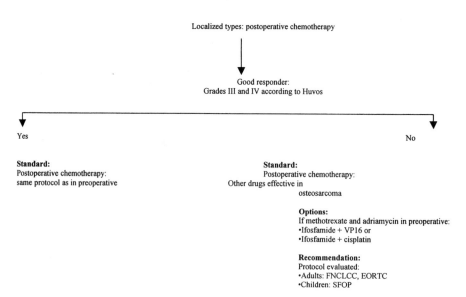

Fig. 7. Treatment options in post-operative localized osteosarcoma.

Chemotherapy

For the majority of patients, neoadjuvant chemotherapy should be initiated as soon as possible after biopsy and staging studies and should be continued for approximately 9 to 12 weeks before definitive surgery of the primary tumor. After surgery, chemotherapy is resumed for an additional 35 to 40 weeks. For patients who receive chemotherapy before surgery, the degree of tumor necrosis observed postoperatively is highly predictive of disease-free survival and overall survival. Assessment of adequacy of bone marrow, and renal, cardiac, and liver function is an essential component of the initial evaluation of all patients undergoing chemotherapy.

Surgery

Both amputation and limb-salvage operations incorporate the basic principle of wide en bloc excision of the tumor and biopsy site through normal tissue planes, leaving a cuff of normal tissue around the periphery of the tumor. Limb-sparing surgery is now the preferred approach for the majority (70–90%) of patients with osteosarcoma, as it achieves a better functional outcome. Reconstruction uses allografts, customized endoprosthetic devices, modular endoprosthetic devices, or combinations. This requires a multidisciplinary team and close cooperation between the chemotherapist and orthopedic oncologist.

Follow-up

Patients with osteosarcomas should be monitored frequently for metastases with radiographic studies for at least 5 years after completion of therapy. The majority of first recurrences appear asymptomatically in the lungs. All patients with recurrent disease should be approached with curative intent, as durable salvage has been reported in 10% to 20% of such patients.

EWING'S FAMILY OF TUMORS

The EFT include Ewing's sarcoma of the bone, primitive neuroectodermal tumors (PNETs), Askin–Rosai tumor (PNET of the chest wall), and extraosseus Ewing's (EOE). Studies using immunohistochemical markers, cytogenetics, and tissue culture indicate that these tumors are all derived from the same primordial stem cell and are distinguished only by the degree of neural differentiation. Epidemiologically, it is remarkable that there is a low incidence in black and Chinese populations. Nearly 12% of patients with Ewing's sarcoma also have associated urogenital anomalies like cryptorchidism, hypospadias, and ureteral duplication.

Symptoms

Ewing's sarcoma accounts for 10% to 15% of all malignant bone tumors; peak incidence is between the ages of 10 and 15 years. Increasing, persistent pain and swelling of the affected area, with impairment of function, is the most common presenting feature. Associated fever and neurologic symptoms including paraplegia suggest metastatic disease and involvement of peripheral nerves, respectively. However, involvement of the lymph nodes, meningeal spread, or central nervous system (CNS) metastases are uncommon at presentation. In comparison to the skeletal distribution of osteogenic sarcoma, the flat bones of the trunk (pelvis, ribs, scapula, and vertebrae) are more often affected. Rib and chest-wall lesions are often associated with pleural effusion. In long bones, Ewing's sarcoma originates from the diaphysis, either centrally or toward the ends. In contrast, osteosarcoma has a typical metaphyseal presentation. Typical radiographic appearance of Ewing's sarcoma often includes a patchy, "moth-eaten" pattern of bone destruction with poorly defined margins and a parallel "onion-skin" periosteal lamellation with a varying degree of soft-tissue extension of tumor.

Diagnosis and Staging

Workup consists of CT and/or MRI of the primary lesion and a search for metastases that includes whole-body radionuclide bone scan, CT scan of the chest, and bone marrow aspiration and biopsy. Approximately 20% of patients have visible metastases at diagnosis. Of these, about 50% have lung metastases, and about 40% have multiple bone involvement and diffuse bone marrow involvement. Serum LDH levels have a prognostic significance and directly reflect tumor burden.

Pathology

Ewing's sarcoma is a malignant bone tumor characterized histologically by a uniform pattern of small cells with round nuclei but without distinct cytoplasmic borders or prominent nucleoli. Routine histopathologic examination is supplemented by invaluable additional diagnostic procedures like immunocytochemistry and molecular genetic characterization of the tumor, leading to the differential diagnosis of the small round-cell tumors of bone and chest wall. A highly specific and recurrent translocation, t(11;22)(q24;q12), is seen in the EFT by conventional cytogenetic evaluation. This translocation results in the formation of a chimeric gene between *EWS* (Ewing's sarcoma gene), a novel putative RNA-binding gene located on chromosome 22q12, and *FLI1*, a member of the erythroblastosis virus transforming sequence (ETS) family of transcription factors located at chromosome 11q24, and has been fully characterized at the molecular genetic level. RT-PCR of the fusion transcripts from the tumor can identify patients with favorable prognosis with localized primary tumors.

Treatment Strategies

Virtually all patients with apparently localized disease at diagnosis have subclinical micrometastatic disease. Hence local disease control with surgery and/or radiation as well as systemic chemotherapy is indicated (Fig. 8).

Surgery

Generally surgery is the preferred approach if the lesion is resectable. Radiation therapy is used for patients who do not have a surgical option that preserves function and for patients whose tumors have been excised but with inadequate margins.

Radiation Therapy

The current recommendation of the Intergroup Ewing's Sarcoma Study (IESS) for patients with gross residual disease is 45 Gy plus a 10.8-Gy boost. For those with microscopic residual disease, the recommendation is 45 Gy plus a 5.4-Gy boost. All patients with pulmonary metastasis should undergo whole-lung radiation at doses between 12 and 15 Gy, even if complete resolution of pulmonary metastatic disease has been achieved with chemotherapy. Metastatic sites of disease in bone and soft tissues should receive radiation therapy of 45 to 56 Gy. Radiation therapy should be delivered in a setting in which stringent planning techniques are applied by those experienced in the treatment of EFT.

Chemotherapy

The two most effective agents are cyclophosphamide and doxorubicin, but vincristine and dactinomycin are also active. Recently dose-intensification studies using ifosfamide and etoposide have shown significant promise. Prognosis was poor before the advent of effective multiagent chemotherapy (5-year survivals of 10–20%, despite good local control) and continues to be dismal in patients with metastatic disease (one recent study reported a 3-year event-free survival of only 26.7% ± 13.2%).

FUTURE DIRECTIONS

Better understanding of the molecular pathogenesis of these tumors by characterization of chromosomal translocations associated with RMS and Ewing's sarcoma can lead to novel therapeutic strategies. Some current investigational approaches include biologic response

Treatment Schema

iii c	iii c	iii c	SR	V		V	V	V	V	I	C
eee a	eee a	eee a	RAD	Dac		Dac		Dac		Dac	E	A
0	3	6	9	11				15		17	20	23

I	C	I	C	I	C	
E	A	E	A	E	A	
26	29	32	35	138	41	44

Induction (weeks 0-6)
i = ifosfamide 2 g/m²/d x 3
e = etoposide 150 mg/m²/d x 3
c = cyclophosphamide 1.5 g/m² d 5
a = doxorubicin 45 mg/m² d 5

Local control (weeks 9-17)
SR = surgical resection
V = vincristine 1.5 mg/m²
Dac = dactinomycin 1.5 mg/m²
RAD-start radiotherapy

Maintenance (week 20-44)
I = ifosfamide 2 g/m²/d x 5
E = etoposide 150 mg/m²/d x 5
C = cyclophosphamide 1.0 OR 1.5 g/m²/d x 2
A = doxorubicin 60 mg/m² continous infusion over 24 hours

Fig. 8. Dose-intensive chemotherapy for children with Ewing's family of tumors (Marina NM et al., 1999).

modifiers, vaccines designed to elicit T-cell immunity with specificity for tumor-specific fusion peptides, and antibody targeting of immunotoxins to tumor cells.

FURTHER READING

1. Wexler LH, Helman LJ. Rhabdomyosarcoma and undifferentiated sarcomas. In: Pizzo, Poplack, eds. *Principles and practice of pediatric oncology.* Philadelphia: Lippincott-Raven, 1997:799–829.
2. Horowitz M, Malawar M, Woo S, Hic ks MJ. Ewing's sarcoma family of tumors. In: Pizzo, Poplack, eds. *Principles and practice of pediatric oncology.* Philadelphia: Lippincott-Raven, 1997:831–863.
3. Link PM, Eilber F. Osteosarcoma. In: Pizzo, Poplack, eds. *Principles and practice of pediatric oncology.* Philadelphia: Lippincott-Raven, 1997:889–920.
4. Arndt CAS, Crist WM. Common musculoskeletal tumors of childhood and adolescence. *N Engl J Med* 1999;342:342–352.
5. NCNN. Pediatric osteosarcoma practice guidelines. *Oncology* 1996;10:1799–1806.
6. Sommelet D, Pinkerton R, Brunat-Mentigny M, et al. Standards, options and recommendations (SOR) for clinical care of rhabdomyosarcoma (RMS) and other soft tissue sarcoma in children [French]. *Bull Cancer* 1998;85:1015–1042.
7. Philip T, Blay JY, Brunat-Mentigny M, et al. Standards, options and recommendations (SOR) for diagnosis, treatment and follow-up of osteosarcoma [French]. *Bull Cancer* 1999;86:159–176.
8. Pinkerton CR. *Clinical challenges in pediatric oncology.* Oxford: ISIS Medical Media, 1999:117–134, 143–156.
9. Marina NM , Pappo AS, Parham DM, et al. Chemotherapy dose-intensification for pediatric patients with Ewing's family of tumors and desmoplastic small round cell tumors: a feasibility study at St. Jude Children's Research Hospital. *J Clin Oncol* 1999;17:180–190.
10. PDQR Cancer Information Summaries. http://cancernet.nci.nih.gov/pdq/pdq_treatment.shtml

SECTION 8

Skin Cancer

21

Skin Cancers and Melanoma

Upendra Hegde and Barry Gause

Medicine Branch, DCS, National Cancer Institute, National Institutes of Health, Bethesda, Maryland

The skin is the largest organ of the human body. Embryologically, it is derived from the neuroectoderm and the mesoderm. It consists of three layers: epidermis, dermis and subcutis. Skin cancers can arise from various cell types and structures in various layers of the skin. The direct exposure of the skin to the environment has special relevance because a wide variety of carcinogens can interact directly with the genetic components of skin cells. Such exposure has increased the incidence of skin cancers. Cell of origin in various types of skin cancers are outlined in Tables 1 and 2. The skin cancers are best divided into melanoma and nonmelanoma.

MELANOMA

This skin tumor originates from the melanocyte, which is derived from the neural crest and migrates during embryogenesis predominantly to skin and less commonly to other tissues like the meninges,the ocular choroid, the mucosa of the respiratory tract, the gastrointestinal tract, and the genitourinary tract, where melanoma has been rarely encountered.

Epidemiology

- Melanoma ranks as the seventh leading cancer in the United States.
- Incidence is increasing faster than that of any other cancer except lung cancer in women.
- Incidence in whites is ten times more than that in the African-American population. Incidence in U.S. whites is 10/100,000, although some geographic areas have higher incidences.
- According to the American Cancer Society, 40,300 new cases of melanoma were diagnosed in the U.S. in 1997, with 7,300 deaths.

TABLE 1. *Cell of origin of tumor types*

Cells of epidermis	Tumor	Incidence
Melanocyte	Melanoma	> 5–7%
Epidermal basal cell	Basal cell carcinoma	60%
Keratinocyte	Squamous cell carcinoma	30%
Merkel cell	Merkel cell tumor	> 1–2%
Langerhans cell	Histiocytosis X	>
Appendage cells	Appendageal tumors	>

TABLE 2. *Cells of dermis and tumor type*

Cells of dermis	Tumor type	Incidence
Fibroblast	Benign and malignant fibrous histiocytic tumors	> <1%
Macrophage	>	
Mast cell	Mast cell tumor	>
Vasculature	Angioma and angiosarcoma	>
	Lymphangioma	>

- Australia has the highest incidence of melanoma in the world, approximately 17 cases per 100,000 per year.
- By the year 2000, the estimated lifetime risk of melanoma in American whites will be 1 in 75.

Etiology

Sunlight exposure: ultraviolet B rays.

1. Intermittent intense exposure.
2. Exposure at a young age.
3. Propensity for sunburns and poor tanners.
4. Fair skin, blue eyes, blonde or red hair.

Age: Higher incidence in young adults and middle-aged persons (except lentigo meligna melanoma in elderly on sun-exposed surface).
Sex: Slightly more common in female than male subjects.
Ethnicity: Higher incidence in northern Europeans than in eastern and southern Europeans.
Familial melanoma: One in ten patients with melanoma has a family history of melanoma.

Following are the characteristic features of familial melanoma

1. Multiple melanomas.
2. Melanoma at young age.
3. Often associated with dysplastic nevi.
4. Locus for melanoma/dysplastic nevus resides in the distal portion of the short arm of chromosome 1.
5. Other genetic loci possible, which include chromosome 9 (loss of 9p21).
   - Precursor lesions:
   - Dysplastic nevi.
   - Congenital nevi.
   - Acquired melanocytic nevi.

Risk Factors for Melanoma

- Xeroderma pigmentosum.
- Familial atypical mole melanoma syndrome (FAMMS).
- Numerous acquired melanocytic nevi.
- Dysplastic nevi.
- Giant congenital nevus.
- Prior melanoma.
- Sun exposure/sun-sensitive phenotype.
- Immunosuppression.
- Melanoma in a first-degree relative.
- Freckling.

Differences between acquired melanocytic nevus and dysplastic nevus are listed in Table 3 and Fig. 1.

TABLE 3. *Differences between acquired melanocytic and dysplastic nevus*

Acquired melanocytic nevus	Dysplastic nevus
Develops in early childhood through fourth decade	Develops throughout life
<5 mm in diameter, sharp borders, evenly pigmented	>6–8 mm in diameter, irregular borders, variegated pigment, topographic asymmetry
If >100 in number, risk of melanoma increased by 10 times	Presence of dysplastic nevus increases the risk of melanoma

Pathophysiology:

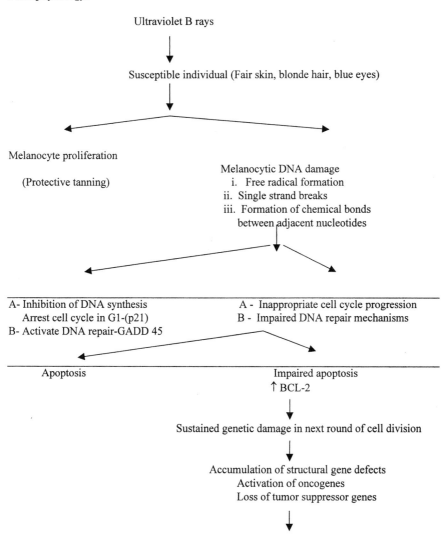

FIG. 1. Acquisition of invasive phenotype.

Common Chromosomal Abnormalities in Malignant Melanoma

Early chromosomal abnormalities:

- Loss of 10q.
- Loss of 9p.

Late chromosomal abnormalities:

- Deletion of 6q.
- Loss of terminal part of 1p.
- Duplication of chromosome 7.
- Deletion of 11q23.

Clinicohistologic Types of Melanoma

The ability to measure the melanoma cells in the dermis and subcutaneous fat is defined in a reproducible way by two groups: Clark et al. and Breslow (Table 4). Clark et al. subdivided the invasion of the papillary dermis into a deep group, in which melanoma cells accumulate at the junction of the papillary and reticular dermis, and a superficial group in which these cells do not accumulate (Fig. 2).

Breslow measured the thickness of melanoma lesions by using an ocular micrometer to measure the vertical thickness from the granular layer of the epidermis or the base of the ulcer to the deepest identifiable contiguous melanoma cell and showed it to be a more reproducible and accurate prognostic parameter than Clark's method of microstaging.

Clark's Method of Microstaging (Level of Invasion)

Clark level

I	Melanoma limited to the epidermis
II	Invasive melanoma with superficial infiltration of the papillary dermis
III	Melanoma extending to the superficial vascular plexus in the dermis
IV	Primary melanoma involving the reticular dermis
V	Melanoma involving the subcutaneous fat

TABLE 4. *Types of melanoma*

Superficial spreading type	Nodular melanoma	Lentigo maligna melanoma	Acral lentiginous melanoma
Most common (70%)	Next most common (15–30%)	4–10% of all melanomas	2–8% of all melanomas
Young to middle age	Young to middle age	Elderly; mean age, 70 yr	Young to middle age
Upper back in men and women; lower extremity in women	Legs and trunk	Sun-exposed areas— head, neck, and arms	Hands, feet, subungual, and periungual skin
Radial growth pattern —early diagnosis	Vertical growth pattern—advanced diagnosis— advanced stage	Radial growth pattern— early diagnosis	Radial and vertical growth patterns— advanced-stage diagnosis
Light-skinned individuals	Light-skinned individuals	Light-skinned individuals	Blacks, Orientals, and Asians

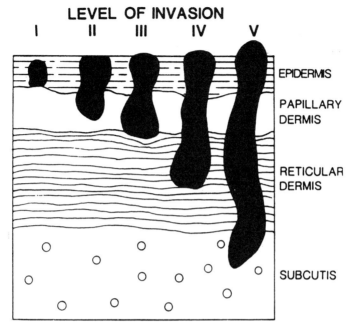

FIG. 2. Schematic of Clark's levels of invasion.

Breslow's Method of Microstaging (Tumor Thickness)

Breslow Tumor Thickness

I	<0.75 mm.
II	0.76 to 1.5 mm.
III	1.51 to 3.99 mm.
IV	4 mm or greater.

Clinical Melanoma Staging

The 1997 AJCC/UICC pTNM staging of Malignant Melanoma.

Stage	Description
IA	Localized melanoma <0.75 mm or level II (T1 N0 M0)
IB	Localized melanoma 0.76 mm to 1.49 mm or level III (T2 N0 M0)
IIA	Localized melanoma 1.5 to 4 mm or level IV (T3 N0 M0)
IIB	Localized melanoma >4 mm or level V (T4 N0 M0)
III	Limited nodal metastasis involving only one regional lymph node basin, *OR* fewer than 5 in transit metastasis without local lymph node metastasis (T any N1 M0)
IV	Advanced regional metastasis (T any N2 M0) *OR* distant metastasis (TNM 1 or 2)

Lesions less than 0.75 mm thick are considered low risk. Lesions more than 4 mm thick are considered high risk. When the thickness and level of invasion criteria do not coincide within a T classification, thickness should take precedence.

Prognostic Factors

Prognostic factors are listed in Table 5 and Fig. 3.

Clinical Features of Malignant Melanoma

Cutaneous melanoma can occur anywhere in the body. The most common sites are the lower extremities in the women and the trunk in men. The classic signs include a pigmented skin lesion

TABLE 5. *Prognostic factors*

Good prognostic factors	Poor prognostic factors
1. Tumor involving an extremity	Melanoma of the skin of the trunk, head, and neck
2. Thin tumor	Thick tumor
3. Nonulcerated tumor	Ulcerated tumor
4. Radial growth pattern	Nodular histology
5. Early stage (stage I and II)	Late stage at presentation (stage III and IV)
6. Absence of foci of regression and satellites of the tumor in the reticular dermis and subcutaneous fat	Presence of foci of regression and/or tumor satellites in reticular dermis and subcutaneous fat
7. Absence of vascular and/or lymphatic invasion	Presence of vascular and/or lymphatic invasion
8. Lower tumor cells mitotic rate	

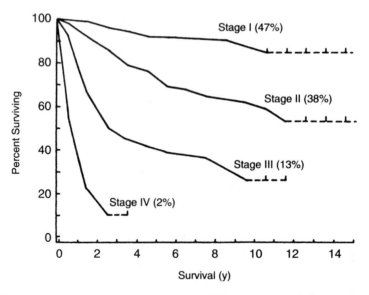

FIG. 3. Fifteen-year survival results for more than 4,000 melanoma patients treated at the University of Alabama at Birmingham and the Sydney Melanoma Unit, staged according to the American Joint Committee on Cancer four-stage system. Distribution of patients is shown in parentheses. Note that patients with clinically localized melanoma (stage I in the original three-stage system) are divided into two stages according to tumor thickness and histologic level of invasion (designated stages I and II). (From Ketcham AS, Moffat FL, Balch CM. Classification and staging. In: Balch C, ed. *Cutaneous melanoma.* 2nd ed. Philadelphia: JB Lippincott, 1992:213–220, with permission.)

that demonstrates change in color or variegated color, a change in lesion size, and irregular borders. Progressive lesions show nodularity and ulceration or bleeding, with or without pruritis.

The majority of lesions are pigmented, although fewer than 1% of lesions lack pigment and are called amelanotic melanomas.

Diagnosis

Types of skin biopsies in the diagnosis of malignant melanoma are listed in Tables 6 and 7. Immunohistologic tests for the diagnosis of malignant melanoma

Antigen	Result
S-100 protein	+
Cytokeratin	-
Premelanosomal protein (HMB-45)	+
Vimentin	+
Nerve growth factor receptor	+
Tyrosinase-related protein-1 (MEL-5)	+

Prognosis

The majority of melanomas are diagnosed in the early stages and are thin. More than 95% of thin melanomas are curable, and approximately 85% of stage I and II melanoma are cured. The prognosis is inversely proportional to the stage of the cancer, and only 40% to 50% of persons with stage III melanoma live for 5 years. Among patients with stage IV melanoma, fewer than 5% live for 5 years.

Table 8 shows a graph depicting the survival in relation to the stage of the melanoma.

TABLE 6. *Diagnosis*

History	Clinical examination	Skin biopsy and histology
1. Details of the skin lesion i. Duration ii. Change in color, size, borders iii. Itching, bleeding, or ulceration iv. Symptoms that suggest 　　distant metastasis 2. Exposure to sunlight and other 　predisposing factors including 　family history of melanoma	Bright light and a hand lens may be useful to 　evaluate the lesion for the following: i.　Asymmetry ii.　Border irregularity iii.　Color variegation iv.　Diameter >6 mm (melanomas smaller 　　　than 6 mm are occasionally seen)	Biopsies should be performed for histologic and immunohistologic evaluation of suggestive lesions

TABLE 7. *Types of skin biopsy*

Types of skin biopsy	Characteristics
Excisional skin biopsy	i. Completely removes the tumor. Curative if the tumor is small, and 　tumor-free margins of 2 mm could be obtained ii. May not be feasible due to anatomic or cosmetic restraints
Incisional skin biopsy	i. Performed if a tumor is large ii. For flat lesions, the darkest area should be sampled. If the lesion 　is raised, the thickest area should be sampled
Shave biopsy	Contraindicated in melanoma because it may not yield adequate 　deep specimen for accurate microstaging

TABLE 8. *Relationship between microstage of primary melanoma, incidence of regional lymph node metastases, and long-term survival in patients from John Wayne Cancer Institute*

	Microstage	Patient number	Lymph node metastases (%)	Ten-year survival (%)
Breslow thickness	<0.75 mm	768	8.3	97
	0.76–1.5 mm	802	20.2	87
	1.51–3.99 mm	765	36.6	67
	≥4 mm	205	40.0	40
Clark level	I/II	622	9.2	97
	III	1,046	23.9	85
	IV	785	35.0	68
	V	87	38.0	46

Management

Algorithm for the management of primary melanoma is reviewed in Figure 4.

Prevention:

- Educate patients about the risk factors for melanoma: ultraviolet light (intense midday sun between 11 a.m. and 1 p.m.). Use of sunblock (SPF >15) and light clothing should be encouraged.
- Educate patients about clinical features of melanoma and precursor lesions and teach them to perform skin self-examination.
- Close surveillance in high-risk patients.

General principles and issues in treatment:

- Surgical excision is the primary treatment of melanoma.
- Regional lymph node dissection for metastasis before any distant spread of the tumor has occurred.
- Adjuvant radiation therapy after lymph node dissection in selected instances.
- Isolated limb perfusion with chemotherapy in selected instances.
- Interferon-α as adjuvant therapy in patients with high-risk resected cutaneous melanomas.
- Combination chemotherapy/chemobiotherapy in metastatic melanoma.
- Newer experimental immunotherapy: role of vaccines.

Surgical Management of Primary Melanoma

Principle: Complete surgical excision confirmed by comprehensive histologic examination of the entire excised specimen is the basis for surgical treatment of primary melanoma.

Pathological stage	Thickness	Margin of excision
PTis	Melanoma in situ	5 mm
PT1 and PT2	0 - 1.5 mm	1 cm
PT3	>1.5 - 4 mm	1 - 2 cm
PT4	>4 mm	2 - 3 cm

Risk of local recurrence was not significantly associated with margin of excision (Table 9).

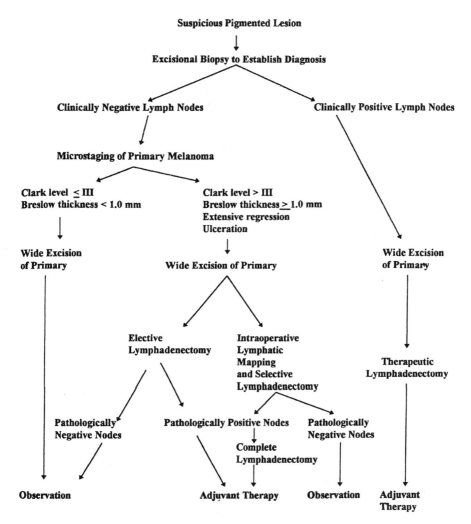

FIG. 4. Algorithm for the management of primary melanoma (AJCC stage I/II).

Ocular Melanoma

Early and limited stage usually managed with close observation. Various methods of treatment include radiation therapy, photoradiation, cryotherapy, ultrasonic hyperthermia, local resection, and enucleation.

Indications for enucleation of the eye in ocular melanoma:

• Tumor growing in a blind eye.
• Melanoma involving more than half of iris.

TABLE 9. *Surgical management of melanoma arising from special sites*

Special site of the melanoma	Management
Face as in lentigo maligna melanoma	Moh's surgery may be effectively used, and plastic surgery may be necessary to tailor the excision to avoid ectropion or a depressed scar
Subungual melanoma	Amputation of the digit proximal to the interphalangeal joint of the thumb or distal interphalangeal joint of the finger. Amputation of the entire finger may be necessary in more extensive melanoma of the nail bed
Desmoplastic melanoma	Wider margin of excision justifiable because of high chances of local recurrences. Sometimes local radiation may be considered as adjuvant to the surgical management
Melanoma of the sole of the foot	Wide excision with the defect filled by a split-thickness graft derived from non–weight-bearing area of the other foot. Important to preserve the deep fascia.
Ear melanoma	Wedge resection of the ear including cartilage

- Involvement of the anterior chamber of the eye by the tumor or extraocular extension.
- Failure of previous local therapy.

Lymph Node Dissection

Invasion of the lymphatics by a vertically growing melanoma causes the tumor to lodge in the local lymph node basin. Uninterrupted at this lymph node basin, the tumor may spread to deeper lymphatics or hematogenously to systemic organs. This principle forms the rationale for complete surgical resection of the tumor from the lymph node basin before the tumor has spread to distant organs, and is considered a potentially curative procedure.

Lymph node dissection can be classified as follows (Table 10):
- Elective: When the lymph nodes that were not clinically palpable are dissected from the lymph node basin because of the high suspicion of melanoma spread to them without evidence of distant spread.
- Therapeutic: When the lymph nodes are clinically palpable and suspected to be involved without distant organ spread.
- Delayed: When initially nonpalpable lymph nodes appear to enlarge over a close follow-up period without distant organ spread.

Sentinel Lymph Node Dissection

Characteristics of a sentinel lymph node:

TABLE 10. *Lymph node dissection*

Advantages	Disadvantages
Helps eradicate occult lymph node metastasis	Overtreatment in 50–60% patients
Correctly stages the tumor	Invasive procedure
Efficacy proved in melanoma of thickness between 1.1 and 2 mm in patients younger than 60 yr	Morbidity of the procedure

- First lymph node in the lymph node basin to which the primary melanoma drains.
- Most at-risk lymph node for metastasis.
- Histology reflects the histology of all lymph nodes in the basin.
- Easily accessible and could be subjected to serial sectioning, immunohistochemistry for markers (like S-100, or HMB 45) and molecular biologic tests to evaluate for tyrosinase mRNA to improve the sensitivity of the procedure to diagnose micrometastasis.
- If negative for metastasis, it spares the patient major surgical morbidity.

Surgical Approach to Obtain a Sentinel Lymph Node

Preoperative lymphoscintigraphy uses vital blue dye and provides a road map of the lymph node basin. Intraoperative lymphoscintigraphy uses radiocolloid injection around the primary tumor, and a gamma camera detects the radioactivity from the involved lymph node, thus acting like a navigator to the involved lymph node. The combination of vital blue dye and technetium-labeled sulfur colloid identifies the sentinel lymph node in 94% of cases.

Isolated Limb Perfusion

Principle: To deliver maximally tolerated chemotherapy doses to a regionally confined tumor area while limiting systemic toxicity. Hyperthermia and oxygenation of the circulation potentiate the tumoricidal effects of the chemotherapeutic agents. Chemotherapeutic agents used in this method of treatment:

- Melphalan.
- Thiotepa (Response rate, 50% to 60%).
- Mechlorethamine.
- These agents with tumor necrosis factor plus interferon-γ: response rate, 91%.

Isolated limb perfusion is described in Table 11.

Indications for isolated limb perfusion:
- Adjuvant to lymph node dissection.
- Recurrent melanoma.
- Bulky symptomatic melanoma of the extremity with bleeding, ulceration, or edema.

Role of radiation therapy in the adjuvant setting: Although melanoma has been considered in general as a "radioresistant tumor," in the following instances, radiation therapy has been found to be of clinical benefit after surgical lymph node resection:

- Head and neck melanomas.
- Multiple large lymph nodes.
- Extracapsular spread.
- Local recurrence in a previously dissected lymph node basin.
- Parotid gland lymph nodes.

TABLE 11. *Isolated limb perfusion*

Advantages	Disadvantages
i. Local control of the disease	i. Expensive
ii. Resolution of edema, bleeding, or ulceration	ii. Invasive
iii. Relieves pain	iii. May cause ischemia of the limb, peripheral neuropathy, and bone marrow suppression

TABLE 12. Use of adjuvant interferon

Study group (accrual)	Treatment regimen	Outcomes analysis
ECOG E1684 (287 patients with stage IBB or stage III malignant melanoma AJCC stage)	Interferon alfa-2b, 20 million Units/m² per dose i.v., 5 days/wk × 4 wk (total dose/wk, 100 million Units/m²), *THEN* Interferon alfa-2b, 10 million Units/m² s.c., 3 times per week for 48 wk (total dose/wk, 30 million Units/m²) V/S Observation	Favored interferon therapy Overall survival, 0.047 Relapse-free survival, p = 0.004 Significant toxicity of interferon observed.
ECOG 1690 (642)	Interferon alfa-2b, 20 million Units/m² per dose i.v., 5 days/wk × 4 wk (total dose/wk, 100 million Units/m²), *THEN* Interferon alfa-2b, 10 million Units/m² s.c., 3 times per week for 48 wk (total dose/wk, 30 million Units/m²) V/S Low-dose interferon Interferon alfa-2b, 3 million Units/m² s.c., 3 times per week for 104 wk (total dose/wk, 9 million Units/m²) V/S Observation	Survival benefit for high-dose interferon • Relapse-free survival p = 0.05 in both node-positive & node-negative patients • greatest in those with 2-3 nodes (p = 0.02) • No overall 5-year survival benefit
ECOG E 1697 (1,444 patients AJCC stage IIA) The aim is to know the impact of interferon on relapse-free survival and overall survival in the adjuvant setting in stage IIA disease	Interferon alfa-2b, 20 million Units/m² per dose i.v. 5 days per week × 4 wk (total dose/wk, 100 million Units/m²), *OR* Observation	Ongoing
UKCCCR Study (1,000 patients AJCC stage II or III)	Interferon alfa-2a, 3 million Units/m² s.c. 3 times per week for 2 years (total dose/wk, 9 million Units/m²), *OR* Observation	Ongoing
EORTC study (18-952) (1,000 patients AJCC stage II or III disease) for interferon in adjuvant setting. The goal is to see the impact of the two lower doses and subcutaneously administered interferon on the disease	Interferon alfa-2b, 10 million Units/m² per dose s.c. 5 days/wk for 4 wk (total dose/wk, 50 million Units/m²), *THEN* Interferon alfa-2b, 10 million Units/m² s.c. 3 times per wk for 1 yr (total dose/wk, 30 million Units/m²), *OR* Interferon alfa-2b, 5 million Units/m² s.c. 3 times per wk for 2 yr (total dose/wk, 15 million Units/m²)	Ongoing

ECOG, Eastern Co-operative Oncology Group; UKCCCR, The UK Coordinating Committee on Cancer Research; EORTC, European Organization for the Research and Treatment of Cancer; i.v. intravenous; s.c., subcutaneous. V/S?

From Kirkwood JM, Strawderman MH, Ernstoff MS, et al. Interferon alfa-2b adjuvant therapy of high risk resected cutaneous melanoma: the Eastern Cooperative Oncology Group trial EST 1684. *J Clin Oncol* 1996;14:7–17, with permission.

- Desmoplastic melanoma with neurotropism.

Studies by Skibber et al. suggested survival benefit of external radiation to the brain after surgical resection of the solitary brain metastasis with malignant melanoma.

Biologic Agents in Malignant Melanoma

Interferon-α was the first recombinant cytokine investigated in phase I/II trials, in the metastatic setting, based on its antiproliferative as well as immunomodulatory effects.

- The response rate in metastatic melanoma was around 16%.
- One third of these responses were complete responses.
- Responses could be observed up to 6 months after the therapy was started.
- Up to one third of the responses were durable.
- Patients with frequent interruptions due to side effects of interferon therapy did less well compared with those who did not require interruptions.
- Patients with small tumor volume did better than those with large-volume tumors.

Interferon in Metastatic Melanoma

The study by Falkson et al. showed a response rate of 53% and median survival of 17.6 months with interferon-α2b combined with dacarbazine compared with a response rate of 20% and median survival of 9.6% months with dacarbazine alone. These results were not reproducible by EORTC studies.

Interferon in the Adjuvant Setting in Malignant Melanoma

Principle: There is a high incidence of relapse among patients with stage III melanoma after therapeutic or elective lymph node dissection and in those with thick melanoma lesions (>4 mm). Interferon's effect on disease-free survival was evaluated in this setting (Table 12).

CONCLUSIONS

- High-dose interferon remains the most active adjuvant agent evaluated to date for high-risk melanoma.
- Prolongs the relapse-free survival, but its impact on overall survival is less clear.

A summary of the management options of melanoma in advanced tumor stage is found in Table 13. Chemotherapy agents and their response rates in metastatic melanoma are listed in Table 14. Combination chemotherapy in metastatic melanoma is described in Table 15.

TABLE 13. *Management options*

Management	Metastatic site	Comments
Combination chemotherapy	Systemic metastasis	Palliative in nature, dacarbazine is the drug of choice
Surgical resection	Brain, soft tissue, lung, or liver	Isolated single legion
Radiation therapy	Brain, bone, symptomatic systemic metastasis	Treatment of symptomatic lesions
Combination chemotherapy + biologic therapy (interleukin-2 and/or interferon alfa)	Systemic metastatic disease	Promising and effective. Regression of visceral metastasis is seen with possible survival advantage.
Immunotherapies	Systemic metastatic disease	Experimental

TABLE 14. *Chemotherapy agents and response rates*

Chemotherapeutic agent	Response rates
Dacarbazine	15–25%
Temozolomide (DTIC analogue)	21%
Nitrosoureas	10–20%
Cisplatin	10–20%
Carboplatin	
Vinca alkaloids	15–25%
Vincristine	
Vinblastine	
Vindesine	
Taxoids	18%
Paclitaxel	
Docetaxel	
Piritrexim	23%

A recent phase III multicenter randomized trial of dacarbazine alone versus the Dartmouth regimen in patients with metastatic melanoma failed to show a statistical difference in survival or tumor response in patients with melanoma (EORTC study).

- Combination of chemotherapy regimen and biologic therapy (Biochemotherapy): Rationale
- Anticancer effects are additive or synergistic.
- Different mechanisms of action.
- Nonoverlapping toxicity.
- No cross resistance.
- Suggestion that biologic agents may produce long-term survivals.

Combination chemotherapy with biologic agents is described in Table 16.

TABLE 15. *Description of chemotherapy regimens*

Chemotherapy regimens	Treatment description	Response rates
CBDT, the "Dartmouth regimen"	Cisplatin, 25 mg/m^2 per day i.v. for 3 days, days 1–3 (total dose/cycle, 75 mg/m^2) Carmustine, 150 mg/m^2 i.v. day 1 on every odd-numbered cycle (i.e., every 43 d) (total dose every two cycles, 150 mg/m^2) Dacarbazine, 220 mg/m^2 per day i.v. for 3 days, days 1–3 (total dose/cycle, 660 mg/m^2) Tamoxifen, 10 mg twice daily p.o. during the therapy • Cycle repeats every 21 days	19–55%
CVD (MD Anderson)	Cisplatin, 20 mg/m^2 per day i.v. for 4 days, days 2–5 (total dose/cycle, 80 mg/m^2) Vinblastine, 1.6 mg/m^2 per day i.v. for 5 days, days 1–5 (total dose/cycle, 8 mg/m^2) Dacarbazine, 800 mg/m^2 i.v. on day 1 (total dose/cycle, 800 mg/m^2) • Cycle repeats every 21 days	24–45%

From Del Prete SA, Maurer LH, O'Donnell I, et al. Combination chemotherapy with cisplatin, carmustine, dacarbazine, and tamoxifen in metastatic melanoma. *Cancer Treat Rep* 1984;68: 1403–1405, with permission.

TABLE 16. *Combination chemotherapy with biologic agents*

Treatment	Response rates
Dacarbazine, 1,000 mg/m² as a continuous infusion over 24 h. (total dose/cycle, 1,000 mg/m²)	22%
Recombinant interleukin-2, administered i.v. over 30 min on an outpatient basis on days 15–19 and days 22–26. The dose of interleukin-2 was 24 MIU/m² for 10 doses, days 1–5 and 8–12 (total dose/cycle, 240 MIU/m²)	
Dacarbazine was repeated once every 28 days, and supportive treatment was given during this protocol	
Dacarbazine, 200 mg/m² i.v. for 5 days, start every week 4	53%
Interferon alfa-2b, 15 MU/m² i.v. daily for 5 days per week for 3 wk, and thereafter, 10 MU/m² s.c. three times per week	
Cycle repeats every 28 days	
Cisplatin, 100 mg/m² i.v. on day 1 (total dose/cycle, 100 mg/m²)	33% overall
Interferon alfa-2a, 10 MU/day s.c. on days 1–5 (total dose/cycle, 50 MU)	response rate
Interleukin-2 given as continuous infusion for 6 days (days 3–8) in a descrescendo schedule, starting on day 3 with 18 MU/m² every 6 h followed by 18 MU/m² every 12 h, 18 MU/m² every 24 h, and a maintenance dose of 4.5 MU/m² every 24 h for 72 h (total dose/cycle, 139.5 MU/m²)	
Cycle repeats every 28 days	
CVD regimen	64% overall
Cisplatin, 20 mg/m² per day i.v. for 4 days, days 2–5 (total dose/cycle, 80 mg/m²)	response rate
Vinblastine, 1.6 mg/m² per day i.v. for 5 days, days 1–5 (total dose/cycle, 8 mg/m²)	
Dacarbazine, 800 mg/m² i.v. on day 1 (total dose/cycle, 800 mg/m²)	
PLUS	
Interleukin-2, 9 million Units/m² per day continuous i.v. infusion for 4 days, days 6–9 (total dose/cycle, 36 million Units/m²)	
Interferon alfa, 5 million Units/m² per dose s.c. for 5 days, days 6–10 (total dose/cycle, 25 million Units/m²)	
Note: The therapy schedule with the biologic agents either immediately precedes or follows the CVD regimen	
Cycle repeats every 21 days	
Cisplatin, 25 mg/m² i.v. 2-h infusion on days 1–3 and 22–25 (total dose/cycle, 175 mg/m²)	55%
Carmustine, 150 mg/m² i.v. 1-h infusion on day 1 (total dose/cycle, 150 mg/m²)	
Dacarbazine, 220 mg/m² i.v. 2-h infusion on days 1–3 and 22–25 (total dose/cycle, 1,540 mg/m²)	
Tamoxifen, 10-mg tablet orally twice a day for 6 weeks and begin on day 1	
Interleukin-2, 1.5 million Units/m² administered i.v. every 8 h, starting day 4 for 15 doses, days 4–8 and 17–21 (total dose/cycle, 45 million Units/m²)	
PLUS	
Interferon alfa-2b, 6 million Units/m² per day s.c. for 10 days, days 4–8 and 17–21 (total dose/cycle, 60 million Units/m²)	
Cycle repeats every 6 weeks	

TABLE 17. *Melanoma-associated antigen epitopes*

Antigen	HLA restriction	Cellular location
MAGE-1	A1/Cw1601	Cytoplasm
MAGE-3	A1/A2	Cytoplasm
MART1/Mela-A	A2	Cytoplasm
Tyrosinase	A2/A24	Melanosomal

Vaccine Therapy in Malignant Melanoma

Immunization principally involves recognition of tumor-specific peptide by cytotoxic T cells when presented by antigen-presenting cells bound to major histocompatibility complex (MHC) molecules. A number of tumor-associated peptide antigens are purified and either administered intradermally with an immune adjuvant, or the peptide is "pulsed" onto autologous antigen-presenting cells, and the combination is injected intradermally. Other approaches include gene therapy for appropriate peptide expression in the antigen-presenting cells, which then process the peptide intracellularly and bind tightly to the appropriate human leukocyte antigen (HLA) molecule for presentation to cytotoxic T cells.

Some of the melanoma-associated antigen epitopes are listed in Table 17. Various studies are in progress, and final results are awaited.

NONMELANOMA SKIN CANCER

There are two major types of nonmelanoma skin cancers: basal cell carcinoma and squamous cell carcinoma. Together they account for nearly one third of all the cancers in the U.S.

Basal Cell Carcinoma

- The most common cancer in the U.S. white population.
- Accounts for 77% of 77,000 new cases of nonmelanoma skin cancers seen in the U.S.

Common clinical presentations of basal cell carcinoma include:

- Shiny skin colored pink with translucent papule with telangiectasia.
- Nodular variant consists of nodule with central depression and rolled margins and may bleed from trauma. Usual location is head and neck area.
- Pigmented basal cell carcinoma: Nodular with brown to black pigment.
- Sclerosing or morphea-type basal cell carcinoma: Yellowish, infiltrated, with indistinct borders, may not be diagnosed for a long time. Moh's surgery may be appropriate for treatment.
- Other less common presentations include hyperkeratotic type: Usually involves head and neck area, sessile growth on the lower trunk, multicentric on face with ulcer and scar tissues, giant exophytic type, and cystic type that presents as a blue–gray nodule on the face.

Squamous Cell Carcinoma

Squamous cell carcinoma involving the skin:

- Usually elderly white men with sun-damaged skin.
- Common sites include back of the hand, forearm, face, and neck, single or multiple lesions.
- Firm, indurated, expanding nodule, often at the site of actinic keratosis.
- The nodule may be ulcerated, and regional lymph nodes may be enlarged.

TABLE 18. *Premalignant lesions of the epidermis*

Actinic keratosis
Chemical keratosis: arsenic, tar, polycyclic aromatic hydrocarbons, thermal keratosis
Radiation dermatitis
Bowen's disease
Erythroplasia of Queret
Bowenoid papulosis
Epidermodysplasia verruciformis
Leukoplakia
Keratoacanthoma

Squamous cell carcinoma of a mucocutaneous site:

- Elderly men with chronic history of smoking, alcohol use, or chewing tobacco or betel nut.
- Common sites include mouth, lower lip.
- Lesions usually start as an erosion or a nodule that ulcerates.

Other sites include:

- Sole of the foot, verrucous form.
- Male genitalia: herpes papillomavirus (HPV) related, underlying condylomata of Buschke–Lowenstein (Table 18).

Table 19 lists the comparative features of basal and squamous cell carcinomas of the skin.

Diagnosis of Nonmelanoma Skin Cancer

History should include duration of the lesion, symptoms like pain/itching, recent changes of the surface:

- History of sun exposure, and recreational and occupational history.
- Ethnic background and the type of the skin.
- History of radiation exposure, arsenic exposure, chronic ulcer/burn scar, or osteomyelitis.

Complete skin examination includes:

- Scalp, ears, palms, soles, interdigital areas, and mucous membranes.

TABLE 19. *Features of basal and squamous cell carcinomas of skin*

Characteristics	Basal cell carcinoma	Squamous cell carcinoma
Incidence	Most common cancer of the skin in whites	Next most common skin cancer in whites
Cell of origin	Basal cells of epidermis and hair follicles	Epidermal keratinocytes
Site of tumor	Sun-exposed areas of head and neck, ear, and extremities	Sun-exposed areas of head, neck, face, forearm, and dorsum of the hand
Ethnic background	Fair skin	Fair skin
Sun exposure	Continuous cumulative exposure	Continuous cumulative exposure
Male female ratio	Common in males	Common in males
Growth and prognosis	Slow growing and good prognosis	Slow growing and good prognosis
Mucosal origin	None	Involves lip and mouth

• Evaluation of the extent of sun damage to skin (solar elastosis, scaling, erythema, telangiectasia, and solar lentigines).

Evaluate for enlargement of the locoregional and distant metastases. Perform skin biopsy, either excisional, when the tumor is small, or incisional, when the tumor is large. A shave biopsy with a scalpel may be used in noduloulcerative, cystic, or superficial type.

Treatment Principles

• Surgery is the primary mode of treatment.
• Excision of the tumor with negative margins of approximately 4 to 6 mm is sufficient.
• The procedure is performed under local anesthesia.
• Locally draining nodes are examined and removed only if they are enlarged.
• Plastic surgery may be needed to close the defects produced by excision of the tumor.
• Mohs' surgery: A progressive excision technique that allows excision of the tumor until the negative margins are achieved. Mohs' micrographic surgery uses the fresh-tissue technique with the use of frozen section and is less time-consuming than the original surgery.

Role of Radiation Therapy

Delivery of x-rays is at a total dose of 2,000 to 3,000 cGy to penetrate up to 2 to 5 mm, where most of the basal cell and squamous cell carcinomas infiltrate. The total dose is divided into multiple fractions, usually over 3 to 4 weeks to reduce side effects (Table 20).
Various other types of treatments are listed in Table 21.

Other Cancers of the Skin

Merkel's cell carcinoma arises from the neoplastic proliferation of the Merkel's cells.

Merkel's cell characteristics:

• Arises from the neural crest cells and is a member of the APUD cell system.
• Situated in the basal layer of the epidermis and hair follicles.
• Important for tactile sensations in lower animals.
• Functions as a mechanoreceptor in humans.

Merkel's cell tumor characteristics:

• Rare tumor seen in elderly whites with sun-exposure history.
• Involves skin of the head and neck and less commonly in the extremities and genitals.

TABLE 20. *Radiation therapy*

Radiation therapy in nonmelanoma skin cancer: Advantages	Common side effects
Most skin tumors are radiosensitive	Loss of hair follicles and sweat glands
Indicated for skin cancer in elderly patients who have high risk for surgery and Large and bulky tumors Tumors located on the nose, eye, lip, eyelid, and inner and outer canthi of the eye as well as skin cancer along the embryonal fusion planes	Skin atrophy and telangiectasia Radiation dermatitis Radiation-induced precancerous lesions of the skin
Cure rate for squamous cell carcinoma and basal cell carcinoma are >90%	

TABLE 21. *Other types of treatment*

Treatment method	Characteristic features

1. Curettage and electrodesiccation preceded by a shave biopsy	Advantages
	  Useful to treat basal cell carcinoma, superficial squamous cell carcinoma, Bowen's disease, and keratoacanthoma actinic keratosis
	  Cure rates in selected patients, 77–97%
	Disadvantages
	  Not suitable for tumors in high-risk areas, histologically aggressive tumors, or morphea-type tumors

2. Cryotherapy Kills tumor cells by freezing Liquid nitrogen (–195.5°C) causes tissue necrosis	Suitable for small tumors of the eyelids, nose, chest, back, or morphea-type basal cell carcinoma Simple procedure; no anesthesia necessary Disadvantages Cannot be used in patients with Raynaud's phenomenon or tumors > 3 cm in diameter.
3. Fluorouracil cream, 1% or 5%, applied topically to cover the lesions twice daily for a few weeks. An inflammatory response is desired; if it does not occur, the drug concentration or frequency of applications or treatment duration should be increased. Typical treatment duration is 2–6 wk or longer	Suitable for basal cell carcinoma on the face and extremities, and on superficial tumors. Disadvantages Photosensitivity, allergic reactions, and not useful in other cancers of skin. Occlusive dressings may increase the incidence of inflammatory reactions in adjacent normal skin. Porous gauze dressings may be used to cover application sites.
4. Fluorouracil plus 2,4-dinitrochlorobenzene	Selected cases of Bowen's disease and *in situ* epidermoid cancer.
5. Combination chemotherapy Fluorouracil plus cisplatin	As a palliative treatment in metastatic skin cancer when surgery is not curative.

- Presents as intracutaneous bluish, firm, and nontender nodule about 0.5 to 1 cm.
- Histologically, a small round cell tumor, containing neurosecretory cytoplasmic granules.
- Neuron-specific enolase positive and anticytokeratin antibody Campath 5.2 positive.
- Differential diagnosis includes small cell carcinoma of lung and lymphoma.
- Early spread by lymphatics and hematogenously to the distant site.
- Surgical excision is the primary treatment, and radiation is used in the adjuvant setting.

Tumors arising from the skin appendages, pilosebaceous complex:

- Hair follicle.
- Sebaceous gland.
- Arrector pili muscle.
- Apocrine sweat gland.
- Majority of the tumors are benign, and carcinomas are rare.
- Significance: Of interest to dermatopathologist.

REFERENCES

1. Balch CM, Reintgen DS, Kirkwood JM, et al. Cutaneous melanoma. In: DeVita VT Jr, Hellman S, Rosenberg SA, eds. *Cancer: principles and practice of oncology.* 5th ed. Philadelphia: Lippincott-Raven, 1997:1947–1994.
2. Santa Cruz DJ, Hurt MA. In: Sternberg SS, ed. *Diagnostic surgical pathology.* 2nd ed. New York: Raven Press, 1999:57–101.

3. Breslow A. Thickness, cross-sectional areas and depth of invasion in the prognosis of cutaneous melanoma. *Ann Surg* 1970;172:902.
4. McCarthy WH, Shaw HM. The surgical treatment of primary melanoma. *Hematol Oncol Clin North Am* 1988;12:797–805.
5. Balch CM, Soong S-J, Bartolucci AA, et al. Efficacy of an elective regional lymph node dissection of 1 to 4 mm thick melanomas for patients 60 years of age and younger. *Ann Surg* 1996;224:255–266.
6. Morton DL. Sentinel lymphadenectomy for patients with clinical stage I melanoma. *J Surg Oncol* 1997;66:267–269.
7. Ghussen F, Nagel K, Groth W, et al. Hyperthermic perfusion with chemotherapy and melanoma of the extremities. *World J Surg* 1989;13:598.
8. Ang KK, Byers RM, Peters LJ, et al. Regional radiotherapy as adjuvant treatment for head and neck malignant melanoma: preliminary results. *Arch Otolaryngol Head Neck Surg* 1990;116:9.
9. Chapman PB, Einhorn LH, Meyers ML, et al. Phase III multicenter randomized trial of the Dartmouth regimen versus dacarbazine in patients with metastatic melanoma. *J Clin Oncol* 1999;17: 2745–2751.
10. Legha SS, Ring S, Papadopoulos N, et al. A prospective evaluation of a triple drug regimen containing cisplatin, vinblastine and dacarbazine (CVD) for metastatic melanoma. *Cancer* 1989;64: 2024–2029.
11. Rosenberg SA, Yang JC, Topalian SL, et al. Treatment of 283 consecutive patients with metastatic melanoma or renal cell cancer using high-dose bolus interleukin 2. *JAMA* 1994;271:907–913.
12. Grob JJ, Dreno B, Salmoniere P, et al. Randomized trial of interferon alfa-2a as adjuvant therapy in resected primary melanoma thicker than 1.5 mm without clinically detectable node metastases. *Lancet* 1998;351:1905–1910.
13. Legha SS, Ring S, Bedikian A, et al. Treatment of metastatic melanoma with combined chemotherapy containing cisplatin, vinblastine and dacarbazine (CVD) and biotherapy using interleukin 2 and interferon alpha. *Ann Oncol* 1996;7:827–835.
14. Rosenberg SA, Yang JC, Schwartzentruber DJ, et al. Immunologic and therapeutic evaluation of a synthetic peptide vaccine for the treatment of patients with metastatic melanoma. *Nat Med* 1998; 4:321–327.
15. Skibber JM, Soong Seng-Jaw, Aushin AC, et al. Cranial irradiation after surgical excision of brain metastasis in melanoma patients. *Ann Surg Oncol* 19 ;3:118–123.
16. Falkson HC. Improved results with the addition of interferon alpha-2b to dacarbazine in the treatment of patients with metastatic malignant melanoma. *J Clin Oncol* 1991;9:1403–1408.

SECTION 9

Hematologic Malignancies

22

The Acute Leukemias

Jame Abraham[*] and [**]Brian P. Monahan

[*]*Medicine Branch, Division of Clinical Sciences, National Cancer Institute,
National Institutes of Health, Bethesda, Maryland
and [**]Division of Hematology and Medical Oncology, Department of Medicine,
Uniformed Services University of the Health Sciences, Bethesda, Maryland*

Adult leukemias consist of acute and chronic leukemias. Acute leukemia is characterized by a block in differentiation, resulting in massive accumulation of immature cells (blasts) in the bone marrow or other organs. Thus bone marrow failure and tissue invasion constitute the clinical features of acute leukemia. Chronic leukemias are due to unregulated proliferation or disordered programmed cell death (apoptosis) and result in marked accumulation of a spectrum of differentiated cells.

Acute leukemia involving myeloid precursors (white cells, red cells, and platelets) is known as acute myeloid leukemia (AML), and leukemia involving cells of lymphoid lineage is known as acute lymphoblastic leukemia (ALL). Acute leukemia is characterized by a rapid clinical course and requires immediate treatment. Advances in the treatment of acute leukemia have resulted in substantial improvement in complete remission and curative potential for selected patients. Untreated acute leukemia is uniformly fatal, with a median survival time less than 3 months. With the available current treatments, most patients will achieve a complete response (CR), many will have a prolonged survival, and some will be cured.

EPIDEMIOLOGY

- In the United States, annual incidence of acute leukemia is 4/100,000 population (AML, 2.5, and ALL, 1.3/100,000).
- AML incidence increases with age, to a peak of 12.6/100,000 adults, age 65 years or older.
- Worldwide incidence is similar to that of the U.S.
- 80% of ALL is seen in children, and only 20% of the cases are reported in adults.
- In adults, AML is by far the most common type of acute leukemia.
- Median age of diagnosis for AML is 65 years, and for ALL is 10 years.

PATHOLOGY

Acute leukemias are a group of clonal disorders of maturation, at an early phase of hematopoietic differentiation. Maturation arrest of myeloblast or promyelocyte is seen in AML and of lymphoblast is seen in ALL.

ETIOLOGY AND RISK FACTORS

For most cases of acute leukemia, the etiology is unknown.

1. Ionizing radiation.
   - It is the most conclusively identified leukemogenic factor in humans.
   - Children exposed to atomic bombs in Japan had 20-fold increased incidence of AML and CML that peaked 5 to 9 years after the explosion.
2. Chemical agents.
   - Occupational chemical exposure has been associated with higher incidence of AML.
   - High-dose occupational benzene exposure (e.g., petroleum products, leather tanning in Third World countries) increases the risk of AML.
   - Use of alkylating agents such as nitrogen mustard, chlorambucil, melphalan and topoisomedrase II inhibitors (etoposide) increases the risk of AML and myelodysplastic syndromes (MDSs).
3. Viruses.
   - Retroviruses like human T-cell lymphoma virus (HTLV-1) cause T-cell lymphoma or leukemia.
4. Genetic Disorders.
   AML:
   - Bloom syndrome.
   - Fanconi's anemia.
   - Diamond–Blackfan anemia.
   - Kostmann's syndrome.
   - Klinefelter's syndrome.
   AML and ALL:
   - Down syndrome.
5. Acquired Disorders.
   - Myelodysplastic syndromes (increased risk for AML).
   - Paroxysmal nocturnal hemoglobinuria (PNH).
   - Myeloproliferative disorders.
   - Polycythemia vera (therapy contributes to risk in case of ^{32}P prior therapy)
   - Primary thrombocytosis (rarely).
6. Secondary Leukemia.
   - Prior chemotherapy increases the risk of acute leukemia, and 90% of these are AML.
   - Reported in survivors of Hodgkin's disease, ALL germ cell tumors, breast cancer, etc.).
   - Chemotherapy agents that can cause secondary leukemia:
       Alkylating agents such as nitrogen mustard, melphalan, cyclophosphamide, chlorambucil, busulfan, thiotepa, CCNU.
       Epipodophyllotoxins (etoposide or teniposide associated with 11q22 deletions).
   - Cytogenetic abnormalities, particularly monosomy 5, 7, 11, and 17 are common in secondary leukemia.
   - Radiation treatment with or without chemotherapy also is a risk factor for secondary leukemia (e.g., pelvic radiotherapy for cervical cancer).

CLINICAL FEATURES

Signs and Symptoms

1. **Bone marrow infiltration with blast cells leading to ineffective hematopoiesis.**
   - Anemia, leading to fatigue and shortness of breath.
   - Thrombocytopenia, causing bleeding and easy bruising.
   - Neutropenia and increased susceptibility for infection.
   - Bone pain from myeloid expansion.

2. **Infiltration of other organs and soft tissues.**
   - Gum hypertrophy (particularly in AML M5).
   - Soft-tissue masses (chloroma) at any location.
   - Hepatomegaly (more common in ALL).
   - Splenomegaly (more common in ALL).
   - Lymphadenopathy (more common in ALL).
   - Testicular involvement (sanctuary site) in ALL.
3. **Central nervous system (CNS) involvement usually restricted to leptomeninges.**
   - Seen in AML M5 and ALL.
   - Features of CNS involvement are headache, radiculopathy or diplopia, cranial nerve palsy, and mental status changes.
4. **Leukocytosis.**
   - Ten percent of all patients may have white blood count (WBC) of >50,000/µL, and it is a poor prognostic factor.
   - They are at increased risk for tumor lysis syndrome and leukostasis.
5. **Leukostasis.**
   - More common in AML than in ALL.
   - Leukocyte thrombi and aggregates are seen in the vasculature of patients with blast count >50,000/µL.
   - It affects the blood flow to the brain and lungs, leading to mental status changes, headache or shortness of breath.
   - Therapy.
       Immediate institution of chemotherapy (e.g., hydroxyurea), even if a final bone marrow biopsy report is not yet available.
       Leukocyte cytoreduction by apheresis.
       Whole-brain XRT if CNS symptoms significant.
6. **Tumor lysis syndrome.**
   - This can be due to spontaneous or treatment-induced cell lysis.
   - It can lead to hyperuricemia, renal failure, acidosis, hyperphosphatemia, hypocalcemia, or coagulopathies.
   - Hyperkalemia can be severe and life threatening.
   - In settings of increasing creatinine levels, prompt hemodialysis is almost always required, and i.v. fluids/allopurinol approaches have limited value.
7. **Disseminated intravascular coagulation (DIC).**
   - Most common in M3 AML (promyelocytic leukemia).
   - Other causes of DIC include septicemia and M4 and M5 AML.
   - Can be confused with the coagulopathy of asparaginase use (results in decreased serum albumin, globulins, coagulation factors).
   - Due to procoagulant release from the leukemic clones' abnormal primary granules, which activate the coagulation cascade, thus decreasing factors II, V, VIII, and X and fibrinogen, and rapidly consuming platelets.
   - M4 and M5 lysozymes released from monoblasts causes are associated with DIC and renal tubular acidosis.

MANAGEMENT OF ACUTE LEUKEMIA

Note on allogeneic stem cell transplantation (SCT): Novel stem cell technologies such as donor lymphocyte infusions after mixed chimerism induction with nonmyeloablative protocols are not considered here but remain of investigational interest. Critically important matters of hyperacute, acute, and chronic graft-versus-host disease identification and management are not discussed here, nor are the very great demands of infrastructure and personnel to achieve the lowest possible treatment-related mortality and morbidity.

Initial Diagnostic Workup for Leukemia

- History and physical examination.
- Complete blood count with differential count.
- Examination of the peripheral blood smear.
- Coagulation studies (PT, aPTT, fibrinogen, D-dimer).
- Serum electrolytes, chemistries with uric acid, calcium, and phosphorus.
- Hepatitis B and C, herpes simplex virus (HSV), cytomegalovirus (CMV), varicella, human immunodeficiency virus (HIV) serologies.
- Bone marrow aspirate for morphology, cytochemistry, cytogenetics, and flow cytometry (many of these studies can be collected from peripheral blood if circulating blast count is high enough). Bone marrow biopsy is needed for cellularity percentage and to evaluate for dysplastic feature.
- Human leukocyte antigen (HLA) typing of patient and siblings if younger than 50 to 55 years.
- Lumbar puncture in all patients with ALL, AML M5, or if otherwise clinically indicated.
- Twelve-lead electrocardiogram for all and ejection fraction estimation if abnormal (echo or MUGA).
- Computed tomography (CT) of the chest (lymphoblastic lymphoma) and abdomen (in mature B-cell ALL).
- Central venous access catheter (dual-lumen catheter preferred). Implanted ports with access needle are not practical. Placement may require plasma or platelet infusion if coagulopathy is present and may be best deferred until later in induction when coagulopathy is less problematic (Fig. 1).

Differentiation of AML from ALL

	AML	ALL
1. Clinical features		
Age groups	Adults (80%)	Adults (20%)
Heptosplenomegaly	±	++
Lymphadenopathy	−	++
Mediastinal Masses	−	T-cell subtypes
Abdominal nodes	−	B-cell subtypes
CNS involvement	±	++
2. Morphology		
Size	Variable	Small
Cytoplasm	Abundant, blue azurophilic granules	Scant
Nucleoli	Distinct, punched-out appearance	Varies by subtype
Auer rods	Present	Absent
3. Cytochemistry		
Myeloperoxidase (MPO)	++	−
Sudan black	++	−
Esterases	+	−
Periodic acid Schiff (PAS)	−	+
Terminal deoxynucleotide transferase (TdT)	−	++
4. Flow cytometry	CD 11, CD13, CD 14, CD 33, HLA DR	CD19, CD20, surface or cytoplasmic IG, CALLA antigens
5. Cytogenetics	t(8;21),t(15;17), inv 16,+8,+21+13	t(4;11),t(1;9),t(8;14), t(9;22),t(4;11)

Emergency management

IV fluids 75–100 mL/h.
Allopurinol 300 mg PO twice daily for 3 days, *then*
Allopurinol 300 mg PO once daily.
Urinary alkalization with IV sodium bicarbonate infusion to
produce a urine pH $\geq$ 7, in selected cases.
Hemodialysis if renal insufficiency is already present.

Anemia

Thrombocytopenia

Mucosal Bleeding

$\downarrow$

Appropriate Blood product

Transfusion
    Sustain Hgb >8-10 g/dL
    Platelets >20,000 if febrile, bleeding, low fibrinogen, prolonged PT or aPTT
    Platelets >10,000 if afebrile, no bleeding or coagulopathy
    Cryoprecipitate for fibrinogen < 125 mg/dl
    FFP for significant PT or aPTT prolongation

Fever and neutropenia

$\downarrow$

Fever work up with blood cultures
and appropriate radiological study.

$\downarrow$

Broad spectrum IV antibiotics
(eg: Ceftazidime 2gm IV q 8 hours)

Fig. 1. Emergency Management.

Identification of Subgroups

Bone marrow should contain more than 20% of nucleated cells as blasts to meet the criteria for diagnosis.

French American British (FAB) classification (Table 1)

- Based on morphology and cytochemistry, and recently, immunophenotyping has been included.
- Depends on identifying the predominant blast population (myeloblast, monoblast, erythroblast, or megakaryoblast) and the degree of their differentiation.
- This classification is applicable only to the material from patients who never received cytotoxic therapy in the past.
- Present classification systems emphasize clinically significant, cytogenetically defined groups rather than FAB.

Risk Stratification in Acute Leukemia

Prognostic Factors in AML

Good prognosis:

- Age: younger than 60 years.
- FAB-M3; t(15;17).

TABLE 1. *The French-American-British (FAB) Classification of AML and Associated Genetic Abnormalities*

FAB Subtype	Common Name (% of Cases)	Results of Staining			Associated Translocation and Rearrangements (% of Cases)	Genes Involved
		MYELOPER-OXIDASE	*SUDAN BLACK*	*NONSPECIFIC ESTERASE*		
M0	Acute myeloblasic leukemia with minimal differentiation (3%)	—	—	—*	inv(3q26) and t(3;3) (1%)	EV11
M1	Acute myeloblastic leukemia without maturation (15–20%)	+	+	—		
M2	Acute myeloblastic leukemia with maturation (25–30%)	+	+	—	t(8;21) (40%), t(6;9) (1%)	AML1-ETO, DEK-CAN
M3	Acute promyelocytic leukemia (5–10%)	+	+	—	t(15;17) (98%), t(11;17) (1%), t(5;17) (1%)	PML-RARα, PLZF-RARα, NPM RARα
M4	Acute myelomonocytic leukemia (20%)	+	+	+	11q23 (20%), inv(3q26) and t(3;3) (3%), t(6;9) (1%)	MLL, DEK-CAN, EV11
M4Eo	Acute myelomonocytic leukemia with abnormal eosinophils (5–10%)	+	+	+	inv(16), t(16;16) (80%)	CBFβ-MYH11
M5	Acute monocytic leukemia (2–9%)	—	—	+	11q23 (20%), t(8;16) (2%)	MLL, MOZ-CBP
M6	Erythroleukemia (3–5%)	+	+	—		
M7	Acute megakaryocytic leukemia (3–12%)	—	—	+†	t(1;22) (5%)	Unknown

*Cells are positive for myeloid antigen (e.g., CD13 and CD33).
†Cells are positive for α-naphthylacetate and platelet glycoprotein IIb/IIIa or factor VIII-related antigen and negative for naphthylbutyrate.

- FAB-M4Eo; inv(16).
- t(8;21).
- t(9;11).

Poor prognosis:

- Age: older than 60 years.
- t(3;3).
- t(4;11).
- t(9;22), -5,-7, (+) 21, +8..
- History of prior myelodysplastic syndromes or secondary leukemia associated with previous chemotherapy or ratiotherapy.
- White cell count >100,000.

Poor Prognostic Factors in ALL

Most adults with ALL have a high risk for recurrence. This may be due to the high incidence of Philadelphia chromosome rearrangement (20–30% of cases).

- High white cell count (730,000/μ1) at the time of diagnosis.
- Age older than 35 years.
- Philadelphia chromosome, t(9:22) rearrangement.
- Prolonged time to achieve remission (>4 weeks from initiation of treatment).
- Leukemic cell immunophenotype.
- T cell has a favorable prognosis.
- Pre B cell has an intermediate prognosis.
- Mature B cell (Burkitt's) has poor prognosis with standard all treatment regimens and requires a specialized chemotherapy and CNS therapy approach.

Treatment of Acute Myeloid Leukemia

Induction chemotherapy alternatives with standard-dose cytarabine (so-called "7 + 3" regimens) (Table 2).

Induction Efficacy Assessment

- Between days 14 and 21, bone marrow aspirate and biopsy are performed to assure that a significant reduction in blast counts has been achieved. If satisfactory, then filgrastim may be initiated (validated efficacy in patients older than 65 years).

TABLE 2. *Induction chemotherapy with standard dose cytarabine*

Regimen	Treatment description	Reference
Cytarabine + daunorubicin	**For patients aged <60 yr** Cytarabine, 100–200 mg/m² per day by continuous i.v. infusion over 24 h for 7 days, days 1–7 (total dose/cycle, 700–1,400 mg/m²), *PLUS* Daunorubicin, 45 mg/m² per day i.v. bolus for 3 days, days 1–3 (total dose/cycle, 135 mg/m²) **For patients aged ≥60 yr** Cytarabine, 100 mg/m² per day by continuous i.v. infusion over 24 h for 7 days, days 1–7 (total dose/cycle, 700 mg/m²), *PLUS* Daunorubicin, 30 mg/m² per day i.v. bolus for 3 days, days 1–3 (total dose/cycle, 90 mg/m²) • Treatment may be repeated in patients who do not achieve a CR after an initial cycle	1
Cytarabine + mitoxantrone	Cytarabine, 100–200 mg/m² per day by continuous i.v. infusion over 24 h for 7 days, days 1–7 (total dose/cycle, 700–1,400 mg/m²), *PLUS* Mitoxantrone, 12 mg/m² per dose i.v. bolus daily for 3 days, days 1–3 (total dose/cycle, 36 mg/m²)	
Cytarabine + idarubicin	Cytarabine, 100–200 mg/m² per day by continuous i.v. infusion over 24 h for 7 days, days 1–7 (total dose/cycle, 700–1,400 mg/m²), *PLUS* Idarubicin, 13 mg/m² per dose i.v. bolus daily for 3 days, days 1–3 (total dose/cycle, 39 mg/m²) • Treatment may be repeated in patients who do not achieve a CR after an initial cycle	2

- If a high blast count remains (e.g., >15%), then an attenuated-duration chemotherapy regimen (cytarabine infusion for 5 days + an anthracycline for 2 days) is initiated immediately. A need for this second attenuated induction course is not considered a case of "induction failure."

- Induction chemotherapy alternatives with high-dose cytarabine (adults younger than 60 years; Table 3) or with etoposide are options for selected patients. These have not been conclusively demonstrated to be superior to idarubicin/cytarabine.

Standard induction therapy. Etoposide may increase induction CR but does not prolong overall survival, while high dose cytabine may improve disease free and overall survival (12).

Post Remission Therapy (Consolidation chemotherapy) (adults, younger than 60 years) is shown in Table 4.

Comments:

- Add prophylaxis with dexamethasone ophthalmic drops to minimize severe keratitis.
- High-dose cytarabine (3,000 mg/m^2) is restricted to patients aged 50 years or younger because risk of CNS toxicity increases with age. Patients require careful monitoring for CNS, hepatic, and pulmonary toxicities. Patients older than 50 years should receive cytarabine, 400 mg/m^2.
- Consolidation is of undetermined value in the setting of secondary AML.

Consolidation chemotherapy (adults, 60 years and older) is outlined in Table 5.

Comments:

- In this age group, cytarabine doses more than 200 mg/m^2/day have not been shown to be superior to standard doses.
- The optimal consolidation treatment in this age group has yet to be defined, due to their much worse prognosis.

TABLE 3. *Induction chemotherapy with high-dose cytarabine*

Regimen	Treatment description	Reference
Cytarabine + daunorubicin	Cytarabine, 3,000 mg/m^2 per dose i.v. over 1 h every 12 h for 12 doses, days 1–6 (total dose/cycle, 36,000 mg/m^2), *PLUS* Daunorubicin, 45 mg/m^2 per day by rapid i.v. infusion, daily for 3 days, days 7–9 (total dose/cycle, 135 mg/m^2)	3
Cytarabine alone	Cytarabine, 3,000 mg/m^2 per dose i.v. over 1 h every 12 h for 12 doses, days 1–6 (total dose/cycle, 36,000 mg/m^2)	
Daunorubicin alone	Daunorubicin, 45 mg/m^2 per day i.v. bolus for 3 days, days 7–9 (total dose/cycle, 135 mg/m^2)	

TABLE 4. *Consolidation chemotherapy with cytarabine*

Treatment description	Reference
Cytarabine, 3,000 mg/m^2 per dose i.v. over 3 h every 12 h for 6 doses, days 1, 3, and 5 (total dose/cycle, 18,000 mg/m^2)	2

TABLE 5. Consolidation chemotherapy

Treatment description	Reference
Cytarabine, 100 mg/m^2 per day by continuous i.v. infusion over 24 h for 5 days, days 1–5 (total dose/cycle, 500 mg/m^2), *PLUS* Daunorubicin, 45 mg/m^2 per day i.v. bolus for 2 days, days 1 and 2 (total dose/cycle, 90 mg/m^2) *OR*	2
Mitoxantrone, 12 mg/m^2 per dose i.v. bolus daily for 2 days, days 1 and 2 (total dose/cycle, 24 mg/m^2) or Cytarabine, 100 mg/m^2 per day by continuous i.v. infusion over 24 h for 5 days, days 1–5 (total dose/cycle, 500 mg/m^2), *PLUS* Idarubicin, 13 mg/m^2 per dose i.v. bolus daily for 2 days, days 1 and 2 (total dose/cycle, 26 mg/m^2)	2

Treatment of M3 AML (Acute Promyelocytic Leukemia; APL)

Induction is described in Table 6. Tretinoin is also known as "all-*trans* retinoic acid."

• Although induction is possible with tretinoin alone, it is seldom used because of a high incidence of retinoic acid syndrome.

Retinoic Acid Syndrome

• Observed in 10% to 20% of patients with APL during induction.
• Symptoms include an abrupt neutrophilia (>20,000/mm^3) between days 5 and 21 accompanied by high fever, respiratory distress, and radiographic evidence of diffuse pulmonary infiltrates, pleural or pericardial effusions ± impaired myocardial contractility, and hypotension.
• Must be differentiated from uncomplicated leukocytosis.
• Requires close monitoring. Manifestations such as unexplained fever and dyspnea indicate discontinuation of tretinoin and immediate intervention with glucocorticoids (e.g., dexamethasone, 10 mg i.v. every 12 hours for 3 or more days or leucocyte apheresis).
• Management may require endotracheal intubation and mechanical ventilation to prevent consequences of progressive hypoxemia.

Post Consultation Maintenance Therapy

Consolidation M3 AML is addressed in Table 7. Maintenance therapy has no demonstrated value in AML.

Response to treatment in AML:

TABLE 6. Induction

Treatment description	Reference
Tretinoin, 22.5 mg/m^2 per dose p.o. twice daily for 45–90 days (total dose/day, 45 mg/m^2) Cytarabine, 100 mg/m^2 per day by continuous i.v. infusion for 7 days, days 1–7 (total dose/cycle, 700 mg/m^2) Daunorubicin, 60 mg/m^2 per day i.v. bolus for three doses, days 1–3 (total dose/cycle, 180 mg/m^2)	9

TABLE 7. Consolidation M3 AML

Treatment description	Reference
Cycle 1	9
Cytarabine, 100 mg/m^2 per day by continuous i.v. infusion for 7 days, days 1–7 (total dose/cycle, 700 mg/m^2)	
Daunorubicin, 60 mg/m^2 per day i.v. bolus for 3 doses, days 1–3 (total dose/cycle, 180 mg/m^2)	
Cycle 2	
Cytarabine, 1,000 mg/m^2 per dose i.v. every 12 h for eight doses, days 1–4 (total dose/cycle, 8,000 mg/m^2)	
Daunorubicin, 45 mg/m^2 per dose i.v. bolus, daily for four doses, days 1–4 (total dose/cycle, 180 mg/m^2)	

- From 50% to 80% of patients achieve a complete remission (CR).
- From 25% to 50% of patients who achieve a CR will have a long-term disease-free survival (DFS).
- Overall 5-year survival is 15% for all groups [favorable cytogenic groups (+8:21), inv(16), +(15:17)] may attain 50–60% long-term survival.

Treatment of relapsed or refractory AML

- All patients should be evaluated for a clinical trial.
- If donors are available, allogeneic bone marrow transplantation (BMT) or matched unrelated donor transplantation should be considered (realize that the long-term survival for refractory induction patients is in the 10% range, and the time for an unrelated donor identification may exceed 3 to 5 months).
- Elderly patients and patients without donors may be considered for autologous BMT, but this is often palliative only.
- Other options are multiagent chemotherapy containing high-dose Ara-C for those younger than 50 years, and supportive care including outpatient transfusion support, oral antibiotics, hydroxyurea, etc. in the elderly.

Stem Cell Transplantation in AML

- There is considerable controversy about the indications and the timing of SCT in AML.
- A recently published study (10) found no significant differences in disease-free survival (DFS) in patients receiving a postinduction course of high-dose cytarabine and those undergoing autologous or allogeneic SCT.
- The treatment-related mortality (TRM) from allogeneic SCT is 20% to 40%. High TRM overwhelms the favorable initial CR rates and limits the overall survival, leading to the equivalent long-term survival in a favorable subset of AML patients treated with chemotherapy consolidation and those treated with BMT in first remission.
- In postconsolidation relapses, the overall survival is so poor for all that the TRM of allogeneic BMT is more acceptable.

Some of the indications for allogeneic SCT in AML:

- Those for whom standard induction therapy fails and who have an identified donor [sibling or matched unrelated donor (MUD)].
- Those who are in first relapse.
- Patients with poor-risk cytogenetics as a postremission therapy in lieu of standard consolidation.

- Patients with an antecedent hematologic disorder in lieu of standard consolidation.
- Patients (young age only) with high-grade myelodysplastic syndrome (trilineage dysplasia with excess blasts) in lieu of standard induction/consolidation.

Autologous SCT in AML

Subject of ongoing clinical trials in risk-adapted protocols.

- Generally considered palliative and of limited value.
- In patients with poor-risk cytogenetics or antecedent hematologic disorder, as a postremission therapy if they have no donors.
- Roles of purging malignant cells from autologous stem cell graft product and timing of transplantation are under investigation.

Treatment of Acute Lymphoblastic Leukemia

Treatment overview:

- Remission induction.
- Consolidation.
- CNS prophylaxis.
- Late intensification.

- Maintenance:
  The "Hoelzer (Berlin-Frankfurt-Munster; "BFM") regimen" is detailed in Table 8, and the "Larson regimen" (5) is described in Table 9.

Special considerations

B-cell ALL (L3):

- Expresses surface immunoglobulin and cytogenetic abnormalities such as t(8;14), t(2;8), and t(8;22).
- Not usually cured with typical ALL treatment regimens.
- Aggressive cyclophosphamide-containing regimens similar to those used in high-grade non-Hodgkin's lymphoma (NHL) have shown higher cure rates.
- Therapy will use an aggressive CNS phase (IT therapy, high-dose methotrexate; e.g., Hoelzer regimen and Magrath regimen).
- No maintenance therapy needed.

Stem Cell Transplantation in ALL

Allogeneic SCT:

- TRM is 20% to 40%. Matched related donor is preferred.
- ALL patients with poor prognostic factors should be considered for allogeneic SCT, if they have a donor (French study).
- ALL patients with Ph+ will benefit from an allogeneic SCT in first remission due to their poor prognosis with standard therapy.
- Otherwise, allogeneic BMT is for patients in second remission.

Autologous SCT:

- Less effective than allogeneic SCT.
- Randomized studies failed to show any survival advantage for autologous BMT over conventional chemotherapy in CR.
- Limited utility of conventional methods leads to opportunities for clinical trials.

TABLE 8. *The Hoelzer regimen*

Treatment description	Reference
Induction phase I	7

Induction phase I
Prednisone, 60 mg/m^2 per dose p.o., daily for 28 doses, days 1–28
(total dose/phase, 1,680 mg/m^2)
Vincristine, 1.5 mg/m^2 per dose i.v. for four doses, days 1, 8, 15, and 22
(total dose/phase, 6 mg/m^2; maximal single dose, 2 mg)
Daunorubicin, 25 mg/m^2 per dose i.v. for four doses, days 1, 8, 15, and 22
(total dose/phase, 100 mg/m^2)
Asparaginase, 5,000 Units/m^2 per dose i.v., daily for 14 doses, days 1–14
(total dose/phase, 70,000 Units/m^2)
• Given during wk 1–4

Induction phase II
Cyclophosphamide, 650 mg/m^2 per dose i.v. for three doses, days 29, 43, and
57 (total dose/phase, 1,950 mg/m^2; maximal single dose, 1,000 mg/m^2)
Cytarabine, 75 mg/m^2 per dose i.v. for 16 doses, days 31–34, 38–41, 45–48,
and 52–55 (total dose/phase, 1,200 mg/m^2)
Mercaptopurine, 60 mg/m^2 per dose p.o., daily for 29 doses, days 29–57
(total dose/phase, 1,740 mg/m^2)
• Given during weeks 5–8

CNS prophylaxis
Cranial irradiation, 24 Gy given with phase II induction
Methotrexate, 10 mg/m^2 per dose i.t. for four doses, days 31, 38, 45, and 52
(total dose/phase, 40 mg/m^2; maximal single dose, 15 mg)
• Given during wk 5–8 when CR is achieved after induction phase I;
otherwise, immediately after induction phase II

Reinduction phase I
Dexamethasone, 10 mg/m^2 per dose p.o. for 28 doses, days 1–28
(total dose/phase, 280 mg/m^2)
Vincristine, 1.5 mg/m^2 per dose i.v. for four doses, days 1, 8, 15, and 22
[total dose/phase, 1.5 mg/m^2 (maximal single dose not specified)]
Doxorubicin, 25 mg/m^2 per dose i.v. for 4 doses, days 1, 8, 15, and 22
(total dose/phase, 100 mg/m^2)
• Given during wk 9–12

Reinduction phase II
Cyclophosphamide, 650 mg/m^2 i.v. day 29
(total dose/phase, 650 mg/m^2; maximal single dose, 1,000 mg/m^2)
Cytarabine, 75 mg/m^2 per dose i.v. for eight doses, days 31–34 and 38–41
(total dose/phase, 600 mg/m^2)
Thioguanine, 60 mg/m^2 per dose p.o., daily for 14 doses, days 29–42
(total dose/phase, 840 mg/m^2)
• Given during wk 13–14

Maintenance
Mercaptopurine, 60 mg/m^2 per dose p.o., daily for 777 doses, during weeks
10–18 and 29–130 (total dose/week, 420 mg/m^2)
Methotrexate, 20 mg per dose p.o. or i.v., weekly for 111 doses, during
weeks 10–18 and 29–130 (total dose/week, 20 mg)

Treatment of Relapsed ALL

• If the patient has a suitable donor, consider for allogeneic SCT, either matched sibling or matched unrelated donor.
• If it is a late relapse (e.g., >12 months), consider reinduction with the initial treatment regimen.
• If it is an early relapse, high-dose cytarabine with mitoxantrone or methotrexate/L-asparaginase can be used.

TABLE 9. *The Larson regimen*

Treatment description	Reference
Course I	8

Induction and early intensification (patients aged <60 yr)
  Cyclophosphamide, 1,200 mg/m^2 i.v. day 1
    (total dose/course, 1,200 mg/m^2)
  Daunorubicin, 45 mg/m^2 per dose i.v. for three doses, days 1–3
    (total dose/course, 135 mg/m^2)
  Vincristine, 2 mg per dose i.v. for four doses, days 1, 8, 15, and 22
    (total dose/course, 8 mg)
  Prednisone, 60 mg/m^2 per dose p.o. or i.v. for 21 doses, days 1–21
    (total dose/course, 1,260 mg/m^2)
  Asparaginase, 6,000 IUnits/m^2 per dose s.c. for six doses, days 5, 8, 11,
    15, 18, and 22 (total dose/course, 36,000 IUnits/m^2)
  • Course duration is 4 weeks
Induction and early intensification (patients aged ≥60 yr)
  Cyclophosphamide, 800 mg/m^2 i.v. day 1
    (total dose/course, 800 mg/m^2)
  Daunorubicin, 30 mg/m^2 per dose i.v. for three doses, days 1–3
    (total dose/course = 90 mg/m^2)
  Vincristine, 2 mg per dose i.v. for four doses, days 1, 8, 15, and 22
    (total dose/course, 8 mg)
  Prednisone, 60 mg/m^2 per dose p.o. or i.v. for seven doses, days 1–7
    (total dose/course = 420 mg/m^2)
  Asparaginase, 6,000 IUnits/m^2 per dose s.c. for six doses, days 5, 8, 11,
    15, 18, and 22 (total dose/course, 36,000 IUnits/m^2)
  • Course duration is 4 weeks
Course II: early intensification course
  Methotrexate, 15 mg i.t. on day 1
    (total dose/course, 15 mg)
  Cyclophosphamide, 1,000 mg/m^2 i.v. day 1
    (total dose/course, 1,000 mg/m^2)
  Mercaptopurine, 60 mg/m^2 per dose p.o. for 14 doses, days 1–14
    (total dose/course, 840 mg/m^2)
  Cytarabine, 75 mg/m^2 per dose s.c. for eight doses, days 1–4 and 8–11
    (total dose/course, 600 mg/m^2)
  Vincristine, 2 mg per dose i.v. for two doses, days 15 and 22
    (total dose/course, 4 mg)
  Asparaginase, 6,000 IUnits/m^2 per dose s.c. for four doses, days 15, 18, 22,
    and 25 (total dose/course, 24,000 IUnits/m^2)
  • Course duration is 4 weeks
  • Course II is repeated once (total, two courses)
Course III: CNS prophylaxis and interim maintenance
  Methotrexate, 15 mg per dose i.t. for five doses, days 1, 8, 15, 22, and 29
    (total dose/course, 75 mg)
  Cranial irradiation, 2,400 cGy in fractionated doses on days 1–12
  • Initiated with the first two doses of intrathecal methotrexate
  Mercaptopurine, 60 mg/m^2 per dose p.o. for 70 doses, days 1–70
    (total dose/course, 4,200 mg/m^2)
  Methotrexate, 20 mg/m^2 per dose p.o. for five doses, days 36, 43, 50, 57,
    and 64 (total dose/course, 100 mg/m^2)
  • Course duration is 12 weeks
Course IV: Late intensification
  Doxorubicin, 30 mg/m^2 i.v. days 1, 8, and 15
    (total dose/course, 90 mg/m^2)

Continued

TABLE 9. *Continued*

Treatment description	Reference
Vincristine, 2 mg per dose i.v. for 3 days, days 1, 8, and 15 (total dose/course, 6 mg)	

Vincristine, 2 mg per dose i.v. for 3 days, days 1, 8, and 15
  (total dose/course, 6 mg)
Dexamethasone, 10 mg/m^2 per dose p.o. for 14 days, days 1–14
  (total dose/course, 140 mg/m^2)
Cyclophosphamide, 1,000 mg/m^2 i.v. day 29
  (total dose/course, 1,000 mg/m^2)
Thioguanine, 60 mg/m^2 per dose p.o. for 14 days, days 29–42
  (total dose/course, 840 mg/m^2)
Cytarabine, 75 mg/m^2 per dose s.c. for 8 days, days 29–32 and 36–39
  (total dose/course, 600 mg/m^2)
• Course duration is 8 weeks
Course V: Prolonged maintenance
Vincristine, 2 mg i.v. on day 1
  (total dose/cycle, 2 mg)
Prednisone, 60 mg/m^2 per dose p.o. for 5 days, days 1–5
  (total dose/cycle, 300 mg/m^2)
Methotrexate, 20 mg/m^2 per dose p.o. for 4 days, days 1, 8, 15, and 22
  (total dose/cycle, 80 mg/m^2)
Mercaptopurine, 60 mg/m^2 per dose p.o. for 28 days, days 1–28
  (total dose/cycle, 1,680 mg/m^2)
• Treatment cycles are repeated every 28 days
• Continues until 24 months after diagnosis

- All patients should be considered for clinical trials.
- Second line therapies have complete response rates in 70+% range, yet 2 yr survival of less than 5%.

Central Nervous System Relapse

- CNS, testis, and eye often have problematic drug delivery (the sanctuary sites) in ALL.
- Standard CNS prophylaxis has reduced the CNS relapse rate from 30% to 10%.
- Patients should be treated with chemotherapy and/or radiotherapy based on considerations for the type of CNS prophylaxis previously given.
- Whole-brain radiotherapy consists of 2,000 to 2,400 cGy with intrathecal methotrexate or cytarabine.
- Chemotherapy alone using an Ommaya reservoir and methotrexate or cytarabine.

Major complications during treatment of acute leukemia

- Tumor lysis syndrome (especially in Burkitt's type or in those with preexisting renal dysfunction).
- Prolonged neutropenia (patient survival is reduced as the duration increases).
- Infections (emerging role of gram-positive pathogens).
- Thrombocytopenia.
- Hemorrhage.
- Coagulopathy (especially in AML M3).
- Retinoic acid syndrome in AML M3 ATRA therapy.

Supportive Care

- Improvement in supportive care has significantly decreased the TRM in acute leukemia.
- Immediate treatment of febrile neutropenia with broad spectrum antibiotics.
- Aggressive blood product support in coagulopathy/thrombocytopenia cases and induction regimens to diminish this high risk in AML M3 cases.
- Careful instructions for central venous catheter care, dental care, and recognition of early signs of infection.
- Ciprofloxacin and norfloxacin have been shown to decrease the incidence of gram-negative infection and time to first fever, in some randomized trials.
- Appropriate transfusion support.
- Use of leukocyte depletion filters with blood products to reduce CMV seroconversion febrile transfusion reactions and subsequent alloimmunization.
- Granulocyte/macrophage–colony-stimulating factor (GM-CSF) or G-CSF decrease morbidity and hospitalization in elderly who are undergoing treatment for acute leukemia.

REFERENCES

1. Dillman RO, Davis RB, Green MR, et al. A comparative study of two different doses of cytarabine for acute myeloid leukemia: a phase III trial of cancer and leukemia: group B. *Blood* 1991;78: 2520–2526.
2. Mayer RJ, Davis RB, Schiffer CA, et al. Intensive postremission chemotherapy in adults with acute myeloid leukemia. *N Eng J Med* 1994;331:896–903.
4. Bishop JF, Matthews JP, Young GA, et al. A randomized study of high-dose cytarabine in induction in acute myeloid leukemia. *Blood* 1996;87:1710–1717.
5. Mayer RJ, Davis RB, Schiffer CA, et al. Intensive postremission chemotherapy in adults with acute myeloid leukemia: cancer and leukemia group B. *N Engl J Med* 1994;331:896–903.
6. Weick JK, Kopecky KJ, Appelbaum FR. et al. A randomized investigation of high-dose versus standard-dose cytosine arabinoside with daunorubicin in patients with previously untreated acute myeloid leukemia: a Southwest Oncology Group study. *Blood* 1996;88:2841–2851.
7. Hoelzer D, Thiel E, Loffler H, et al. Prognostic factors in a multicenter study for treatment of acute lymphoblastic leukemia in adults. *Blood* 1988;71:123–131.
8. Larson RA, Dodge RK, Burns CP, et al. A five-drug remission induction regimen with intensive consolidation for adults with acute lymphoblastic leukemia: cancer and leukemia group B study 8811. *Blood* 1995;85:2025–2037.
9. Fenaux P, Wattel E, Archimbaud E, et al. Prolonged follow-up confirms that all-trans retinoic acid followed by chemotherapy reduces the risk of relapse in newly diagnosed acute promyelocytic leukemia: the French APL Group. *Blood* 1994;84:666–667.
10. Cassileth PA, Harrington DP, Appelbaum FR, et al. Chemotherapy compared with autologous or allogeneic bone marrow transplantation in the management of acute myeloid leukemia in first remission. *N Engl J Med* 1998;339:1649–1656.
11. Edenfield WJ, Gore SD. Stage-specific application of allogeneic and autologous marrow transplantation in the management of acute myeloid leukemia. *Semin Oncol* 1999;26:21–34.
12. Lowenberg B, Downing JR, Burnett A. Acute myeloid leukemia. *N Eng J Med* 1999;341:1051–1062.

23

Chronic Leukemias

William Jawien and John Chute

National Naval Medical Center, National Institutes of Health, Bethesda, Maryland

Chronic lymphocytic leukemia (CLL) accounts for more than one third of all leukemias and because of its prevalence in hematologic practice, it is the focus of this chapter. Additional chronic leukemias discussed in this chapter include prolymphocytic leukemia (PLL) and hairy cell leukemia (HCL) (Tables 1 and 2).

DIAGNOSIS

Various diagnostic criteria have been proposed for CLL; two of the most commonly used are the National Cancer Institute–sponsored Working Group (NCI-WG) guidelines and those of the International Workshop on CLL (IWCLL). The NCI-WG guidelines require (a) an absolute lymphocytosis ($\geq 5 \times 10^3/\mu L$) with cells having a morphologically mature appearance sustained for 4 weeks; (b) ($\geq 30\%$ lymphocytes in a normocellular or hypercellular bone marrow; and (c) monoclonal B-cell phenotype with a low-level surface immunoglobulin expression expressing CD5. The IWCLL recommends similar criteria but requires $\geq 10 \times 10^3/\mu L$ lymphocytes if facilities to obtain phenotyping are not available.

STAGING

There also are several staging methods for CLL. The three most commonly used are the Rai, modified Rai, and the Binet staging systems (Table 3).

TREATMENT

CLL is clearly an indolent hematologic malignancy often not requiring treatment at diagnosis. In general, treatment is initiated after the occurrence of one of the following complications: (a) significant and persistent fatigue; (b) weight loss; (c) fever without infection; (d) night sweats; (e) significant anemia (Hgb, <10 g/dL); (f) thrombocytopenia ($<10 \times 10^3/\mu L$); and (g) disfiguring or bulky lymphadenopathy and/or significant splenomegaly. Usually the level of lymphocytosis is not an absolute indication for treatment. However, treatment is usually initiated for a lymphocytosis $>200 \times 10^3/\mu L$. The most common initial systemic therapies used are chlorambucil and fludarabine. Use of the anti-CD20 monoclonal antibody therapy also is increasing in popularity, probably because of the possibility of its less severe side-effect profile as compared with standard chemotherapy. In Table 4, we describe several of the treatments available for CLL and particular comments related to those therapies.

Complications can occur as an intrinsic component of the disorder or a result of therapy. Table 5 is a summary of such complications.

TABLE 1. *Chronic lymphocytic leukemia*

CLL	Comments
CLL	B-cell malignancy (>95%)
Incidence	10,000 cases annually in U.S.
Median age	55 yr
M:F	2:1
Etiology	No known causes, slight increased risk of CLL and B-cell malignancies in family members
Molecular	Accumulation of clonal lymphocytes, possibly a result of overexpression of bcl-2, which can interfere with apoptosis
Cytogenetic abnormalities	Trisomy 12; abnormalities in long arm of 6, 13, and 14 also identified

TABLE 2. *Clinical and laboratory features*

	Comments
Symptoms	Fatigue, weight loss, fever in the absence of active infection, night sweats, unusually severe local reactions to insect bites, increased frequency of bacterial and viral infections
Physical examination	Lymphadenopathy, splenomegaly
Laboratory features	Lymphocytosis (5–500 × 10^3/μL), appear as normal lymphocytes by light microscopy with presence of scant cytoplasm; mature nuclear chromatin, and poorly developed endoplasmic reticulum, low mitotic index; presence of smudge cells (artifact of blood smear preparation); absolute neutrophil count can be low, normal, or increased; anemia or thrombocytopenia may be present
Bone marrow	Demonstrates nodular or diffuse infiltration of small- to medium-sized lymphocytes with mature features and normal myeloid components
Lymph nodes	Infiltrates of small- to medium-sized lymphocytes with condensed mature-appearing chromatin and an occasional nucleolus; larger lymphocytes with more prominent nucleoli are usually present and are termed prolymphocytes, can be clustered as pseudofollicles
Immunologic features	Expression of single light chain on the surface of the cell, light and heavy chain immunoglobulin gene rearrangements are usually identified, the majority of cases also demonstrate heavy chain on surface (usually mu); rare individual cases can be found to secrete immunoglobulin in sufficient quantity to identify a monoclonal gamma globulin spike; flow cytometry is found to be positive for CD19, CD20, CD21, CD23, CD5 with variable results for CD25 and CD11c

TABLE 3. *Staging*

Rai	Modified Rai	Criteria
0	Low risk	Lymphocytosis only ($\geq$15 × 10^3/μL in peripheral blood)
1	Intermediate risk	Lymphocytosis with enlarged nodes
2	Intermediate risk	Lymphocytosis with increased splenic or hepatic size
3	High risk	Lymphocytosis with anemia (Hgb <11 g/dL)
4	High risk	Lymphocytosis with thrombocytopenia (<100 × 10^3/μL)

TABLE 4. *Therapies*

Therapy	Comments
Chlorambucil	Well tolerated, can be administered low dosage (2–8 mg/day), or high-dose intermittent (30–60 mg/m^2) p.o. over 1–3 days q 2–4 wk
Fludarabine	25 mg/m^2 i.v. daily for 5 days q 4 wk, consider precautions against tumor lysis during first cycle; cumulative toxicity includes myelosuppression and prolonged immunosuppression
Cyclophosphamide	2–3 mg/kg/day p.o. for 5 days q 3 weeks, or 600 mg/m^2 q 3–4 wk
Cladribine	0.1 mg/kg i.v. continuous infusion for 7 days q wk, or 0.14 mg/kg daily over 2 h for 5 days q 4 wk
CVP	Cyclophosphamide, 300 mg/m^2 p.o. days 1–5, or 800 mg/m^2 on day 1, vincristine, 1 mg/m^2 on day 1, and prednisone, 40 mg/m^2 p.o. days 1–5 given monthly, effective in some patients refractory to chlorambucil
Rituximab	375 mg/m^2 i.v. infusion q wk for 4 wk
Corticosteroids	May have a lymphocytolytic effect at 40–80 mg/day given for several weeks, high-dose prednisone, 40–60 mg/m^2 also useful for treatment of immune-mediated hemolysis and thrombocytopenia
Radiation therapy	Potentially beneficial in hypersplenism and symptomatic splenomegaly; nodal radiation may also be beneficial to relieve local symptoms and in treatment of organ dysfunction
Splenectomy	Potential benefit in chemotherapy-unresponsive disease, hypersplenism and autoimmune anemia, appropriate presplenectomy vaccinations
Leukopheresis	Rarely used in CLL; consider for leukocyte counts >500 × 10^3/μL or when symptoms or signs of hyperviscosity are present.
Investigational	Current investigational protocols should be investigated and discussed with patient

TABLE 5. *Complications*

Complication	Comments
Anemia	May be secondary to a suppressive effect of CLL or secondary to autoimmune hemolytic anemia (AIHA); AIHA may require high-dose prednisone and/or splenectomy for treatment
Thrombocytopenia	Also can be secondary to marrow suppression or an autoimmune nature
Granulocytopenia	Secondary to either CLL or chemotherapy
Hypogammaglobulinemia	Suggested by frequent sinopulmonary infections, CLL patients often have an inadequate humoral response to infections and immunizations; infections with encapsulated organisms and gram-negative bacteria constitute the major etiologies of mortality and morbidity in CLL
Pure red cell aplasia	Possibly caused by a suppressive effect of suppressor cytotoxic T cells; cyclosporine has been used successfully as treatment, with a reticulocyte response seen within 2 weeks after starting therapy
Paraneoplastic pemphigus	Autoantibody-induced oral mucocutaneous lesions
Transformation	Transformation to more aggressive malignancies occurs in 10% of cases; these transformations include prolymphocytic, Richter's syndrome (large B-cell lymphoma), ALL, and multiple myeloma

PROGNOSIS

Prognosis is outlined in Table 6.

T-cell CLL

T-cell CLL occurs in 2% to 5% of patients with CLL. A large amount of variability exists with respect to the clinical findings and clinical course. PLL is shown in Table 7 and HCL in Table 8.

TABLE 6. *Prognosis*

Modified Rai stage	Median survival (yr)
Low risk	>10
Intermediate risk	7
High risk	3

TABLE 7. *Prolymphocytic leukemia*

	Comments
Morphology	Large cells with abundant cytoplasm and prominent nucleolus within a convoluted nucleus with immature chromatin
Immunology	High-density immunoglobulin, CD19, CD20, and CD22, with absence of CD5
Cytogenetics	t(11:14), which represents the translocation of the bcl-1 oncogene in proximity to the Ig heavy chain gene
Clinical findings	High blast counts with splenomegaly, usually lacking significant adenopathy, occurs as a terminal finding in up to 10% of CLL
Treatment	Fludarabine, cladrabine, CHOP
T-cell PLL	20% of PLL cases, usually a more aggressive course than the B-cell form, expression of CD3, CD4, occasionally CD8, with rearrangement of the T cell–receptor gene, treatment commonly involves pentostatin

TABLE 8. *Hairy cell leukemia*

	Comments
Clinical findings	Male predominance, pancytopenia, splenomegaly, lymphadenopathy is uncommon, necrotizing vasculitis, opportunistic infections, lytic bone abnormalities
Morphology	Lymphocytes with cytoplasmic projections, tartrate-resistant acid phosphatase (TRAP) stain positive
Bone marrow	Aspiration frequently unsuccessful secondary to fibrosis; marrow biopsy reveals "hairy" cells and classic "fried-egg" appearance
Immunology	High-intensity sIg, CD19, 20, 21, 22, 11c, 25, PCA-1 and Bly7, light and heavy chain Ig rearrangements
Treatment indications	Life-threatening infections, vasculitis, bony involvement, symptomatic splenomegaly, neutropenia (<0.5–1.0 × 10^9/mL), anemia (hgh, <8–10 g/dL), thrombocytopenia (<50–100 × 10^9/mL), leukocytosis with a significant number of hairy cells
Treatment	2-Chlorodeoxyadenosine provides a >95% response, given at 0.1 mg/kg/d by CI over 7 days, 2'-deoxycofomycin produces response rates of 40–80% and is administered at 4 mg/m² every other week for 3–6 months, interferon-α produces a >70% response rate and is adminstered 3 times per week s.c. at 2 million units/m², splenectomy is currently reserved for those with thrombocytopenia and bleeding or those for whom systemic chemotherapy has failed

REFERENCES

1. Harris NL, Jaffe ES, Stein H, et al. A revised European-American classification of lymphoid neoplasms: a proposal from the International Lymphoma Study Group. *Blood* 1994;84:1361–1392.
2. International Workshop on Chronic Lymphocytic Leukemia. Chronic lymphocytic leukemia: recommendations for diagnosis, staging, and response criteria. *Ann Intern Med* 1989;110:236–238.
3. Rai KR, Sawitsky A, Cronkite EP, et al. Clinical staging of chronic lymphocytic leukemia. *Blood* 1975;46:219–234.
4. Binet JL, Auquier A, Dighiero G, et al. A new prognostic classification of chronic lymphocytic leukemia derived from a multivariate survival analysis. *Cancer* 1981;48:198–206.
5. Sawitsky A, Rai KR, Glidewell O, et al. Comparison of daily versus intermittent chlorambucil and prednisone therapy in the treatment of patients with chronic lymphocytic leukemia. *Blood* 1977;50: 1049–1059.
6. O'Brien S, Katarjian H, Beran M, et al. Results of fludarabine and prednisone therapy in 264 patients with chronic lymphocytic leukemia with multivariate analysis-derived prognostic model for response to treatment. *Blood* 1993;82:1695–1700.
7. Maloney DG, Grillo-Lopez AJ, White CA, et al. IDEC-C2B8 (Rituximab) anti-CD20 monoclonal antibody therapy in patients with relapsed low-grade non-Hodgkin's lymphoma. *Blood* 1997;90: 2188–2195.
8. Merl SA, Theodorakis ME, Goldberg J, et al. Splenectomy for thrombocytopenia in chronic lymphocytic leukemia. *Am J Hematol* 1983;15:253–259.
9. Ferrant A, Michaux JL, Sokal G. Splenectomy in advanced chronic lymphocytic leukemia. *Cancer* 1986;58:2130–2135.
10. Chikkappa G, Pasquale D, Phillips PG, et al. Cyclosporin-A for the treatment of pure red cell aplasia in a patient with chronic lymphocytic leukemia. *Am J Hematol* 1987;26:179–189.
11. Robertson LE, Pugh W, O'Brien S, et al. Richter's syndrome: a report on 39 patients. *J Clin Oncol* 1993;11:1985–1989.
12. Flandrin G, Sigaux F, Sebahoun G, et al. Hairy cell leukemia: clinical presentation and follow-up of 211 patients. *Semin Oncol* 1984;11:458–471.
13. Golomb HM, Catovsky D, Golde DW. Hairy cell leukemia: a clinical review based on 71 cases. *Ann Intern Med* 1978;89:677–683.
14. Piro LD, Carrera CJ, Carson DA, et al. Lasting remissions in hairy-cell leukemia induced by a single infusion of 2-chlorodeoxyadenosine. *N Engl J Med* 1990;322:1117–1121.
15. Cassileth PA, Cheuvart B, Spiers ASD, et al. Pentostatin induces durable remissions in hairy cell leukemia. *J Clin Oncol* 1991;9:243–246.
16. Keating MJ, Kantarjian M, Talpaz J, et al. Fludarabine: A new agent with major activity against chronic lymphocytic leukemia, *Blood* 1989;74:19–25.
17. Juliusson G, Liliemark J. High complete remission rate from 2-chloro-2'-deoxyadenosine in previously treated patients with B-cell chronic lymphocytic leukemia: Response predicted by rapid decrease of blood lymphocyte count. *J Clin Oncol* 1993;11:679–689.
18. Raphael B, Anderson JW, Silber R, et al. Comparison of chlorambucil and prednisone versus cyclophosphamide, vincristine, and prednisone as initial treatment for chronic lymphocytic leukemia: Long-term follow-up of an Eastern Cooperative Oncology Group randomized clinical trial. *J Clin Oncol* 1991;9:770–776.
19. Byrd JC, Waselenko JK, Maneatis TJ, et al. Rituximab therapy in hematologic malignancy patients with circulating blood tumor cells: Association with increased infusion-related side effects and rapid blood tumor clearance. *J Clin Oncon* 1999;17:791–795.
20. Huguley CM. Treatment of chronic lymphocytic leukemia. *Cancer Treat Rev* 1977;4:261–273.
21. Estey EH, Kurzrock R, Kantarjian HM, et al. Treatment of hairy cell leukemia with 2-chlorodeoxyadenosine (2-CdA). *Blood* 1992;79:882–887.
22. Kraut EH, Bouroncle BA, Grever MR. Pentostatin in the treatment of advanced hairy cell leukemia. *J Clin Oncol* 1989;7:168–172.

24

Chronic Myeloid Leukemia

Yogen Saunthararajah and Johnson M. Liu

National Heart Lung and Blood Institute, National Institutes of Health, Bethesda, Maryland

EPIDEMIOLOGY

Chronic myeloid leukemia (CML) has an incidence in the United States of one to two cases per 100,000 per year, with the median age at diagnosis of 50 years. More than 80% of patients are diagnosed in the chronic phase, often incidentally during routine tests. CML rarely occurs in children (2–3% of childhood leukemias).

PATHOPHYSIOLOGY

The hallmark of CML is the Philadelphia chromosome (Ph-chromosome), a reciprocal translocation between the long arms of chromosomes 9 and 22 [i.e., t(9;22)]. The translocation results in the transfer of the Abelson (abl) gene to an area of chromosome 22 termed the breakpoint cluster region (bcr). The fusion product of this translocation, a protein with tyrosine kinase activity, is believed to play a pathogenic role in this disease.

STAGING AND PROGNOSIS

CML typically progresses over time from its chronic phase to an accelerated phase and then a blastic phase (see Table 1).

- Blast crisis: An abrupt transition to a blastic phase is known as a blast crisis. Features of a blast crisis include fever, malaise, progressive and painful splenomegaly and/or hepatomegaly, bone pain, worsening anemia and thrombocytopenia, and thrombotic or bleeding complications.

TABLE 1. *CML stages and prognosis*

Stage	Features	Median survival
Chronic phase	<5% blasts and promyelocytes in PB or BM	5–6 yr
Accelerated phase	Increasing symptoms such as fever or bone pain, progressive splenomegaly, >5% blasts and promyelocytes in PB or BM, worsening thrombocytopenia, cytogenetic clonal evolution, >20% peripheral basophils	<1 yr
Blastic phase	>30% blasts and promyelocytes in the PB and BM with features of accelerated phase as described earlier	A few months

Accelerated and blastic phase definitions are vague; PB, peripheral blood; BM, bone marrow.

TABLE 2. *Modified Sokal's risk index*

Risk category	Median survival
Low risk, score ≤780 (good responses with interferon-α)	98 mo
Intermediate risk, score ≤1,480	65 mo
High risk, score >1,480	

Score = (0.6666 × age [0 when age <50 y; 1 otherwise] + 0.420 × spleen size [cm below costal margin] + 0.0584 × blasts [%] + 0.0413 × eosinophils [%] + 0.2039 × basophils [0 when basophils <3%; 1, otherwise] + 1.0956 × platelet count [0 when platelets <1,500 × 10°/L; 1, otherwise]) × 1,000.

• Prognosis: The chronic phase typically lasts 3 to 4 years, with the annual rate of progression to a blastic phase of 5% to 10% in the first 2 years and 20% in subsequent years. The prognosis for the patient in the chronic phase is 5 to 6 years, with some patients surviving as long as 10 years. For patients in the accelerated phase, survival is usually less than 1 year, and for blast crisis, a few months. A shorter chronic phase may be predicted by features at diagnosis such as older age, male sex, increased lactate dehydrogenase (LDH), multiple cytogenetic abnormalities, a high percentage of immature myeloid cells, basophilia, eosinophilia, thrombocytosis, and anemia. A useful predictive model using these multiple risk factors is the Sokal's risk index. A recently modified version of this index that predicts patients who do best with chemotherapy or interferon-α is illustrated in Table 2.

DIAGNOSIS AND CLINICAL FEATURES

Symptoms

• Early chronic phase may have no symptoms.
• Fatigue.
• Anorexia.
• Weight loss.
• Dyspnea on exertion.

Signs

• The most common finding is splenomegaly, which can be massive (in about 10% of patients, the spleen is not enlarged, even on splenic scan).

Laboratory Studies

• Increased white count (usually greater than $25 \times 10^3/\mu L$).
• Increased platelet count in approximately 50% of cases.
• Myeloid cells at all stages of maturation in the peripheral smear (the percentage of immature myeloid cells in the blood or bone marrow can indicate the phase of the disease, as described earlier).
• Marked marrow myeloid hyperplasia.
• Leukocyte alkaline phosphatase (LAP) activity of CML neutrophils is markedly diminished from the 20% reactivity of normal neutrophils (or leukoerythroblastic reaction).
• Diagnosis confirmed through detection of the t(9;22) abnormality on cytogenetic analysis or polymerase chain reaction (PCR) detection of the bcr-abl fusion in white cells from

peripheral blood [about 10% of patients will be negative for the t(9;22) on standard karyotypic analysis].

Differential Diagnoses

• Leukoerythroblastic reaction in response to infection or malignancy (see Table 1 in Chapter 25 for features to distinguish CML from other myeloproliferative disorders).
• Chronic myelomonocytic leukemia (CMML).
• Atypical CML.
• Idiopathic myelofibrosis.
• Essential thrombocytosis.
• Polycythemia rubra vera.

TREATMENT

The treatment options for CML can be divided into:

• Related and unrelated stem cell transplantation.
• Interferon-α with or without chemotherapy (cytarabine or hydroxyurea).
• Chemotherapy alone (hydroxyurea).
• Specific tyrosine kinase inhibitors.

Stem Cell Transplantation

Although interferon-α–containing regimens and hydroxyurea alone can prolong survival, it is generally accepted that the only curative option for CML remains allogeneic stem cell transplantation. As such, this remains the treatment of choice for patients younger than 50 years with a matched sibling donor (about 20% of patients). In patients older than 50 years with a matched donor, nonmyeloablative stem cell transplantation is currently being evaluated in clinical trials. A matched unrelated donor (MUD) may be found in an additional 10% of patients without a matched related donor; however, MUD stem cell transplantation has a significantly higher transplant-related mortality and morbidity. This increased up-front risk in unrelated stem cell transplantation must be weighed against the potential benefit of cure and against the risk–benefit ratios for other treatment options such as interferon-α and chemotherapy combinations. In formal decision analysis comparing early unrelated transplantation, delayed unrelated transplantation, and no transplantation as the options for a hypothetical 35-year-old patient with intermediate-prognosis chronic phase CML, transplantation within the first year appeared to provide the greatest quality-adjusted survival. In this analysis, the benefit of early unrelated transplantation decreased with increasing age, almost disappearing for a hypothetical patient aged 45 years.

Hydroxyurea

Hydroxyurea is very effective in producing hematologic remissions (>90%; see also Table 3), but cytogenetic studies show persistence of the Ph-chromosome abnormality.

Interferon-α with and without Chemotherapy

Interferon-α (see also Table 3) given alone requires prolonged periods to produce a hematologic remission, but results in partial (<34% Ph-positive metaphases) or complete cytogenetic responses in approximately 20% of patients. These cytogenetic responses are associated with more prolonged survival. Combining chemotherapy with interferon-α may allow a greater reduction in the burden of abnormal clonal cells: interferon-α in combination with

TABLE 3. *Suggested regimens, toxicities, and response rates*

Drug	Treatment plan	Toxicity	Response Rate
Hydroxyurea	Hydroxyurea, 500–2,000 mg p.o. daily	Leukopenia common, anemia, thrombocytopenia, nausea, rash	90% hematologic remission; 34–44% 5-yr survival
Interferon α-2a/b	Interferon α-2a/b, 5 × 10^6 Units/m^2 per day s.c.	Fever, myalgia, rashes, depression, leukopenia, anemia, thrombocytopenia	19% cytogenetic responses; 52–79% 5-yr survival[a]
Interferon α-2a/b + Cytarabine	Interferon α-2a/b, 5 × 10^6 Units/m^2 per day s.c.; cytarabine, 20 mg/m^2 s.c. single daily dose for 10 days (d 1–10; total dose/cycle = 200 mg/m^2) Cytarabine cycle is repeated monthly Discontinue cyterabine after complete cytogenetic response is achieved	Nausea, vomiting, diarrhea, mucositis, weight loss, leukopenia, anemia, thrombocytopenia	41% cytogenetic response rate; 86% 3-yr survival[a]
HLA-matched sibling stem cell transplantation	Busulfan, 4 mg/kg/day in divided doses orally on days −7, −6, −5, and −4 Cyclophosphamide, 60 mg/kg i.v. on days −3 and −2 *Or* TBI, 10 Gy with lung shielding and cyclophosphamide as above	Graft-vs.-host disease, infections, mucositis	50–70% 5-yr survival
HLA-matched unrelated stem cell transplantation	Regimens differ from center to center	Graft-vs.-host disease, infections, mucositis	57% 5-yr survival reported by Seattle

[a]<34% ph-positive metaphases on cytogenetic analyses.

cytarabine produced greater long-term survival and more major cytogenetic responses compared with interferon-α alone. Patients in this randomized study received induction therapy with interferon-α and hydroxyurea at a daily dose of ≤50 mg/kg (depending on the patient's white count) until hematologic remission before randomization to the interferon-alone or interferon-with-cytarabine arms. The purpose of this induction therapy was to avoid the long delay to hematologic remission seen with interferon-α alone. There was significant gastrointestinal and hematologic toxicity in the patients treated with interferon-α and cytarabine.

Other chemotherapies being used to intensify interferon-α therapy include hydroxyurea, idarubicin, and cytarabine in moderate dosage as well as high-dose chemotherapy with autologous transplantation.

Specific Tyrosine Kinase Inhibitors

A tyrosine kinase inhibitor specific for the abl tyrosine kinase component of the bcr-abl fusion protein (STI 571) is in clinical trials. In the phase I dose-exploratory trial, this agent produced a 100% complete hematologic remission rate at a dose of 300 mg/day in 31 patients with chronic-phase CML. There was no dose-limiting toxicity. Longer follow-up is required to determine the curative potential (cytogenetic remission rate, proportion of patients rendered negative for bcr-abl on PCR analysis) of this agent. In combination with other agents, possibly interferon-α, STI 571 may also have a future role in the management of blastic-phase CML.

Treatment of Blastic-phase CML

Treatment in this phase is usually unsuccessful. The approximately 30% of cases with a blastic phase having lymphoid features (tdt or CD10 positive) may respond to regimens used for acute lymphoblastic leukemia. See also the earlier section on specific tyrosine kinase inhibitors.

REFERENCES

1. Lee SJ, Kuntz KM, Horowitz MM, et al. Unrelated bone marrow transplantation for chronic myelogeneous leukemia: a decision analysis. *Ann Intern Med* 1997;127;1080–1088.
2. Guilhot F, Chastang C, Michallet M, et al. Interferon alfa-2b combined with cytarabine versus interferon alone in chronic myelogenous leukemia. *N Engl J Med* 1997;337:223–229.
3. Sawyers CL. Chronic myeloid leukemia. *N Engl J Med* 1999;340:1330–1339.
4. Drucker BJ. Lyndon NB. Lesson learned from the development of an abl tyrosine kinase inhibitor for chronic myelogenom leukemia. *J Clin Invest* 2000;105:3–7.

25

Myeloproliferative Diseases

Yogen Saunthararajah and Johnson M. Liu

National Heart Lung and Blood Institute, National Institutes of Health, Bethesda, Maryland

The myeloproliferative diseases (MPDs) of polycythemia vera (PV), essential thrombocythemia (ET), idiopathic myelofibrosis (MF, also known as agnogenic myeloid metaplasia), and chronic myeloid leukemia (covered in a separate chapter), earn their designation through increased production of one or more mature blood cell lineages by an abnormal hematopoietic stem cell. Diagnosis depends on exclusion of secondary causes of increased blood counts and distinguishing between the various MPDs (prompted by the particular blood cell lineage that appears to be in excess, and then by identifying characteristic biochemical or cytogenetic abnormalities) (see Table 1). Treatment for PV, ET, and MF is generally directed toward minimizing morbidity and prolonging survival through the prevention of complications such as hemorrhage and thrombosis, in the case of PV and ET, and alleviating anemia and symptoms associated with the splenomegaly of MF. As these are clonal disorders, there is a risk of transformation to acute leukemia. This risk is highest for MF; thus bone marrow transplantation is a potentially curative option that should be considered for this disease.

TABLE 1. *Distinguishing features of the MPD*

	CML	PV	ET	MF
Hematocrit	N or ↓	↑↑	N	↓
WBC	↑↑↑	↑	N	↑ or ↓
Platelet count	↑ or ↓	↑	↑↑↑	↑ or ↓
Splenomegaly	+++	+	+	+++
Cytogenetic abnormality	Ph chromosome	±	−	±
LAP score	↓	↑↑	N or ↑	N or ↑
Marrow fibrosis	±	± or ↓	±	+++ (Dry tap)
Marrow cellularity	↑↑↑ myeloid	↑↑	↑↑ megakaryocytes	N or ↓
Basophils ≥2%	+	±	±	Usually +

N, normal; LAP, leucocyte alkaline phosphatase score (see CML chapter); PV, polycythemia vera; MPD, myeloproliferative disease; ET, essential thrombocytopenia; CML, chronic myeloid leukemia.

EPIDEMIOLOGY AND RISK FACTORS

Annual incidence per 100,000 population

- 0.5 to 1.7 in PV.
- Approximately 2.5 in ET.
- Approximately 1.4 in MF.

Median age at diagnosis

- Late middle age for all three disorders.

Risk Factors

Some studies have suggested radiation exposure or occupational exposure to solvents and glues as risk factors, but these findings have not been confirmed.

ETIOLOGY AND PATHOPHYSIOLOGY

Clonal Hematopoiesis

The etiology of these disorders remains unclear. PV and MF are disorders of an early stem cell or progenitor, as all three blood lineages are derived from the same clone. Careful clonal studies in clinically diagnosed ET, however, demonstrate clonal hematopoiesis in only about half of the cases. The clinical significance of this finding is currently unclear. The marrow fibroblasts in MF are not derived from an abnormal clone. As a result of clonal hematopoiesis, all the MPDs have a tendency to transform to acute leukemia, although the probability of this occurrence differs considerably among the disorders.

Growth Factor or Growth Factor–receptor Mutations

Studies that have sought to implicate erythropoietin (EPO) levels or EPO receptor (EPO-R) involvement in PV have thus far demonstrated EPO-R involvement only in some cases of familial polycythemias. EPO levels tend to be low in PV. In contrast, thrombopoietin (TPO) levels can be high in ET, and molecular abnormalities of the TPO gene have been identified in certain families with an autosomal dominant form of hereditary thrombocytosis. Mutations of the TPO receptor have not been demonstrated in ET. Increased platelet-derived growth factor and other cytokines secreted by megakaryocytes and platelets are believed to play a role in the marrow fibrosis of MF.

PROGNOSIS

Median survivals

- Untreated PV, 1.5 years.
- PV treated with phlebotomy, 3.5 years.
- PV treated with myelosuppression, 7 to 13 years.
- ET, more than 10 years.
- MF, 3 to 5 years.

Rate of transformation to acute leukemia

- PV, 1% to 5% (1.5% with phlebotomy alone, 5.9% with hydroxyurea, 10% to 13.5% with chlorambucil or ^{32}P).

- ET, 3% to 5% (transformation to MF and acute leukemia).
- MF, 10%.

The major cause of death in PV is thrombosis (cerebral, cardiac, pulmonary, mesenteric); the major causes of death in ET are thrombosis and hemorrhage.

Spent Phase

Both PV and ET may progress to a "spent phase" resembling MF and characterized by cytopenia, splenomegaly, and marrow fibrosis.

Risk Factors for Thrombosis

- In PV, hematocrit greater than 45%. Avoid surgery until a hematocrit less than 45% has been maintained for >2 months.
- In ET, older than 60 years, and the presence of other cardiovascular risk factors (e.g., smoking, previous thrombosis).

In ET, an association between platelet count and thrombosis has not been established, but platelet cytoreduction with hydroxyurea is associated with a lower risk.

Risk Factors for Hemorrhage

- In ET, platelet count greater than $2 \times 10^6/\mu l$.

DIAGNOSIS AND CLINICAL FEATURES

Excluding Secondary Causes of Polycythemia or Thrombocytosis

The Polycythemia Vera Study Group (PVSG), an international study group, has established diagnostic criteria for PV and ET (see Tables 2 and 3). Establishing these diagnostic criteria in a particular case helps exclude secondary causes of polycythemia or thrombocytosis or apparent erythrocytosis (increased hematocrit but normal red cell mass). Thirty percent of patients with PV may have an abnormal karyotype such as del(20q); such a finding excludes secondary polycythemia.

TABLE 2. *Suggested criteria for diagnosis of PV*

Category A		Category B	
A1	Red cell mass >36 mL/kg (male) or 32 mL/kg (female) or >25% above mean normal predicted value	B1	Thrombocytosis (platelets >400 × 10³/μL)
A2	Normal arterial pO₂ (saturation >92%)	B2	Neutrophilia (neutrophils >10 × 10³/μL)
A3	Palpable splenomegaly	B3	Splenomegaly on nuclear med or CT or ultrasound scan
A4	Clonality: e.g., abnormal karyotype	B4	Hyperresponsive CFU-E/BFU-E growth or low-serum EPO

Diagnosis: A1 + A2 + A3 or A4; A1 + A2 and any two from category B. (Ref: Fruchtman SM, et al. 1998)

TABLE 3. *Diagnostic criteria for ET*

1	Platelets >600 × 10³/μL
2	Hct <40% or normal RBC mass
3	Stainable iron in marrow, or normal ferritin, or normal MCV
4	No Ph chromosome or bcr/abl rearrangement, or MDS-type cytogenetic abnormality
5	No marrow fibrosis or marrow fibrosis <1/3 of biopsy and no more than minimal splenomegaly and no leukoerythroblastic cells in the peripheral blood
6	No other cause for reactive thrombocytosis

Distinguishing between the Myeloproliferative Disorders

All the MPDs can present as a result of incidentally noted abnormal blood counts (Table 1). Otherwise, PV can demonstrate symptoms attributable to the increased red blood cell mass, such as headaches, vertigo, tinnitus, and blurred vision. A distinctive symptom in PV is that of pruritus aggravated by hot water. Cerebrovascular ischemia, digital ischemia, erythromelalgia, and spontaneous abortions resulting from arterial thrombosis are more commonly seen with ET. MF may have symptoms related to anemia or with abdominal fullness or early satiety from splenomegaly. Hypermetabolic symptoms such as weight loss and sweating can be seen with all the MPDs. ET is diagnosed after excluding PV; MF is diagnosed after excluding PV and ET, as marrow fibrosis can be a sequela of the other MPDs. The thrombotic episodes seen with all the MPDs can occur in unusual locations such as the hepatic vein (Budd–Chiari syndrome) and portal vein. Platelet function tests or bleeding times have little utility in diagnosis or in guiding management of the MPDs.

TREATMENT

PV

Maintenance of a hematocrit of less than 45% dramatically decreases the incidence of thrombotic complications (in PV, 35% of initial thrombotic events are fatal). This can be achieved through phlebotomy, myelosuppressive oral chemotherapy, or interferon-α (IFNα). Selection among these options is guided by data from the Polycythenia Vera Study Group (PVSG) studies.

PVSG studies (Phlebotomy and Chemotherapy)

PVSG-01 randomized more than 400 patients to either phlebotomy, chlorambucil, or ³²P. The thrombosis rate with phlebotomy alone was significantly higher than that for myelosuppression with chlorambucil or ³²P. Median survival was more than 10 years in the ³²P and phlebotomy groups and 9 years in the chlorambucil group, with an excess of leukemic deaths with chlorambucil and ³²P. In PVSG-05, aspirin, 325 mg 3 times a day, added to phlebotomy did not decrease the risk of life-threatening thrombosis but increased hemorrhagic complications. PVSG-08 studied the nonalkylating myelosuppressive agent hydroxyurea (HU), in the hope that this agent would not have an association with leukemic transformation, as was noted for ³²P and chlorambucil in PVSG-01. HU, with supplemental phlebotomy as needed, was found to have a significantly lower risk of thrombosis compared with phlebotomy alone. However, a statistically nonsignificant higher risk of transformation to acute leukemia also was observed in the HU-treated group.

A reasonable treatment approach based on the results of the PVSG studies is as follows:

- In patients younger than 70 years, maintain the hematocrit less than 45% with phlebotomy (250–500 mL qod) unless they have thrombosis, hemorrhage, severe pruritus, painful splenomegaly, or B symptoms, in which case HU or IFN-α in a clinical trial should be considered.

- HU is the agent of first choice to decrease the hematocrit to less than 45% in of patients older than 69 years. Busulphan or ^{32}P are reasonable alternatives in this age group.
- Aspirin is generally not indicated in patients with PV. IFN-α remains an experimental therapy for PV; the potential benefits compared with HU include possible inhibition of platelet-derived growth factor (PDGF), and hence myelofibrosis, and a lower likelihood of triggering leukemic transformation.
- Spent phase. Options to alleviate cytopenia from massive splenomegaly include HU, IFN-α, and erythropoietin. Analgesia may be required for splenic infarct pain. Cytopenia associated with marrow fibrosis and massive splenomegaly is difficult to treat. Splenectomy can be followed by progressive hepatomegaly and eventual transformation to acute leukemia. In such patients, allogeneic transplantation may be an appropriate experimental approach.
- Pruritus. This symptom often responds to chemotherapy. Additional agents to try as symptomatic treatments include antihistamines, cholestyramine, and PUVA.
- Hyperuricemia. Allopurinol should be started before chemotherapy to decrease the risk of urate nephropathy (300–800 mg/day in divided doses given orally; dose reduction needed in renal insufficiency).

ET

Treatment in ET must be qualified by the fact that life expectancy in this condition is nearly normal and that platelet reduction with HU may be associated with an increased risk for leukemic transformation. Treatment is directed at preventing thrombosis and hemorrhage in those deemed to be at risk of these complications. These are patients with a history of thrombosis, associated cardiovascular risk factors such as smoking, age older than 60 years, and patients with a platelet count greater than $2 \times 10^6/\mu L$.

For platelet cytoreduction, see Table 4.

- A randomized trial of HU in 114 high-risk patients showed a significant reduction of thrombotic events in the treatment arm (3.6% vs. 24%). The HU dose was adjusted to achieve a platelet count of $600 \times 10^3/\mu L$. Anagrelide is a nonmutagenic orally active agent that produces selective platelet cytoreduction by interfering with megakaryocyte maturation. IFN-α also can effectively cause platelet cytoreduction. The HU study has provided the precedent for a platelet count of $600 \times 10^3/\mu L$ as the therapeutic target with anagrelide or IFN-α therapy. Plateletpheresis is used as emergency therapy when ongoing thrombosis cannot be adequately managed with chemotherapy and antithrombotic agents.
- Antiplatelet agents. Aspirin can exacerbate the bleeding tendency in patients with ET and other MPDs and should be used selectively. Low-dose aspirin (81 mg/day orally) may benefit ET patients with cerebral or digital ischemia. It is contraindicated in those who have had previous episodes of hemorrhage and is unnecessary in asymptomatic patients.

MF

- Palliative therapy for MF is directed toward alleviating anemia and painful splenomegaly. For anemia, androgens (oxymethalone, 1–5 mg/kg/day orally, may take 3 to 6 months for a response) can produce responses in about 30% of patients. Transfusion support (with iron chelation when indicated) may be necessary. Splenectomy as performed in experienced centers is associated with an operative mortality of less than 10%, and besides alleviating pain, discomfort, and early satiety, can improve anemia. Increasing white counts and platelet counts after splenectomy may necessitate HU therapy. IFN-α is an experimental therapy for MF.
- Curative therapy. Allogeneic transplantation should be considered for young patients (younger than 55 years) with MF; 5-year survivals with a related or unrelated matched transplant are 54% and 48%, respectively, as determined by the European Group for Blood and

TABLE 4. *Chemotherapeutic agents used in the therapy of the MPDs*

Drug	Treatment plan	Indications	Toxicity	Reference
Hydroxyurea	Start with hydroxyurea, 1,000–2,000 mg p.o. daily. In PV, adjust to keep Hct <45% without producing thrombocytopenia or neutropenia. Augment with phlebotomy if necessary. In ET, adjust dose to maintain plt counts <600 × 10³/μL; long-term therapy is necessary.	All PV pts >69 yr of age; younger patients with thrombosis, hemorrhage, severe pruritis, painful splenomegaly, or B symptoms. ET pts who require therapy (see text). MF pts requiring cytoreduction after splenectomy	Increased risk of acute leukemic transformation or myelodysplastic syndrome with a chromosome 17p deletion; leg ulceration	
Anagrelide	Anagrelide, 0.5–1 mg p.o. 4 times daily. Prolonged treatment is necessary	Generally used as a second-line agent for decreasing plt counts. Consider using as primary therapy for young pts with ET requiring therapy	Fluid retention, congestive heart failure symptoms, postural hypotension, headaches, dizziness, nausea, and diarrhea	
Interferon-α 2a/b	Start with interferon-α 2a/b 3 × 10⁶ Units s.c. 3 times/wk. Adjust the dose against response and adverse effects. Long-term treatment is necessary	Experimental therapy in PV (refer for clinical trials). Consider for young pts as an alternative to phlebotomy. A second-line plt-lowering agent in ET	Flu-like symptoms, altered mental status, depression	

Hct, hematocrit; plt, platelets; pts, patients; p.o., oral administration; s.c., subcutaneous administration.

Marrow Transplantation (EBMT). A recommendation for transplantation is not clear-cut in asymptomatic patients without cytogenetic abnormalities and no cytopenia, as the median survival in this group is greater than 14 years with palliative therapy alone. Although the outcome with transplantation also is adversely affected by these features, poor prognostic features such as a hemoglobin less than 10 g/dL white cell count less than $4 \times 10^3/\mu L$ or greater than $30 \times 10^3/\mu L$, greater than 10% circulating blasts, promyelocytes, or myelocytes or abnormal cytogenetics should prompt consideration for transplant. Although not necessary in every patient, pretransplant splenectomy is associated with faster engraftment and can be considered in those with massive splenomegaly. Marrow fibrosis is reversible with transplantation.

REFERENCES

1. Fruchtman SM, Mack K, Kaplan ME, et al. From efficacy to safety: a polycythemia vera study group report on hydroxyurea in patienta with polycythemia vera. *Semin Hematol* 1997;34:17–23.
2. Berk PD, Goldberg JD, Donovoun PB, et al. Therapeutic recommendations in polycythemia vera based on Polycythemia Vera Study Group protocols. *Semin Hematol* 1986;23:132–143.
3. Kaplan ME, Mack K, Goldberg JD, et al. Long term management of polycythemia vera with hydroxyurea: a progress report. *Semin Hematol* 1986;23:167–171.
4. Silver RT. Interferon-alpha: effects of long-term treatment for polycythemia vera. *Semin Hematol* 1997;34:40–50.
5. Guardiola P, Anderson JE, Bandini G, et al. Allogeneic stem cell transplantation for agnogenic myeloid metaplasia: a European Group for Blood and Marrow Transplantation, Societe Francaise de Greffe de Moelle, Gruppo Italiano per il Trapianto del Midollo Osseo, and Fred Hutchinson Cancer Research Center Collaborative Study. *Blood* 1999;93:2831–2838.
6. Cortelazzo S, Finazzi G, Ruggeri M, et al. Hydroxyurea for patients with essential thrombocythemia and a high risk for thrombosis. *N Engl J Med* 1995;332:1132–1136.

26

Multiple Myeloma

Yogen Saunthararajah and Johnson M. Liu

National Heart Lung and Blood Institute, National Institutes of Health, Bethesda, Maryland

EPIDEMIOLOGY AND RISK FACTORS

Incidence

- About four per 100,000 per year in the United States.
- Incidence among African-Americans is twice that in whites and 3 times that in Asians and Pacific Islanders.

The mean age at diagnosis is 61 years. An increased incidence in atomic bomb survivors implicates excessive radiation as a risk factor, but there is little evidence to implicate other environmental causes. The role of the human herpesvirus 8 (HHV-8) in myeloma pathogenesis is controversial and has yet to be established. Familial clustering has been reported in some cases.

Pathophysiology

Multiple myeloma is caused by the malignant proliferation of a relatively differentiated B cell, as indicated by advanced immunoglobulin gene rearrangement in the malignant clone (Fig. 1). The extent of somatic mutation in the complementarity-determining regions (the antigen-binding portions) of the variable gene segment suggests that the proliferation of the clone was at some point antigen driven, although the identity of the antigen or antigens is unknown. Chromosomal translocations mostly involving the heavy chain locus on chromosome 14 can be identified with techniques such as fluorescence *in situ* hybridization (FISH), although no characteristic molecular abnormality has yet been identified. The clinical features of multiple myeloma are a result of bone marrow infiltration by the clone, the secretion of osteoclast-activating factors, high levels of clonal immunoglobulin, and altered immunity.

STAGING AND PROGNOSIS

Durie–Salmon clinical staging system

- Not a very good guide to prognosis, more often used to categorize patients for protocol purposes than to guide clinical decisions (See Table 1).

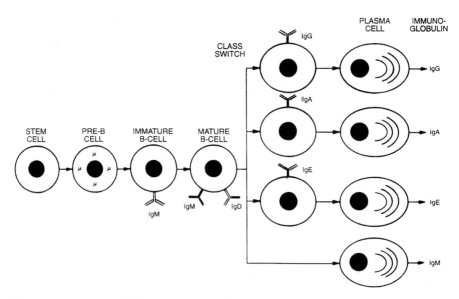

FIG. 1. Differentiation of B lymphocytes and plasma cells. A pleiotropic stem cell gives rise to the pre–B cell that has acquired the capacity to synthesize heavy chains (μ). The immature B cell can synthesize light chains, so that a complete immunoglobulin M (IgM) molecule is formed and expressed on the cell surface. Mature B cells express both IgM and IgD on their surfaces. These cells can either mature into IgM-secreting plasmacytoid lymphocytes, or undergo a class switch to express IgG, IgA, or IgE on their surfaces. The latter cells can undergo terminal differentiation into IgG- or IgE-secreting plasma cells. From Stamatovannopoulos G, Nienhuis AW, Leder P, et al., eds. *The molecular basis of blood diseases.* Philadelphia: WB Saunders, 1987, with permission.

Plasma cell labeling index and β2-microglobulin levels

• Correlate best with prognosis in untreated patients.

Median survival

• Less than 1 year in untreated myeloma.
• Two to 3 years with melphalan and prednisone.

TABLE 1. *Durie Salmon staging system*

Stage I (myeloma mass, <0.6 × 10¹² cells/m²)	All of the following: Hgb, >10 g/dL; serum Ca, ≤12 mg/dL; ≤1 lesion on skeletal survey; IgG M protein, <50 g/L; IgA M protein, <30 g/L; urinary light chains, <4 g/24 h
Stage II (myeloma mass, 0.6–1.2 × 10¹² cells/m²)	Results fit neither stage I nor stage III
Stage III (myeloma mass, >1.2 × 10¹² cells/m²)	Any of the following: Hgb, ≤8.5 g/dL; serum Ca, >12 mg/dL; >1 lesion on skeletal survey; IgG M protein, >70 g/L; IgA M protein, >50 g/L; urinary light chain excretion, >12 g/24 h
Subclassification A	Serum creatinine, <2 mg/dL
Subclassification B	Serum creatinine, ≥2 mg/dL

DIAGNOSIS AND CLINICAL FEATURES

In addition to a history and physical, the workup of a patient with suspected multiple myeloma should include the following:

- Complete blood count (CBC).
- Electrolytes.
- Blood urea nitrogen (BUN)/creatinine.
- Calcium.
- Urate.
- β_2-Microglobulin.
- Lactate dehydrogenase (LDH).
- Serum protein electrophoresis (SPEP).
- Urine protein electrophoresis (UPEP).
- Quantitative immunoglobulins.
- Unilateral bone marrow aspirate and biopsy.
- Radiographic skeletal survey.

An SPEP alone is inadequate, as some myeloma clones secrete only light chains, which are rapidly cleared from the plasma to the urine (Fig. 2). A nuclear medicine bone scan may not detect the purely lytic lesions of multiple myeloma and should not be used. The plasma cell labeling index measures the proportion of plasma cells actively synthesizing DNA and is useful in prognostication.

Most patients with myeloma have bone pain (commonly induced by movement) and fatigue. In a patient with clinical features that suggest myeloma, the following minimal criteria for diagnosis have been established:

- 10% plasma cells in the bone marrow or a plasmacytoma and one of the following:
  (a) >3 g/dL of serum monoclonal protein (M protein) *OR*
  (b) urine M protein *OR*
  (c) lytic bone lesions.

Pallor is the most common physical finding. A normochromic, normocytic anemia is common; 25% of patients have renal insufficiency; 20% have hypercalcemia. Circulating plasma cells are present in fewer than 1% of cases. The circulating monoclonal protein is immunoglobulin G (IgG) in 50%, IgA in 20%, light chain only (Bence Jones proteinemia) in 20%, IgD in 2%, and biclonal in 1%. As bone marrow involvement may be focal rather than diffuse, repeated bone marrow sampling may be needed before more than 10% plasma cells are identified. Radiologic changes include punched-out lytic lesions, osteoporosis, and fractures. Amyloidosis is clinically evident in fewer than 5% of patients.

The minimal criteria for diagnosis help exclude the differential diagnoses of:

- Monoclonal gammopathy of unknown significance (MGUS).
- Smoldering multiple myeloma (SMM).
- Primary amyloidosis.
- Lymphoma.
- Metastatic carcinoma.

An incidental M protein detection of less than 3 g/dL in an asymptomatic patient with less than 10% bone marrow plasma cells and no other features of multiple myeloma suggests the diagnosis of MGUS. If in the asymptomatic patient, the M spike is greater than 3 g/dL and there are more than 10% bone marrow plasma cells, but no other features of multiple myeloma, SMM should be considered. Both SMM and MGUS can remain benign for many years, and close follow-up without treatment is indicated for both these conditions until progression to typical multiple myeloma (about 1% per year for MGUS) or symptoms intervene.

Renal insufficiency may be caused by hypercalcemia or light chain deposition in the kidneys (myeloma kidney). In some patients amyloidosis can cause a nephrotic syndrome.

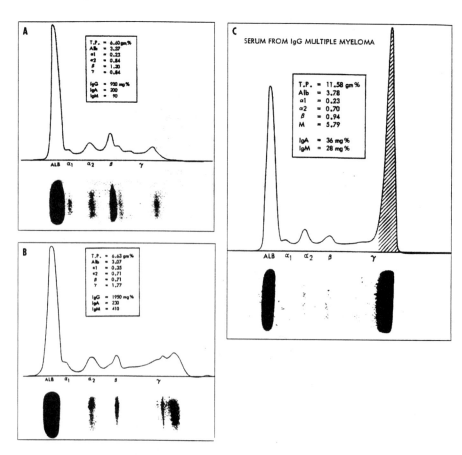

FIG. 2. Electrophoretic pattern of **(A)** normal human serum, **(B)** hypergammaglobulinemia, and **(C)** immunoglobulin G (IgG) multiple myeloma. From Lee GR, Bithell TC, Foerster J, et al., eds. *Wintrobe's clinical hematology.* Philadelphia: Lea & Febiger, 1993, with permission.

Acquired Fanconi's syndrome with glycosuria, phosphaturia, and aminoaciduria can occur. Infections are an important cause of morbidity and mortality in multiple myeloma.

TREATMENT

The treatment options (Table 2; Fig. 3) can be divided into six groups:

- Melphalan and prednisone.
- Combination chemotherapy.
- Infusional chemotherapy without an alkylating agent.
- High-dose chemotherapy with autologous stem cell transplantation.
- Allogeneic stem cell transplantation.
- Interferon-α.

In addition to chemotherapy and transplantation, there is an important role for pamidronate and local radiation for control of bone pain.

TABLE 2. *Treatment options*

Regimen	Treatment description	Toxicities	Response rate	Reference
Combination chemotherapy Age 65–70 yr with Sxs; Do not use in young pts being considered for HDT/auto SCT				
Melphalan + prednisone (MP)	Melphalan, 10 mg/m² per day p.o. for 4 days (d 1–4; total dose/cycle, 40 mg/m²) + Prednisone, 60 mg/m² per day p.o. for 4 days (d 1–4; total dose/cycle, 40 mg/m²) Cycle duration, 4–6 wk Treatment continues until approximately 4 mo of plateau phase (see text for explanation of plateau phase)	Myelosuppression Start at low doses and increase if tolerated. Decrease doses if myelo-suppression is prolonged. Secondary myelodysplasia and leukemias	50–70% Rare CR	1
Combination chemotherapy Age >65 yr with Sxs, good PS, and poor prognostic features (controversial). Age <65 yr as induction before consolidation with HDT/auto SCT				
VBAP	Vincristine, 1 mg/m² i.v. day 1 (total dose/cycle, 1 mg/m²) Carmustine (BCNU), 30 mg/m² i.v. day 1 (total dose/cycle, 30 mg/m²) Doxorubicin, 30 mg/m² i.v. day 1 (total dose/cycle, 30 mg/m²) Prednisone, 100 mg orally days 1 to 4 Cycle repeats every 3 wk for 12 mo or for 4–6 cycles before HDT/auto SCT	Myelotoxicity, neurotoxicity, cardiotoxicity	50–70% Rare CR	2
VCAP	Vincristine, 1 mg/m² i.v. day 1 (total dose/cycle, 1 mg/m²) Cyclophosphamide, 125 mg/m² per day p.o. for 4 days (d 1–4; total dose/cycle, 500 mg/m²) Doxorubicin, 30 mg/m² i.v. day 1 (total dose/cycle, 30 mg/m²) Prednisone, 60 mg/m² per day p.o. for 4 days (d 1–4; total dose/cycle, 240 mg/m²) Cycle repeats every 3 wk for 12 mo or for 4–6 cycles before HDT/auto SCT			
VMCP	Vincristine, 1 mg/m² i.v. day 1 (total dose/cycle, 1 mg/m²) Melphalan, 6 mg/m² per day p.o. for 4 days (d 1–4; total dose/cycle, 24 mg/m²)			

Continued

311

TABLE 2. *Continued*

Regimen	Treatment description	Toxicities	Response rate	Reference
	Cyclophosphamide, 125 mg/m² orally on days 1 to 4 Prednisone, 60 mg/m² per day p.o. for 4 days (d 1–4; total dose/cycle, 240 mg/m²) Cycle repeats every 3 wk for 12 mo or for 4–6 cycles before HDT/auto SCT			
Infusional therapy Age >65 yr with disease refractory to alkylating agents Consider dexamethasone alone if PS is poor Age <65 yr: induction in pts before consolidation with HDT/auto SCT				
VAD	Vincristine, 0.4 mg/day continuous i.v. infusion for 4 days (d 1–4; total dose/cycle, 1.6 mg) Doxorubicin, 9 mg/m² per day continuous i.v. infusion for 4 days (d 1–4; total dose/cycle, 36 mg/m²) Dexamethasone, 40 mg per day p.o. for 4 days, repeated every 8 days (d 1–4, 9–12, and 17–20; total dose/cycle, 480 mg) Cycle repeats every 25 days, four additional cycles after maximal reduction in myeloma protein levels Administer four cycles before consolidation with HDT/auto SCT	GI and myelotoxicity	30% in disease refractory to alkylating agents	4
High-dose chemotherapy and autologous stem cell transplantation (HDT/auto CST) Age <65 yr with good PS				
	Conditioning regimen: Melphalan, 200 mg/m² i.v. (total dose/cycle, 200 mg/m²) as a single agent, *OR* Melphalan, 140 mg/m² i.v. + TBI, 800 cGy delivered in four daily fractions for 4 days	5% transplant-related mortality	80% overall 20% CR	

Continued

312

TABLE 2. *Continued*

Regimen	Treatment description	Toxicities	Response rate	Reference
Allogeneic stem cell transplantation Age <55 yr with Durie Salmon stage I on protocol				
	TBI, 1,000 cGy with lung shielding + Cyclophosphamide, 60 mg/m^2 per day i.v. for 2 days (d 1 and 2; total dose, 120 mg/m^2)	40–50% transplant-related mortality	50% CR with 30% 5-yr survival for pts who achieved CR	
Interferon-α 2a/b Monotherapy during plateau phase after chemotherapy or HDT/auto SCT				
	Interferon-α 2a/b, 3 million Units/m^2 s.c., three doses/wk (total dose/wk, 9 million Units/m^2)	CNS toxicity, cytopenias, fever and myalgia, GI toxicity	3- to 7-mo overall survival advantage	
Pamidronate For all pts with myeloma				
	Pamidronate, 90 mg i.v. infusion over 2–4 h, monthly (total dose/month, 90 mg)	Fever, nausea, hypokalemia, hypocalcemia	Decreased bone pain and skeletal events; small survival benefit	

CR, complete response; HDT/auto SCT, high-dose chemotherapy and autologous stem cell transplantation; i.v., intravenously; p.o., orally; PS, performance status; pts, patients; s.c., subcutaneously;
GI, gastrointestinal; TBI, total body irradiation; CNS, central nervous system.

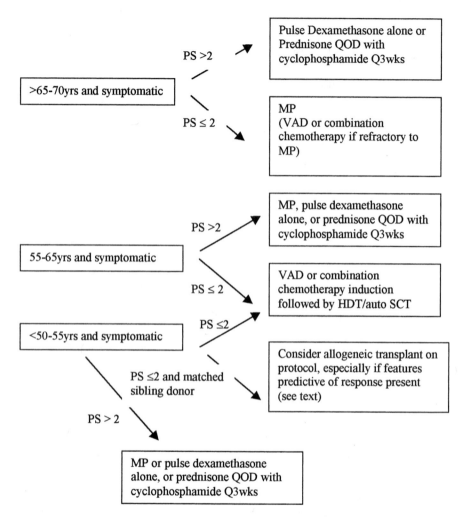

FIG. 3. A suggested treatment algorithm. All patients should receive supportive care, be considered for bisphosphonate treatment and clinical trials.

Choice of Therapy

To date, there is no curative therapy available for multiple myeloma. With therapy, patients may achieve a plateau phase characterized by a stable M-protein level, persistent bone marrow plasma cells, but an absence of symptoms. The goal of standard therapy is to improve quality of life and to delay disease progression. With these goals in mind, the choice of therapy (What intensity therapy? When to start?) is guided by consideration of symptoms, prognosis, age, and performance status. Eligible patients should always be considered for enrollment in clinical trials such as those investigating the use of vaccines.

Melphalan and Prednisone

Melphalan and prednisone (MP) has been the standard treatment for multiple myeloma for many decades and remains so for patients in whom high-dose chemotherapy and autologous stem cell transplantation (HDC/auto SCT) is not appropriate.

Combination Chemotherapy

Combination chemotherapy regimens containing an alkylator, steroid, doxorubicin, and vincristine such as VCMP, VBAP, and VCAP have shown no significant survival benefit, although they may have a higher initial response rate than does melphalan with prednisone. Infusional therapy with vincristine, doxorubicin, and dexamethasone (VAD) has a high response rate (30%) in disease refractory to alkylating agents. The absence of an alkylating agent in this regimen makes this the appropriate induction regimen in patients for whom high-dose chemotherapy followed by autologous stem cell transplantation is being considered for consolidation.

High-Dose Chemotherapy and Autologous Stem Cell Transplantation

A large randomized trial has established the role of HDC/auto SCT for the treatment of multiple myeloma in patients older than 65 years. Two hundred patients with Durie–Salmon stage II or III disease were randomized to receive high-dose melphalan and total body irradiation or further cycles of VMCP/BVAP after four to six induction cycles of VMCP/BVAP. Both arms received maintenance therapy with interferon-α until progression. In an intention-to-treat analysis, 22% of the patients in the HDT/auto SCT arm had a complete remission versus 5% in the conventional chemotherapy arm. In the HDT/auto SCT arm, the overall response rate was 88%, and at 5 years, the event-free survival was 28%, and overall survival, 52%. In the conventional chemotherapy arm, the overall response rate was 75%, and at 5 years, the event-free survival was 10%, and overall survival, 12%. In the HDT/auto SCT arm, response to treatment correlated with survival; patients who achieved complete remission or very good partial remission did significantly better than patients who achieved only partial remission or did not respond. The lack of a plateau in the survival curves in both arms of this study indicates that neither conventional chemotherapy nor HDT/auto SCT is curative.

Allogeneic Stem Cell Transplantation

Data from Europe and Seattle show that allogeneic transplantation induces a complete remission in about 50% of patients with multiple myeloma. Unfortunately, it is associated with a high rate of transplant-related mortality (TRM), between 40% and 50%. Although the relapse rate remains high (~50% at 5 years), it appears to be lower than that in autologous transplantation. The 5-year survival for patients who enter complete remission is 30%, inferior to the 5-year survival with HDT/auto SCT. Predictors of response include female sex, Durie–Salmon stage I at diagnosis, low β_2-microglobulin at diagnosis, IgA multiple myeloma, one line of treatment before transplant, and chemoresponsiveness at transplantation. Strategies such as lower-than-standard-dose conditioning regimens, selective T-cell depletion, peripheral blood stem cell transplantation, aggressive infectious disease management, donor lymphocyte infusions, and idiotype vaccination may decrease the TRM and relapse rate associated with allogeneic transplantation. Graft-versus-myeloma effects offer the promise of cure with allogeneic transplant, and young patients with favorable features, as listed earlier, and a matched sibling donor should be considered for allogeneic bone marrow transplant protocols.

Interferon-α

The use of interferon-α in multiple myeloma remains controversial. It has been extensively studied as a single agent for induction, in combination with chemotherapy for induction, for maintenance of chemotherapy-induced remission, and in combination with steroids in the treatment of refractory disease. Meta-analyses of the data suggest small but significant advantages for maintenance and in combination with chemotherapy for remission induction. However, these small benefits must be balanced against high treatment-associated toxicity and costs. There are no general recommendations for interferon-α use, and decisions are made on a case-by-case basis.

Biphosphonate Therapy

Biphosphonates have become part of the standard armamentarium against multiple myeloma and are generally thought to be beneficial in all patients with myeloma. Intravenous pamidronate given monthly reduced bone pain and the incidence of pathologic fractures, and the need for surgery or irradiation to the bone in patients with Durie–Salmon stage III myeloma. Longer term follow-up of these patients also suggested a survival benefit. Two large randomized studies of oral clodronate versus placebo have shown decreased hypercalcemia, beneficial effects on bone disease, and improved survival, even for patients without overt skeletal disease. These beneficial effects of the biphosphonates may be a result of their effects on bone resorption as well as a direct antitumor effect.

SUPPORTIVE MEASURES

Supportive measures in myeloma include adequate analgesia for bone pain, local radiation for bone pain, radiation or surgery for cord compression, surgery for impending pathologic fractures, treatment of hypercalcemia, a high fluid intake of around 3 L/day to maintain renal function, and dialysis if necessary.

REFRACTORY OR RELAPSED DISEASE

In a patient who progresses during MP or combination chemotherapy (refractory disease), or who relapses within 6 months of stopping induction therapy, VAD is a suitable second-line regimen. If the patient progressed on MP, combination chemotherapy regimens such as VMCP/VBAP can be considered. In a treatment-refractory patient with significant cytopenia, pulse dexamethasone alone or alternate-day prednisone (100 mg p.o. every 48 h) with cyclophosphamide, 800 to 1,200 mg orally every 3 weeks, can be considered. Interferon-α has also been used in combination with corticosteroids. Recently oral thalidomide at doses of 200 to 800 mg/day has been reported to produce a decrease in myeloma protein in patients refractory to other therapies including high-dose chemotherapy. The overall response rate to thalidomide as a single agent in this group of patients was 32%. Ongoing studies seek to explore the role of thalidomide in combination with other chemotherapy agents as an initial therapy for multiple myeloma.

REFERENCES

1. Gregory WM, Richards MA, Malpas JS. Combination chemotherapy versus melphalan and prednisolone in the treatment of multiple myeloma: an overview of published trials. *J Clin Oncol* 1992; 10:334–342.
2. Attal M, Harousseau JL, Stoppa AM, et al. A prospective randomized trial of autologous bone marrow transplantation and chemotherapy in multiple myeloma. *N Engl J Med* 1996;335;91–97.

3. Bjorkstand B, Ljungman P, Svensson H, et al. Prognostic factors in autologous stem cell transplantation for multiple myeloma: an EBMT registry study. *Leuk Lymphoma* 1994;15:265–272.
4. Gahrton G, Tura S, Ljungman P, et al. Allogeneic bone marrow transplantation in multiple myeloma. *N Engl J Med* 1991;325;1267–1272.
5. Berenson J, Lichtenstein A, Porter L, et al. Efficacy of pamidronate in reducing skeletal events in patients with advanced multiple myeloma. *N Engl J Med* 1996;334:488–493.
6. McCloskey EV, Maclennan ICM, Drayson M, et al. A randomized trial of the effect of clodronate on skeletal morbidity in multiple myeloma. *Br J Haematol* 1998;100:317–325.
7. Singhal S, Mehta J, Desikan R, et al. Antitumor activity of thalidomide in refractory multiple myeloma. *N Engl J Med* 1999;21:1565–1571.

27

Non-Hodgkin's Lymphoma

Martin Gutierrez and Wyndham H. Wilson

Medicine Branch, DCS, National Cancer Institute, National Institutes of Health, Bethesda, Maryland

The non-Hodgkin's lymphomas (NHLs) are a group of entities that vary in clinical behavior and morphologic appearance. The various types of NHLs are thought to represent neoplastic lymphoid cells arrested at different stages of normal differentiation. Based on their natural history, NHLs can be clinically classified as indolent, aggressive, and highly aggressive.

EPIDEMIOLOGY

Since 1950, the incidence of NHL has steadily increased at approximately 4% per year, which represents 55,000 new cases annually. Mortality has similarly increased.

PATHOPHYSIOLOGY

- Cytogenetics, gene rearrangement, and oncoproteins are important molecular markers of histologic subtype and mechanisms of lymphomagenesis.

TABLE 1. *Molecular characteristics of B-cell lymphomas*

Histology	Cytogenetics	Oncogene/protein	Immunoglobulin gene rearrangements	
			Heavy	κλ
CLL/SLL[a]	t(14;19)	Bcl-3	+	
	Trisomy 12, 13q			+
Lymphoplasmacytoid lymphoma			+	+
Follicular center cell grade I and II	t(14;18)	Bcl-2	+	
Marginal zone[b]	Trisomy 3			
	t(11;18)		+	
Mantle cell lymphoma	t(11;14)	Bcl-1/Cyclin-D1	+	
Follicular center cell grade III[c]	t(14;18)	Bcl-2	+	
Large B-cell[d]	t(3;22)(q27;q11)	Bcl-6		+
		Bcl-2		
Lymphoblastic lymphoma/leukemia			+	+/−
Burkitt's lymphoma,	t(8;14)(q24;q32)	c-*myc*	+	
Burkitt's-like	t(2;8)(11p;q24)			λ+
	t(8;22)(q24;q11)			κ+

[a]Trisomy 12 is seen in 30% of cases, and abnormalities in 13q are present in 25% of patients.
[b]Cytogenetic abnormalities have been seen in extranodal marginal zone NHL.
[c]t(14;18) is present in 75% to 95% of FCC NHL.
[d]Bcl-2 is present in 30% of cases and c-*myc* is uncommon.

TABLE 2. *Molecular characteristics of T-cell lymphomas*

Histology	Cytogenetics	Oncoprotein	TCR gene rearrangements
T-CLL/T-PLL	Inv14(q11;q32), Trisomy 8q	Bcl-3	+
Mycosis fungoides			+
Peripheral T-cell lymphoma			+/–
Angiocentric		EBV+	+
Angioimmunoblastic[a]	Trisomy 3 or 5	EBV+	+
ATLL		HTLV I integration +	+
Enteropathy T cell		EBV–	β+
Hepatosplenic γ/δ			δγ+
ALCL[b,c]	T(2;5)	Alk+	+
Precursor T-lymphoblastic lymphoma/leukemia	T(7;9)	Tcl-4	Variable

[a]TCR gene rearrangement is present in 75% and IgH in 10%.
[b]TCR gene rearrangement in 60%+.
[c]Alk, Anaplastic lymphoma kinase gene.

- Tumor clonality may be assessed by immunoglobulin (Ig) gene rearrangement in B cells and T cell–receptor (TCR) rearrangement in T cells. Cytogenetics and/or oncogene rearrangement by polymerase chain reaction (PCR) also may be useful to assess clonality. However, the absence of evidence for clonality does not exclude the presence of a malignant lymphoid process (Tables 1 and 2).

Staging for Non-Hodgkin's Lymphoma

- Staging evaluation usually includes chest radiograph (CXR), whole-body computed tomography (CT) scans, and bone marrow (BM) biopsies. Lumbar puncture with cytol-

TABLE 3. *Staging system in NHL*

Stage	Ann Arbor/AJCC and Cotswolds	St. Jude lymphoblastic NHL	Mycosis fungoides
I	Single node region or lymphoid structure	Single tumor (extranodal) or single anatomic area (nodal), excluding mediastinum or abdomen	Confined to the skin
II	Two or more nodes on same side of diaphragm or single extranodal site and adjacent node	Single tumor (extranodal) with regional node involvement Primary gastrointestinal tract tumor (usually iliocecal) +/– mesenteric nodes	Clinically positive nodes
III	Node regions or lymphoid structure on both side of the diaphragm III₁ Limited to spleen/hilar nodes, celiac, or portal nodes III₂ Paraaortic, iliac, or mesenteric nodes plus structures in III₁	Node regions or lymphoid structures on both sides of the diaphragm All primary intrathoracic tumor (mediastinal, pleural, thymic) All extensible primary intraabdominal disease; unresectable All primary paraspinal or epidural tumors regardless of other site	Histologically proven nodes
IV	Extranodal site(s) beyond those designated as "E"	Any of the above with initial CNS or BM involvement	Visceral disease

CNS, central nervous system; BM, bone marrow; NHL, non-Hodgkin's lymphoma.

ogy should be performed in patients at risk of central nervous system (CNS) disease [i.e., aggressive NHL with elevated lactate dehydrogenase (LDH) and more than one extranodal site and/or positive BM biopsy]. Baseline gallium or positron emission tomography (PET) scans are useful for staging and for comparison with posttreatment scans during response assessment.
- The Ann Arbor/American Joint Commission for Cancer (AJCC) and Cotswolds staging systems are applicable to all histologies except lymphoblastic and mycosis fungoides (Table 3).
- **Definitions:**
    B-symptoms: Unexplained weight loss more than 10% of body weight over the past 6 months, fever, and "drenching" night sweats.
    X: Bulky disease (10 cm maximal dimension.
    E: (extranodal disease).
    Single E site proximal to or contiguous with a nodal site.
    Single E site so limited in extent/location that it can be subjected to definitive treatment with radiation.

CLASSIFICATION OF NHL

- The Revised European–American Classifications of Lymphoid Neoplasms (REAL) is the currently accepted classification. It was developed in 1994 based on assessment of morphology, immunophenotype (Tables 4 and 5), and genetic and clinical features of lymphomas. The REAL was further refined by the World Health Organization (WHO) classification of hematologic malignancies in 1997.
- To facilitate the description of each histologic entity for the reader, they are grouped by general clinical behavior into indolent, aggressive, or highly aggressive lymphomas.

TABLE 4. *B-cell immunophenotype*

Histology	SIg	CIg	CD 5	10	11	15	23	30	34	43	45
CLL/SLL[a]	+/−	−/+	+	−	−/+		+			+	
Lymphoplasmacytoid[a]	+	+	−	−	−/+		−			+/−	
Follicular center cell grade I–II[ab]	+	−	−	+/−	−		−/+			−	
Marginal zone[ac]	+	+	−	−	+/−		−			−/+	
Mantle cell lymphoma[ad]	+	−	+	−/+	−		−			+	
Follicular center cell grade III[a]	+	−	−	+/−	−		−/+			−	
Diffuse large cell[a]	+/−	−/+	−/+	−/+			−				+/−
Primary mediastinal large cell[ae]	−	−	−/+	−/+		−	−	−/+			+/−
Precursor B lymphoblastic lymphoma/leukemia[af]	−	−/+		+/−					+/−		
Burkitt's lymphoma[a]	+		−	+			−				
Burkitt's-like lymphoma[a]											

[a]Positive B-cell–associated antigens: CD19, CD20, CD22, and CD79.
[b]SIg+: IgM+/−, IgD > IgG > IgA.
[c]SIg M > G > A and IgD−; CIg+ in 40%.
[d]SIgM+ usually IgD+, κ > λ, and CD11c−.
[e]M > G > A and IgD−; CIg+ in 40%.
[f]TdT+, HLA-Dr+, and CD20−/+.

TABLE 5. *T-cell immunophenotype*

Histology	1a	2	3	4	5	7	8	25	56	TdT
					CD					
T-CLL/T-PLL[a]		+	+	+	+	+	+	−		
Mycosis fungoides		+	+	+	+	−/+	−	−		
Peripheral T-cell lymphoma[b]	+/−	+/−	+	+/−	−/+	+/−				
Angiocentric		+	−	+	+/−	+/−	+		+	
Angioimmunoblastic		+	+	+	+					
Adult T-cell lymphoma/ leukemia		+	+	+	+	−	−	+		
Enteropathy T cell[c]			+	−		+	+/−			
Hepatosplenic γ/δ			+	−			−		+	
Anaplastic large-cell lymphoma[d]			−/+					+/−		
Precursor T lymphoblastic lymphoma/leukemia	+/−	+/−	+	+	+/−	+	+			+

[a]T-CLL: 60% are CD4+ and 21% CD4+8+, rare cases are CD4−8+ and CD25−.
[b]Peripheral T cells are most commonly CD4 > CD8, can be CD4−8−, CD45RA may be + and CD45RA−.
[c]Intestinal T cell is CD103+.
[d]ALCL are CD30+, CD45+, EMA+, and CD15+.

Indolent Lymphomas

B Cell

- **B-chronic lymphocytic leukemia (CLL)/Small lymphocytic lymphoma (SLL).** These diseases affect older patients (median age, seventh decade) and often involve the BM, peripheral blood (PB), lymphadenopathy (LN), liver, and spleen. SLL represents the non-leukemic equivalent of CLL. They are incurable and have median survivals of approximately 10 years. They can transform to more aggressive prolymphocytic leukemia (PLL) or large B-cell NHL (Richter's syndrome), which have median survivals of less than 1 year.
- **Lymphoplasmacytoid.** This lymphoma affects primarily older patients (median age, seventh decade). Sites of involvement include BM, LN, and spleen; rarely PB or extranodal sites are involved. Paraproteinemia with IgM and hyperviscosity symptoms may occur. When disseminated, this entity is incurable and has a median survival of approximately 8 to 10 years.
- **Follicular center cell (FCC) grades I and II.** The median occurrence of this lymphoma is in the sixth decade. It is the second most common subtype of NHL, comprising approximately 40% of lymphomas. FCC lymphomas are graded based on the proportion of small and large cells; grade I contains predominantly small B cells, and grade II contains mixed small and large B cells. It commonly has LN and BM involvement, and splenomegaly, extranodal involvement, and a clinical leukemic phase also are seen. Advanced stage disease is incurable in the vast majority of patients, and has a median survival of 8 to 10 years. Histologic transformation to an aggressive large B-cell lymphoma occurs in a fourth of patients.
- **Marginal zone (MZ).** These have two major clinical presentations: extranodal and nodal types. Extranodal types are associated with autoimmune diseases like Sjögren's syndrome or Hashimoto's thyroiditis, or *Helicobacter pylori* gastritis. Recent evidence suggests that proliferation in some mucosa-associated lymphoid tissue (MALT) lymphomas may be antigen driven such as *H. pylori* gastritis, and eradication of the antigen may result in tumor

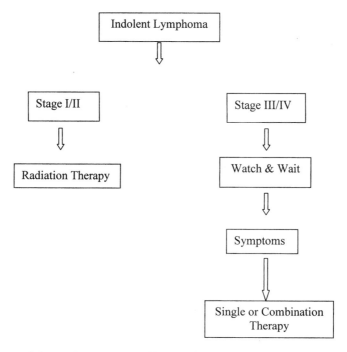

FIG. 1. Indolent non-Hodgkin's lymphoma treatment principles.

regression. Median age of occurrence of MZ lymphomas is in the seventh decade. They are usually quite indolent but incurable, and have a median survival of 10 years. Nodal types may represent nodal dissemination of extranodal types. However, isolated nodal types occur, and although usually indolent, are less so than the extranodal types.

T Cell

- **T-CLL/T-PLL.** These lymphomas comprise 1% of CLL but up to 20% of PLL. Patients often have high white counts (e.g., >100,000/mm^3) and may have cutaneous or mucosal infiltrates. They are more aggressive than their B-cell counterparts and have a median survival of 8 years.
- **Mycosis fungoides (MF).** Mycosis fungoides is a cutaneous T-cell lymphoma that often has multiple cutaneous plaques, nodules, and/or generalized erythroderma. Nodal involvement and leukemic phases (S...zary syndrome) are late occurrences. Large-cell lymphoma may develop as a terminal event. The disease may be relatively indolent over prolonged periods and has a median survival of 10.2 years, but in the worse prognostic group (patients older than 65 years and stage IVB) have a median survival of 1.1 years.

TREATMENT PRINCIPLES

Patients with early-stage FCC and MZ lymphomas are potentially curable with radiation treatment. In stage I FCC lymphoma, radiation treatment (e.g., 30–50 Gy) has a 54% to 88% disease-free survival at 10 years (Fig. 1). In advanced-stage patients, the Stanford group

TABLE 6. *Indolent lymphoma treatment*

	Treatment description	Reference
Combination chemotherapy		
CVP	Cyclophosphamide, 400 mg/m² p.o. daily for 5 days, days 1–5 (total dose/cycle, 2,000 mg/m²)	9
	Vincristine, 1.4 mg/m² i.v. on day 1 (maximum dose/cycle, 2 mg; total dose/cycle, 1.4 mg/m²)	
	Prednisone, 100 mg/m² p.o. daily for 5 days, days 1–5 (total dose/cycle, 500 mg/m²)	
	Treatment is repeated every 21 days	
Single agents		
Fludarabine	Fludarabine, 25 mg/m² per day i.v. for 5 days, days 1–5 (total dose/cycle, 125 mg/m²)	6–8
	Treatment is repeated every 28 days	
Rituximab	Rituximab, 375 mg/m² i.v. weekly (total dose/week, 375 mg/m²)	10

showed no difference in survival between watching until medical symptoms required treatment (called "watch and wait") and early intervention. Based on this approach, therapy is often not begun until symptoms or impending organ compromise occurs, or there is transformation to an aggressive subtype. Selection of treatment is based on the clinical situation. Generally, radiation may be used to palliate local disease, whereas cytotoxic or monoclonal antibody therapies are used in disseminated disease. The choice of agents is dependent on the cell type (B vs. T cell), histology, and treatment history (Table 6).

Aggressive NHL

B Cell

- **Mantle cell lymphoma** primarily occurs in older patients (median age, seventh decade) with a high male-to-female ratio. It demonstrates splenomegaly, BM, LN, and extranodal sites, particularly the gastrointestinal tract (lymphomatous polyposis) in 20% of cases. Unlike other aggressive lymphomas, it is incurable and has a short median survival of 3 to 5 years. The blastic variant is more aggressive, with a propensity for CNS involvement (25%) and shorter survival.
- **Follicular center cell (FCC)** grade III. FCC lymphomas with predominantly large cells, termed grade III, are potentially curable. Among all FCC lymphomas, grade III compose around 15%. This subtype usually has predominantly LN involvement.
- **Diffuse large B cell (DLBC)** constitutes up to 30% to 40% of adult lymphomas and is the single most common type. Like other lymphomas, the median age is in the sixth decade. Patients frequently have a rapidly enlarging mass or acute onset of symptoms. Extranodal involvement is seen in 40% of cases. DLBC is curable with combination chemotherapy and should be treated promptly and aggressively. The overall survival (OS) and progression-free survival (PFS) are approximately 50% and 32%, respectively, at 5 years.
- **Primary mediastinal (thymic) large cell.** This recently recognized subtype is believed to arise in thymic tissue and commonly forms a large anterior mediastinal mass. It occurs most commonly in young women in their fourth decade, and often involves extranodal sites such as the kidney, lung, and liver. The OS and PFS are similar to other large B-cell lymphomas.
- **HIV-associated B-cell lymphomas.** The incidence of lymphoma is 60 times higher than expected among human immunodeficiency virus (HIV)-infected individuals. The median age of occurrence is in the fourth decade, compared with the sixth decade in non–HIV-

related lymphomas. Most patients have advanced-stage disease and often have extranodal involvement, including the gastrointestinal tract, BM, and CNS. Involvement of the CNS may be the only site, as in primary CNS lymphoma, or part of systemic disease. Histologically, these lymphomas are aggressive B cells, and are divided between large B-cell ($\approx$ 70%) and Burkitt's subtypes.

T Cell

- **Peripheral T-cell lymphomas (PTLs)** are uncommon, composing fewer than 15% of lymphomas in the West, with a higher incidence in other parts of the world. Patients typically have generalized disease and may have pruritis and eosinophilia. They frequently involve LN, skin (subcutis), liver, and spleen. In general, PTLs have an aggressive clinical course, although some may be relatively indolent. Compared with large B-cell lymphomas, T-cell lymphomas have a lower rate of cure and higher rate of relapse, with an OS and FFS of 25% and 18%, respectively, at 5 years.
- **Intestinal T-cell lymphoma.** Adult patients often have a history of gluten-sensitive enteropathy, or uncommonly there may be no evidence of an underlying enteropathy. Its geographic distribution is that of intestinal enteropathies, and hence is rare in Western countries. Patients may have abdominal pain and jejunal perforation.
- **Angiocentric lymphoma.** These lymphomas are seen most commonly in Asia, where they usually occur in the nasopharyngeal area with symptoms of obstruction and pain. Nasal angiocentric lymphoma, the most common type, is caused by T/natural killer cells that express Epstein–Barr antigens. Treatment for localized disease is primarily radiation, and the role of chemotherapy is unclear. At relapse, and less commonly at presentation, the disease may disseminate to extranodal sites such as the lungs and skin.
- **Angioimmunoblastic T-cell lymphoma.** This subtype is commonly known as angioimmunoblastic lymphadenopathy with dysproteinemia (AILD). It occurs in older patients who often have fever, rash, diffuse adenopathy, and polyclonal hypergammaglobulinemia. It used to be considered to be primarily a reactive condition, but recent studies have shown that the majority of cases have clonal T-cell rearrangements. The course is quite aggressive but very responsive to steroids and chemotherapy. However, most patients relapse and die of disease.
- **Adult T-cell Lymphoma/Leukemia (ATLL)** is most common in areas with endemic HTLV-1 infection such as Japan and the Caribbean basin. The disease is an aggressive T-cell lymphoma caused by HTLV-1 infection. The clinical presentation includes high white blood cell count, hypercalcemia, hepatosplenomegaly, and lytic bone lesions. Clinically, ATLL has been separated into four distinct clinical presentations termed smoldering, chronic, lymphomatous, and acute, with clinical behaviors that range from indolent to highly aggressive.
- **Anaplastic large-cell lymphoma.** There are two clinical entities: systemic and primary cutaneous. The systemic form occurs in both children and adults. It has either a T-cell or null phenotype; true anaplastic large-cell lymphomas with a B-cell phenotype are very rare. It may involve lymph nodes or extranodal sites, including the skin, and half of patients may have B symptoms and advanced stages at presentation. It is highly responsive to chemotherapy and curable, with an OS and FFS of 75% and 60%, respectively, at 7 years. The primary cutaneous form occurs mostly in adults and has isolated skin nodules. The clinical behavior is indolent, and the skin lesions may spontaneously regress. Systemic disease is uncommon and a late occurrence. This entity appears to be incurable, and some cases appear to be within the spectrum of lymphomatoid papulosis type A.

Treatment Principles

- Many subtypes of aggressive lymphomas are potentially curable with appropriate therapy. However, histologic subtype and prognostic factors influence their curative potentials.

TABLE 7. *International Prognostic Index for NHL*

Risk factors	Definition	Predictive Model
Age	>60 yrs	
LDH	>1× normal	
ECOG performance status	>1	⇓
Stage	III/IV	
Extranodal sites	>1	

Risk category	No. of risk factors	% Cases	CR	DFS of CR[a]	Overall survival[a]
Low	0–1	35	87%	70%	73%
Low intermediate	2	27	67%	51%	51%
High intermediate	3	22	55%	49%	43%
High	4–5	16	44%	42%	26%

[a]DFS, Disease-free survival at 5 years.

Among the various histologies, the aggressive B-cell lymphomas have a better PFS than do T-cell lymphomas, with the exception of anaplastic lymphoma, which is among the most curable subtypes. It is important to recognize that some T-cell subtypes, such as ATLL and primary cutaneous anaplastic lymphoma, have no curable potential and should be approached in a palliative mode. Other T-cell subtypes such as angioimmunoblastic and PTL have low curative potential with conventional-dose treatment and should be considered for trials targeting high-risk patients. Prognostic factors are helpful for identifying patients at various risk levels for cure. The International NHL Prognostic Factor Project evaluated 3,273 patients from 16 institutions to develop a validated prognostic model. Known as the International Prognostic Index (IPI), the model identified five adverse prognostic factors, which, based on the number of factors, could stratify patients into low, low-intermediate, high-intermediate, and high-risk groups (Table 7). Clinically this model can be used to identify patients at high risk of failure who should be considered for more aggressive therapy, preferably in a clinical trial.

• For patients with curable lymphomas, early and appropriate treatment will improve outcome. Among patients with advanced-stage disease, doxorubicin-containing combination chemotherapy should be used, the standard being cyclophosphamide, hydroxydaunomycin, vincristine (Oncovin), and prednisone (CHOP); second- and third-generation regimens were shown to be equivalent to CHOP but were more costly and toxic (Table 8). Patients should be restaged after four and six cycles of treatment. Patients in complete response (CR) or stable minimal residual disease (i.e., unconfirmed CR) after four cycles usually received two to four more cycles. However, patients with persistent disease after six cycles should receive

TABLE 8. *Comparison of CHOP and three intensive regimens for advanced NHL*

Regimen	Number of patients	FFS[a]	OS[a]
CHOP	225	41%	54%
m-BACOD	223	46%	52%
ProMACE-CytaBOM	223	46%	50%
MACOP-B	218	41%	50%

[a]Failure-free survival (FFS) and overall survival (OS) estimated at 3 years.

TABLE 9. *Chemotherapy regimens for NHL*

Combination chemotherapy	Treatment description	Reference
CHOP	Cyclophosphamide, 750 mg/m^2 i.v. day 1 (total dose/cycle, 750 mg/m^2) Doxorubicin, 50 mg/m^2 i.v. day 1 (total dose/cycle, 50 mg/m^2) Vincristine, 1.4 mg/m^2 i.v. day 1 (maximal dose/cycle, 2 mg; total dose/cycle, 1.4 mg/m^2) Prednisone, 50 mg/m^2 per day p.o. for 5 days, days 1–5 (total dose/cycle, 250 mg/m^2) Treatment is repeated every 21 days	1

TABLE 10. *Salvage chemotherapy regimens is aggressive NHL*

Combination chemotherapy	Treatment description	Reference
EPOCH (dose adjusted)[a]	Etoposide, 50 mg/m^2 per day by continuous i.v. infusion for 4 days, days 1–4 (total dose/cycle, 250 mg/m^2) Doxorubicin, 10 mg/m^2 per day by continuous i.v. infusion for 4 days, days 1–4 (total dose/cycle, 40 mg/m^2) Vincristine, 4 mg/m^2 per day by continuous i.v. infusion for 4 days, days 1–4 [total dose/cycle, 1.6 mg/m^2 (no cap)] Prednisone, 60 mg/m^2 per dose p.o. every 12 h for 5 days, days 1–5 (total dose/cycle, 600 mg/m^2) Cyclophosphamide, 750 mg/m^2 i.v. day 5 (total dose/cycle, 750 mg/m^2) Filgrastim, 5 µg/kg per day s.c. starting day 6; continues until ANC >5,000 cells/mm^3 Treatment is repeated every 21 days Cotrimoxazole (800 mg sulfamethoxazole + 160 mg trimethoprim), 1 dose p.o. 3 times weekly (e.g., Monday, Wednesday, Friday) given continuously throughout antineoplastic treatment	2
DHAP	Cisplatin, 100 mg/m^2 by continuous i.v. infusion for 24 h on day 1 (total dose/cycle = 100 mg/m^2) Cytarabine, 2,000 mg/m^2 per dose i.v. over 3 h every 12 h for two doses on day 2 (total dose/cycle, 4,000 mg/m^2) Dexamethasone, 40 mg per day p.o. or i.v. for 4 days, days 1–4 (total dose/cycle, 160 mg/m^2) Treatment is repeated every 21–28 days	3
ESHAP	Etoposide, 40 mg/m^2 per day over 1 h i.v. for 4 days, days 1–4 (total dose/cycle, 160 mg/m^2) Methylprednisolone 250–500 mg per day i.v. for 5 days, days 1–5 (total dose/cycle, 1,250–2,500 mg) Cytarabine, 2,000 mg/m^2 i.v. over 2 h on day 5 (total dose/cycle, 2,000 mg/m^2) Cisplatin, 25 mg/m^2 per day by continuous IV infusion for 4 days, days 1–4 (total dose/cycle, 100 mg/m^2) Treatment is repeated every 21–28 days	4
CEPP(B)[b]	Cyclophosphamide, 600 mg/m^2 per dose i.v. for two doses, days 1 and 8 (total dose/cycle, 1,200 mg/m^2) Etoposide, 70 mg/m^2 per day i.v. for 3 days, days 1–3 (total dose/cycle, 210 mg/m^2) Prednisone, 60 mg/m^2 per day p.o. for 10 days, days 1–10 (total dose/cycle, 600 mg/m^2) Procarbazine, 60 mg/m^2 per day p.o. for 10 days, days 1–10 (total dose/cycle, 600 mg/m^2) Bleomycin, 15 U/m^2 i.v. on days 1 and 15 (total dose/cycle, 30 U/m^2)	5

[a]Etoposide, cyclophosphamide, and doxorubicin dosages may be increased by 20% from the previous cycle's dosage if there was no evidence of absolute neutropenia (ANC, <500/mm^3) or thrombocytopenia (platelet count, <25,000/mm^3).

[b]Increments in the doses of cyclophosphamide by 50 mg/m^2 and etoposide by 15 mg/m^2 each cycle are allowed if patient could tolerate without significant neutropenia.

salvage treatment. Including all risk groups, CHOP was shown to produce 44% CRs, with an overall survival of 54% and PFS of 41% at 3 years. Patients with early-stage disease (i.e., stage I and nonbulky stage II) should receive combined-modality treatment with four cycles of a doxorubicin-containing regimen followed by involved radiation therapy. With this approach, the 5-year estimates of overall survival and PFS are 82% and 77%, respectively.

- Salvage therapy. Patients with potentially curable lymphomas who are refractory or who have relapsed after standard treatment may still be curable with salvage approaches. High-dose therapy with autologous transplantation has been shown to be superior to conventional-dose salvage therapy with DHAP and is now a standard of care. The curative potential of transplantation, however, is influenced by multiple factors including disease responsiveness (i.e., sensitive vs. resistant relapse), number of prior regimens, and bulky (≥10 cm) disease. Depending on the study, the long-term survival of patients after autologous transplantation ranges from 20% to 50%, depending on prognostic factors and length of follow-up. Patients at high risk of salvage failure should be considered for experimental approaches such as allogeneic transplantation. Patients who are not candidates for transplantation or who have relapsed thereafter may be effectively palliated with single-agent or combination chemotherapy or radiation.
- Chemotherapy regimens for NHL are listed in Tables 9 and 10). The approach of aggressive NHL treatment is shown in Fig. 2.

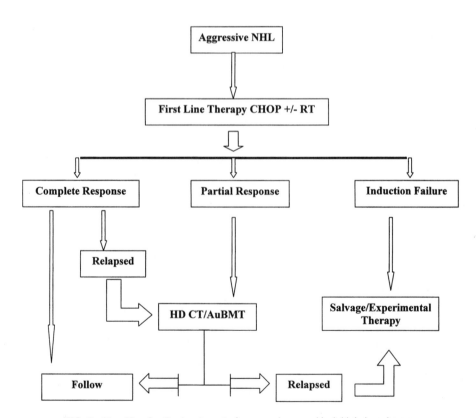

FIG. 2. Algorithm for the treatment of aggressive non-Hodgkin's lymphoma.

HIGHLY AGGRESSIVE

B Cell

- **Precursor B lymphoblastic lymphoma/leukemia** is mostly a disease of children and presents as leukemia in 80% and as lymphoma in 20% of cases. Involvement of nodes, skin, bone and/or bone marrow may be seen. Poor prognostic factors include translocations of t(1;19), t(9;22), 11q13 abnormalities, and tumors that lack expression of CD10, CD34, and CD24. Cases with more than 50 chromosomes have a better prognosis. The event-free survival (EFS) at 5 years is 85% and 64% for localized and advanced disease, respectively.
- **Burkitt's lymphoma** occurs primarily in children, although occasional cases, which are often called Burkitt's-like, are seen in adults. Burkitt's and Burkitt's-like lymphomas are believed to be similar diseases, with the latter showing some "atypical" pathologic features. The disease was initially identified in equatorial Africa, where it was found to be associated with Epstein–Barr virus (EBV) and translocation of the c-*myc* oncogene, and is regarded as the endemic form. In the West, a sporadic "nonendemic" form mostly occurs, which is infrequently associated with EBV. In the West, Burkitt's often involves mesenteric lymph nodes and the distal ileum and cecum. With aggressive chemotherapy, Burkitt's is highly curable, with PFS greater than 90%.

T Cell

- **Precursor T-lymphoblastic lymphomas/leukemias** are most common in young adult men in their third third decade. In pediatrics, they constitute 40% of all lymphomas and 15% of lymphoblastic leukemias. Patients often have a rapidly enlarging mediastinal mass, with or without peripheral lymph node involvement. The distinction between lymphoma and leukemia is based on the percentage involvement of the bone marrow, with 25% to 30% defining the disease as a leukemia. The EFS at 5 years is 85% and 64% for localized and advanced disease, respectively.

Treatment Principles

Most highly aggressive lymphomas are curable with chemotherapy and should be treated expeditiously and with appropriate therapy. A number of aggressive regimens have shown equal results and are outlined in Tables 11 and 12. The aggressive treatment of adults with Burkitt's lymphoma has achieved results similar to those obtained in children, and justify the higher toxicity associated with these regimens. However, older patients often poorly tolerate these aggressive regimens.

TABLE 11. *Outcome in adults and children with Burkitt's and Burkitt's-like lymphoma with CODOX-M/IVAC regimen*

	Number	CR	EFS at 2 yr
Children	21	90%	85%
Adults	20	100%	100%
Total	41	95%	92%

From ref. 23, with permission.

TABLE 12. *Childhood non-Hodgkin's lymphoma therapy: COMP or LSA$_2$L$_2$*

	EFS		OAS	
	COMP	LSA$_2$L$_2$	COMP	LSA$_2$L$_2$
Localized disease[a]	83%	85%	87%	
Advanced Disease[b]	34%	64%	45%	67%

[a]Lymphoblastic and large cell, nonstatistically significant difference between COMP and LSA$_2$L$_2$.
[b]Statistically significant in lymphoblastic only.
From reference 24, with permission.

SUGGESTED READING

1. McKelvey EM, Gottlieb JA, Wilson HE, et al. Hydroxydaunomycin combination chemotherapy in malignant lymphoma. *Cancer* 1976;38:1484– 1493.
2. Wilson WH, Bryant G, Bates S, et al. EPOCH chemotherapy: toxicity and efficacy in relapsed and refractory non-Hodgkin's lymphoma. *J Clin Oncol* 1993;11:1573–1582.
3. Valasquez W, Cabanillas F, Salvador P, et al. Effective salvage therapy for lymphoma with cisplatin in combination with high-dose Ara-C and dexamethasone (DHAP). *Blood* 1988;71:117–122.
4. Valasquez W, McLaughlin P, Tucker S, et al. ESHAP: an effective chemotherapy regimen in refractory and relapsing lymphoma: a 4-year follow up study. *J Clin Oncol* 1994;12:1169–1176.
5. Chao NJ, Rosenberg SA, Horning SJ. CEPP (B): an effective and well-tolerated regimen in poor-risk, aggressive non-Hodgkin's lymphoma. *Blood* 1990;76:1293–1298.
6. Danhauser L, Plunkett W, Keating M, et al. 9-'-D-arabinofuranosyl-2-fluoroadenine 5'-monophosphate pharmacokinetics in plasma and tumor cells of patients with relapsed leukemia and lymphoma. *Cancer Chemother Pharmacol* 1986;18:145–152.
7. Hutton JJ, Von Hoff DD, Kuhn J, et al. Phase I clinical investigation of 9-'-D-arabinofuranosyl-2-fluoroadenine 5'-monophosphate (NSC 312887): a new purine antimetabolite. *Cancer Res* 1984;44: 4183–4186.
8. Hersh MR, Kuhn JG, Phillips JL, et al. Pharmacokinetic study of fludarabine phosphate (NSC 312887). *Cancer Chemother Pharmacol* 1986;17:277–280.
9. Bagley CM, DeVita VT, Berard CW, et al. Advanced lymphosarcoma: intensive cyclical combination chemotherapy with cyclophosphamide, vincristine and prednisone. *Ann Intern Med* 1972;76: 227–234.
10. McLaughlin P, Grillo-Lopez A, Link B, et al. Rituximab chimeric anti-CD20 monoclonal antibody therapy for relapsed indolent lymphoma: half of the patients respond to 4-dose treatment program. *J Clin Oncol* 1998;16:2825–2833.
11. Armitage JO, Vose JM, Bierman PJ. Salvage therapy for patients with non-Hodgkin's lymphoma. *J Natl Cancer Inst* 1990;10:39–43.
12. Chabner BA, Longo D. *Cancer chemotherapy and biotherapy principles and practice.* 2nd ed. Philadelphia: Lippincott-Raven, 1996:1–16.
13. Reed JC. Dysregulation of apoptosis in cancer. *Cancer J Sci Am* 1999;4:S8—S13.
14. Kitada S, Andersen J, Reed JC, et al. Expression of apoptosis-regulating proteins in chronic lymphocytic leukemia: correlations with in vitro and in vivo chemoresponses. *Blood* 1998;91:3379–3389.
15. Goldstein L, Galaski H, Fojo A, et al. Expression of a multidrug resistance gene in human cancers. *J Natl Cancer Inst* 1989;81:116–120.
16. Lai G-M, Chen Y-N, Mickley LA, et al. P-glycoprotein expression and schedule dependence of Adriamycin cytotoxicity in human colon carcinoma cell lines. *Int J Cancer* 1991;49:696–697.
17. Legha SS, Benjamin RS, MacKay B, et al. Reduction of doxorubicin cardiotoxicity by prolonged continuous intravenous infusion. *Ann Intern Med* 1982;96:133–139.
18. Dana B, Dahlberg S, Miller T, et al. m-BACOD treatment for intermediate- and high-grade malignant lymphomas: a Southwest Oncology Group phase II trial. *J Clin Oncol* 1990;8:1155–1162.
19. Klimo P, Connors J. MACOP-B chemotherapy for the treatment of diffuse large cell lymphoma. *Ann Intern Med* 1985;102:596–602.

20. Weick J, Dahlberg S, Fisher R, et al. Combination chemotherapy of intermediate-grade and high-grade non-Hodgkin's lymphoma with MACOP-B: a Southwest Oncology Group study. *J Clin Oncol* 1991;9:748–753.
21. Cabanillas F, Hagemister F, McLaughlin P, et al. Results of MIME salvage regimen for recurrent or refractory lymphoma. *J Clin Oncol* 1987;5:407–412.
22. Non-Hodgkin's Lymphoma Classification Project: A clinical evaluation of the international lymphoma study group classification of non-hodgkin's lymphoma. *N Eng J Med* 1993;329:987.
23. Magrath I, Adde M, Shad A, et al. Adults and children with small noncleaved cell lymphoma have a similar excellent outcome when treated with the same chemotherapy regiment. *J Clin Oncol* 1996;14:925–934.
24. Anderson JR, Jenkins RD, Wilson JF, et al. Long term follow-up of patients treated with COMP or LSA2L2 therapy for childhood non-hodgkin's lymphoma: a report of CCG-551 from the children cancer group. *J Clin Oncol* 1993;11:1024–1032.

28

Hodgkin's Lymphoma

Jame Abraham and Wyndham H. Wilson

Medicine Branch, DCS, National Cancer Institute, National Institutes of Health, Bethesda, Maryland

Hodgkin's lymphoma (HL) is a neoplastic disorder of the lymphoid system characterized by the presence of multinucleated giant cells, known as Reed–Sternberg (RS) cells. In 1832, Thomas Hodgkin reported his observations from autopsies of six patients with unusually enlarged lymph nodes, and 60 years later, Sternberg and Reed described the pathognomonic giant cells called Reed–Sternberg (RS) cells of Hodgkin's lymphoma. It is one of the few malignancies in which modern diagnostic and treatment modalities have made dramatic advancements. Currently more than 75% of newly diagnosed patients with HL are cured with radiation therapy and/or combination chemotherapy.

EPIDEMIOLOGY

Hodgkin's lymphoma is among the most common malignancies of young adults. It constitutes approximately 1% of all malignancies and 18% of all lymphomas, and in the United States, three of every 100,000 people develop this condition. In Europe and North America, there is a bimodal age distribution, with an increasing frequency between the second and third decades, and a second peak in the seventh decade. In contrast to other lymphomas, the overall incidence of HL is stable in the Western Hemisphere.

ETIOLOGY AND RISK FACTORS

- The etiology of HL is unclear and may be multifactorial.
- Same-sex siblings of patients with HL have a 10 times higher risk of developing HL. This association may be due to genetic factors and/or environmental factors.
- From 40% to 50% of the cases of "classic" HL have clonal integration of Epstein–Barr virus (EBV) in the Reed–Sternberg cells.

PATHOLOGY

HL has a unique cellular composition, usually composed of a minority of neoplastic cells (RS cells) in an inflammatory background.

The pathologic diagnosis of HL requires an adequate tissue biopsy of an enlarged lymph node. Generally needle biopsies are suboptimal for a proper diagnosis. RS cells or their variants should be present, and the tissue should have an appropriate immunophenotype.

RS Cells or Variants

- The RS cell is a lymphoid cell, and in most cases studied, it is a clonal B cell.
- Cytologically, the RS cell is a multinucleated giant cell with large eosinophilic inclusion-like nucleoli, with a thick, well-defined nuclear membrane and pale-staining chromatin.
- The classic RS cell has two mirror-image nuclei, which are often described as "owl's eyes."
- A background of lymphocytes, eosinophils, and histiocytes is usually present (Fig. 1).

Pathologic Classification

In 1994, the International Lymphoma Study Group introduced a new classification, incorporating new immunologic and molecular data as part of a Revised European-American Lym-

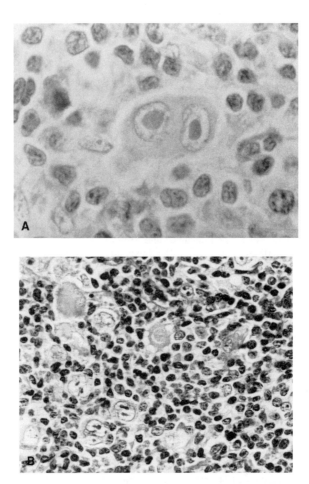

FIG. 1. A: Diagnostic Reed–Sternberg cell, seen in classic types of Hodgkin's lymphomas (mixed cellularity, nodular sclerosis, lymphocyte depletion). B: Variants of Reed–Sternberg cells seen in nodular lymphocyte-predominant Hodgkin's lymphomas: popcorn cells or L and H cells (lymphocytic or histiocytic predominance). Reed–Sternberg cells of the classic type generally are not seen in a nodular lymphocyte-predominant Hodgkin's lymphoma.

TABLE 1. *Classification systems*

REAL Classification, 1994	Rye Classification, 1965
Lymphocyte predominance	**Lymphocyte predominance,**
Classic Hodgkin's lymphoma	**nodular**
Lymphocyte-rich classic HL	Lymphocyte predominance, diffuse (most cases)
	Lymphocyte predominance, nodular (some cases)
Nodular sclerosis	Nodular sclerosis
Mixed cellularity	Mixed cellularity
Lymphocyte depletion	Lymphocyte depletion

TABLE 2. *Immunophenotypes*

Cells/Antigen	Classic HL	Lymphocyte predominance
Diagnostic RS cells	Always present	Rare to absent
Background		
Lymphocytes	T > B cells	B > T cells
CD30 (Ki-1)	Usually positive	Often positive
CD15 (Leu M1)	Usually positive	Negative
CD45 (LCA)	Usually negative	Positive
CD20 (L26)	Usually negative	Usually positive
EBV	Often positive	Usually negative

phoma classification (REAL) for HL. The REAL classification has replaced the older Rye classification (Table 1).

- REAL clasification distinguishes two types of HL: classic HL (CHL) and lymphocyte predominance (LPHL).
- LPHL closely resembles a low-grade B-cell lymphoma.

The immunophenotypes for classic HL and LPHL are described in Table 2.

CLINICAL FEATURES

- More than 80% of patients have cervical lymph node enlargement, and more than 50% will have mediastinal adenopathy.
- Lymph nodes are usually nontender, firm, and rubbery.
- Constitutional symptoms ("B" symptoms):
  - Unexplained fever (temperature, >38°C).
  - Drenching night sweats.
  - Unexplained weight loss (>10% of body weight, over 6 months before the diagnosis).
- Other symptoms include fatigue, weakness, anorexia, alcohol-induced nodal pain, and pruritus.

Staging (Ann Arbor/AJCC and Cotswold) is outlined in Table 3.

Pretreatment Evaluation

1. Biopsy and diagnosis.
2. History with attention to B symptoms.
3. Complete physical examination.

TABLE 3. *Staging*

Stage I	Involvement of single lymph node region or lymphoid structure (spleen, thymus, Waldeyer's ring), or involvement of a single extralymphatic site (IE)
Stage II	Involvement of two or more lymph node regions on the same side of the diaphragm (II), which may be accompanied by localized contiguous involvement of an extralymphatic organ or site (IIE). The number of anatomic sites may be indicated by numeric subscript
Stage III	Involvement of lymph node regions on both sides of the diaphragm (III), which may also be accompanied by localized involvement of an associated extralymphatic organ or site (IIIE), by involvement of the spleen (IIIS), or both (IIIE+S)
Stage IV	Disseminated involvement of one or more extralymphatic organs, with or without associated lymph node involvement, or isolated extralymphatic organ involvement with distant (nonregional) nodal involvement

Each stage is divided into A and B categories: B for those with defined systemic symptoms, and A for those without

X	A mass >10 cm or a mediastinal mass larger than one third of the thoracic diameter
E	Involvement of a single extranodal site contiguous to a known nodal site
CS	Clinical staging
PS	Pathologic staging

4. Laboratory tests include
   - Complete blood count (CBC), erythrocyte sedimentation rate (ESR).
   - Biochemical tests of liver function, renal function, and serum uric acid.
5. Radiologic studies.
   - Chest radiograph and computed tomography (CT) scan of the chest, abdomen, and pelvis.
   - Gallium or positron emission tomography (PET) scans are useful but not mandatory.
   - Bone scan or radiographs if bone pain or tenderness is present.
6. Bone marrow biopsy of the posterior iliac crest for those with abnormal CBC or clinical stage IIB, III, or IV.
7. Lymphangiogram for patients considered for a staging laparotomy.
8. Staging laparotomy and splenectomy for patients with early-stage disease, above the diaphragm, who are being considered for definitive radiation treatment and are at significant risk for occult advanced-stage disease.

Unfavorable Prognostic Features

- Advanced stage (IIIB and IV).
- Presence of B symptoms (primarily fever and weight loss).
- Size of the mass, particularly in the mediastinum (more than one third of chest diameter).
- Extranodal involvement (liver, spleen, and bone marrow).
- Older than 60 years.
- Increased ESR (B symptoms + ESR > 30, or no B symptoms and ESR > 70).
- Unfavorable histology (mixed cellularity and lymphocyte depletion vs. lymphocyte predominant and nodular sclerosis).

MANAGEMENT OF NEWLY DIAGNOSED HL

Advances in the treatment of HL have dramatically improved the response rate and survival. This is mainly due to careful staging, understanding of the pattern of spread, and advances in radiation and chemotherapy.

The goal of therapy for HL is cure. In general, the management of HL with radiation therapy consists of treating regions of known disease plus adjacent nodal groups. Whereas radiation therapy is reserved for the early stages of HL, chemotherapy with or without radiation is reserved for the advanced stages.

- Treatment selection is influenced by stage, prognostic factors, and toxicity.
- Staging laparotomy is becoming infrequent:
  - Risk paradigms can identify early-stage patients with low incidence of occult advanced-stage disease who are candidates for radiation alone.
  - It is unnecessary for patients receiving combination chemotherapy.
  - Risks of surgical morbidity should be considered.
  - The primary role of laparotomy is to perform a pathologic staging.

Tumor debulking is not indicated.

1. **Radiation treatment.**
   - Radiation is the most effective single "agent" treatment for HL. Failures are usually in unirradiated sites.
   - Radiation therapy is delivered to three major fields, known as the mantle, paraaortic, and pelvic or inverted-Y fields. Extended field (EF) radiation refers to the inclusion of adjacent clinically negative nodal sites (Table 4; Fig. 2).
2. **Chemotherapy.**
   Aggressive chemotherapy produces long-term disease-free remissions in advanced HL. The first "curative regimen" was mechlorethamine, Oncovin, procarbazine, prednisone (MOPP), which resulted in a 70% complete remission in stage III and stage IV patients. Subsequently many regimens have been developed, including MOPP variants, doxorubicin (Adriamycin), bleomycin, vinblastine, and dacarbazine (ABVD) and its variants, and hybrids of MOPP/ABVD. Chemotherapy is usually administered for two cycles beyond complete response or stable disease, for a minimum of six cycles.
   - ABVD and MOPP contain different agents. Studies have shown that ABVD is less toxic and more effective than MOPP, with a higher freedom from progression and overall survival. At 10 years, the risk of developing treatment-related leukemia with the MOPP regimen is 2% to 3%, whereas it is 0.7% with ABVD.

Choosing between MOPP, ABVD, and MOPP/ABVD

Historically, MOPP was considered the standard treatment for advanced HL. Because of considerable controversy regarding the best regimen, cooperative groups in North America and Europe address this issue. In a randomized study, the Cancer and Leukemia Group B (CALGB) compared leading regimens with an 8-year follow-up (Table 5).

The results indicate that ABVD alone or MOPP/ABVD was superior to MOPP alone, in terms of remission, freedom from progression, and survival.

ABVD is currently the standard treatment in North America (Table 6).

Combined-Modality Treatment

In an attempt to reduce toxicity and increase progression-free survival, combined treatment with reduced doses of chemotherapy and radiotherapy are being explored in patients with unfavorable clinical stage I and II disease (Table 7).

Primary treatment of HL is addressed in Table 8.

TABLE 4. *Radiation guidelines*

Tumoricidal dose	40–45 Gy at the rate of 10 Gy/wk
Clinically negative nodal regions	35 Gy
Consolidation (after chemotherapy)	15–20 Gy

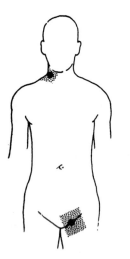 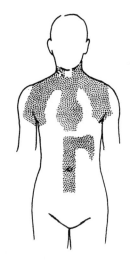

A Involved field irradiation   **B** Subtotal nodal irradiation
including mantle and spade fields

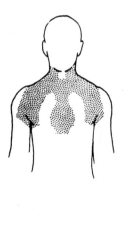 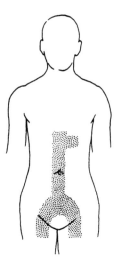

C Mantle field irradiation   **D** Inverted-Y field irradiation

FIG. 2. Radiation therapy fields used in treating Hodgkin's disease. When the fields shown in **C** and **D** are combined, this is commonly called total nodal irradiation (TNI). From Haskell CM. *Cancer Treatment*. 4th ed. Philadelphia: WB Saunders, 1995:965, with permission.

TABLE 5. *CALGB study comparing combination treatments*

Regimen	Complete response rate	Survival rate
MOPP	67%	64%
ABVD	82%	72%
MOPP/ABVD	83%	73%

TABLE 6. *Commonly used treatment regimens*

ABVD
   Doxorubicin, 25 mg/m^2 per dose i.v. push for two doses, days 1 and 15
      (total dose/cycle, 50 mg/m^2)
   Bleomycin, 10 Units/m^2 per dose i.v. push for two doses, days 1 and 15
      (total dose/cycle, 20 Units/m^2)
   Vinblastine, 6 mg/m^2 per dose i.v. push for two doses, days 1 and 15
      (total dose/cycle, 12 mg/m^2)
   Dacarbazine, 375 mg/m^2 per dose i.v. infusion for two doses, days 1 and 15
      (total dose/cycle, 750 mg/m^2)
   Treatment cycle repeats every 28 days
MOPP
   Mechlorethamine, 6 mg/m^2 per dose i.v. push for two doses, days 1 and 8
      (total dose/cycle, 12 mg/m^2)
   Vincristine, 1.4 mg/m^2 per dose i.v. push for two doses, days 1 and 8
      (total dose/cycle, 2.8 mg/m^2)
   Procarbazine, 100 mg/m^2 per day p.o. for 14 doses, days 1–14
      (total dose/cycle, 1,400 mg/m^2)
   Prednisone, 40 mg/m^2 per day p.o. for 14 doses, days 1–14 (cycles 1 and 14 only)
      (total dose/cycle, 560 mg/m^2)
   Treatment cycle repeats every 28 days
Alternating MOPP/ABVD
   Alternate MOPP and ABVD cycles by 28 days
MOPP/ABV hybrid
   Mechlorethamine, 6 mg/m^2 i.v. push day 1 (total dose/cycle, 6 mg/m^2)
   Vincristine, 1.4 mg/m^2 i.v. push day 1
      (total dose/cycle, 1.4 mg/m^2; maximal dose, 2 mg)
   Procarbazine, 100 mg/m^2 per day p.o. for 7 doses, days 1–7 (total dose/cycle, 700 mg/m^2)
   Prednisone, 40 mg/m^2 per day p.o. for 14 doses, days 1–14 (total dose/cycle, 560 mg/m^2)
   Doxorubicin, 25 mg/m^2 i.v. push day 8 (total dose/cycle, 25 mg/m^2)
   Hydrocortisone, 100 mg i.v. day 8, before bleomycin (total dose/cycle, 100 mg)
   Bleomycin, 10 Units/m^2 i.v. push day 8 (total dose/cycle, 10 Units/m^2)
   Vinblastine, 6 mg/m^2 i.v. push day 8 (total dose/cycle, 6 mg/m^2)
   Treatment cycle repeats every 28 days

TABLE 7. *Combined-modality treatment*

Study group	Cytotoxic regimen	Radiation
NCI, Milan	ABVD, four cycles	36 Gy to involved sites and 30 Gy to uninvolved sites
Sanford V	Doxorubicin	36 Gy to initial sites of bulky disease
	Methochloroethamine	
	Vinblastine	
	Vincristine	
	Bleomycin	
	Etoposide	
	Prednisone	

TABLE 8. *Primary treatment*

Stage I and II
a) Very favorable
   Female: IA, IIA NSHL and/or ≤3 nodal sites above diaphragm
   Male: IA LPHL, neck or groin
   ESR < 50
   Treatment
     EF RT
     Consider: ABVD ×6 cycles for smokers and females <27
b) Favorable
     >3 nodal sites above the diaphragm
     ESR < 50
   Treatment
     EF RT after negative lap; or ABVD ×6 cycles
     Consider: ABVD ×4 cycles + mantle (IF) RT
     ABVD ×6 for smokers and females <27
c) Unfavorable
     >3 nodal sites above the diaphragm
     LMA or bulky (≥10 cm) adenopathy
     ESR < 50
     B symptoms
     Bilateral hilar adenopathy
     Involvement of pericardium, pleura, lung, or bone
     Gross lymphatic permeation and obstruction
   Treatment
     ABVD ×6 cycles Or ABVD ×6–8 cycles + mantle for LMA
     Consider: ABVD ×4 + mantle (IF) RT except for LMA
IIIA
     ABVD ×6–8 cycles
     Consider ABVD ×4 with IF RT
IIIB and IV
     ABVD ×6–8 cycles
     Consider RT to sites of bulky disease

RT, radiation therapy; EF RT, extended-field radiation; IF RT, Involved-field radiation; LAG, lymphangiogram; Lap, laparotomy; LMA, large mediastinal adenopathy.

COMPLICATIONS OF THERAPY

Radiation Therapy

Early complications:

- Mantle field radiation may cause mouth dryness, pharyngitis, cough, and dermatitis.
- Subdiaphragmatic radiation may cause anorexia and nausea.
- Radiation can cause myelosuppression or thrombocytopenia.

Late complications:

- Hypothyroidism.
- Pericarditis and pneumonitis.
- Lhermitte's sign: 15% of the patients receiving mantle radiation may experience electric shock sensation radiating down the back of the legs when the head is flexed, 6 to 12 weeks after the treatment. May be due to transient demyelinization of the spinal cord, and it usually resolves spontaneously.
- Coronary artery disease (CAD): Increased risk in patients who received cardiac radiation. Patients should be monitored and evaluated for other risk factors for CAD.

- **Secondary neoplasms** (lung, breast, stomach, and thyroid).
- Lung cancer: twofold to eightfold increase in lung cancer is observed more than 5 years after the radiation treatment and persists through the second decade.
- The increase in lung cancer occurs mostly in smokers.
- Smokers should be encouraged stop smoking.
- **Breast cancer** is inversely proportional to the age at radiation treatment. The relative risk (RR) is 136 if the patient is younger than 15 years. RR is 19 for age group 15 to 24 years. RR is 7 for age group 24 to 29 years.
- The high risk is restricted to women irradiated before age 30 years.
- Average interval between radiation and diagnosis of breast cancer is 15 years.
- Breast examination should be part of follow-up for women at risk.
- Routine mammography should begin about 8 years after completion of the radiation.

Chemotherapy

Early complications:

- Nausea and vomiting.
- Alopecia.
- Myelosuppression.
- Infection.

Late complications:

- Sterility (primarily with MOPP-based regimens).
- Neuropathy (primarily with vincristine).
- Cardiomyopathy (doxorubicin).
- Pulmonary fibrosis (bleomycin).
- Secondary leukemia (MOPP ± radiation).

TREATMENT OF HODGKIN'S LYMPHOMA IN RELAPSE

For successful management of patients with relapsed HL, one should have a clear understanding of:

1. Sites of relapse.
2. Time since the last treatment.
3. Details of previous treatment.
   - If the relapse is due to inadequate initial treatment, retreatment with chemotherapy or radiation is considered.
   - Relapse after primary radiation is best managed with chemotherapy.
   - Generally relapse after primary combination chemotherapy should be consolidated with autologous stem cell transplant.

Prognostic factors in relapse (Stanford study):
1. Stage at relapse is important in radiation failures.
   For 10-year DFS:
   - Stage IA, 88%.
   - Stage IIA and IIIA, 58%.
   - Stage IV or B symptoms, 34%.
2. Histology is important.
   For 10-year DFS:
   - LPHL and NSHL, 67%.
   - MCHL and LPHL, 44%.
   - Duration of remission less than 12 months is a poor prognostic finding.

Potentially curative treatment approach

1. High-dose chemotherapy with autologous stem cell transplantation.
2. Combination chemotherapy.
3. Extended-field radiation therapy.

Palliative treatment

1. Investigational treatment.
2. Radiation treatment.
3. Sequential single-agent chemotherapy.

REFERENCES

1. Connors JM. An update on the Vancouver experience in the management of advanced Hodgkin's disease treated with the MOPP/ABV hybrid program. *Semin Hematol* 1988;25:34–40.
2. Klimo P, Connors JM. MOPP/ABV hybrid program: combination chemotherapy based on early introduction of seven effective drugs for advanced Hodgkin's disease. *J Clin Oncol* 1985;3: 1174–1182.
3. Connors JM, Klimo P. MOPP/ABV hybrid chemotherapy for advanced Hodgkin's disease. *Semin Hematol* 1987;24:35–40.
4. Connors JM, Klimo P, Adams G, et al. Treatment of advanced Hodgkin's disease with chemotherapy: comparison of MOPP/ABV hybrid regimen with alternating courses of MOPP and ABVD: a report from the National Cancer Institute of Canada clinical trials group [published erratum appears in *J Clin Oncol* 1997;15:2762]. *J Clin Oncol* 1997;15:1638–1645.
5. Lister TA, Crowther D, Suteliffe SB, et al. Report of a committee convened to discuss the evaluation and staging of patients with Hodgkin's disease: Cotswolds meeting. *J Clin Oncol* 1989;7:1630–1636.
6. Mauch P, Larson D, Osteen R, et al. Prognostic factors for positive surgical staging in patients with Hodgkin's disease. *J Clin Oncol* 1990;8:257–265.
7. Urba WJ, Longo DL. Hodgkin's disease. *N Engl J Med* 1992;326:678–687.
8. Sears JD, Greven KM, Ferree CR, et al. Definitive irradiation in the treatment of Hodgkin's disease: analysis of outcome, prognostic factors, and long term complications. *Cancer* 1997;79:145–151.
9. Swerdlow AJ, Douglas AJ, Hudson GV, et al. Risk of second primary cancers after Hodgkin's disease by type of treatment: analysis of 2846 patients in the British National Lymphoma Investigation. *BMJ* 1992;304:1137–1143.
10. Canellos GP, Anderson JR, Propert KJ, et al. Chemotherapy of advanced Hodgkin's disease with MOPP, ABVD, or MOPP alternating with ABVD. *N Engl J Med* 1992;327:1478–1484.
11. Bonfante V, Santoro A, Viviani S, et al. ABVD in the treatment of Hodgkin's disease. *Semin Oncol* 1992;19(2 suppl 5):38–45.
12. Mauch PM. Controversies in the management of early stage Hodgkin's disease. *Blood* 1994;83: 318–329.
13. Viviani S, Bonnadonna G, Santoro A, et al. Alternating versus hybrid MOPP and ABVD combinations in advanced Hodgkin's disease: ten year results. *J Clin Oncol* 1996;14:1421–1430.
14. Armitage JO, Bierman PJ, Vose JM, et al. Autologous bone marrow transplantation for patients with relapsed disease. *Am J Med* 1991;91:605–611.
15. Aisenberg AC. Problems in Hodgkin's disease management. *Blood* 1999;93:761–779.
16. Harris NL. Hodgkin's disease: classification and differential diagnosis. *Modern Pathol* 1999;12: 159–176.

29

Hematopoietic Stem Cell Transplantation

Jame Abraham and Michael R. Bishop

Medicine Branch, National Cancer Institute, National Institutes of Health, Bethesda, Maryland

Hematopoietic stem cell transplantation (HSCT) is an increasingly effective treatment for leukemia, several other malignant and nonmalignant conditions, and for selective solid tumors. About 30,000 autologous and 17,000 allogeneic stem cell transplants were performed in 1997 throughout the world. With the development of improved supportive care measures and a better understanding of transplant immunology, the mortality and morbidity associated with transplants have been significantly reduced.

RATIONALE OF STEM CELL TRANSPLANTATION

- Both lymphoid and myeloid cells are derived from a single pleuripotent stem cell that is capable of both self-renewal and differentiation.
- Many malignancies exhibit a steep dose–response relation to chemotherapy or radiotherapy, but the dose-limiting toxicity for most of the chemotherapeutic agents is myelosuppression.
- Dose intensity and marrow rescue with infusion of hematopoietic stem cells, obtained either from the peripheral blood or from the bone marrow, are the primary biologic rationales of autologous HSCT.
- High-dose chemotherapy rarely completely eradicates malignancy.
- The therapeutic benefit in allogeneic HSCT is largely due to the immune-mediated graft-versus-malignancy effect.
- In hematopoietic disorders (e.g., leukemia), the HSCT replaces the defective clone with a normal stem cell or replaces a missing hematopoietic or lymphoid component in disorders such as aplastic anemia or severe combined immune deficiency (SCID).

TYPES OF TRANSPLANTATION

Autologous

- Patient's own bone marrow or peripheral blood stem cells (PBSCs) are collected before administration of high-dose chemotherapy (HDCT).
- The stored cells are reinfused after HDCT for enhancement of bone marrow recovery.

Allogeneic

Stem cells can be collected from:
- Matched related human leukocyte antigen (HLA)-identical sibling of the patient.
- Partially matched sibling or parent of the patient.

TABLE 1. *Indications for HSCT*

Malignant	Nonmalignant	Congenital
Acute myeloid leukemia	Aplastic anemia	Immunodeficiencies
Acute lymphocytic leukemia	Paroxysmal nocturnal	Hematologic defects
Chronic myeloid leukemia	hemoglobinuria (PNH)	Mucopolysaccharidoses
Non-Hodgkin's lymphoma	Myelodysplastic syndrome	Mucolipidoses
Hodgkin's lymphoma		Other lysosomal diseases
Multiple myeloma		
Hairy cell leukemia		
Chronic lymphocytic leukemia		
Cancer of the breast		

- Matched unrelated donor selected through a search of the computer files of various international registries, including National Marrow Donor Program (NMDP).
- Bone marrow, PBSCs, or umbilical cord blood may be used as a stem cell source.

Syngeneic

- Marrow or PBSCs are collected from an identical twin.

Indications for HSCT are listed in Tables 1 and 2.

TABLE 2. *Indications for Hematopoietic stem cell transplantation*

Condition	Preferred type of transplant	5-yr DFS (%)
CML	Sibling or unrelated allogeneic	
Chronic phase		40–80
Accelerated phase		25–45
Blast crisis		10–20
AML		
First remission	Sibling or URD or autologous	45–65
Early relapse	Sibling or URD	20–30
Second or greater Remission	Sibling or URD or autologous	20–45
ALL		
Second or greater remission	Sibling or URD or autologous	25–55
NHL		
Initial treatment	Autologous or sibling allogeneic	60–80
Relapsed but responsive	Autologous or sibling allogeneic	30–70
Hodgkin's disease		
Relapse or responsive	Autologous or sibling allogeneic	25–65
Neuroblastoma		
High-risk initial therapy	Autologous or sibling allogeneic	40–60
Aplastic anemia	Sibling allogeneic	40–80
Congenital immunodeficiencies	Sibling or unrelated allogeneic haploidentical	40–75
Hemoglobinopathies	Sibling allogeneic	50–95
Multiple myeloma	Autologous or sibling allogeneic	17–54

URD, unrelated donor; CML, chronic myeloid leukemia; AML, acute myeloid leukemia; ALL, acute lymphoid leukemia; NHL, non-hodgkins lymphoma.

PRETRANSPLANT EVALUATION

Patient Evaluation

Discuss in detail about the HSC transplantation including its rationale, risks, benefits, and alternative therapeutic options with the patient, donor, and family.

1. Complete medical history.
   - Diagnosis.
   - History of previous treatments, responses, and duration of responses.
   - List of chemotherapeutic agents used in the past with cumulative doses.
   - Complications of prior treatment.
   - Other medical problems.
   - Transfusion history.
   - Psychosocial evaluation
2. Complete physical examination.
3. Confirmation of original diagnosis.
4. Confirmation of metastatic spread and appropriate restaging.
5. Organ evaluation.
   - Renal function evaluation.
   - Hepatic function and hepatitis serology.
   - Pulmonary evaluation with chest radiograph and pulmonary function test.
   - Cardiac assessment with electrocardiogram (ECG), ECHO, or multiple-gated acquisition (MUGA).
6. Review the infectious disease risk factors.
   - Hepatitis
   - Cytomegalovirus (CMV).
   - Human immunodeficiency virus (HIV).
7. HLA testing.
8. Transfusion support planning.
   - ABO typing of the patient.
   - Evaluation of allogeneic sensitization.
   - Transfusion reactions.
9. Discussion about sterility and sperm banking in younger patients.

Donor Evaluation

1. HLA typing.
2. Blood grouping.
3. Donor safety for bone marrow procurement or apheresis.
   - History of coronary artery disease (CAD) is risk for both apheresis and general anesthesia for bone marrow procurement.
   - History of complications with anesthesia.
   - History of lung disease.
   - Back or spine problems.
   - Medications [especially angiotensin-converting enzyme (ACE) inhibitors, aspirin, nonsteroidal antiinflammatory drugs (NSAIDs), and coumadin].
4. Product safety.
   - History of high-risk behavior for sexually transmitted disease (STD).
   - History of HIV, hepatitis, CMV.
   - History of pregnancy.

ALLOGENEIC TRANSPLANTATION

Donor Selection

The success of allogeneic transplantation depends on the degree of donor–recipient matching at the Human Leukocyte Antigen (HLA) or major histocompatibility complex (MHC) locus. Genes encoding for HLA are located on chromosome 6, and they are codominantly expressed. HLA class I antigens are A, B, and C, and class II antigens are DP, DQ, and DR. Even when a donor–recipient pair is related and completely genotypically matched for HLA, the incidence of graft-versus-host disease (GVHD) in allogeneic transplant is about 50%.

Histoincompatibility can cause increased incidence of Graft Versus Host Disease (GVHD), graft failure, or graft rejection.

Related donor

- The probability of HLA-identity between any two given siblings is 25%.
- In the United States, the chance of having an HLA-matched sibling is about 35%.
- HLA typing is done on blood samples from the patient and the donor.
- Both serologic and molecular methods are used for HLA typing.
- For allogeneic transplantation, the most important HLA antigens are:
    Class I (*A, *B) and class II (*DRB1).
    Most transplant centers prefer a 6/6 match or a minimum 5/6 match.

Unrelated donor

If the patient has no donors in the family:

- A search can be done in the National Marrow Donation Program (NMDP).
- About 20% to 30% of the searches through the NMDP result in transplant.
- The median time to transplant from the initiation of search is 208 days.
- The phone number of the NMDP is 1-800-627-7692.
- Because of the high incidence of GVHD, the mortality and morbidity associated with matched unrelated transplant can be high.

Stem Cell Collection in Allogeneic Transplantation

Peripheral Blood Stem Cell (PBSC) Collection

Stem cells can be mobilized to the periphery by growth factors and collected through an apheresis procedure.

- Usually GCSF, 5 to 16 μg/kg s.c. per day is given for 5 days.
- Stem cells are collected through an apheresis procedure on day 5 or 6.
- Stem cell dose varies with protocol (2–8×10^6 cells/kg of CD34$^+$ cells).
- This is increasingly becoming the preferred mode of stem cell collection.
- Less chance of complication and morbidity for the donor.
- Early engraftment is seen with PBSC transplantation.
- Possibility of collecting a higher number of CD34$^+$ cells exists.

Bone Marrow Harvest

- Marrow can be aspirated from the posterior iliac crest through multiple aspirations while the donor is under general anesthesia.
- Usually a marrow of 10 to 15 mL/kg of the donor weight is aspirated.
- Complications of the donors are anemia, pain, and neuropathies.
- Life-threatening complications occur in only 0.27% of the procedures.

T-Cell Depletion

- To decrease the incidence of GVHD.
- Complete depletion of T cells increases the risk of relapse and graft rejection.
- Selective depletion is the commonly accepted mode.
- Commonly done with monoclonal antibodies with or without complement.
- Magnetic beads coated with monoclonal antibodies are used.

Stages of Allogeneic Transplantation

Conditioning

Conditioning regimens are used for two main purposes: immunosuppression of the recipient to prevent graft rejection and allow engraftment, and eradication of malignant disease or an abnormal cell population. Conditioning regimens are chosen according to the particular clinical situation, the disease under treatment, the age and health of the patient, and the source of stem cells (Table 3, Fig. 1).

Transplantation Phase

After the conditioning regimen, the patient receives stem cells as an intravenous infusion. Usually this is a well-tolerated procedure. The day of transplant is considered day 0.

Engraftment

The rate of engraftment depends on the source of stem cells, use of hematopoietic growth factor, and choice of prophylaxis against GVHD. Most rapid engraftment is seen in SCT, in which granulocyte recovery occurs by day 10 to 12. This is accelerated by use of filgrastim (G-CSF) or sargramostim (GM-CSF) after the transplant.

Post Transplant Phase

Most important events in the post transplant period are multiple complications including mucositis, nausea, vomiting, infection, hemorrhage, GVHD, graft failure, and relapse of the disease. Supportive care and prevention of GVHD and of graft failure are the major considerations of this period.

Supportive Care

Patients require intensive supportive care during this period for several complications including:

Infections.

Neutropenic fever: see Chapter 37 for details of management of fever with neutropenia.

Cytomegalovirus (CMV) infection
- Major cause of morbidity and mortality.

TABLE 3. *Commonly used regimens*

Total body irradiation (TBI) and high-dose cyclophosphamide
Busulfan and high-dose cyclophosphamide
TBI and antithyomcyte globulin (ATG)
Cyclophosphamide and total lymphoid irradiation (TLI)

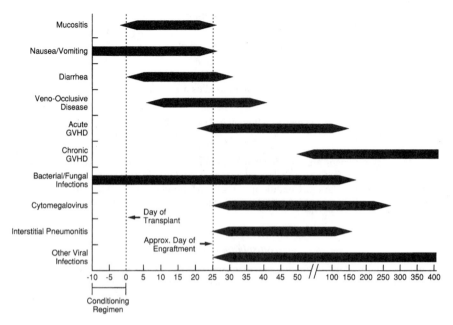

FIG. 1. Time course of complications in stem cell transplantation. The bars represent the period in which each complication may occur but should serve only as a general guide. Patients with severe graft-versus-host disease have much more prolonged immunosuppression and may develop serious bacterial, fungal, and viral infections, even after the period of greatest risk shown. (Adapted from Schiffman RJ. *Hematopathology.* Philadelphia: Lippincott Williams and Wilkins, 1998.)

- From 5% to 10% of death in the posttransplant period is due to CMV interstitial pneumonia.
- Pneumonia usually occurs 7 to 10 weeks after transplantation.
- CMV infection is treated with ganciclovir, 5 mg/kg b.i.d. for 3 weeks, and i.v. immunoglobulin (IVIG).

Hematologic complications:

- All patients require both red cell and platelet transfusions for 3 to 4 weeks, and then intermittently.
- All blood products should be irradiated to prevent GVHD and filtered to prevent CMV infection and febrile reaction.
- Platelet count is usually kept at more than 10,000 to 20,000 cells/mm^3.

Other complications:

- Mucositis
- Hemorrhagic cystitis: can be due to cyclophosphamide or viruses like adenovirus and BK virus.
- Veno-occlusive disease (VOD) of the liver occurs in 20% to 30%.
- Clinical features of VOD are right upper quadrant pain, hepatomegaly, jaundice, and ascites.
- Treatment is supportive care.

TABLE 4. *Organ-specific classification of acute graft-versus-host disease*

Level of injury	Skin	Liver (bilirubin)	Intestinal tract
1	Maculopapular rash <25% of body surface	2–3 mg/dL	500–1,000 mL liquid stool/day
2	Maculopapular rash 25–50% of body surface	>3–6 mg/dL	>1,000 and <1,500 mL liquid stool/day
3	Generalized erythroderma	>6–15 mg/dL	>1,500 mL liquid stool/day
4	Generalized erythroderma with bullae and desquamation	>15 mg/dL	>1,500 mL liquid stool/day; severe abdominal pain with or without ileus

	Level of injury		
Clinical grade	Skin	Liver	Intestinal tract
I	1 or 2	0	0
II	1–3	1	1
III	2 or 3	2 or 3	2 or 3
IV	2–4	2–4	2–4

Graft-Versus-Host Disease

- Immunologically competent donor T-lymphocytes react against recipient tissues, which leads to GVHD.
- Acute GVHD is usually seen before 100 days, and chronic GVHD after 100 days.
- It is seen in about 40% to 80% of the allogeneic transplantations.
- The incidence of GVHD increases with age.
- Clinical manifestations are usually seen in liver, gastrointestinal (GI) tract and skin (Tables 4 and 5).

Management of GVHD

Treatment (Table 6)

- Methylprednisone, 1 to 2 mg/kg/day in divided doses (30% to 50% will respond):

TABLE 5. *Risk factors for acute graft versus host disease*

Recipient
    Increased age
    Infection with DNA viruses (HSV, VZV)
    Intensive conditioning
    Low progenitor cell dose
Donor
    Previous transfusions
    Previous pregnancies
    Increased age
Donor–recipient matching
    Sex mismatch
    HLA-A, B, DR mismatch
    Unrelated donor

HSV, herpes simplex virus; VZV, varicella zoster virus; HLA, human leukocyte antigen.

TABLE 6. *Commonly used agents for prophylaxis*

T-cell depletion of the donor cells
Prednisone
Cyclosporine
Methotrexate
Antithymocyte globulin (ATG)
Tacrolimus (FK 506)
Azathioprine
Mycophenolate mofetil

- ATG, 30 mg/kg/day i.v. (25% to 30% response).
- Cyclosporine, 5 mg/kg/day p.o.
- Mycophenolate mofetil, 500 to 1,000 mg/day p.o.
- PUVA therapy for skin GVHD.

Chronic Graft-Versus-Host Disease

- Occurs usually after day 100.
- Pathology of chronic GVHD (cGVHD) is different from that of acute GVHD.
- Diagnosis is made by clinical presentation.
- Management is the same as for acute GVHD.

Graft Versus Leukemia

- Major challenge is to separate the adverse effects of GVHD from the beneficial effects of GVL.
- Allogeneic transplantation with T cell–depleted bone marrow has increased relapse risk.
- Greatest GVL effect is seen in chronic myelogenous leukemia (CML), intermediate in AML, and the least in ALL.
- GVL occurs more in recipients of mismatched family or unrelated donors, and less in HLA-identical siblings.

AUTOLOGOUS STEM CELL TRANSPLANTATION

Usually PBSCs are collected through an apheresis procedure. Bone marrow harvest is rarely used in autologous transplantation because of concerns about tumor cell contamination.

Before the apheresis, the patient receives two or more cycles of chemotherapy with growth factors for cytoreduction and mobilization of the stem cells.

Because autologous stem cells can be potentially contaminated with malignant cells (gene-marking studies showed that relapse could be from infused marrow in AML), different purging methods are being extensively studied. After collecting, the autologous stem cells are stored in dimethyl sulfoxide (DMSO).

Conditioning regimens are meant for cytoreduction and mobilization of the stem cells.

The hematologic and infectious complications during transplant and posttransplant phases are similar to those of allogeneic transplantation. Mucositis can be severe in autologous transplantation. GVHD and VOD are not that common.

FUTURE DIRECTIONS

Nonmyeloablative Transplantation

- Conventional myeloablative transplant causes high morbidity and mortality, and can be used only in young patients without comorbid conditions.

- In nonmyeloablative transplant, the conditioning regimen is designated not to eradicate the malignancy, but rather to produce immunosuppression to achieve engraftment and development of graft-versus-malignancy effect.
- Encouraging results are reported in CML, CLL, and renal cell carcinoma.
- At present, it is an active area of research.

Donor Lymphocyte Infusion (DLI)

Infusions of lymphocytes obtained from the original donor represent a new approach for treating patients who have relapsed after an allogeneic transplantation. The purpose of DLI is to use the graft-versus-leukemia effect from the T cells of the donor.

- In patients who relapsed after allogeneic transplantation, DLI induces complete remission in 70% of CML, 30% of AML, and 30% of MDS patients.
- DLI is associated with GVHD in 90% of the patients who achieved remission.

Cord Blood Transplantation (CBT)

Cord blood transplantation (CBT) is an active area of research. The first CBT was performed in 1988. By now, more than 1,000 cord blood transplants have been performed worldwide.

Advantages of Cord Blood Transplantation

1. The cord blood is a rich source of the most primitive form of stem cells. The properties of hematopoietic stem cells from cord blood give them a proliferative advantage and should compensate for the relatively low number of stem cells in a single unit of cord blood.
2. The incidence and severity of GVHD may be less in CBT because the immune system at birth is immature.
3. The main practical advantages of cord blood as an alternative source of stem cells are the:
   - Relative ease of procurement.
   - No side effects for mothers and donors.
   - Reduced incidence of transmission of infection, especially CMV.
   - The ability to store it fully tested and HLA matched.

SUGGESTED READING

1. Champlin R, Khouri I, Kornblau S, et al. Allogeneic hematopoietic transplantation as adoptive immunotherapy: induction of graft-versus-malignancy as primary therapy. *Hematol Oncol Clin North Am* 1999;13:1041–1057.
2. Przepiorka D, Smith TL, Folloder J, et al. Risk factors for acute graft-versus-host disease after allogeneic blood stem cell transplantation. *Blood* 1999;94:1465–1470.
3. Lazarus HM, Rowlings PA, Zhang MJ, et al. Autotransplants for Hodgkin's disease in patients never achieving remission: a report from the Autologous Blood and Marrow Transplant Registry. *J Clin Oncol* 1999;17:534–545.
4. Henslee-Downey PJ, Gluckman E. Allogeneic transplantation from donors other than HLA-identical siblings. *Hematol Oncol Clin North Am* 1999;13:1017–1039.
5. Childs R, Epperson D, Bahceci E, et al. Molecular remission of chronic myeloid leukaemia following a non-myeloablative allogeneic peripheral blood stem cell transplant: in vivo and in vitro evidence for a graft-versus-leukaemia effect. *Br J Haematol* 1999;107:396–400.
6. Ferrara JL, Levy R, Chao NJ. Pathophysiologic mechanisms of acute graft-vs.-host disease. *Biol Blood Marrow Transplant* 1999;5:347–356.
7. Popplewell L, Forman SJ. Allogeneic hematopoietic stem cell transplantation for acute leukemia, chronic leukemia, and myelodysplasia. *Hematol Oncol Clin North Am* 1999;13:987–1015.

8. Bennett C, Waters T, Stinson T, et al. Valuing clinical strategies early in development: a cost analysis of allogeneic peripheral blood stem cell transplantation. *Bone Marrow Transplant* 1999;24:555–560.

9. Bensinger WI, Clift R, Martin P, et al. Allogeneic peripheral blood stem cell transplantation in patients with advanced hematologic malignancies: a retrospective comparison with marrow transplantation. *Blood* 1996;88:2794–2800.

10. Lee SJ, Weller E, Alyea EP. Efficacy and costs of granulocyte colony-stimulating factor in allogeneic T-cell depleted bone marrow transplantation. *Blood* 1998;92:2725–2729.

11. Pavletic ZS, Bishop MR, Tarantolo SR, et al. Hematopoietic recovery after allogeneic blood stem-cell transplantation compared with bone marrow transplantation in patients with hematologic malignancies. *J Clin Oncol* 1997;15:1608–1616.

12. Bredeson C, Malcolm J, Davis M, et al. Cost analysis of the introduction of PBPC for autologous transplantation: effect of switching from bone marrow (BM) to peripheral blood progenitor cells (PBPC). *Bone Marrow Transplant* 1997;20:889–896.

SECTION 10

Other Malignancies

30

AIDS-Related Malignancies

Muhammad Wasif Saif and *Richard F. Little

*Medicine Branch, and *HIV and AIDS Malignancy Branch, DCS,
National Cancer Institute, National Institutes of Health, Bethesda, Maryland*

Individuals with human immunodeficiency virus (HIV) infections are at increased risk of developing neoplastic disease. The clinical behavior of specific malignancies is often markedly altered in HIV infection relative to the HIV-negative counterpart.

- Three neoplasms are acquired immunodeficiency syndrome (AIDS)-defining conditions when they occur in HIV-infected patients: Kaposi's sarcoma (KS), non-Hodgkin's lymphoma (both aggressive peripheral lymphomas and primary central nervous system lymphomas), and cervical cancer.
- A number of other cancers that are not considered AIDS defining occur with increased frequency in HIV-infected patients, including Hodgkin's disease, angiosarcoma, multiple myeloma, brain cancer, lung cancer, and seminoma.
- Since the advent of potent antiretroviral therapy (PAT) for HIV infection, the incidence of KS and AIDS-associated primary central nervous system lymphoma (AIDS-PCNSL) appear to have decreased. However, it is less clear whether the incidence of other malignant conditions has changed over the same period.
- Treatment of neoplastic disease in HIV-infected patients can be complex and requires expertise in both oncology and HIV disease. Goals of cancer therapy (e.g., curative vs. palliative) should be determined on the basis of both the cancer and the status of the HIV disease.

KAPOSI'S SARCOMA

Epidemiology

- KS, first described in 1872 by Moritz Kaposi, is the most common tumor associated with HIV infection. The risk of KS is highest (>100,000-fold greater than in the HIV-negative population) among individuals who acquire HIV from men who have sex with other men.
- Other risk groups for HIV infection have increased risk of KS compared with the background HIV-negative population, but to a somewhat lesser extent.
- The incidence of KS as an AIDS-defining event has declined from 30% of HIV-infected gay men in 1982 to about 11% in 1996.
  1. The case definition of AIDS was changed in 1992 to include a CD4 cell count less than 200 cells/mm^3: KS reporting is not required among patients with a previous AIDS-defining diagnosis.
  2. Safer-sex practices among high-risk groups have led to relatively lower rates of transmission of the virus that causes KS: the Kaposi's sarcoma–associated herpes virus (KSHV), also known as human herpes virus-8 (HHV-8).

3. There are anecdotal reports that PAT can result in improvement in AIDS-KS, possibly due to better control of HIV and improved immune function resulting from such therapy.

Pathophysiology

- KS lesions are highly vascular, hyperpigmented tumors arising simultaneously in multiple nonmetastatic sites on the skin and virtually any internal organ. Lesions can be flat or nodular and can sometimes take on a symmetric appearance. Lymphadenopathy and edema may be present in the absence of cutaneous involvement.
- Microscopically, the lesions comprise predominantly spindle-shaped cells, most likely of vascular endothelial origin. Development of KS is characterized by endothelial cell hyperproliferation in response to proangiogenic factors such as oncostatin-M, basic fibroblast growth factor (bFGF), and vascular endothelial growth factor (VEGF).
- KSHV/HHV-8, which was discovered in 1994, is the etiologic agent for KS, although not all KSHV/HHV-8–infected persons will develop KS. Co-infection with HIV and KSHV/HHV-8 substantially increases the risk of KS development. KSHV/HHV-8 is found in essentially all patients with KS (AIDS-related as well as non-AIDS KS). KSHV/HHV-8 can induce the production of a number of virally encoded mimics of human cytokines and other factors involved in KS pathogenesis, including human interleukin-6 (IL-6), macrophage inhibitory protein, and interferon regulatory factor, and upregulates VEGF.
- Routes of KSHV/HHV-8 transmission have not been established but may include mother-to-infant transmission and sexual transmission. It does not appear to be efficiently transmitted by transfusion of blood products.

Diagnosis

- A 4- to 6-mm skin punch biopsy can often establish the diagnosis of KS. It must be distinguished from bacillary angiomatosis, melanoma, granulomatous conditions, and prominent vascularity in the lymph nodes.

Clinical Presentation

- The clinical course of AIDS-KS can be quite variable, from indolent waxing and waning of minimal cutaneous involvement to relentless progression of lesions with severe tumor-associated edema, pain, and disfigurement.
- Minimal KS may require no treatment unless the psychological impact, which can be severe, warrants therapy.
- KS commonly involves the internal organs [primarily the lungs and gastrointestinal (GI) tract] and can cause substantial morbidity and death. Pulmonary involvement may be associated with a particularly poor prognosis (median survival <7 months in the pre-PAT era).

Staging of KS

- The most widely used staging system for KS is the TIS staging system (Table 1), which was devised by the AIDS Clinical Trials Group Oncology Committee. Patients are scored based on the extent of tumor involvement (T), the immune status of the patient (I), and other AIDS-related systemic illness (S) in an attempt to stratify risk of poor prognosis. The TIS system stages patients as being overall either good risk, designated with a subscript 0, or poor risk, designated by the subscript 1, the summary taking the form $T_{0 \text{ or } 1} I_{0 \text{ or } 1} S_{0 \text{ or } 1}$.
- The staging of KS includes (a) enumeration and bidirectional measurement of cutaneous and oral lesions; (b) baseline chest radiograph: if abnormal, computed axial tomography (CT) of the chest should be performed; (c) CD4 cell count; (d) endoscopy if symptoms referable to the GI tract are present.

TABLE 1. *Revised ACTG staging classification for Kaposi's sarcoma*

	Good risk (0) (All of the following)	Poor risk (1) (Any of the following)
Tumor (T)	Confined to skin and/or lymph nodes and/or nonnodular oral disease confined to the palate	Tumor-associated edema or ulceration Extensive oral KS Nonnodal viscera
Immune system (I)	CD4 cells $\geq 150/mm^3$	CD4 cells $<150/mm^3$
Systemic illness	No history of opportunistic infection or thrush No "B" symptoms (unexplained fever, night sweats, >10% involuntary weight loss, or diarrhea) persisting >2 weeks Performance status ≥ 70 (Karnofsky)	History of opportunistic infections and/or thrush; "B" symptoms present Performance status <70 Other HIV-related opportunistic illness

KS, Kaposi's sarcoma; HIV, human immunodeficiency virus.
Based on reference 1, with permission.
The revised CD4 cutoff of 150 cells/mm^3 is lower than the original proposal of 200 cells/mm^3.
Example of staging: A patient with only nodular oral KS, CD4 count of 175 cells/mm^3, and a history of *Pneumocystis carinii* pneumonia would be $T_1 S_0 T_1$.

- Lesions should be characterized as flat or nodular; presence of tumor-associated edema should be noted. If there are more than 50 cutaneous lesions, representative areas containing at least 20 lesions are designated for individual lesion assessment for response to therapy.
- Abnormalities on chest CT may indicate pulmonary involvement by KS. Bronchoscopic evaluation can establish the diagnosis of pulmonary KS if lesions are visualized in the airways. Endobronchial or open-lung biopsy should be avoided, as there is a risk of severe hemorrhage. Pulmonary symptoms without radiographic findings should prompt evaluation for infectious versus malignant etiology.

Prognostic Factors

Response to KS therapy may be related to a variety of factors:

- Tumor extent.
- Performance status.
- CD4 cell count: patients with more than 150 to 200 CD4 cells/mm^3 have a better prognosis.
- Degree of HIV replication. Better control of HIV may result in a more indolent course of KS. The HIV viral load also predicts the rate of progressive immunosuppression.

Management of KS

- Therapy can be local or systemic.
- The goal of treatment in KS is palliation. Frequently KS will progress when therapy is suspended.
- Optimize antiretroviral therapy. There are reports of KS responses to PAT. For patients with minimal, slowly progressing KS, optimization of antiretroviral therapy may be considered before definitive therapy.
- Local therapy: most useful for patients with limited cutaneous disease that is cosmetically disturbing to the patient. A limitation is the extent of the disease, as well as inadequate cosmetic outcome in some cases.

1. Surgical excision of small lesions can yield acceptable cosmetic results in areas where scarring is likely not to be cosmetically problematic.
2. Cryotherapy is useful for small lesions, but permanent destruction of melanocytes may sometimes yield unacceptable cosmetic outcome, particularly in dark-skinned individuals. An advantage to cryotherapy is its ease of administration, and it can be accomplished without local anesthesia.
3. Photodynamic therapy has the advantage over other local therapies in that 40 to 50 lesions can be treated during a single session. It is frequently associated with moderate pain and then photosensitivity for a number of weeks after the treatment.
4. Intralesional injection or iontophoresis of low-dose vinblastine (0.1 mL of 0.1 mg/mL) or 3% sodium tetradodecyl sulfate injection (0.1–0.3 mL) causes a nonspecific necrosis or sclerosis of mucocutaneous tissue with reasonable cosmetic outcome for small lesions.
5. Topical 9-*cis*-retinoic acid (Panretin Gel), recently Food and Drug Administration (FDA) approved for use in KS, may result in responses in more than 45% of lesions but can cause local inflammation and lightening of the skin, yielding inadequate cosmesis in some cases.
6. Radiotherapy is useful as adjunctive therapy in severe disease. Areas of painful involvement may respond rapidly, and thus radiation therapy is useful when it is deemed that the potentially slower responses to systemic therapy may compromise the outcome. For example, oral lesions causing poor nutritional intake may best be treated with radiotherapy in some patients. However, oral radiotherapy can sometimes result in severe mucositis. Tolerance to radiation may be decreased among AIDS–KS patients, particularly on the mucosal surfaces. Radiotherapy also is useful for cosmetic purposes, such as involvement of the eyelid or conjunctiva, when other local therapies are not practical. Applied doses vary between 800 rad given over one fraction to 3,000 rad given over 10 fractions, depending on the site of involvement. Reappearance of KS in the area of previous irradiation can occur. Residual radiation-induced pigmentation or telangiectasia, which can at times be severe, may compromise the cosmetic outcome. Radiation therapy can be used for palliation of visceral disease, including pulmonary involvement, and may be reasonably well tolerated in some circumstances.
7. The use of carbon dioxide laser therapy to remove a tumor of the mouth, oropharynx, or larynx may result in immediate improved oral intake and with less toxicity than is sometimes seen with radiation to the oral cavity.

- Systemic therapy:
  1. Immunotherapy: Interferon-α (dose escalation to $5–10 \times 10^6$ U/day or 3 times weekly) can be effective in KS, with responses most likely to be seen in patients with CD4 cell counts more than 200/mm^3 receiving antiretroviral therapy. Toxicity may include flu-like symptoms and depression, resulting in decreased quality of life.
  2. Cytotoxic chemotherapy: Monotherapy with liposomal anthracyclines or paclitaxel (Table 2) represents important recent therapeutic advances in KS therapy. Better palliation and lower toxicity are possible with these agents than with previous combination chemotherapy regimens. Another advantage of the use of single-agent KS regimens is that it may simplify administration of concurrent complicated antiretroviral regimens during chemotherapy administration.
     - Liposomal daunorubicin (DaunoXome) has been approved by the United States FDA as first-line KS therapy.
     - Second-line therapy for KS:
     - Liposomal doxorubicin (Doxil).
     - Paclitaxel (Taxol): for particularly severe disease, many oncologists use paclitaxel as first-line therapy (even though this may deviate from the FDA labeling of the drug), based on high response rates seen in phase II trials.

TABLE 2. *Commonly used standard therapies in KS*

	Doses	Response rates
Standard KS therapy		
Liposomal anthracyclines		
Doxorubicin	20 mg/m^2 q 2–3 wk	59%
Daunorubicin	40–60 mg/m^2 q 2 wk	25%
Paclitaxel	135 to 175 mg/m^2 q 3 wk	59%–71%
	100 mg/m^2 q 2 wk	
	105 mg/m^2 c.i.v. for 96 h	
Alternative therapies		
Doxorubicin/bleomycin/ vinca alkaloids (ABV)	ABV q 2–4 weeks Doxorubicin, 10–40 mg/m^2 Bleomycin, 15 U Vincristine, 1 mg (**OR** vinblastine, 6 mg/m^2)	24–88% (higher response rates with higher doxorubicin doses, but greater toxicity)
Vincristine/vinblastine	Vincristine, 1 mg, alternating with vinblastine, 2–4 mg q wk	45%
Bleomycin/vinca alkaloids	Bleomycin, 10 U and vincristine, 1 mg **OR** vinblastine, 2–4 mg weekly	23%

Adapted from reference 2, with permission.

- Before development of these newer single-agent KS regimens, combination doxorubicin, bleomycin, and vinca alkaloid (either vincristine or vinblastine) (ABV) was used as the standard of care. Response rates range from 28% to 84%, depending on the dose of doxorubicin administered as part of the regimen. The higher doses tended to be associated with unacceptable toxicity owing to pronounced myelosuppression.
- Because KS requires long-term treatment, there is strong interest in pathogenesis-based therapies, which may have less associated toxicity. Ongoing research includes clinical investigations into the use of antiangiogenesis therapies and antiviral therapies.

AIDS-ASSOCIATED LYMPHOMAS

Epidemiology

- In 1985, the Centers for Disease Control (CDC) modified the case definition of AIDS to include aggressive non-Hodgkin's lymphoma of high-grade pathologic type (diffuse, undifferentiated) and of B-cell or unknown immunologic phenotype, diagnosed by biopsy.
- Non-Hodgkin's lymphoma (NHL) is the second most frequently occurring AIDS-associated malignancy. It is the AIDS-defining diagnosis in approximately 3% of HIV-infected patients. Estimated incidences up to 10% per year with a prevalence of 4.5% to 25% have been documented in certain patient populations. The true incidence is not known, as lymphoma is not a reportable condition among patients already defined as having a prior AIDS-indicating condition, such as fewer than 200 CD4 cells/mm^3.
- The excess risk of developing AIDS-NHL appears to be independent of the particular risk group for HIV acquisition or life-style factors such as drug use. The risk, however, does vary with age. The excess risk of NHL in HIV is reported to be approximately 360-fold for the age group younger than 19 years (although it is quite rare in this age group), and 20-fold for the age group older than 60 years. NHL is the most frequent AIDS-related malignancy among hemophiliacs, as KS appears so rarely in this group.
- There are somewhat conflicting data on the impact of PAT on the incidence of AIDS-NHL.

- 1. In the Australian AIDS-registration data, NHL has decreased by 37.5% as an AIDS-defining diagnosis since 1994, coincident with the introduction of PAT as common anti-HIV therapy, and the French data base has suggested a 44% decrease in NHL.
- 2. Other studies have found less evidence of substantial impact on the incidence of peripheral lymphoma. An analysis of data from the Multicenter AIDS Cohort Study showed that the incidence of NHL as an AIDS-defining condition has remained fairly constant over time.
- 3. PCNSL, which most commonly develops in patients with fewer that 50 CD4 cells/mm^3, clearly appears to have decreased in incidence since the introduction of PAT, and is consistent with the observation that PAT can profoundly increase the CD4 cell count.

Classification of AIDS-NHLs

There are three major categories of HIV-associated B-cell lymphomas based on anatomic site of presentation:

- Systemic (nodal/extranodal).
- Primary central nervous system lymphoma.
- Primary effusion lymphomas (PELs), also termed body-cavity lymphomas, which occur rarely.

The Revised European–American Classification of Lymphoid (REAL) Neoplasms groups these as:

- Burkitt and Burkitt-like lymphomas, including SNCCL, and accounting for about 20% of the cases.
- Diffuse large B-cell lymphoma (DLCL), which includes the large non–cleaved cell and large cell–immunoblastic plasmacytoid types and accounts for approximately 60% of cases and includes AIDS-PCNSL and PEL. The World Health Organization classifies PEL as a unique lymphoma type.

Pathology of Systemic AIDS-associated Non-Hodgkin's Lymphomas

There appear to be distinct genetic pathways for the lymphoma subtypes that correlate with a number of clinical features distinguishing these groups of tumors (Table 3).

TABLE 3. *Genetic and clinical features of systemic AIDS/NHLs*

Feature	Systemic lymphoma subtypes		
	Burkitt/Burkitt-like	Immunoblastic	Primary effusion lymphoma
Presentation	++CNS	+++CNS	Effusions
	+Systemic	+++GI/	(May be relatively resistant
		Extranodal	to cytotoxic chemotherapy)
	++Bone marrow	±Bone marrow	
Prior AIDS	<30%	>75%	>75%
CD4 cells	Usually normal	Decreased	Decreased
Epstein–Barr virus	30%–50%	90%	>90%
	−LMP-1, −EBNA2	+LMP-1, +EBNA	
HHV-8	Negative	Negative	100%

CNS, central nervous system; GI, gastrointestinal; AIDS, acquired immunodeficiency syndrome; NHL, non-Hodgkin's lymphoma; HHV, human herpesvirus.

Presentation of Systemic AIDS-NHL

- Peripheral AIDS-NHL frequently is seen as advanced stage 3 or 4 disease.
- Frequently behaves aggressively with unusual patterns of organ involvement.
- The majority of patients will have either a rapidly growing mass lesion or the development of systemic "B" symptoms (unexplained fever, drenching night sweats, or unexplained weight loss in excess of 10% of the normal body weight).
- Extranodal involvement is common, including the bone marrow (25–40%), GI tract (26%), and the CNS (17–32%).
- PEL presents as lymphomatous effusions of the pleural spaces, but can occasionally present initially as nodal.

Presentation of AIDS-PCNSL

- PCNSL comprises about 19% of AIDS-NHLs (in non–AIDS-NHL, it is about 1%).
- The frequency of PCNSL is more than 3,000-fold higher in patients with AIDS than in the general population, occurring in up to 12% of HIV-infected individuals.
- From 20% to 30% of CNS lesions in patients with AIDS are ultimately found to be PCNSL.
- PCNSL is the second most common mass lesion found in patients with AIDS and the most common brain tumor in this population.
- AIDS-PCNSL occurs most frequently when the CD4 cell count is less than $50/mm^3$.
- Patients can have signs and symptoms of mass lesions such as altered mental status and lateralizing signs, depending on the location of the mass. They may be asymptomatic or exhibit only subtle personality changes, decreased alertness, or headache. Seizures are seen in approximately 10% of cases of CNS lymphoma.

Diagnosis of AIDS-PCNSL

Definitive diagnosis of focal brain lesions in AIDS patients requires biopsy, and there is often some reluctance to do this procedure. In many medical centers, it has become standard practice to treat AIDS patients with focal brain lesions and antitoxoplasmosis antibodies empirically with antitoxoplasmosis therapy, reserving biopsy for those patients who are seronegative for antitoxoplasma antibodies or who fail to respond to treatment. However, delay in diagnosis can adversely affect survival in AIDS-PCNSL.

Strategies to make reasonably accurate diagnosis of AIDS-PCNSL without biopsy are in early development.

- Preliminary studies suggest that ^{18}F-fluoro-2-deoxyglucose and positron emission tomography (FDG-PET) and thallium-201 single-photon emission computed tomography (^{201}Tl SPECT) may have some utility in distinguishing malignant and nonmalignant conditions.
- Recently it has been shown that detection of cerebrospinal fluid (CSF) Epstein–Barr virus (EBV)-DNA by polymerase chain reaction (PCR) in HIV-infected patients is reliably associated with PCNSLs. The basis for this approach is the observation that nearly all HIV-associated PCNSLs are associated with EBV infection. In a study of this approach, the sensitivity and specificity of PCR for EBV-DNA detection in lumbar CSF were 80% and 100%, respectively. An even higher diagnostic confidence of AIDS-related focal brain lesions has been reported by using combined CSF EBV DNA detection by PCR with SPECT.

Staging of AIDS-NHL

- Systemic AIDS-NHL:
  - History and physical examination.
  - Clinical laboratory assessment of organ function.

- CD4 cell count.
- Bilateral bone marrow biopsies.
- CT of the chest, abdomen, and pelvis.
- All patients should undergo radiologic imaging of the brain and cytologic evaluation of the CSF to assess for potential CNS involvement. CT of the brain with contrast is adequate to assess for parenchymal brain lesions, but magnetic resonance imaging (MRI) with gadolinium has the potential advantage of revealing evidence of leptomeningeal involvement by lymphoma.

AIDS-PCNSL Staging

- Staging of PCNSL includes evaluation for potential peripheral lymphoma because its occurrence by definition indicates central lesions to be of metastatic origin.
- Because ocular involvement is frequent, an ophthalmologic examination with slit-lamp should be included in the evaluation, and its findings should be interpreted as part of the CNS involvement.

Prognosis of Systemic AIDS-NHL

- The factor most correlated with prognosis is the CD4 cell count. With standard therapy, patients with fewer than 100 CD4 cells/mm^3 have a median survival of about 4 months, whereas those with 100 or more CD4 cells/mm^3 have a median survival of 11 months.
- Other factors associated with poor outcome are age older than 35 to 40 years, high lactate dehydrogenase (LDH), presence of extranodal sites, intravenous drug use, and preexisting AIDS diagnosis. The international prognostic index for lymphoma is thus of some utility in AIDS-lymphomas, although its use is not widely reported.
- With PAT, it is quite possible that overall prognosis in AIDS-NHL will improve.

Treatment of Peripheral AIDS-associated Non-Hodgkin's Lymphomas

- Optimal therapy for AIDS-NHL remains incompletely defined (Table 4). It is difficult to compare AIDS-NHL clinical trial results conducted at different times owing to the rapid recent improvements in therapy for the underlying HIV infection.

TABLE 4. *Selected regimens and outcomes for AIDS-associated non-Hodgkin's lymphoma*

Course of therapy	Number of evaluable patients	Median CD4 cells/mm^3 at baseline	Complete response rate (%)	Median overall/ disease-free survival	Author
Low or standard dose m-BACOD	175	100 (low) 107 (standard)	41 (low) 52 (standard)	8 mo/8 mo	Kaplan et al.
ACVB/LNH84	141	227	63	9 mo/16 mo	Gisselbrecht et al.
Low or standard dose CHOP plus HAART	53	119	35 (low) 37 (standard)	Not available	Ratner et al.
Infusional CDE	21	87	62	18 mo/not available	Sparano et al.
Dose-adjusted EPOCH	23	255	79	Medians not yet reached but are 72%/83% at 23 mo	Little et al.

- Overall survival appears to be similar in groups treated with reduced or standard-dose chemotherapy. However, in general, studies have not been designed to determine if a subset of patients with better prognostic characteristics would benefit from standard-dose chemotherapy.
- A large randomized trial comparing standard- to low-dose m-BACOD was completed in 1997. This trial showed equivalent results in both groups, with complete responses ranging from 41% to 52%. There was a lower incidence of febrile neutropenia in the low-dose group.
- Studies comparing dose-reduced with standard-dose CHOP have generally shown equivalent efficacy, although the numbers are relatively small for assessment.
- In a prospective multicenter study using intensive combination chemotherapy in patients with favorable prognostic features, patients were treated with three cycles of doxorubicin, 75 mg/m^2; cyclophosphamide, 1,200 mg/m^2; vindesine, 2 mg/m^2 for 2 days; bleomycin, 10 mg for 2 days; and prednisolone, 60 mg/m^2 for 5 days (ACVB), followed by a consolidation phase of high-dose methotrexate plus leucovorin, ifosfamide, etoposide, asparaginase, and cytarabine (LNH84) and CNS prophylaxis with intrathecal methotrexate. Of these, 63% achieved complete remission and at a median follow-up of 28 months median survival and disease-free survival were 9 and 16 months, respectively. This study, conducted in the era before PAT, demonstrates that a subset of patients with AIDS-NHL was able to tolerate aggressive antilymphoma therapy, and appeared to do reasonably well in terms of disease-free survival.
- Routine CNS prophylaxis is considered important in AIDS-NHL, as a high percentage (15–20%) of HIV-associated lymphomas have involvement of the CNS at presentation. Thus CNS prophylaxis with intrathecal methotrexate or ARA-C should be considered standard practice for AIDS-NHL.
- All patients receiving combination antilymphoma chemotherapy should receive prophylaxis for *Pneumocystis carinii* pneumonia (PCP), regardless of the CD4 count. Prophylaxis should be given for *Mycobacterium avium* complex (MAC) prophylaxis for at-risk patients (CD4 cell count <50–100/mm^3). The CD4 cell count should be periodically monitored during chemotherapy, as cytotoxic chemotherapy in itself can cause a profound decrease in CD4 cell counts.
- Investigators have begun to administer newer antiretroviral regimens along with the chemotherapy regimens to explore whether such approaches are feasible. This is a complicated issue and as yet only scant data exist to guide best use of antiretroviral drugs during chemotherapy. Preliminary results suggest that HIV viral loads can be suppressed during cytotoxic chemotherapy, but that complicated pharmacokinetic interactions can occur when antiviral therapy and combination cytotoxic chemotherapy are administered concomitantly. Such interactions may lead to changes in the toxicity and therapeutic profiles of the various drugs. Care should always be taken to refer to appropriate drug information manuals when considering the therapeutic plan.
- Preliminary reports using six 21-day cycles of dose-adjusted EPOCH chemotherapy with filgrastim [etoposide, 50 mg/m^2/day c.i.v., days 1–4; vincristine, 0.4 mg/m^2/day c.i.v., days 1–4; doxorubicin, 10 mg/m^2/day c.i.v., days 1–4; prednisone, 60 mg/m^2 p.o., days 1–5; and cyclophosphamide (given by conventional i.v. bolus on day 5 and initially dosed according to CD4 count: 187 mg/m^2 for CD4 cells <100/mm^3, 375 mg/m^2 if CD4 cells ≥100/mm^3, and then adjusted up or down each cycle by 187 mg/m^2 to a maximum of 750 mg/m^2, depending on the neutrophil nadir)] have been encouraging, with a complete response rate of 79% in 24 patients treated. Antiretroviral therapy (ART) is suspended until the sixth cycle of chemotherapy is completed. The median progression-free survival and overall survival have not been reached, but are 83% and 79%, respectively, at 22.5 months as of this writing. Febrile neutropenia occurred in only 12% of the cycles administered. No new opportunistic infections developed in these patients despite the withdrawal of ART on initiation of chemotherapy (PCP prophylaxis was administered to all patients, and MAC prophylaxis to at-risk patients).

Treatment and Prognosis of AIDS-PCNSL

- If biopsy is to be performed, corticosteroids should be withheld until a diagnosis is made, unless the patient is in immediate danger of herniation, as corticosteroids can obscure the pathologic diagnosis because of brisk tumor response.
- Treatment modalities for immunocompetent patients are applied to patients with AIDS-PCNSL, but with greater toxicity and poorer results.
    1. The median overall survival is 2 to 5 months.
    2. PCNSL is highly responsive to whole-brain irradiation, and most patients can be expected to have complete tumor eradication.
    3. There is a high rate of recurrent lymphoma and opportunistic infection, leading to poor outcome.
    4. Relapse can occur remote from the primary site, but also within the radiation port.
    5. Recent experience of combining chemotherapy with radiotherapy suggests that a small subgroup of patients can benefit from this approach, with survival reaching longer than 1 year. However, this is still shorter than survival in non-AIDS patients.
    6. Surgery has no therapeutic role in PCNSL because microscopic tumor infiltration into brain parenchyma extends from the site of primary involvement.

HIV-associated Hodgkin's Disease

- Several features of Hodgkin's disease support its association with HIV infection, although it is not presently considered an AIDS-defining condition.
- The most common histologic subtype in HIV-associated Hodgkin's disease (HIV-HD) is mixed cellularity, followed by lymphocyte depleted, whereas in HIV-negative (primary HD) patients, the most common histologic subtype is nodular sclerosing HD.
- EBV infection appears to be more predominant among cases of HIV-HD (78–100% of cases) than in cases of primary HD (15–48% of cases).
- Patients with HIV-HD generally are first seen at a younger age, with higher-stage disease, with less frequent mediastinal involvement, more frequent involvement of extranodal sites of disease, and more frequent occurrence of B symptoms compared with their HIV-negative counterparts. These differences are more than can be accounted for by the overrepresentation of the mixed cellularity histologic subtype in HIV-HD.
- Prognosis is generally poorer for HIV-HD than for primary HD, even though patients often have relatively well-preserved CD4 cell counts (median >275 CD4 cells/mm^3 in some series).

Treatment of HIV-HD

Many oncologists advocate the use of systemic chemotherapy for all clinically staged patients with HIV-HD.

- Patients frequently have a number of features that have been associated with poor prognosis in primary non–HIV-associated HD, including male sex, large number of sites involved, and mixed cellularity or lymphocyte-depleted histology.
- In general, complete response rates are relatively high with systemic chemotherapy (50% to >80%), but have also been reported as low as 14%.
- Relapse of HD and progression of AIDS are common, contributing to poor overall survival.
- Patients with a CD4 cell count less than 20 to 250 CD4 cells/mm^3 have a median survival of less than 11 months, whereas higher CD4 cell counts are associated with somewhat better outcome.
- Most patients do not have an AIDS diagnosis when they develop HIV-HD, but 48% to 71% develop AIDS within 3 years after treatment for HIV-HD. This rate of progression to AIDS

appears to be more rapid compared with most other HIV-infected patients with similar CD4 cell counts. This emphasizes the need for adequate management of the underlying HIV with potent therapy.

Conventional Hodgkin's disease treatments [e.g., radiotherapy, mechlorethamine, vincristine, procarbazine, and prednisone (MOPP), doxorubicin, bleomycin, vinblastine, and dacarbazine (ABVD), or alternating MOPP/ABVD, epirubicin, bleomycin, vinblastine, and prednisone (EBVP) or combined-modality therapy] are most often used in AIDS-associated HD. The CNS is rarely involved, so CNS prophylaxis is not commonly used.

ANOGENITAL CANCERS IN HIV INFECTION

Overview

- Cervical cancer was added to the CDC list of AIDS-defining conditions in 1993.
- Anal cancer is also relatively prevalent among HIV-infected women and homosexual and bisexual men with HIV infection, although it is not an AIDS-defining condition.
- These cancers are associated with human papillomavirus (HPV) infection and appear to be more aggressive in HIV-infected than in non–HIV-infected individuals.

Screening

- It is recommended that HIV-infected women undergo regular periodic cervical Papanicolaou (Pap) testing. The CDC has recommended cytologic screening as part of the initial evaluation when HIV seropositivity is diagnosed. If the initial Pap smear is normal, at least one additional evaluation should be repeated within 6 months. If the repeat is normal, then reevaluation should be done at least annually. If the initial or follow-up Pap smear shows severe inflammation with reactive squamous cellular changes, another Pap smear should be collected within 3 months. If the initial or follow-up Pap smear shows squamous intraepithelial lesions (SILs) or atypical squamous cells of undetermined significance, the woman should be referred for a colposcopic examination of the lower genital tract and, if indicated, undergo colposcopically directed biopsies.
- HIV infection is not an indication for colposcopy among women with normal Pap smears.
- HPV-associated cytologic abnormalities are common in the anal mucosa of both HIV-infected women and homosexual men. Some experts have suggested that routine periodic cytologic examination of the anal mucosa also should also be considered in high-risk individuals.

Cervical Cancer

Epidemiology

- SILs, vulvovaginal condyloma acuminata, and anal intraepithelial neoplasia are seen with approximately fivefold increase in HIV-infected women above that seen in women not infected with HIV.
- The prevalence of cervical intraepithelial neoplasia has been reported to be from 11% to 29% overall for HIV-infected women.
- Among sexually active women, HIV-infected women have a substantially higher rate of persistent HPV infections of the types most strongly associated with intraepithelial lesions and invasive cervical cancer (i.e., HPV-16– or HPV-18– associated viral types).
- HPV infection is associated with development of SILs, and increased prevalence of HPV infection among HIV-infected women may explain the increased incidence of SILs in this population.

- Women with a CD4 cell count less than 500/mm^3 appear to be at greater risk for poor outcome.
- The incidence of invasive cervical cancer appears unchanged since the advent of PAT.
- It is unclear whether this is due to reduced use of these medications among the women at highest risk for both HIV and HPV, or some other factor.

Therapy

- Standard therapy for preinvasive cervical neoplasia, including cryotherapy, laser therapy, cone biopsy, and loop excision, is used.
- Recurrence is at least twice as high among HIV-infected women (even among those with high CD4 cell counts) as in HIV-seronegative women. The lower the CD4 count, the higher the risk for recurrence. Preliminary data suggests that early preinvasive lesions can regress with effective antiretroviral therapy, and that potent antiretroviral therapy reduces recurrence and progression after standard excisional therapy.
- Invasive cervical cancer should be approached with the same principles of oncologic management that guide treatment of cervical cancer in HIV-negative patients.
- Patients with well-controlled HIV infection and relative immune preservation can be expected to have outcomes similar to those of HIV-negative women.
- Patients with advanced HIV disease may be more intolerant of the myelosuppressive effects of radiation therapy and combination chemotherapy.
- After surgery, recurrence is common.
- When antineoplastic therapy is administered concomitant with antiretroviral therapy, potential for overlapping toxicity of the various agents should be considered in the therapeutic plan.

Anal Cancer

- HPV infection of the anal canal and anal cancer and the immediate precursor lesion, high-grade anal intraepithelial neoplasia, is common among HIV-infected women and among men who have sex with men, especially those with HIV or immunosuppression.
- The prevalence of cytologically abnormal anal epithelium has been reported to be as high as 39%, and the incidence of high-grade anal intraepithelial lesions has been reported to be as high as 15% among HIV-seropositive men.
- Anal squamous intraepithelial lesions do not appear to regress in patients receiving PAT, except perhaps in some with high CD4 cell counts.
- For invasive anal cancer, standard combined chemotherapy and radiation appears to control disease effectively in most patients.
- Patients with CD4 counts less than 200/mm^3 appear more likely to suffer treatment-related toxicity including cytopenias, intractable diarrhea, moist desquamation requiring hospitalization, or a colostomy either for a therapy-related complication or for salvage.
- Patients with CD4 of 200/mm^3 or greater appear to have better disease control with acceptable morbidity.

REFERENCES

1. Krown SE, Testa MA, Huang J. AIDS-related Kaposi's sarcoma: prospective validation of the AIDS Clinical Trials Group staging classification: AIDS Clinical Trials Group Oncology Committee. *J Clin Oncol* 1997;15:3085–3092.
2. Yarchoan R. Therapy for Kaposi's sarcoma: recent advances and experimental approaches. *J Acquir Immune Defic Syndr* 1999;21(suppl 1):S66–S73.
3. Grulich AE, Wan X, Law MG, et al. Risk of cancer in people with AIDS. *AIDS* 1999;13:839–843.

4. Biggar RJ, Rosenberg PS, Cote T, et al. Multistate AIDS/Cancer Match Study Group [published erratum appears in *Int J Cancer* 1997;17:727]. *Int J Cancer* 1996;68:754–758.
5. Goedert JJ, Cote TR, Virgo P, et al. Spectrum of AIDS-associated malignant disorders. *Lancet* 1998;351:1833–1839.
6. Little RF, Pluda JM, Feigal E, et al. The challenge of designing clinical trials for AIDS-related Kaposi's sarcoma. *Oncology (Huntingt)* 1998;12:871–877, 881–883; discussion 883–884.
7. Volm MD, von Roenn JH. Treatment strategies for epidemic Kaposi's sarcoma. *Curr Opin Oncol* 1995;7:429–436.
8. Yarchoan R, Little R. Optimizing combination chemotherapy for Kaposi's sarcoma. *Cancer J Sci Am* 1997;3:268–270.
9. Yarchoan R, Little R. AIDS-associated malignancies. In: Vincent T, DeVita J, Hellman S, Rosenberg SA, eds. *Cancer: principles and practice of oncology.* Philadelphia: Lippincott-Raven, 2000.
10. Knowles DM. Molecular pathology of acquired immunodeficiency syndrome-related non-Hodgkin's lymphoma. *Semin Diagn Pathol* 1997;14:67–82.
11. Kaplan LD, Straus DJ, Testa MA, et al. Low-dose compared with standard-dose m-BACOD chemotherapy for non-Hodgkin's lymphoma associated with human immunodeficiency virus infection: National Institute of Allergy and Infectious Diseases AIDS Clinical Trials Group. *N Engl J Med* 1997;336:1641–1648.
12. Straus DJ, Huang J, Testa MA, et al. Prognostic factors in the treatment of human immunodeficiency virus-associated non-Hodgkin's lymphoma: analysis of AIDS Clinical Trials Group protocol 142—low-dose versus standard-dose m-BACOD plus granulocyte-macrophage colony-stimulating factor: National Institute of Allergy and Infectious Diseases. *J Clin Oncol* 1998;16:3601–3606.
13. Antinori A, De Rossi G, Ammassari A, et al. Value of combined approach with thallium-201 single-photon emission computed tomography and Epstein-Barr virus DNA polymerase chain reaction in CSF for the diagnosis of AIDS-related primary CNS lymphoma. *J Clin Oncol* 1999;17:554–560.
14. Little RF, Pearson D, Steinberg S, et al. Dose-adjusted EPOCH chemotherapy (CT) in previously untreated HIV-associated non-Hodgkin's lymphoma (HIV-NHL), American Society of Clinical Oncology 35th Annual Meeting, Atlanta: May 15–18, 1999.
15. Gisselbrecht C, Oksenhendler E, Tirelli U, et al. Human immunodeficiency virus-related lymphoma treatment with intensive combination chemotherapy: French-Italian Cooperative Group. *Am J Med* 1993;95:188–196.
16. Ratner L, Redden D, Hamzeh F, et al. Chemotherapy for HIV-NHL in combination with HAART, 3rd National AIDS Malignancy Meeting, Bethesda, Maryland, 1999.
17. Sparano JA, Wiernik PH, Strack M, et al. Infusional cyclophosphamide, doxorubicin and etoposide in HIV-related non-Hodgkin's lymphoma: a follow-up report of a highly active regimen. *Leuk Lymphoma* 1994;14:263–271.
18. Tirelli U, Errante D, Dolcetti R, et al. Hodgkin's disease and human immunodeficiency virus infection: clinicopathologic and virologic features of 114 patients from the Italian Cooperative Group on AIDS and Tumors. *J Clin Oncol* 1995;13:1758–1767.
19. Northfelt DW. Cervical and anal neoplasia and HPV infection in persons with HIV infection. *Oncology (Huntingt)* 1994;8:33–37; discussion 38–40.
20. Northfelt DW, Swift PS, Palefsky JM. Anal neoplasia: pathogenesis, diagnosis, and management. *Hematol Oncol Clin North Am* 1996;10:1177–1187.
21. Palefsky JM. Human papillomavirus infection and anogenital neoplasia in human immunodeficiency virus-positive men and women. *J Natl Cancer Inst Monogr* 1998;23:15–20.

31

Pediatric Malignancies

V. Koneti Rao and *Ian T. McGrath

*Medicine Branch, DCS, National Cancer Institute, National Institutes of Health, Bethesda, Maryland; and *International Network for Cancer Treatment and Research (INCTR), Institut Pasteur, Brussels, Belgium*

Although rare, cancer is the leading cause of death from disease in children younger than 15 years in the United States. Advances have been made in treating these patients over the last three decades by delivering therapy in the context of appropriate, well-designed clinical trials at major medical centers with expertise in treating children. This dramatic improvement in outcome has led to the estimates that in the year 2000, one in every 1,000 young adults between the ages 20 and 29 years would have been a survivor of childhood cancer. This represents a large cohort nationally that, with maturation, may be increasingly beset by the medical and social consequences of cancer and its treatment. Increased awareness of these potential consequences of curative cancer therapy in children has prompted tailoring of the therapy to ensure optimal survival and quality of life. A team approach that incorporates the skills of the primary care physician, surgeon, radiation oncologist, pediatric hematologist/oncologist, rehabilitation specialist, pediatric nurse specialist, and social worker is imperative to ensure that all patients receive treatment, supportive care, and rehabilitation with maximal efficacy and minimal morbidity. It is equally important that strong lines of communication be maintained between specialists directing the patient's care and the referring primary care physician in the community, to optimize any urgent or interim care that may be required when the child is at home. An overview of incidence, diagnosis, prognosis, and treatment options for the common and curable childhood malignancies is presented here; constraints of space permit only a very brief synopsis of the less-common tumors. Some of the medical consequences of cure in long-term survivors are also outlined.

CHILDHOOD ACUTE LEUKEMIAS

Acute Lymphoblastic Leukemia

Diagnosis

An extensive initial work-up should start with a history, including family history, and a detailed physical examination followed by assessment of bone marrow and spinal fluid, and a chest radiograph. Extramedullary disease at diagnosis involving central nervous system (CNS), mediastinum, or testes carries an adverse prognosis. Although simple bone marrow morphology remains the cornerstone of diagnosis of leukemia, specialized studies such as cytochemical and immunophenotypic evaluation of cells in peripheral blood and bone marrow, cytogenetics, and molecular features [e.g., reverse transcription–polymerase chain reaction (RT-PCR) study of unique fusion transcripts] of the leukemia are being increasingly used for determination of prognosis and management.

TABLE 1. *Prognostic variables in childhood ALL*

Prognosis	Risk factors	Specific details of risk factors
Poor prognosis (high risk)	High WBC	≥50,000/μL
	Age	≥10 yr and ≤1 yr
	Gender	Male
	CNS leukemia at diagnosis	CNS-2 (<5 cells/μL); CNS-3 (≥5 cells/μL)
	Bulky disease at presentation	Mediastinal mass, massive organomegaly, massive adenopathy
	Poor early response to therapy	Persistent blasts (>5% M2 and >25% M3) on day 14 bone marrow.
	Cytogenetics	Near haploid chromosome number (24–29) t(4;11): MLL gene rearrangement in 11q23 t(9;22): Philadelphia chromosome
Good prognosis (standard risk)	Low WBC	≤50,000/μL
	Age	1.0–9.99 yr
	Gender	Female
	No CNS leukemia at diagnosis	CNS-1 (no blasts)
	Immunophenotype	Precursor B cell
	Early response to therapy	<5% (M1) blasts on day 14 bone marrow
	DNA content (ploidy)	DNA index (DI) >1.16 by flow cytometry
	Cytogenetics	High hyperdiploid chromosome number (50–59) t(12;21): tel-AML-1 fusion

All prognostic factors are ultimately dependent on the treatment administered. For instance, B-cell ALL has a very poor prognosis with standard ALL therapy but an excellent prognosis when treated like Burkitt's lymphoma.

ALL, acute lymphocytic leukemia; WBC, while blood cell; CNS, central nervous system.

- Worldwide, approximately 240,000 new cases of childhood acute lymphoblastic leukemia are diagnosed annually, and 75% of them live in developing countries. In the U.S. alone, approximately 2,500 children are diagnosed with acute lymphoblastic leukemia (ALL), and 500 children with acute myeloid leukemia (AML) on a yearly basis.
- ALL is the most common childhood cancer, and AML is the most common secondary malignancy.
- Approximately 70% of children with ALL are cured with current protocol-based treatments. Survival of children with Down's syndrome and ALL has greatly improved in the most recent period and is comparable to that in children without Down's syndrome.
- Numerous prognostic factors have been identified and incorporated into risk-classification systems used to assign treatment for children with ALL. Use of uniform age/white blood cell (WBC) criteria as well as biologic characteristics to define prognosis will facilitate comparisons of different therapeutic approaches and permit tailoring treatment intensity to prognosis (Table 1).

Treatment Option Overview

Clinical trials in pediatric leukemia are designed to compare potentially better therapy with therapy that is currently accepted as standard. Because treatment entails many potential complications and requires aggressive supportive care (transfusions; management of infectious complications; and emotional, financial, and developmental support), all children with cancer should be treated in tertiary care centers with all of the necessary pediatric supportive care facilities available. Only 3% of patients have detectable CNS involvement at diagnosis. However, unless specific therapy is directed toward the CNS (intrathecal medication, cranial irradiation, high-dose systemic chemotherapy with methotrexate or Ara-C), 50% of children will eventually develop overt CNS leukemia.

- Treatment is divided into phases: remission induction, CNS prophylaxis, consolidation, intensification, and maintenance. Intensity of immediate postinduction chemotherapy varies considerably, but some form of late intensification is advisable for all patients.
- In children with standard-risk disease, there has been an attempt to limit exposure to drugs with an increased risk of late toxic effects or to use only low cumulative dosages of anthracyclines and alkylating agents.
- Average duration of maintenance therapy for children with ALL ranges between 2 and 3 years. The backbone of maintenance therapy is daily oral mercaptopurine, preferably given in the evening, and weekly methotrexate. It is imperative to carefully monitor children receiving maintenance therapy for both drug-related toxicity and compliance.
- Infants with ALL represent a distinct category of children at higher risk for treatment failure, those with mixed lineage leukemia (MLL) gene rearrangement on chromosome 11q23 having the poorest prognosis.
- In high-risk groups, such as patients with t(9;22) and t(4;11), intensified treatment approaches, including bone marrow transplantation in first remission, are frequently used.

Recurrent Childhood ALL

Prognosis for a child with recurrent ALL depends on the time and site of relapse. If the recurrence occurs either during front-line therapy or shortly after discontinuation of initial therapy, the prognosis for long-term survival in patients with marrow relapse is poor (20%). However, 40% to 50% long-term disease-free survival can be achieved if the relapse occurs more than a year after completion of initial therapy. The incidence of isolated extramedullary (CNS and testicular) relapse is less than 10%. Aggressive systemic and intrathecal therapy combined with craniospinal irradiation has improved the outlook for children with isolated CNS relapse, especially those who have not received prior cranial irradiation, with 5-year estimated disease-free survival of 70% ± 11% in one report. The 3-year event-free survival (EFS) of boys with overt testicular relapse during therapy is 39%. However, 4-year EFS for occult testicular relapse discovered in boys at the end of treatment and late overt testicular relapse are 55% and 85%, respectively.

Late Sequelae

1. Each year approximately 1,500 childhood ALL patients become long-term survivors of their disease in the U.S. alone. A better understanding of the pattern and magnitude of the late complications is important not only for pediatric oncologists, but also for the primary care physicians who care for these patients in their later life.
2. Children who received cranial irradiation at age 5 years or younger are most susceptible to brain tumors, neuropsychological deficits, and endocrine dysfunction resulting in obesity, short stature, precocious puberty, and osteoporosis.
3. Secondary AML is linked to the use of epipodophyllotoxins.
4. Anthracyclines, especially given to young girls at high cumulative doses, has been associated with cardiomyopathy.
5. Intensive use of methotrexate and glucocorticoids has led to an increased frequency of neurotoxicity and aseptic necrosis of bone.

Acute Myeloid Leukemia

Diagnosis and Prognosis

In contrast to ALL, very few clinical, laboratory, or treatment factors have been consistently predictive of the prognosis for children with AML.

1. FAB subtypes.
   - Of children with AML, 50% to 60% can be assigned to FAB subtypes M1, M2, M3, M6, or M7.
   - Approximately 40% have M4 or M5 subtypes. About 80% of children younger than 2 years with AML have an M4 or M5 subtype.
   - The response to cytotoxic chemotherapy among children with different subtypes of AML is relatively similar. One exception is FAB subtype M3, acute promyelocytic leukemia (APL), for which all-*trans*-retinoic acid (ATRA) followed by chemotherapy achieves remission and cure (>2 year survival of 70–80%) in the majority of children. ATRA is given orally at a dose of 45 mg/M^2/day for 30 to 45 days.
2. Cytogenetics: Use of molecular probes and cytogenetic techniques like fluorescent *in situ* hybridization (FISH) can detect cryptic abnormalities that are not evident by standard cytogenetic banding studies and help in diagnosis when APL is suspected but the specific t(15;17) is not identified by routine cytogenetic evaluation. The presence of the Philadelphia chromosome in children with AML most likely represents chronic myelogenous leukemia (CML) that has transformed to AML rather than *de novo* AML. Children with AML who have a WBC greater than 100,000/mm^3, secondary AML, and leukemia cells with a monosomy 7 karyotype have low remission induction rates, whereas children with leukemia cell chromosomal abnormalities t(8;21) and inv 16 have a high likelihood of achieving remission and a decreased likelihood of relapse. Translocations of chromosomal band 11q23, as seen in most AML secondary to epipodophyllotoxin administration, are generally unfavorable for remission duration.
3. In several studies, M4 and M5 FAB subtype, a WBC greater than 20,000/mL^3, and a requirement of more than one cycle to achieve remission, predicted a short duration of remission.
4. Children with Down's syndrome have an increased risk of leukemia with a ratio of ALL to AML typical for childhood acute leukemia, except during the first 3 years of life, when AML (especially M7) predominates. Neonates with Down syndrome may manifest a transient myeloproliferative syndrome (TMS). This disorder mimics congenital AML but improves spontaneously within 4 to 6 weeks. Retrospective surveys indicate that as many as 30% of infants with Down syndrome and TMS will develop AML before age 3 years. Interestingly, the majority of children with Down syndrome and AML can be cured of their leukemia. Appropriate therapy for these children is less intensive than current AML therapy. and bone marrow transplant (BMT) is not indicated in first remission. A significant proportion of patients with marrow-failure syndromes such as Fanconi's anemia also develop AML.

Treatment Option Overview

Between 75% and 85% of children with AML can achieve complete remission after appropriate induction chemotherapy with an event-free 5-year survival rate of approximately 40%. The two most effective drugs used to induce remission in children with AML are cytarabine and anthracycline, which are sometimes given in conjunction with etoposide and thioguanine. It is usually necessary to induce profound bone marrow aplasia to achieve a complete remission. This may lead to severe myelosuppression and significant morbidity and mortality from infection or hemorrhage. The presence of CNS leukemia at diagnosis is more common in childhood AML (especially M4 and M5 AML with inv 16 or 11q23 chromosomal abnormalities) than in childhood ALL. Therefore high-dose cytarabine and some form of specific CNS treatment (intrathecal chemotherapy with or without cranial irradiation) has been incorporated into most protocols. A major challenge in the treatment of children with AML is to prolong the duration of initial remission with additional intensive postremission chemotherapy. Treatment approaches include high-dose cytarabine, etoposide, and anthracycline; and/or allogenic BMT. Nearly 60% of children who undergo allogenic BMT from a human leukocyte antigen

(HLA)-identical sibling donor during their first remission achieve long-term (>3 years) remissions without severe graft-versus-host disease. The role of alternate sources of bone marrow (matched unrelated donors and cord blood) in AML is under investigation. There is no conclusive evidence of significant prolongation of remission duration by use of maintenance chemotherapy given after intensive postremission chemotherapy in AML.

HODGKIN'S AND NON-HODGKIN'S LYMPHOMA

Pediatric lymphomas are the third most common group of malignancies in children (after acute leukemias and brain tumors) and account for nearly 12% of all newly diagnosed childhood cancers in affluent countries. Approximately 60% of pediatric lymphomas are non-Hodgkin's lymphomas (NHLS), with the remainder being Hodgkin's disease.

Non-Hodgkin's Lymphoma

About 500 new cases of pediatric NHLs are diagnosed annually in the U.S. Incidence of NHL appears to be much higher among children in developing countries. It is unusual in children younger than 3 years, but NHL is the most common malignancy in young children with AIDS, and hence screening for HIV should be considered for all children with NHL. Intensification of conventional chemotherapy treatment approaches coupled with improved supportive care have resulted in marked improvements in EFS with rates approximating more than 90% in patients with B-cell lymphomas, and only slightly lower in patients with T-cell lymphomas.

Diagnosis and Staging

In contrast to adult lymphomas, childhood NHL is almost never "low grade"-indolent or follicular and occurs predominantly in the chest and abdomen rather than in peripheral nodal areas. The histologic spectrum of childhood NHL is considerably narrower than that in adults and falls into three broad categories: lymphoblastic lymphoma, Burkitt's lymphoma, and large cell lymphoma. All are diffuse, rapidly growing lymphomas with very high growth fractions. Almost two thirds of the children have widespread disease at the time of diagnosis, which may involve the bone marrow, CNS, or both. When there is replacement of more than 25% of the bone marrow with tumor cells, the disease is traditionally assigned a diagnosis of ALL. But "acute B-cell leukemia" is equivalent to "Burkitt's leukemia" in children and should be treated as Burkitt's lymphoma (Tables 2 and 3).

Treatment Option Overview

NHL in children is generally considered to be widely disseminated from the outset, even when apparently localized; as a result, combination multiagent chemotherapy is recommended for all patients. Two potentially life-threatening clinical situations are often seen in children with NHL: superior vena cava syndrome (or mediastinal tumor with airway obstruction), most often seen in lymphoblastic lymphoma; and tumor lysis syndrome, most often seen in Burkitt's and Burkitt's-like NHL. These emergency situations should be anticipated, although sometimes they may arise even before a diagnosis is made in children with NHL, and addressed immediately.

Superior Vena Cava Syndrome (Mediastinal Tumor with Airway Obstruction)

Patients with large mediastinal masses are at risk of cardiac or respiratory arrest during general anesthesia or heavy sedation, needing a careful physiologic and radiographic evaluation. Least-invasive procedures like a bone marrow aspirate and biopsy should always be performed early in the work-up of patients with lymphoblastic lymphoma and can often be used

TABLE 2. *Characteristics of four major categories of childhood NHL*

Histology	Immunophenotype	Cytogenetics	Molecular genetics of the fusion transcripts	Incidence
BL and BLL[a] (Burkitt's and Burkitt's-like lymphoma)	B	t(8;14), t(8;22) t(2;8)	IgH/c-*myc* Igkappa/c-*myc* Iglambda/c-*myc*	40–50% (~20% contain EBV genome)
DLBCL[a] (including thymic B-cell lymphoma)	B	Nonrecurrent		25% (10%)
Lymphoblastic lymphoma	Immature T Pre-B	t(10;14), t(11;14) t(1;14), t(1;19)	*TCR-TAL1* *TCR-RHOM2* *TCR-LCK*	30%
Anaplastic LCL (CD30+, Ki-1+, ALK+)	T, Null	t(2;5)(p23;q35) and variants t(1;2)(p23;q25) Inv(2)(p23q35) t(2;13)(p23;q34) t(2;3)(p23;q21)	*NPM-ALK* *TPM3-ALK* *ATIC-ALK*	10–15%

[a]Distinctions between Burkitt's lymphoma, Burkitt's-like lymphoma, and diffuse large B-cell lymphomas (DLBCL) are subjective and difficult to reproduce. EBV, Epstein-Barr virus; LCL, large cell lymphoma.

to establish the diagnosis of lymphoma. If a pleural effusion is present, a cytologic diagnosis is frequently possible with thoracentesis. In those children with peripheral adenopathy, a lymph node biopsy under local anesthesia and in an upright position may be possible. In situations in which these diagnostic procedures are not fruitful, consideration of a CT-guided core-needle biopsy should be contemplated. This procedure can frequently be carried out with light sedation and local anesthesia before proceeding to more invasive procedures.

TABLE 3. *Clinical presentation of childhood NHL*

Lymphoma subtype	Commonest clinical features
Precursor T-cell lymphoblastic lymphomas	Mediastinal mass, pleural effusion, supradiaphragmatic lymphadenopathy, airway obstruction, superior vena caval obstruction, bone marrow involvement
B-cell Burkitt's and Burkitt's-like lymphoma (sporadic)	Abdominal pain, iliac mass, changes in bowel habits, intussusception, gastrointestinal bleeding and rarely perforation, ascites and pleural effusion, CNS and bone marrow involvement
Endemic Burkitt's lymphoma (e.g., Africa)	Jaw tumors (70%), orbital and paraspinal tumors, and CNS involvement with cranial nerve palsies; abdominal mass
Diffuse large B-cell lymphoma and its variant thymic B-cell lymphoma	Commoner in females. Abdominal mass and mediastinal mass presenting as superior vena cava syndrome. Pleural effusion less common than in lymphoblastic lymphoma. Relapses mainly in extranodal sites
Anaplastic large cell lymphoma (CD30+, Ki-1+)	Systemic symptoms (fever and weight loss), involve lymph nodes and a variety of extranodal sites including skin, bone, lung, and muscle. Bone marrow and CNS involvement uncommon

CNS, central nervous system.
We thank Dr. Elaine S. Jaffe for kindly reviewing tables 2 and 3.

Tumor Lysis Syndrome

Tumor lysis syndrome results from rapid breakdown of malignant cells, resulting in a number of metabolic abnormalities, most notably hyperuricemia, hyperphosphatemia, and hyperkalemia. Hyperhydration (using potassium-free alkalinizing i.v. fluids such as D5 1/4 NS + $NaHCO_3$, 50–100 mEq/L, 3–6 L/m^2) to maintain urine-specific gravity at less than 1.010, and allopurinol or i.v. urate oxidase are essential components of therapy in all patients with extensive disease. Hyperuricemia and tumor lysis syndrome, particularly when associated with ureteral obstruction (requiring hemodialysis and rarely percutaneous nephrostomy), frequently result in life-threatening complications. Therefore NHL patients should be managed only in institutions having pediatric tertiary care facilities.

Treatment Options

The most widely used chemotherapy regimens are listed later. Regimens for lymphoblastic lymphoma are based on protocols designed for ALL, and these are intensive protocols that use combinations of eight to 10 drugs and include prophylactic intrathecal chemotherapy given over an extended period ranging from 9 to 18 months. Most protocols for B-cell lymphomas today consist of short-duration, intensive, alkylating agent (cyclophosphamide, ifosfamide) therapy, coupled with other agents active in lymphomas and accompanied by intrathecal CNS prophylaxis. Therapy regimens in use worldwide are listed in Table 4.

Childhood Hodgkin's Disease

Only salient feature relevant to diagnosis and management of children with Hodgkin's disease are discussed here.

- Incidence: An early peak in incidence before adolescence, markedly in boys younger than 10 years, occurs in developing countries, although HD is rare before age 5 years in industrialized countries. The majority of these cases from developing countries in children younger than 5 years are associated with the presence of Epstein–Barr virus in Reed–Sternberg cells.
- Prognosis and risk-adapted therapy regimens: More than 90% of all children and adolescents with newly diagnosed HD are curable with modern risk-adapted combined-modality

---

TABLE 4. *Regimens*

BFM (Berlin, Frankfurt, Munster) regimen:
    prednisone, vincristine, daunorubicin, asparaginase, cyclophosphamide, cytarabine,
      methotrexate, and mercaptopurine
NCI-89-C-0041F:
    cyclophosphamide, vincristine, doxorubicin, methotrexate (Codox-M) alternating with
      cytarabine, etoposide, and ifosfamide (IVAC)
French LMB-89:
    high-dose cyclophosphamide, high-dose methotrexate/leucovorin, cytarabine, vincristine,
      prednisone, doxorubicin, lomustine, hydrocortisone
Total-B (St. Jude's regimen):
    high-dose cyclophosphamide, high-dose methotrexate, cytarabine, and POG-9317:
      modified "total B" (no doxorubicin) with or without ifosfamide/etoposide
Patients with limited disease need two to three cycles of less-intensive therapy:
    a) COMP: cyclophosphamide, vincristine, methotrexate, prednisone
    b) CHOP plus MTX: cyclophosphamide, doxorubicin, vincristine, and prednisone,
      alternating with infusional methotrexate
    c) Vincristine, doxorubicin, cyclophosphamide, prednisone, mercaptopurine, methotrexate

---

TABLE 5. *Late complications of therapy*

Patients	Radiation	Chemotherapy
Both boys and girls	Solid tumors (e.g., sarcomas) Damage to thyroid, heart, and lungs Renal dysfunction after irradiation of the paraaortic nodes and splenic pedicle (can be prevented by placement of titanium clips at the splenic hilum to shield the left kidney) Localized growth abnormalities (the neck may have a smaller circumference or the upper chest may be poorly developed if these areas are irradiated) Long-term risk (20%) of bacterial sepsis due to splenectomy	Hematopoietic malignancies (such as acute myeloid leukemia and non-Hodgkin's lymphoma) Sterility and infertility, reversible in girls Carotid stenosis
Girls	Risk of breast cancer for girls between the ages of 10 and 16 years who are treated with radiation therapy is especially high (cumulative risk is 35% at age 40 years) and is dose related. Ten-fold increase in risk of breast cancer after therapy in all females aged <30 years Infertility and early menopause (decreased by oophoropexy to move gonads out of the radiation therapy field during laparotomy if pelvic irradiation is planned)	Hematopoietic malignancies

regimens prescribing low-dose (2,000–2,500 Gy), involved-field radiotherapy, and a small number of cycles of multiagent chemotherapy. With improved cure rates, increasing attention is focused on minimizing the early and late complications of therapy. Modifying therapy to reduce late effects while maintaining high cure rates has been the goal of pediatric oncologists in recent years.

- Late complications of therapy: The risk of sterility; damage to the thyroid, heart, and lungs, and second malignancies must be considered. Consequently, the dose of radiation administered to patients in the younger age group has tended to be lower than that classically given to adult patients. Combination chemotherapy may be used as part of the treatment or, in selected cases, as the only treatment of early-stage disease (Table 5).

Changes in Therapy

- Radiation therapy has been decreased in dose, duration, and fields and can even be completely omitted in some patients.
- Chemotherapy regimens have been developed that limit alkylating agents and anthracyclines to decrease the risk of second neoplasms, loss of fertility, and late cardiopulmonary toxicity, and substitute etoposide for procarbazine in boys to avoid sterility. Latest German DAL-HD-90 studies using the OEPA regimen [vincristine, etoposide, prednisone, and doxorubicin (Adriamycin)] have shown 98% 5-year overall survival, with decreased incidence of testicular dysfunction. It offers a favorable risk/benefit ratio, combining excellent disease control, moderate acute toxicity, and reduced long-term toxicity.
- In the patient who is still growing (that is, patients who are younger than 13 years or who have not attained sexual maturity), every attempt is made to preserve the integrity of bony and connective tissue structures.
- In sexually mature boys who will undergo combination chemotherapy or pelvic irradiation, consideration should be given to storing sperm, because seminiferous tissue is often irreparably damaged by chemotherapy or scattered irradiation.

OVERVIEW OF CHILDHOOD BRAIN TUMORS

Primary brain tumors are a diverse group of diseases that together constitute the most common solid tumor of childhood in most world regions. Brain tumors are classified according to histology, but tumor location and extent of spread are important factors that affect treatment and prognosis. Immunohistochemical analysis and measures of mitotic activity have been used in tumor diagnosis and classification.

- Infratentorial tumors constitute approximately 50% of brain tumors in children. Three fourths of these are located in the cerebellum or fourth ventricle. Common infratentorial (posterior fossa) tumors include
  1. Cerebellar astrocytoma (usually pilocytic but occasionally invasive or high-grade).
  2. Medulloblastoma (primitive neuroectodermal tumor).
  3. Ependymoma.
  4. Brainstem glioma (often diagnosed neuroradiographically without biopsy; may be high- or low-grade).
- Supratentorial tumors include those tumors that occur in the sellar or suprasellar region and/or other areas of the cerebrum, and compose approximately 20% of childhood brain tumors.

Sellar/suprasellar Tumors

Common sellar/suprasellar tumors include the following:
1. Craniopharyngioma.
2. Diencephalic (chiasm, hypothalamic, and/or thalamic) low-grade gliomas.
3. Germinoma.

Other Supratentorial Tumors

1. Low-grade astrocytoma or glioma (grade 1 or grade 2).
2. High-grade or malignant astrocytoma (anaplastic astrocytoma, glioblastomas).
3. Mixed glioma multiforme (grade 3 or grade 4).
4. Oligodendroglioma.
5. Primitive neuroectodermal tumor (cerebral neuroblastoma).
6. Ependymoma.
7. Meningioma.
8. Choroid plexus tumors (papilloma and carcinoma).
9. Pineal parenchymal tumors (pineoblastoma, pineocytoma, or mixed pineal parenchymal tumor).
10. Neuronal and mixed neuronal glial tumor (ganglioglioma, desmoplastic infantile gangli-oglioma, dysembryoplastic neuroepithelial tumor).

- Important general concepts that should be understood by those caring for children with brain tumor include the following:
  1. Selection of appropriate therapy can be made only if the correct diagnosis is made and the stage of the disease is accurately determined. Functional outcome and quality-of-life issues are critical to overall success.
  2. Children with primary brain tumors represent a major therapy challenge that, for optimal results, requires the coordinated efforts of pediatric specialists in fields such as neuro-surgery, neurology, rehabilitation, neuropathology, radiation oncology, pediatric oncology, neuroradiology, endocrinology, and psychology.
  3. More than half of children diagnosed with brain tumors will survive 5 years from diagnosis. In some subgroups of patients (e.g., children with medulloblastoma), a 60% to 80% survival is seen after aggressive surgery; irradiation, including the entire subarach-

noid space or neuraxis plus a boost to the posterior fossa and chemotherapy (typically consisting of cisplatinum, vincristine, cyclophosphamide, or lomustine).

4. Each child's treatment should be approached with curative intent, and the possible long-term sequelae of the disease and its treatment should be considered when therapy is begun. Aggressive total resection involving the lower brainstem may result in a morbid posterior fossa syndrome (with mutism, pharyngeal dysfunction, and ataxia). Near-total removal with minimal residual tumor (<1.5 cm^2) appears to confer equivalent survival benefit.

- Staging system: Until recently, the most commonly used staging system was that proposed by Harisiadis and Chang. This system rates the tumor by an intraoperative evaluation of both size and extent, as well as by the presence of metastatic disease. Alternative postoperative staging systems are now being used that are based on surgical impression and postoperative imaging studies. Factors that may portend an unfavorable outcome include disseminated disease at diagnosis, younger age, brainstem involvement, subtotal resection, and a non–posterior fossa tumor. The prognostic importance of brainstem involvement is still being debated.
- Prognostic variables must be evaluated in the context of the treatment received. Two major subclassifications are now being used:
- Average risk: Children older than 3 years with posterior fossa tumors; tumor is totally or "near-totally" (<1.5 cc of residual disease) resected; no dissemination.
- Poor risk: Children younger than 3 years or those with metastatic disease and/or subtotal resection (>1.5 cc of residual disease) and/or nonposterior fossa location.
- Challenges and future directions:

1. Identification of biologic differences may indicate subsets of children appropriately addressed with more- or less-aggressive treatment regimens. Biologic markers, such as tumor-cell ploidy and cytogenetic and molecular genetic findings, are being evaluated, and the subcategories of disease may change over time.
2. New technologies like introduction of three-dimensional planned conformal radiation therapy, including stereotactic radiosurgery, augmenting irradiation by single fraction boost to focal areas of disease visible on postoperative imaging, and hyperfractionated craniospinal irradiation, offer potential advantages in improved efficacy with diminished neurotoxicity.
3. New experimental chemotherapeutic agents improving the efficacy of available cytotoxic drugs, such as the use of bradykinin B$_2$ agonist RMP7 in combination with carboplatin. This allows chemotherapy dose intensification by increasing the delivery of hydrophilic compounds across the blood–tumor barrier.

NEUROBLASTOMA

Neuroblastoma is derived from the primordial neural crest cells forming the sympathetic chain and adrenal medulla. It is the most common extracranial solid tumor of childhood, accounting for 8% to 10% of childhood cancers, and is the most common neoplasm of infants. More than 90% of the 500 cases diagnosed annually in the U.S. involve children younger than 5 years. Many of these children escape detection because of spontaneous regression or maturation into benign lesions. Localized, regional, 4S neuroblastoma rarely evolves into the lethal stage IV pattern. Despite progress in outcomes of neuroblastoma in infants and children with localized disease, there has been only nominal improvement in cure rates ($<20\%$) of children with disseminated disease, which includes nearly 50% of cases, in the last 30 years.

Diagnosis and staging are addressed in Tables 6 through 10.

Treatment Approach

1. Low-risk neuroblastoma: Patients with stage I disease plus hyperdiploidy but without N-*myc* amplification may be treated with surgical resection alone.
2. Intermediate-risk neuroblastoma: Patients having stage II or III disease without N-*myc* amplification may be treated with either surgery alone or biopsy followed by chemotherapy followed by second-look surgery.

TABLE 6. *Presenting syndromes associated with neuroblastoma*

Eponym	Syndrome features
Pepper syndrome	Massive involvement of the liver with metastatic disease with or without respiratory distress
Horner's syndrome	Unilateral ptosis, myosis, and anhydrosis associated with a thoracic primary tumor. Symptoms do not recover with tumor removal.
Hutchinson's syndrome	Limping and irritability in the young child associated with bone and bone marrow metastases
Opsomyoclonus	Myoclonic jerking and random eye movement, with or without cerebellar ataxia. May be associated with a differentiated, favorable-outlook tumor, but symptoms may or may not resolve after tumor removal.
Kerner–Morrison syndrome	Intractable secretory diarrhea associated with a biologically favorable tumor that secretes vasointestinal peptides. Symptoms always resolve with tumor removal.
"Racoon eyes"	Noted when there is periorbital hemorrhage secondary to metastatic tumor

TABLE 7. *The International Neuroblastoma Staging System (INSS) minimum recommended studies for determining extent of disease*

Tumor location	Diagnostic studies
Primary	Computed tomography (CT) scan, magnetic resonance imaging (MRI), or both, with three-dimensional measurements[a] metaiodobenzylguanidine scan, if available[b]
Metastases	Bilateral posterior iliac crest bone marrow aspirates and trephine (core) bone marrow biopsies necessary to exclude marrow involvement. A single positive site documents marrow involvement. Core biopsies must contain at least 1 cm of marrow (excluding cartilage) to be considered adequate.
	Bone radiographs and either scintigraphy by technetium-99 scan or MIBG scan, if available, are recommended.
	Abdominal and liver imaging by CT scan or MRI with three-dimensional measurements[a]
	Chest radiography (anteroposterior and lateral). Chest CT scan or MRI necessary only if the chest radiograph is positive, or if abdominal mass or lymph node disease extends into chest

[a]Ultrasound imaging is considered suboptimal for accurate three-dimensional measurements.
[b]The MIBG scan is applicable to all sites of disease.
MIBG *meta*-iodo-benzyleguanidine.

TABLE 8. *The International Neuroblastoma Staging System (INSS)*

Stage 1:	Localized tumor confined to the area of origin; complete gross resection, with or without microscopic residual disease; identifiable ipsilateral and contralateral lymph node negative for tumor
Stage 2A:	Unilateral with incomplete gross resection; identifiable ipsilateral and contralateral lymph node negative for tumor
Stage 2B:	Unilateral with complete or incomplete gross resection; with ipsilateral lymph node positive for tumor; identifiable contralateral lymph node negative for tumor
Stage 3:	Tumor infiltrating across midline with or without regional lymph node involvement; or unilateral tumor with contralateral lymph node involvement; or midline tumor with bilateral lymph node involvement
Stage 4:	Dissemination of tumor to distant lymph nodes, bone marrow, liver, or other organs except as defined in stage 4S
Stage 4S:	Localized primary tumor as defined in stage 1 or 2, with dissemination limited to liver, skin, or bone marrow

Less than 10% of nucleated marrow cells are tumor cells.

TABLE 9. *Genetic and clinical subsets of neuroblastoma*

Feature	Type 1	Type 2	Type 3
N-*myc* gene	Normal	Normal	Amplified
Karyotype/ploidy	Hyperdiploid	Near-diploid	Near-diploid
	Triploid	Near-tetraploid	Near-tetraploid
1p LOH	Absent	Present	Present
*trk*A expression	High	Variable (low)	Low or absent
Age	<1 yr	≥1 yr	1–5 yr
INSS stage	1, 2, 4S	3, 4	3, 4
3-yr survival	~95%	25%–50%	~5%

LOH, loss of heterozygosity; INSS, International Neuroblastoma Staging System.

3. High-risk and very-high-risk neuroblastoma: These patients include stage IV patients diagnosed after the first birthday, patients at any age with stage IIB, III, or IVS disease and N-*myc* amplification. Therapy of these patients includes chemotherapy (using cyclophosphamide, cisplatin, doxorubicin, etoposide, and vincristine), second-look surgery and radiation therapy to sites of residual disease, consolidation with myeloablative chemotherapy, and/or total body irradiation followed by stem cell rescue. Targeted radioimmunotherapy using iodine 131–labeled MIBG (*meta*-iodo-benzyl-guanidine) or monoclonal antibody have shown 10% to 57% responses in pilot studies.

4. Biologic therapy of minimal residual disease using retinoic acid and anti-G_{D2} monoclonal antibodies have been under investigation and are yet to complete evaluation in clinical trials.

TABLE 10. *Risk group and protocol assignment schema: POG and CCG*

INSS Stage	Age (yr)	N-*myc* status	Shimada histology	DNA ploidy	Risk group/study
1	0–21	Any	Any	Any	Low
2A and 2B	<1	Any	Any	Any	Low
	≥1–21	Nonamplified[a]	Any	NA	Low
	≥1–21	Amplified[b]	Favorable	NA	Low
	≥1–21	Amplified	Unfavorable	NA	High
3	<1	Nonamplified	Any	Any	Intermediate
	<1	Amplified	Any	Any	High
	≥1–21	Nonamplified	Favorable	NA	Intermediate
	≥1–21	Nonamplified	Unfavorable	NA	High
	≥1–21	Amplified	Any	NA	High
4	<1	Nonamplified	Any	Any	Intermediate
	<1	Amplified	Any	Any	High
	≥1–21	Any	Any	NA	High
4S	<1	Nonamplified	Favorable	>1	Low
	<1	Nonamplified	Any	1	Intermediate
	<1	Nonamplified	Unfavorable	Any	Intermediate
	<1	Amplified	Any	Any	High

[a]N-*myc* copy number ≤10.
[b]N-*myc* copy number >10.
POG, Pediatric Oncology Group; CCG, Children's Cancer Group; INSS, International Neuroblastoma Staging System; NA, not applicable.

Wilms' Tumor

Wilms' tumor is an embryonal neoplasm of the kidney, accounting for 6% to 7% (400 new cases annually) of all childhood malignancies in the U.S. It is a curable disease in the majority of affected children. More than 90% of patients survive 4 years after diagnosis. Prognosis is related to the stage of disease at diagnosis, the histopathologic features of the tumor, patient age, and tumor size. Previous clinical trials have in part been designed to evaluate whether reduced therapy is sufficient to control disease in patients with early-stage, favorable-histology Wilms' tumor. Ongoing clinical trials are addressing the duration and refinement of therapy.

- Wilms' tumor is derived from primitive metanephric blastema and has a triphasic composition of blastemal, epithelial, and stromal cells. Only a small group (15%) of tumors exhibits unfavorable histology in the form of anaplasia and sarcomatous features. Clear cell sarcoma and rhabdoid tumor of the kidney are now recognized as separate entities from Wilms' tumor, and the latter respond poorly to all current treatment regimens.
- Specific germ-line mutations in one of the genes (Wilms' tumor gene-1, WT1) located on the short arm of chromosome 11 (band 11p13) not only are associated with both hereditary and sporadic Wilms' tumor but also cause a variety of genitourinary abnormalities such as cryptorchidism, hypospadias, and the rare Denys–Drash syndrome. A gene that causes aniridia is located near the WT1 gene on chromosome 11p13, and deletions encompassing the WT1 and aniridia genes may explain the association between aniridia and Wilms' tumor. Consequently patients with aniridia or hemihypertrophy should be screened with ultrasound every 3 months until they are 10 years old.
- A second Wilms' tumor gene is located at or near the Beckwith–Wiedemann gene locus on chromosome 11p15, and children with Beckwith–Wiedemann syndrome are at increased risk for developing Wilms' tumor. It is recommended that these patients be screened with ultrasound every 3 months until they are 7 years old (Table 11).

TABLE 11. *National Wilms' Tumor Study Clinicopathologic Staging System*

Stage I:	Tumor limited to kidney and completely excised. The surface of the renal capsule is intact. Tumor was not ruptured before or during removal. There is no residual tumor apparent beyond the margins of resection.
Stage II:	Tumor extends beyond the kidney but is completely removed. There is regional extension of the tumor (i.e., penetration through the outer surface of the renal capsule into the perirenal soft tissues). Vessels outside the kidney substance are inflated or contain tumor thrombus. A biopsy of the tumor may have been taken or there has been local spillage of tumor confined to the flank. There is no residual tumor apparent at or beyond the margins of excision.
Stage III:	Residual nonhematogenous tumor confined to the abdomen: 1. Lymph nodes on biopsy are found to be involved in the hilus, the periaortic chains, or beyond. 2. There has been diffuse peritoneal contamination by tumor, such as spillage of tumor beyond the flank before or during surgery or tumor growth that has penetrated through the peritoneal surface. 3. Implants are found on the peritoneal surface. 4. The tumor extends beyond the surgical margins either microscopically or grossly. 5. The tumor is not completely resectable because of local infiltration into vital structures.
Stage IV:	Hematogenous metastases. Deposits beyond stage III (e.g., lung, liver, bone, and/or brain)
Stage V:	Bilateral renal involvement at diagnosis. An attempt should be made to stage each side according to the previous criteria on the basis of the extent of disease before biopsy.

From Green GM, D'Angio GL, Beckwith JB, et al. Wilms' tumor. *CA Cancer J Clin* 1996;46:46, with permission.

Treatment Overview

- Patients with stage I favorable histology, stage I anaplasia, or stage II favorable histology need only postnephrectomy chemotherapy with vincristine and actinomycin D.
- Stage III patients with favorable histology benefit from the addition of doxorubicin and abdominal irradiation (1,000 cGy) to these two drugs.
- Stage IV patients receive abdominal and whole-lung irradiation (1,200 cGy) in addition to the three drugs vincristine, actinomycin D, and doxorubicin.
- Addition of a fourth drug, cyclophosphamide, may benefit patients with stages II to IV diffuse anaplasia.
- Bilateral Wilms' tumor (stage V) is seen in 5% of patients. Therapy in these and patients with tumors in the horseshoe kidney is individualized and comprises initial bilateral renal biopsy followed by chemotherapy with vincristine and actinomycin D. Optimally tumor resection with significant renal preservation is attempted after 5 weeks. Advances in dialysis and transplantation programs for young children offer the potential for a marked improvement in the prognosis for patients with bilateral Wilms' tumor, especially when associated with nephropathy in those with Denys–Drash syndrome.

Late Effects

- Doxorubicin coupled with mediastinal and whole-lung irradiation for metastatic Wilms' tumor causes cardiomyopathy, significant reduction of total lung capacity and vital capacity, with a cumulative 1.7% of children developing congestive heart failure in NWTS-2 and 3 at 15 years after diagnosis.
- Veno-occlusive disease has been reported in 3.1% of children treated with actinomycin D and vincristine.
- Renal hyperfiltration injury, decreased creatinine clearance, proteinuria, and hypertension have been noted 10 to 20 years after nephrectomy, local irradiation, and chemotherapy for Wilms' tumor.

HEPATOBLASTOMA AND HEPATOCELLULAR CARCINOMA

- Incidence and prognosis: Liver cancer, a rare malignancy in children and adolescents, is divided into two groups: hepatoblastoma and hepatocellular carcinoma. The age at onset of liver cancer in children is related to the histology of the tumor. Hepatoblastomas usually occur before age 3 years, whereas the incidence of hepatocellular carcinoma in the U.S. varies little with age between 0 and 19 years. The overall survival rate for children with hepatoblastoma is 70% but is only 25% for hepatocellular carcinoma. If the tumor is completely removed, the majority of patients survive, but only a minority of patients have lesions amenable to complete resection at diagnosis.
- Tumor marker: The majority of patients with either hepatoblastoma or hepatocellular carcinoma have a serum tumor marker, α-fetoprotein, that parallels disease activity. Lack of a significant decrease of α-fetoprotein levels with treatment predicts a poor response to therapy. Absence of elevated α-fetoprotein may be a poor prognostic sign in hepatoblastoma; it is associated with the small-cell (anaplastic) histologic variant, which responds very poorly to therapy. Occasionally hepatoblastomas produce β-human chorionic gonadotropin, resulting in isosexual precocity. Severe osteopenia is not uncommon.
- Hepatoblastoma is part of the constellation of findings associated with the Beckwith–Wiedemann syndrome. Loss of the allele of maternal origin at the 11p15.5 familial Beckwith–Wiedemann syndrome locus occurs in many hepatoblastomas. About 2% of children with hepatoblastoma have hemihypertrophy.
- There is a clear association between hepatoblastoma and familial adenomatous polyposis (FAP); children in families that carry the FAP gene are at an increased risk for hepatoblas-

toma, although it occurs in fewer than 1% of FAP family members. Childhood hepatoblastomas frequently have mutations in the β-catenin gene, the function of which is closely related to FAP.

- Several specific types of nonviral liver injury and cirrhosis in children are associated with hepatocellular carcinoma: tyrosinemia, biliary cirrhosis, and α_1-antitrypsin deficiency.
- Prevention: Hepatocellular carcinoma is associated with perinatally acquired hepatitis B and C infection. Therefore widespread hepatitis B immunization carried out in endemic populations of Taiwan has been shown to decrease the incidence of hepatocellular carcinoma.
- Treatment options:
  1. In recent years, virtually all children with advanced-stage hepatoblastoma have been treated with chemotherapy, consisting of four courses of cisplatin/vincristine/fluorouracil or cisplatin/doxorubicin followed by attempted complete tumor resection. If the tumor is completely removed, two postoperative courses of the same chemotherapy should be given. If the tumor is not resectable after four courses of chemotherapy, alternative therapies should be considered.
  2. In some centers, even children with resectable hepatoblastoma are treated with preoperative chemotherapy, which may reduce the incidence of surgical complications at the time of resection.
  3. In contrast, the current Intergroup protocol for treatment of children with hepatoblastoma does not include chemotherapy for stage I tumors of purely fetal histology unless they develop progressive disease, and resection at the time of diagnosis is encouraged for all tumors amenable to resection without undue risk.
  4. Liver transplantation has been used with some success to treat unresectable primary hepatic, presumably nonmetastatic, tumors in children.

RETINOBLASTOMA

Incidence

Retinoblastoma is the most common ocular embryonal tumor in children younger than 2 years, with an incidence of 1 in 15,000 to 20,000 births. Two thirds of these tumors are unilateral, and one third are bilateral. The majority of the latter are inherited and associated with constitutional anomaly of the RB1 gene situated at 13q1.4. It is a model disease for a tumor caused by loss of an anti-oncogene.

Prognosis

1. Most patients have tumors confined to the eye, with an excellent prognosis (5-year disease-free survival > 90%). However, DFS for patients with extraocular disease, 5-year (DFS) is less than 10%.
2. Patients with the hereditary type of retinoblastoma have a markedly increased frequency of second malignant neoplasms (SMNs). The cumulative incidence is about 26% ± 10% in nonirradiated and 58% ± 10% in irradiated patients by 50 years after diagnosis of retinoblastoma. Most of the SMNs are osteosarcomas, soft-tissue sarcomas, or melanomas. In irradiated patients, two thirds of the second cancers occur within irradiated tissue, and one third outside the radiation field. The risk for SMNs in the field of radiation is dependent on the patient's age at the time the external-beam radiation is given. This risk may be less for patients older than 12 months. Second malignancies should also be treated with curative intent.
3. There is no clear increase in second malignancies in patients with nonhereditary retinoblastoma.
4. Genetic counseling should be an integral part of the therapy for a patient with retinoblastoma, whether unilateral or bilateral. All siblings of patients with retinoblastoma should

be examined periodically, and studies suggest that DNA polymorphism analysis may be used to predict which persons are at risk and warrant close follow-up. Cytogenetic abnormalities (e.g., deletion on the long arm of chromosome 13) are sometimes observed.

Treatment Outline

The goals of therapy are twofold: to cure the disease and to preserve as much vision as possible. Treatment options for the involved eye include the following:

1. Enucleation, if the tumor is massive or if there is little expectation of useful vision
2. External-beam radiation with doses ranging from 3,500 to 4,600 cGy. Because of the need to sedate young children and the intricacies of field planning, special expertise in pediatric radiation therapy is important.
3. Photocoagulation is used for posteriorly located tumors that are smaller than four disc diameters in size, distinct from the optic nerve head and macula, and without involvement of large nutrient vessels or choroid involvement. In patients with early stages of disease, light coagulation is usually used in addition to radiation therapy or when there is limited recurrence after radiation therapy.
4. Cryotherapy, in addition to radiation or in place of photocoagulation for lesions smaller than four disc diameters in size in the anterior portion of the retina
5. Brachytherapy with radioactive plaques for either focal unilateral presentations or recurrent disease after previous external-beam irradiation
6. Under investigation is the use of systemic chemotherapy to reduce tumor volume (chemoreduction) and to avoid the long-term effects of radiation therapy for patients with bilateral tumors or intraocular tumors that are not amenable to treatment with cryotherapy or photocoagulation alone.

PEDIATRIC EXTRACRANIAL GERM CELL TUMORS

Extracranial germ cell tumors (particularly testicular germ cell tumors) are more common among patients age 15 to 19 years and rare in younger children, accounting for only 2% to 3% of cancers in this age group. The germ cell tumors that arise in children younger than 5 years have different biologic characteristics from those that arise in adolescents and young adults.

Pathogenesis and Clinical Presentation

1. These germ cell tumors originate in pluripotent germ cells and are composed of elements from at least one of the three embryonic germ layers, and usually contain tissues foreign to the anatomic site of origin. In general, germ cell tumors encompass a variety of histologic diagnoses including teratomas and malignant germ cell tumors. The teratomas can be further classified as mature or immature and can be either pure or a component of a mixed malignant germ cell tumor.
2. Childhood extracranial germ cell tumors most commonly arise in midline extragonadal sites (including but not limited to the retroperitoneum, sacrococcygeal area, mediastinum, neck, and pineal gland), but also can occur at gonadal sites in either the ovaries or testes. Their typical midline location hypothetically relates to the deposition of primordial germ cells along their migration pathway from the hind gut–yolk sac region into the embryonic genital ridge.
3. The signs and symptoms produced by these tumors will vary according to their anatomic location. Generally, sacrococcygeal tumors can cause constipation and urinary retention; testicular tumors usually present as painless swelling or a mass, whereas ovarian tumors tend to cause increasing abdominal girth and pain. Very little is known about the poten-

tial genetic or environmental factors associated with childhood extracranial germ cell tumors. However, patients with Klinefelter's syndrome appear to be at increased risk for mediastinal germ cell tumors, whereas patients with Swyer's syndrome appear at increased risk for gonadoblastomas and germinomas.

4. Malignant germ cell tumors usually contain frankly malignant tissues of germ cell origin (e.g., yolk sac carcinoma, embryonal carcinoma, germinoma, or choriocarcinoma) or rarely of somatic origin. Yolk sac carcinomas produce AFP, whereas choriocarcinomas produce β-human chorionic gonadotropin (bHCG), resulting in elevation of these markers in the serum, which can serve as tumor markers. In addition, germinomas also can produce elevation of serum bHCG but not to the levels associated with choriocarcinoma. Most children with germ cell tumors will have a component of yolk sac tumor and have elevations of AFP, which is serially monitored during treatment and helps assess response to therapy.

5. Primary site and the stage of disease appear to be the most important prognostic factors identified in patients with childhood extracranial germ cell tumors.

Subtypes

Biologically distinctive subtypes of germ cell tumors include the following:

1. Testicular germ cell tumors of early childhood: These germ cell tumors commonly have yolk sac tumor (endodermal sinus tumor) histology and are generally diploid or tetraploid and lack the isochromosome of the short arm of chromosome 12 that is characteristic of testicular cancer in young adults. Deletions of chromosomes 1p and 6q are reported as recurring chromosomal abnormalities for this group of tumors.

2. Extragonadal, extracranial germ cell tumors: These tumors typically are first seen during early childhood. The majority of these tumors are benign teratomas occurring in the sacrococcygeal region. However, malignant yolk sac tumor histology occurs in a minority of these tumors, with cytogenetic abnormalities similar to those observed for tumors occurring in the testes of young males.

3. Extragonadal, extracranial germ cell tumors of older children and adults: The most common primary sites for these tumors are within the mediastinum. Some, although not all, mediastinal germ cell tumors have an isochromosome of the short arm of chromosome 12. Hematologic malignancies associated with germ cell tumors may exhibit isochromosome 12p.

4. Ovarian germ cell tumors: These tumors occur primarily in adolescents and young adults. They show greater biologic diversity than do germ cell tumors arising in the testes, and include benign mature teratomas, immature teratomas, and malignant germ cell tumors (dysgerminomas, yolk sac tumors, and mixed germ cell tumors). The latter, like their testicular counterparts, commonly show increased copies of the short arm of chromosome 12.

Treatment Option Overview

Because of the exquisite chemosensitivity of these tumors, cure rates are very high, even in the event of relapse and recurrent disease. A watch-and-wait policy is advocated, if complete microscopic surgical resection can be accomplished. Chemotherapy has dramatically improved the outcome for these patients, even in advanced-stage disease, with 5-year survival rates increasing to 60% to 90%. The standard chemotherapy regimen for both adults and children with malignant nonseminomatous germ cell tumors includes carboplatin/cisplatin, etoposide, and bleomycin (PEB).

REFERENCES

1. PDQ(r)CancerInformationSummaries: http://cancernet.nci.nih.gov/pdq/pdq_treatment.shtml
2. Pinkerton CR. *Clinical challenges in pediatric oncology.* Oxford: ISIS Medical Media, 1999.
3. Pizzo, and Poplack, eds. *Principles and practice of pediatric oncology.* Philadelphia: Lippincott-Raven Press, 1997.
4. Michael IP, guest ed. *Pediatr Clin North Am* Philadelphia: 1997;44:4.
5. Smith M, Arthur D, Camitta B, et al. Uniform approach to risk classification and treatment assignment for children with acute lymphoblastic leukemia. *J Clin Oncol* 1996;14:18–24.
6. NCCN. Pediatric acute lymphoblastic leukemia practice guidelines. *Oncology* 1996;10:1787–1794.
7. Rubnitz JE, Look AT. Molecular genetics of childhood leukemias. *J Pediatr Hematol/Oncol* 1998; 20:1–11.
8. Linet MS, Ries LAG, Smith MA, Tarone RE, Devesa SS. Cancer surveillance series: recent trends in childhood cancer incidence and mortality in the United States. *J Natl Cancer Inst* 1999;91: 1051–1058.
9. Schwartz CL. Long-term survivors of childhood cancer: the late effects of therapy. *Oncologist* 1999; 4:45–54.
10. Raimondi S, Chang MN, Ravindranath Y, et al. Chromosomal abnormalities in 478 children with acute myeloid leukemia: clinical characteristics and treatment outcome in a cooperative pediatric oncology group study-POG8821. *Blood* 1999;94:3707–3716.
11. Ablin AR, ed. *Supportive care of children with cancer.* The Johns Hopkins University Press, 1997.
12. Schellong G, Potter R, Brämswig J, et al. High cure rates and reduced long-term toxicity in pediatric Hodgkin's disease: the German-Austrian multicenter trial DAL-HD-90. *J Clin Oncol* 1999;17:3736–3744.

32

Carcinoma of Unknown Primary

Hung T. Khong and *Stan Lipkowitz

*Surgery Branch and *Medicine Branch, National Cancer Institute, Bethesda, Maryland*

DEFINITION

Carcinoma of unknown primary (CUP) is defined as the detection of one or more metastatic tumors for which routine evaluation, including history and physical, routine blood work, urinalysis, chest radiograph (CXR), and histologic evaluation, fails to identify the primary site.

EPIDEMIOLOGY

- Incidence: 3% of all diagnosed oncologic cases.
- Gender: male/female ratio is approximately equal.
- Age: highest incidence in the sixth decade of life.

CLINICAL FEATURES AND PROGNOSIS

Clinical features:

- At presentation, most patients (97%) typically complain of symptoms at metastatic site(s). Common presenting sites and common metastatic sites are listed in Tables 1 and 2.

TABLE 1. *Common presenting sites*

Site	%	Range (%)
Lymph node	26	14–37
Lung	17	16–19
Bone	15	13–30
Liver	11	4–19
Brain	8	7–10
Pleura	7	2–12
Skin	5	0–22
Peritoneal	4	1–6

Only the metastatic site that was first apparent or first symptomatic in each patient was counted. Data were collected from three series involving a total of 611 patients. (From Refs. 10,11,12.)

387

TABLE 2. *Common metastatic sites*

Site	%	Range (%)
Lymph nodes	41	20–42
Liver	34	33–43
Bone	29	29
Lung	27	26–31
Pleura	11	11–12
Peritoneal	9	—
Brain	6	6
Adrenal	6	4–6
Skin	4	—
Bone marrow	3	—

All principal metastatic sites in each patient were counted. Data collected from two series involving a total of 1,051 patients. Data reported from subspecialty practices were excluded. (From Refs. 13,14.)

- Nonspecific constitutional symptoms also are common: anorexia, weight loss, and fatigue.
- At diagnosis, more than half of patients (59%) have multiple sites (more than two) of metastatic involvement.

Prognosis:

- As a group, the median survival time is 3 to 4 months; however, some recent studies have reported a median survival duration of 5 to 12 months.
- Most (55–85%) die within 1 year; 5% to 10% survive at 5 years (Fig. 1)

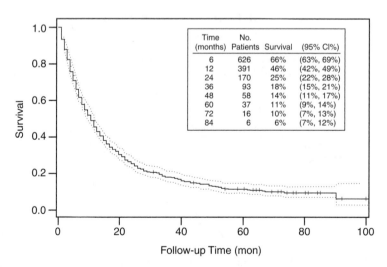

Time (months)	No. Patients	Survival	(95% CI%)
6	626	66%	(63%, 69%)
12	391	46%	(42%, 49%)
24	170	25%	(22%, 28%)
36	93	18%	(15%, 21%)
48	58	14%	(11%, 17%)
60	37	11%	(9%, 14%)
72	16	10%	(7%, 13%)
84	6	6%	(7%, 12%)

FIG. 1. Kaplan–Meier survival curve of 1,000 consecutive patients with cancer of unknown primary (CUP). Median survival, 11 months (95% CI, 10–12 months).

TABLE 3. *Median survival in some prognostic subgroups*

Median survival time (mo)			
40	24	5	5
<3 metastatic organ sites; nonadenocarcinoma; no involvement of liver, bone, adrenal, or pleura	Liver mets and neuroendocrine histology	Liver mets; nonneuroendocrine histology; age >61.5 yr	Adrenal mets

The median survival for all patients in this study was 11 mo.
mets, metastasis.

Poor prognostic factors

- Male.
- Adenocarcinoma histology.
- Increasing number of involved organ sites.
- Hepatic involvement.
- Supraclavicular lymphadenopathy.

Advantageous prognostic factors

- Nonsupraclavicular lymphadenopathy.
- Neuroendocrine histology.
- A recent study of 1,000 patients (from M.D. Anderson) revealed several prognostic subgroups. Some are shown in Table 3.

DIAGNOSIS

- Recommended initial evaluation is listed in Table 4.
- Generous tissue samples should be obtained at the first biopsy.
- Accurate pathologic evaluation is critical.
  - Light microscopic examination: four major histologic subtypes can be identified by the initial light microscopic examination (Fig. 2).

TABLE 4. *Initial evaluation*

Complete H & P (attention to breast and pelvic exam in women; prostate and testicular exam in men; head/neck and rectal exam in all patients)
CBC
Chemistry profiles
Urinalysis
Stool testing for occult blood
CXR

H & P, history and physical; CBC, complete blood count; CXR, chest radiograph.

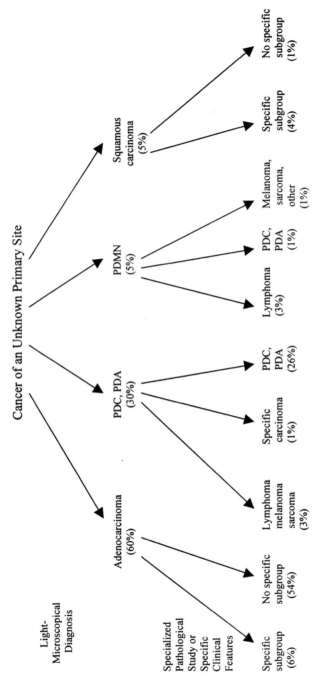

FIG. 2. Relative size of various clinical and histologic subgroups of patients with cancer of an unknown primary site as determined by optimal clinical and pathologic evaluation. Potentially treatable subgroups are indicated in italics and compose approximately 40% of patients. *PDC*, poorly differentiated carcinoma; *PDA*, poorly differentiated adenocarcinoma; *PDMN*, poorly differentiated malignant neoplasm. Reprinted from Hainsworth JD, Greco FA. Treatment of patients with cancer of an unknown primary site. *N Engl J Med* 1993;329:257–263, with permission.

TABLE 5. *Immunoperoxidase staining in the differential diagnosis of carcinoma of unknown primary site*

Tumor type	Immunoperoxidase stains				
	Cytokeratin	Leukocyte common antigen	S100 protein, HMB 45	Neuron-specific enolase, chromogranin	Vimentin desmin
Carcinoma	+	−	−	±	−
Lymphoma	−	+	−	−	−
Melanoma	−	−	+	±	−
Sarcoma	−	−	−	−	+
Neuroendocrine	+	−	−	+	−

- Immunoperoxidase staining (IPS) should be performed in all CUP cases of poorly differentiated carcinomas. Table 5 lists some immunoperoxidase stains that are most useful.
- Electron microscopy should be considered if the tumor cannot be identified by IPS.
- Most common primary sites are listed in Table 6.

TABLE 6. *Primary sites (diagnosed during life or at autopsy)*

Primary sites	%
Lung	23.7
Pancreas	21.1
Ovary	6.4
Kidney	5.5
Colorectal	5.3
Gastric	4.6
Liver	4.3
Prostate	4.1
Breast	3.4
Adrenal	2.2
Thyroid	2.2
Urinary tract/bladder	1.9
Esophagus	1.5
Lymphoma	1.5
Gallbladder/biliary tree	1.2
Testicular germ cell	1
Mesothelioma	0.5
Uterus	0.3
Others	9.3
Total	100

Data collected from nine series involving a total of 1,453 patients with CUP. A diagnosis was made either during life or at autopsy in 582 patients. Excluded in the calculation are head/neck primary and data from subspecialty practices (to avoid artifactual representation of certain cancers such as the high rates of pancreatic primary reported by clinics specializing in GI malignancy).
CUP, cancer of unknown primary; GI, gastrointestinal.

WELL OR MODERATELY DIFFERENTIATED ADENOCARCINOMA OF UNKNOWN PRIMARY

Clinical Features

- Typically elderly patients.
- Metastatic tumors at multiple sites.
- Poor performance status (PS) at diagnosis.
- Common metastatic sites are lymph nodes, liver, lung, and bone.
- Most common primary sites identified are the lung and pancreas (45%) (Table 6).
- Poor prognosis (median survival of 3 to 4 months).
- Primary site rarely found (<15% before death); an exhaustive search is not indicated.

Further Work-up

Additional studies that should be performed include prostate specific antigen (PSA) serum level and/or immunoperoxidase stain (IPS) for men, mammography, serum CA 15-3, serum CA 125, and ER/PR (IPS) for women. CT scan of the abdomen can identify a primary site in approximately 30% of cases.[1]

Treatment

- Most cases (90%) of well or moderately differentiated adenocarcinoma of unknown primary have low response rates and few complete responses with systemic chemotherapy.
- Poor prognosis.
- Empiric chemotherapy (Table 7)
- However, the following are subsets of patients for whom useful therapy can be given:

Peritoneal carcinomatosis in women

Characteristics:

- Typical of ovarian cancer.
- Occasionally associated with cancers from the gastrointestinal (GI) tract or breast.
- Serum CA125 often elevated.

Treatment:

- Treat as stage III ovarian cancer (laparotomy with surgical cytoreduction, followed by paclitaxel and cisplatin-based combination chemotherapy) (see Chapter 16). Note: About 20% have CR, and 16% have prolonged disease-free survival (5).

Women with axillary lymph node metastases

Characteristics:

- Think breast cancer!
- Check ER/PR.
- Occult breast primary found in 55% to 75% of cases

---

[1]In CUP patients with metastatic adenocarcinoma to the axillary lymph nodes and a negative mammogram, a primary breast cancer was detected on breast MRI in nine (75%) of 12 patients in one study (15) and 19 (86%) of 22 patients in a second study (16).

TABLE 7. *Empiric chemotherapy for CUP*

Drug regimen	Treatment description	Cycle
EP[a]		
Cisplatin	60–100 mg/m^2 i.v., day 1	21 days
Etoposide	80–100 mg/m^2 i.v., days 1–3	
FAM[b]		
Fluorouracil	600 mg/m^2 i.v., days 1, 8, 29, 36	8 wk
Doxorubicin	30 mg/m^2 i.v., days 1, 29	
Mitomycin	10 mg/m^2 i.v., day 1	
Paclitaxel[c]	200 mg/m^2 i.v. over 1 h, day 1 followed by	21 days
Carboplatin	Dose calculated by Calvert formula to AUC 6 i.v., after paclitaxel	
Etoposide	50 mg p.o. qd alternating with 100 mg p.o. qd, days 1–10	

[a]Ref. 17.
[b]Ref. 5.
[c]Ref. 18.
In this study, there was an overall response rate (RR) of 47%, with 13% complete responses, and median survival of 13.4 months. Activity was seen in both well-differentiated adenocarcinoma (45% RR) and poorly differentiated carcinoma (48% RR).

Treatment:

- Treat as stage II breast cancer.
- Modified radical mastectomy has been recommended.
- Alternatively, radiation therapy (XRT) to the breast after axillary node dissection.
- Adjuvant systemic chemotherapy should also be considered (see Chapter 16).
- Patients with metastatic sites besides the axillary nodes should be treated for metastatic breast cancer (see Chapter 11).

Men with elevated PSA or osteoblastic bone metastasis

- If the PSA serum level or tumor staining is positive, a trial of hormonal therapy as for metastatic prostate cancer (see Chapter 13) should be started.
- If osteoblastic bone metastases are present, start an empiric hormonal trial, regardless of PSA levels.

Patients with a single metastatic site

- Surgical excision and/or XRT.

POORLY DIFFERENTIATED CARCINOMA/ADENOCARCINOMA OF UNKNOWN PRIMARY

Introduction

- 30% of CUP (poorly differentiated carcinoma: two thirds of cases; poorly differentiated adenocarcinoma: one third of cases).
- Poor response to fluorouracil-based chemotherapy, and a short survival.
- Some patients have neoplasms highly responsive to platinating chemotherapy-based combination treatments. Some long-term survivors and cures have been described.

Clinical Features

- Younger median age (about 40 years).
- Rapid progression of symptoms.
- Evidence of rapid tumor growth.
- Most common sites of metastatic involvement (50% of cases): lymph nodes, mediastinum, and retroperitoneum.

Pathologic Evaluation

- Immunoperoxidase (IP) staining is useful.
- Electron microscopy should be performed if tumor cannot be identified by IP stains.
- Genetic analysis may be useful (e.g., i(12p), del(12p), or multiple copies of (12p) are diagnostic of germ cell tumor).

Further Workup

- Additional workup should include CT scan of chest and abdomen, and serum β-human chorionic gonadotropin (bHCG) and α-fetoprotein (AFP).

Treatment

1. **Extragonadal germ cell cancer syndrome.**
   - Young men.
   - Predominantly midline tumors (mediastinum or retroperitoneum).
   - Elevated bHCG, AFP, or both.
   - Genetic analysis may be diagnostic (e.g., abnormalities in chromosome 12).
   - Treat as a germ cell tumor (see Chapter 15).
2. **Poorly differentiated neuroendocrine carcinoma.**
   - High-grade tumors.
   - Multiple metastatic sites.
   - Highly responsive to cisplatin-based chemotherapy.
   - Overall response rate of 71% (33 of 46 patients treated with combination chemotherapy), with a CR of 13 (28%) of 46; eight (17%) of 46 had durable disease-free survival.
   - Patients in this group should be treated with a trial of combination chemotherapy including a platinating agent and etoposide (Table 7). Note: Other patients with poorly differentiated carcinoma or poorly differentiated adenocarcinoma should receive an empiric trial of platinating agent-based chemotherapy (Table 7). (In a prospective study of 220 patients, the overall response rate was 62%, with a complete response rate of 26%. Thirteen percent of patients were considered cured.)

POORLY DIFFERENTIATED MALIGNANT NEOPLASMS OF UNKNOWN PRIMARY

- 5% of all patients with CUP.
- After specialized pathologic study, 35% to 65% found to be lymphomas; carcinomas account for most of the remaining cases. Fewer than 15% are melanoma and sarcoma.

SQUAMOUS CELL CARCINOMA OF UNKNOWN PRIMARY
Cervical Node Involvement
High Cervical Node(s)

- Work up and treat as for primary head and neck cancer (see Chapter 1).
- High long-term survival rates (30–70%) have been reported after local treatment.
- Role of chemotherapy is undetermined.

Low Cervical or Supraclavicular Node(s)

- Histology can be either squamous, adenocarcinoma, or poorly differentiated tumors.
- Poorer prognosis (particularly adenocarcinoma histology) because lung and GI tract are frequent primary sites.
- If no other sites of disease found, a minority of patients (10–15%) will have long-term disease-free survival with aggressive local therapy (surgery and/or XRT).
- Role of chemotherapy is undetermined.

Inguinal Lymph Node(s)

- A primary site in the genital or anorectal areas is often identified in most patients.
- Curative therapy is available for some of these patients.
- If no primary found, surgical node dissection (with or without radiation therapy) can offer long-term survival.

REFERENCES

1. Abbruzzese JL, Abbruzzese MC, Hess KR, et al. Unknown primary carcinoma: natural history and prognostic factors in 657 consecutive patients. *J Clin Oncol* 1994;12:1272–1280.
2. Bataini JP, Rodriguez J, Jaulerry C, et al. Treatment of metastatic neck nodes secondary to an occult epidermoid carcinoma of the head and neck. *Laryngoscopy* 1987;97:1080–1089.
3. Ellerbroek N, Holmes F, Singletary E, et al. Treatment of patients with isolated axillary nodal metastases from an occult primary carcinoma consistent with breast origin. *Cancer* 1990;66:1481–1491.
4. Eltabbakh GH, Piver MS. Extraovarian primary peritoneal carcinoma. *Oncology* 1998;12:813–819.
5. Greco FA, Hainsworth JD. Cancer of unknown primary site. In: DeVita VT Jr, Hellman S, Rosenberg SA, eds. *Cancer: principles and practice of oncology.* 5th ed. Philadelphia: Lippincott-Raven, 1997: 2423–2443.
6. Greco FA, Oldham RK, Fer MF. The extragonadal germ cell cancer syndrome. *Semin Oncol* 1982;9:448–455.
7. Hainsworth JD, Johnson DH, Greco FA. Cisplatin-based combination chemotherapy in the treatment of poorly differentiated carcinoma and poorly differentiated adenocarcinoma of unknown primary site: results of a 12-year experience. *J Clin Oncol* 1992;10:912–922.
8. Sporn JR, Greenberg BR. Empirical chemotherapy in patients with carcinoma of unknown primary. *Am J Med* 1990;88:49–55.
9. http://cancernet.nci.nih.gov/clinpY_of_unknown_primary_Physician.html.
10. Le Chevalier T, Cvitkovic E, Caille P, et al. Early metastatic cancer of unknown primary origin at presentation. A clinical study of 302 consecutive autopsied patients. *Arch Intern Med* 1988;148(9):2035-2039
11. Kirsten F, Chi CH, Leary JA, Ng AB, Hedley DW, Tattersall MH. Metastatic adeno or undifferentiated carcinoma from an unknown primary site-natural history and guidelines for identification of treatable subssets. *Q J Med* 1987;62(238):143–161.

12. Lyman GH, Preisler HD. Carcinoma of unknown primary: natural history and response to therapy. *J Med* 1978;9(6):445–459.
13. Shildt RA, Kennedy PS, Chen TT, Athens JW, O'Bryan RM, Balcerzak SP. Management of patients with metastatic adenocarcinoma of unknown origin: a Southwest Oncology Group study. *Cancer Treat Rep* 1983;67(1):77–79.
14. Hess KR, Abbruzzese MC. Lenzi R, Raber MN, Abbruzzese JL. Classification and regression tree analysis of 1000 consecutive patients with unknown primary carcinoma. *Clin Cancer Res* 1999;5(11):3403–3410.
15. Morris EA, Schwartz LH, Dershaw DD, van Zee KJ, Abramson AF, Liberman L. MR imaging of the breast in patients with occult primary breast carcinoma. *Radiology* 1997;205(2):437–440.
16. Orel SG, Weinstein SP, Schnall MD, et al. Breast MR imaging in patients with axillary node metastases and unknown primary malignancy. *Radiology* 1999;212(2):543–549.
17. Goldberg RM, Smith FP, Ueno W, Ahlgren JD, Schein PS. 5-fluorouracil, adriamycin, and mitomycin in the treatment of adenocarcinoma of unknown primary. *J Clin Oncol* 1986;4(3):395–399.
18. Shepherd FA. Treatment of advanced non-small cell lung cancer. *Semin Oncol* 1994;21:7–18.

33

Central Nervous System Tumors

Patrick J. Mansky and J. Michael Hamilton

National Cancer Institute, National Institutes of Health, Bethesda, Maryland

Primary brain tumors represent a diverse spectrum of diseases that uniformly pose a unique problem to the practitioner based on their intracranial location. Brain tumors represent the second most common neurologic cause of death after stroke, but only the tenth most common cancer cause of death. The majority of adult brain tumors occur in the cerebral hemispheres, but two thirds of all pediatric brain tumors are infratentorial.

Metastatic brain tumors can be found in 25% to 30% of patients with systemic cancer in autopsy series. With the advancement of computed tomography (CT) and magnetic resonance imaging (MRI), early detection and accuracy of diagnosis have markedly improved. In spite of this, the prognosis for malignant brain tumors remains poor, with a median survival of 1 to 3 years. The mainstays of therapy remain surgery and radiation, whereas chemotherapy is of benefit only in a selected group of tumors.

EPIDEMIOLOGY

According to SEER registry for 1973 through 1987, the range of incidence is two to 19 cases per 100,000 persons per year, depending on age at diagnosis.
- Peak: age 0 to 4 years, 3.1/100,000 persons.
- Plateau: 65 to 79 years, 17.9 to 18.7/100,000 persons.
- 17,000 to 20,000 new cases per year.
- Primary brain tumors comprise 2% of newly diagnosed malignancies per year in the United States.

Distribution

The most common central nervous system (CNS) tumors are derived from glial precursors. The age distribution of tumor frequency by age is demonstrated in Table 1.

Mortality

There are an estimated 13,000 deaths from primary brain tumors per year. CNS tumors are the most prevalent solid tumors in childhood. In children younger than 15 years, brain tumors are reported to represent the second most frequent cancer-related cause of death. In the age group 15 to 59 years, CNS tumors are the third leading cause of cancer-related death. However, 80% of all primary brain tumor–related deaths occur beyond the age of 59 years.

TABLE 1. *Age distribution of tumor frequency by age*

Histology	Age (yr)						
	0–9	10–19	20–29	30–39	40–49	50–59	60–74
Astrocytoma	60%	59%	76%	81%	86%	87%	91%
Low grade	10%	7%	5%	5%	3%	2%	2%
Anaplastic	47%	43%	51%	55%	48%	39%	40%
GBM	1%	7%	14%	18%	33%	44%	51%
Mixed glioma	3%	4%	5%	6%	6%	4%	2%
Oligodendroglioma	1%	4%	5%	6%	6%	4%	2%
Ependymoma	9%	3%	4%	2%	1%	1%	1%
Medulloblastoma	21%	10%	6%	2%	1%	0%	0%
Embryonal/teratoid	1%	1%	0%	0%	0%	0%	0%
Meningioma	0%	0%	1%	2%	1%	2%	2%

Data adapted from DeVita VT Jr, Hellman S, Rosenberg SA, eds. *Cancer: principles and practice of oncology.* Philadelphia: Lippincott-Raven, 1997, with permission.

CLINICAL DIAGNOSIS

Common symptoms (by decreasing frequency):

- Headache.
- Seizure.
- Cognitive/personality changes.
- Focal weakness.
- Nausea/vomiting.
- Speech abnormalities.
- Altered consciousness.

Common signs (by decreasing frequency):

- Hemiparesis.
- Cranial nerve palsies.
- Papilledema.
- Cognitive dysfunction.
- Sensory deficits.
- Hemianesthesia.
- Hemianopia.
- Dysphasia (Fig. 1).

DIFFERENTIAL DIAGNOSIS

Tumors of the cerebrum may be differentiated by location according to age at onset of symptoms (Table 2).

Acute Complications of Intracranial Tumors

As the skull's rigid nature does not allow for processes associated with intracranial expansion, brain lesions routinely result in structural displacement and life-threatening consequences. Following the path of least resistance, tentorial or foramen magnum herniation may ensue. Neurologic findings are described in Tables 3 and 4.

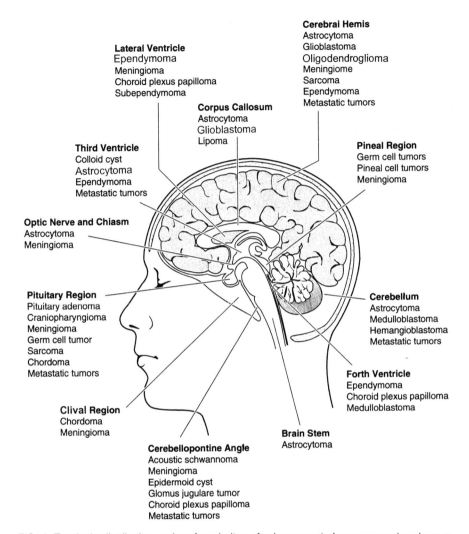

Cerebral Hemis
Astrocytoma
Glioblastoma
Oligodendroglioma
Meningiome
Sarcoma
Ependymoma
Metastatic tumors

Lateral Ventricle
Ependymoma
Meningioma
Choroid plexus papilloma
Subependymoma

Corpus Callosum
Astrocytoma
Glioblastoma
Lipoma

Pineal Region
Germ cell tumors
Pineal cell tumors
Meningioma

Third Ventricle
Colloid cyst
Astrocytoma
Ependymoma
Metastatic tumors

Optic Nerve and Chiasm
Astrocytoma
Meningioma

Pituitary Region
Pituitary adenoma
Craniopharyngioma
Meningioma
Germ cell tumor
Sarcoma
Chordoma
Metastatic tumors

Cerebellum
Astrocytoma
Medulloblastoma
Hemangioblastoma
Metastatic tumors

Forth Ventricle
Ependymoma
Choroid plexus papilloma
Medulloblastoma

Clival Region
Chordoma
Meningioma

Brain Stem
Astrocytoma

Cerebellopontine Angle
Acoustic schwannoma
Meningioma
Epidermoid cyst
Glomus jugulare tumor
Choroid plexus papilloma
Metastatic tumors

FIG. 1. Topologic distribution and preferred sites of primary central nervous system tumors. From Burger PC, Scheithauer BW, Vogel FS. *Surgical pathology of the nervous system and its coverings.* 3rd ed. New York: Churchill Livingstone, 1991, with permission.

TABLE 2. *Differential diagnosis*

Location	Adult	Child
Supratentorial	Metastatic disease	Astrocytoma
	Glioblastoma	Glioblastoma
	Astrocytoma	Oligodendroglioma
	Meningioma	Sarcoma
	Oligodendroglioma	Neuroblastoma
	Mixed glioma	Mixed glioma
Infratentorial	Metastatic disease	Astrocytoma
	Astrocytoma	Medulloblastoma
	Glioblastoma	Ependymoma
	Ependymoma	Brainstem glioma
	Brainstem glioma	
Sellar/parasellar	Pituitary tumor	Craniopharyngioma
	Meningioma	Optic glioma
		Epidermoid
Base of skull	Neurinoma	
	Meningioma	
	Chordoma	
	Carcinoma	
	Dermoid/epidermoid	

TABLE 3. *Neurologic findings*

Tentorial/temporal lobe herniation
Pupillary dilatation
Ptosis
Ipsilateral hemiplegia
Contralateral hemiplegia
Homonymous hemianopia
Midbrain syndrome
Coma with rising blood pressure/bradycardia

TABLE 4. *Neurologic findings*

Cerebellar/foramen magnum herniation
Head tilt
Stiff neck
Neck paresthesias
Tonic tensor spasms of limbs and body
Coma
Respiratory arrest

PRIMARY BRAIN TUMORS

Gliomas

Three major types of gliomas have been recognized according to the existing types of glial cells:

- Astrocytes.
- Oligodendrocytes.
- Ependymal cells.

TABLE 5. *Epidemiology*

Type	Percentage
Glioblastoma	55
Astrocytoma	20.5
Ependymoma	6.0
Medulloblastoma	6.0
Oligodendroglioma	5.0
Choroid plexus papilloma	2.0
Colloid cyst	2.0

Epidemiology

Gliomas comprise 45% of all intracranial tumors with peak age in the seventh decade. The frequency of the pathologic subtypes is shown in Table 5 in relation to other more common primary brain tumors.

Grading

A pathologic grading system proposed by the World Health Organization (WHO) incorporated the following criteria:

- Cellular atypia.
- Mitotic activity.
- Degree of cellularity.
- Vascular proliferation.
- Degree of necrosis.

Grade I, none of above.
Grade II, one feature.
Grade III, two features.
Grade IV, three or more features or any two plus necrosis.

Accordingly, gliomas can be graded as:

Grade 1
- Pilocytic astrocytoma.
- Giant cell astrocytoma.
- Ganglioglioma.
- Dysembryoplastic neuroepithelial tumors.

Grade 2
- Well-differentiated low-grade astrocytomas.
- Oligodendrogliomas.
- Ependymomas.

Grade 3
- Anaplastic astrocytomas (AAs).
- Anaplastic oligodendrogliomas.
- Anaplastic ependymal tumors.

Grade 4
- Glioblastoma multiforme (GBM).
- Embryonal tumors.

TABLE 6. *Molecular genetics of gliomas*

Genetic alteration	Anaplasia	Glioma variant
TP53 mutation	Low grade	Low-grade astrocytoma
PDGF overexpression		
Loss of chromosome 17p and 22q		
CDKN2/p16 deletion		Anaplastic astrocytoma
RB mutation		
CDK4 amplification		
Loss of chromosome 9p, 19q, 11p		
MDM2 amplification/overexpression	High grade	GBM
EGFR amplification rearrangements		
PTEN mutation		
Loss of chromosome 10		

GBM, glioblastoma multiforme.

Molecular Genetics of Gliomas

Genetic alterations form a continuum of progressive anaplasia in gliomas (Table 6). Whereas secondary or progressive gliomas seldom show epidermal growth factor receptor (EGFR) amplification, primary or *de novo* glioblastoma multiforme (GBM) usually lack TP 53 mutations and contain an amplified EGFR. However, none of the molecular parameters has demonstrated any significant association with patient survival in GBM.

Glioblastoma Multiforme

- Most common adult supratentorial neoplasm, 10% to 15% of intracranial tumors.
- Peak incidence, age 45 to 55 years; overall, two to three per 100,000; sex distribution, male/female = 3:2.
- Median survival, 6 months.

Localization

- Mostly frontal lobe.
- Characteristic bihemispheric presentation with "butterfly" distribution.

Development

Development is *de novo* or as a progression from a lower grade precursor lesion.

Genetics

- p53 mutations.
- EGFR amplification.
- Loss of heterozygosity (LOH) chromosome 10.
- LOH chromosome 17p.

Imaging Characteristics on MRI

- Heterogeneous mass with contrast enhancement.
- Hypervascular appearance.
- Calcifications rare.

- Poorly identified tumor margins.
- Multifocal in 5%.

Differential Diagnosis

- Brain metastasis.
- Radiation necrosis.
- Single photon emission CT (SPECT) and MR cerebral perfusion imaging may be used to distinguish radiation necrosis (hypovascular) from recurrence (hypervascular).

Gliosarcoma is a variant with a mesenchymal component and a greater tendency for dural invasion, cerebrospinal fluid (CSF) seeding, and distant metastasis. GBM characteristically appears infiltrative within brain parenchyma and may cross layers (dura, leptomeninges, ependyma, subarachnoid space), but rarely shows extracerebral metastasis.

Therapy

Current treatment recommendations for malignant gliomas (i.e., high-grade astrocytomas and GBM) include surgical resection, adjuvant radiotherapy, and in selected patients, the addition of chemotherapy. Because of the infiltrative growth characteristics of malignant gliomas, the majority of tumors recur even after gross total primary resection.

An analysis of several Radiation Therapy Oncology Group (RTOG) trials was able to create the survival categories by patient characteristics shown in Table 7.

Radiation therapy has demonstrated a clear survival benefit in several randomized clinical trials, increasing the median survival from 20 to 36 weeks. Irradiation usually includes the contrast-enhanced tumor volume or peritumoral edema with a margin of 2 to 3 cm. A total dose of 60 Gy is delivered in 30 to 33 fractions. Palliative courses provide treatment to 30 Gy in 10 fractions over 2 weeks.

The role of chemotherapy in the treatment of malignant gliomas was established by the Brain Tumor Study Group (BTSG) in several phase III trials, introducing nitrosoureas as effective agents. At a carmustine (BCNU) dose of 80 mg/m^2 given daily for 3 days, repeated every 6 weeks, median survival increased from 38 to 51 weeks in patients with GBM. The role of multiagent chemotherapy versus single-agent therapy with BCNU remains controversial. The most commonly used regimen is PCV (Table 8), which has demonstrated durable responses of more than 50% in anaplastic oligodendrogliomas. Anaplastic astrocytomas, mixed gliomas, and recurrent oligodendrogliomas also have shown favorable responses to this regimen.

New treatment strategies are shown in Table 9. Other treatment strategies currently under investigation include farnesyl-transferase inhibitors, gene therapy, antisense oligonucleotides,

TABLE 7. *Survival categories by patient characteristics*

Patient characteristics	Tumor	Median survival (mo)
Age <50 yr, normal mental status Age >50 yr, KPS >70, symptoms >3 mo	Anaplastic astrocytoma	40–60
Age <50 yr, abnormal mental status Age >50 yr, symptoms <3 mo	Anaplastic astrocytoma	11–18
Age <50 yr Age >50 yr, KPS >70	Glioblastoma	11–18
Age >50 yr, KPS <70 or abnormal mental status	Glioblastoma	5–9

KPS, Karnofsky performance status.

TABLE 8. *PCV regimen: Procarbazine, lomustine (CCNU), vincristine*

Procarbazine, 60 mg/m^2 per day p.o. for 14 days, on cycle days 8–21 (d 8–21;
  total dose/cycle, 840 mg/m^2)
Lomustine (CCNU), 110 mg/m^2 p.o. day 1 (d 1; total dose/cycle, 110 mg/m^2)
Vincristine, 1.4 mg/m^2 per dose i.v. on days 8 and 29 (d 8 and 29; total dose/cycle, 2.8
  mg/m^2)
Cycle duration is 6 weeks; may be extended to 8 weeks for hematologic recovery

From Levin VA, Silver P, Hannigan J, et al. Superiority of post-radiotherapy adjuvant chemotherapy with CCNU, procarbazine, and vincristine (PCV) over BCNU for anaplastic astrocytoma: NCOG 6G61 final report. *Int J Radiat Oncol Biol Phys* 1990;18:321–324, with permission.

and adoptive immunotherapy. A main prognostic factor for treatment outcome and survival is age at diagnosis.

Astrocytoma

Astrocytomas compose 25% to 30% of all hemispheric gliomas.

Low-grade Diffuse Astrocytoma

- Grade II.
- Approximately 5% of primary brain tumors.
- Mean age, 34 years.
- Distribution: mostly cerebral hemispheres but also brainstem.
- Imaging characteristics on MRI:
  - Little edema/mass effect.
  - Difficult to distinguish from nonmalignant infarct/cerebritis/demyelination.
  - Rare calcifications.
  - Large area of white/gray matter changes.
  - Differential diagnosis: infarct, cerebritis.

TABLE 9. *New treatment strategies*

	Study	Response	Tumor	Comment
Chemotherapy				
Temozolomide	Phase I/II	PR 9–43%	AA, GBM	
Irinotecan	Phase I/II	PR 12–20%	AA, GBM	Now in phase II
Topotecan	Phase II	PR 10%	AA, GBM	Excellent BBB penetration
Oxaliplatin	Phase I/II	PR 33%, CR 11%	GBM	Small numbers
Biologic therapy				
Tamoxifen	Phase I/II	PR 0–80%	AA, GBM	Dose dependence
Antiangiogenesis				
Marimastat	Phase III	Pending	Malig. glioma	MMP inhibitor
Thalidomide	Phase II	PR 2/32	Malig. glioma	
Drug delivery				
RMP-7	Phase II	Surv. hazard ratio 2	Malig. glioma	Increases BBB penetration for carboplatin

AA, anaplastic astrocytoma; GBM, glioblastoma multiforme; BBB, blood–brain barrier.

Median survival after surgery of 19% to 32% at 5 years, and 10% at 10 years are surpassed by 36% to 55% after 5 years and 26% to 43% after 10 years for patients treated with surgery and postoperative irradiation. Radiation doses of greater than 53 Gy appear to improve survival. Pilocytic astrocytoma can be cured, with long-term survival, by complete surgical therapy alone. It represents the most common childhood astrocytic tumor. Clinically and histopathologically it is distinct from diffuse fibrillary astrocytoma of adulthood. Frequent association with neurofibromatosis-1 (NF1) has been noted. Several trials are ongoing, but the role of chemotherapy has not been established. The combination of radiosensitizers with postradiation PCV chemotherapy in small studies has shown improved survival rates.

High-grade Diffuse Astrocytoma

- Grade III.
- Approximately 5% of primary brain tumors; mean age, 41 years.
- Macroscopically indistinguishable from low-grade astrocytomas.
- Survival, 2 to 5 years.

Therapy

Early trials established the role of postoperative radiation therapy at a dose of approximately 60 Gy, increasing median survival times from 14 to 36 weeks. The introduction of postoperative chemotherapy with nitrosourea-based regimens like PCV significantly increased survival, particularly in anaplastic astrocytoma, with 50% of patients alive at 157 weeks.

Cerebellar Astrocytomas

- Predominantly younger than 20 years, mostly low-grade tumors, often pilocytic.
- Overall prognosis is better than that of cerebral astrocytomas.
- Primary therapy is surgery with curative intent of complete removal of the tumor via posterior fossa craniotomy. Irradiation of 50 to 60 Gy is used for incompletely resected tumors.

Brainstem Gliomas

Brainstem gliomas predominantly occur in the pediatric population as a group of diffuse fibrillary astrocytomas, comprising astrocytomas, glioblastomas, and ependymomas.

The clinical course is often malignant, with a typical initial unilateral presentation of cranial nerve VI and VII palsies.

Management

- Surgery: preferentially stereotactic needle biopsy for diagnosis. Complete resection is contraindicated because of localization of tumor.
- Radiation therapy: 60 to 72 Gy, with some evidence emerging that hyperfractionation may have a benefit in a subgroup of patients.
- Chemotherapy: regimens including lomustine (CCNU), PCV, 5-fluorouracil, and hydroxyurea have been tested without clear survival benefits.

Other Gliomas

Desmoplastic cerebral astrocytoma and desmoplastic infantile ganglioglioma are benign, large, superficial astrocytomas with often cystic appearances, typically in children during the first 2 years of life. Adult gangliogliomas are benign lesions that lack EGFR amplification or other genetic abnormalities characteristic of malignant gliomas.

Oligodendrogliomas and Oligoastrocytomas (Mixed Gliomas)

- Diffuse, mostly cerebral tumors; often appear with prominent areas of calcification on CT scan.
- From 5% to 10% of all gliomas, clinically and biologically closely related to diffuse fibrillary astrocytomas, uncommon.
- Better prognosis than astrocytomas: low-grade, mean survival, 10 years.
- Chemosensitive, particularly anaplastic oligodendroglioma; most promising regimen is PCV.
- May progress to grade III anaplastic oligodendroglioma/oligoastrocytoma or grade IV GBM.

Prognosis

- Pure oligodendrogliomas, 10-year survival, 46%.
- Mixed gliomas, 10-year survival, 33%.
- High-grade mixed gliomas, 10-year survival, 25%.

EPENDYMOMA

Ependymomas comprise a spectrum of tumors ranging from aggressive childhood intraventricular tumors to benign adult spinal cord lesions. Typical locations according to the cell of origin are the white matter surrounding the ventricular surface and the filum terminale.

Epidemiology

- From 2% to 7.8% of all CNS neoplasms.
- 75% benign.
- 50% occur before age 5 years.
- Intracranial tumors: 60% infratentorial, 40% supratentorial, with 50% intraventricular.
- Overall incidence of spinal seeding, approximately 7% to 15.7% for high-grade infratentorial lesions, increased in patients with uncontrolled primary lesions.

Imaging

CT and MRI scanning are considered adequate to make the anatomic diagnosis before treatment. Fourth ventricle calcifications are characteristic, but not diagnostic.

Management

Surgery

Survival benefit is noted only for complete resections confirmed by neuroimaging.

Radiotherapy

- Infratentorial ependymomas are treated to the entire posterior fossa.
- Supratentorial ependymomas are treated with wide local fields, margins of 2 to 3 cm.
- Treatment with 45 Gy, with 55- to 65-Gy boost to area of residual disease after surgery.
- Craniospinal irradiation for evidence of seeding by CSF cytology or radiographic studies or for anaplastic ependymoma.

Chemotherapy

Multiple chemotherapeutic regimens have been tested in recurrent and anaplastic ependymomas, with responses of 22% to 82% and time to progression of 3.8 to 21.6 months.

The role of chemotherapy in this disease remains investigational for older children and adults.

Prognosis

- Low-grade tumors: 5-year survival, 60% to 80%.
- Anaplastic ependymoma: 5-year survival, 10% to 47%.
- With surgery alone: long-term survival, 17% to 27%.
- Surgery plus radiation: long-term survival, 40% to 87%.
- Age is dominant prognostic factor; infants do poorly.

CHOROID PLEXUS TUMORS

These tumors mostly occur in ventricles; in adults, predominantly in the fourth ventricle. The spectrum ranges from aggressive supratentorial childhood tumors to benign cerebellopontine angle tumors of adulthood. An association with Li–Fraumeni syndrome and von Hippel–Lindau disease has been described.

Diagnosis

- Signs of increased intracranial pressure.
- Fourth ventricle focal findings: ataxia, nystagmus.
- Anaplastic histologic changes warrant CSF examination for increased risk of disseminated disease.

Management

Surgery

Complete resection is the goal.

Radiation Therapy/Chemotherapy

Radiation therapy has been used with some benefit for choroid plexus carcinoma and anaplastic tumors also in conjunction with chemotherapy. Combinations of doxorubicin, cyclophosphamide, vincristine, and nitrosoureas have been used, as well as intraventricular methotrexate and cytarabine. Studies to evaluate these approaches have not been performed.

MEDULLOBLASTOMA

Malignant, "small, blue, round cell tumor" of CNS.

Epidemiology

- Forms 25% of all pediatric tumors, found predominantly in posterior fossa in children.
- Rare in adults.
- From 30% to 50% isochromosome 17q.
- Associated with Gorlin syndrome, Turcot's syndrome.

Clinical Presentation

Most frequently, signs of increased intracranial pressure, also cerebellar and bulbar signs. From 20% to 50% have CSF dissemination at diagnosis, with 10% systemic metastasis, frequently to bone; 40% have brainstem infiltration.

Risk Stratification

• Average: localized disease at diagnosis, total or near-total resection achieved.
• High: disseminated disease and/or partial resection.

Imaging

Typically, contrast-enhancing posterior fossa midline lesion on CT or MRI, most frequently arising from cerebellar vermis.

Staging

• Chang staging system (Table 10) for posterior fossa medulloblastoma most widely used with prognostic significance.
• Evaluation according to size, local extension, presence of metastasis.
• CSF and spinal axis should be evaluated for metastasis with lumbar puncture and contrast-enhanced MRI scan.

Management

• Surgery: goal is complete resection.
• Radiation therapy: postoperative 35 Gy whole brain with 15- to 20 Gy boost to posterior fossa. Average-risk patients may be cured with radiation alone.
• In children with nondisseminated disease, evidence is emerging that 23.4 Gy to the craniospinal axis, supplemented by 31Gy local irradiation, in conjunction with vincristine, 1.5

TABLE 10. *Chang staging system*

Stage	Description
T1	Tumor <3 cm in diameter, limited to midline position in the vermis, the roof of the fourth ventricle, and less frequently to the cerebellar hemisphere
T2	Tumor >3 cm, further invading one adjacent structure or partially filling the fourth ventricle
T3a	Tumor invading two adjacent structures or completely filling the fourth ventricle with extension into aqueduct of Sylvius, foramen of Magendie, or foramen of Luschka, producing marked hydrocephalus
T3b	Tumor arising from the floor of the fourth ventricle or brainstem and filling the fourth ventricle
T4	Tumor further spreading through the aqueduct of Sylvius to involve the third ventricle or midbrain, or extending to the upper spinal cord
M0	No evidence of gross subarachnoid or hematogenous metastasis
M1	Microscopic tumor cells found in cerebrospinal fluid
M2	Gross nodule seedings demonstrated in cerebellar cerebral subarachnoid space or in the third or lateral ventricles
M3	Gross nodule seedings in the spinal subarachnoid space
M4	Extraneuraxial metastasis

mg/m^2 for eight doses, followed by adjuvant lomustine (CCNU), 75 mg/m^2 p.o., and cis-platin, 75 mg/m^2 i.v. every 6 weeks, with vincristine weekly × 3 for six cycles total, showed equivalent overall survival compared with using a regimen including 36-Gy craniospinal radiation, with less long-term intellectual sequelae. Progression-free survival at 5 years was 79%.
- Chemotherapy most commonly used: adjuvant lomustine (CCNU), 75 mg/m^2 p.o.; cisplatin, 75 mg/m^2 i.v. every 6 weeks; vincristine, 1.5 mg/m^2 weekly during radiation for eight doses, and then weekly × 3 during adjuvant chemotherapy cycles.

Prognosis

Progression-free survival after chemotherapy and radiation:

- High risk: 25% to 85%.
- Average risk (localized, posterior fossa disease): 65% to 91%.

MENINGIOMAS
Epidemiology

Common, composing up to 39% of primary CNS tumors, usually benign.

Genetics

- Monosomy 22, with frequent mutation of *NF2* gene on 22q.
- Malignant meningiomas frequently show loss of 1p, 10, 14q.
- Predisposition: Female sex, ionizing irradiation, NF2, breast carcinoma.

Clinical Presentation

- Most common areas of presentation are parasagittal, cerebral convexity, and sphenoidal ridge.
- Signs and symptoms: seizures, hemiparesis, visual field loss, and other focal findings.

Management
Surgery

- Treatment goal is complete resection.
- Surgical mortality, 7% to 14%.
- 10-year survival rate, 43% to 77%.
- Recurrence rate after complete resection, 7% at 5 years, 20% at 10 years.

Radiotherapy

- Adjuvant irradiation reduces recurrence after subtotal resection by 30%, increases median time to recurrence from 5 to 10 years.
- In benign meningiomas, increase of 10-year survival with adjuvant irradiation from 50% to 80%.
- Malignant meningiomas: mean survival increases from 7.1 months after resection to 5.1 years with adjuvant radiation.
- 20% recurrence reduction with adjuvant irradiation after complete resection.
- Dosing: benign, 54 Gy in 1.8- to 2.0 Gy fractions; malignant, dose increase to 60 Gy.

PRIMARY BRAIN LYMPHOMA

Intracerebral lymphoma most frequently presents as parenchymal lymphoma; however, other anatomic sites such as the eye, meninges, or ependymal nodules may be found.

Primary CNS lymphoma is a rare tumor, accounting for fewer than 2% of all primary brain tumors. There has been a dramatic increase in the frequency of this tumor over the last few decades in immunocompetent patients, currently exceeding the incidence rate of NHL per year.

Risk Factors

• Acquired immunodeficiency syndrome (AIDS).
• Immunosuppression for organ transplantation.
• Autoimmune disease.
• Congenital immunodeficiencies like Wiscott–Aldrich syndrome.

Clinical Presentation

• Symptoms of intracranial mass with headaches, signs of increased intracranial pressure (ICP).
• Frontal lobe is most frequently involved site, often multiple lesions; personality changes, decreased level of alertness are common.
• Multifocal disease; 42% leptomeningeal seeding at diagnosis.

Clinical Diagnosis

A tissue diagnosis is paramount.

Staging studies should include:

• MRI of brain with gadolinium.
• Lumbar puncture.
• Bone marrow examination.
• Ophthalmologic evaluation.
• Abdominal CT scan.
• Chest radiograph.

Management

Approximately 40% of tumors are highly steroid sensitive; therefore, steroids should be withheld if at all possible until a tissue diagnosis has been established. A ring-enhancing lesion that "disappears" after starting steroids is strongly suggestive of a CNS lymphoma.

Surgery

For confirmation of diagnosis, but without role in therapy.

Radiotherapy

Radiotherapy yields 80% clinical and radiographic complete response (CR), commonly dosed at 40 to 50 Gy to tumor; median survival, 12 to 18 months.

Chemotherapy

Chemotherapy is detailed in Table 11. Immunocompromised patients may benefit from chemotherapy, but generally tolerate therapy poorly.

TABLE 11. *Chemotherapy*

Regimen	Median survival (mo)	5-yr survival rate (%)
HD MTX	42	30
CHOP/CHOD	9.5–16	14 (3 yr)
MACOP-B	14	10 (3 yr)

CHOP, cyclophosphamide/Adriamycin/vincristine/prednisone; CHOD, cyclophosphamide/Adriamycin/vincristine/dexamethasone; MACOP-B, meclorethamine/Adriamycin/cyclophophamide/vincristine/prednisone/bleomycin; HD MTX, high-dose methotrexate.

GERM CELL TUMORS

Epidemiology

CNS germ cell tumors (GCTs) are typically located in the pineal region. The most common histologic type is germinoma, composing 30% to 50% of all pineal tumors. Overall, however, this group of tumors represents a rare subgroup of less than 1% of all intracranial tumors.

Diagnosis

As the pineal region involves an area close to the center of the brain, symptoms are generally related to increased ICP and ocular pathway cranial nerve palsies.

- Obstructive hydrocephalus: headache, nausea, vomiting, lethargy.
- Cranial nerve palsies: diplopia, upward-gaze paralysis.
- Serum tumor marker elevations: α-fetoprotein (AFP), β-human chorionic gonadotropin (bHCG), placental alkaline phosphatase (PLAP).

Management

Surgery

- Microsurgical infratentorial supracerebellar approach or supratentorial under occipital lobe to establish diagnosis and attempt resection in radioresistant tumors.

Radiation therapy

Germinomas are exquisitely radiosensitive.

- Localized germinomas: 24 Gy to ventricular system, 26 Gy to tumor.
- Disseminated germinoma: 20 to 35 Gy to craniospinal axis in addition to systemic chemotherapy.
- Nongerminomatous germ cell tumors: after chemotherapy. Localized tumors: 24 Gy to ventricular system, 54- to 60-Gy boost to tumor. Disseminated tumors: craniospinal irradiation with 54 to 60 Gy to tumor, 45 Gy to ventricles, 35 Gy to spinal cord.

Chemotherapy

- Used primarily for nonseminomatous GCTs.
- Commonly used regimens include cisplatin/etoposide/bleomycin (PEB), carboplatin/etoposide/vinblastine in doses used for extragonadal germ cell tumors.
- Teratoma: treatment primarily surgical, possibly with radiation.

Prognosis

Germinomas: 5-year survival greater than 80% with radiation only.

Nonseminomatous GCT:

- The 5-year survival with small resection/radiation: less than 25%.
- With multimodality treatment, 5-year survival approximately 60% overall.
- Low survival for mixed germ cell tumors.
- High survival in mature teratomas.

BRAIN METASTASES

Epidemiology

Brain metastases represent the most frequent intracranial malignancy. With an estimated incidence of 80,000 to 170,000 cases per year in the U.S., compared with 17,000 to 20,000 newly diagnosed primary brain tumors, the importance of diagnosis and management of this disease is well understood.

From 10% to 30% of adults and 6% to 10% of children with cancer develop brain metastases, with lung and breast cancers being the most common primary cancers in adults. In pediatric metastatic brain disease, sarcomas, neuroblastomas, and germ cell tumors appear to be most common (Tables 12–15).

TABLE 12. *Frequency of brain metastases*

Primary tumor	Frequency (%)
Lung cancer	50
Breast cancer	15–20
Unknown primary	19–15
Melanoma	10
Colon cancer	5

TABLE 13. *Distribution by location*

Location	Frequency (%)
Hemispheres	80
Cerebellum	15
Brainstem	5

TABLE 14. *Diagnosis: clinical signs*

Sign	Frequency (%)
Hemiparesis	44
Mental status changes	35
Gait ataxia	13
Hemisensory loss	9
Papilledema	9

TABLE 15. *Diagnosis: clinical symptoms*

Symptom	Frequency (%)
Headache	42
Mental changes	31
Focal deficit	27
Seizure	20
Gait ataxia	17
Speech disturbance	10
Sensory problems	6

Differential Diagnosis

- Primary brain tumors.
- Abscess.
- Demyelination.
- Cerebral infarction.
- Cerebral hemorrhage.
- Progressive multifocal leukoencephalopathy.
- Radiation necrosis.

The false-positive rate for single brain metastasis is approximately 11%. Nonmetastatic brain lesions are equally divided between primary brain tumors and infections. In patients with primary breast cancer with a dural-based brain lesion, meningioma must be considered, as the frequency of this primary brain tumor is increased in breast cancer.

Imaging

Contrast-enhanced MRI is the diagnostic imaging modality of choice. Features on MRI that favor the diagnosis of brain metastasis include:

- Multiple lesions.
- Location at gray–white matter junction.
- Low degree of margin irregularity.
- High ratio of vasogenic edema to tumor size.

If imaging modalities and clinical history do not provide sufficient information to render a diagnosis, a biopsy of the lesion is indicated.

Brain Metastasis with Unknown Primary

A chest radiograph should be obtained in any patient with a new brain mass, as 60% of patients with brain metastasis of unknown primary have a lung mass from a pulmonary malignancy or pulmonary metastasis of a primary in a different location. A CT scan of the chest significantly increases the likelihood of finding a lung mass if the chest radiograph is nondiagnostic.

To determine the extent of metastatic disease, CT scans of abdomen and pelvis and a bone scan should be performed.

Management

Symptomatic Therapy

Reduction of symptomatic edema: Dexamethasone, 10 mg loading dose, followed by 4 mg four times a day.

- Symptomatic improvement should be expected within 24 to 72 hours.
- Imaging studies may not show a decrease of cerebral edema for up to 1 week.
- Steroid taper after completion of irradiation or earlier if cerebral edema minimal.

Seizure Management

Because infratentorial metastases carry a very low risk for seizures, anticonvulsant therapy is usually not indicated. The role of prophylactic anticonvulsant therapy remains controversial in unoperated-on patients with supratentorial brain metastasis without prior seizures. After seizure activity has occurred or a patient has undergone craniotomy, phenytoin therapy generally is initiated. Close monitoring is advised because dexamethasone and phenytoin mutually increase their clearance, and the number of reports suggesting a correlation between Stevens–Johnson syndrome and palliative whole-brain irradiation in patients taking phenytoin is increasing.

Surgery

Factors influencing the decision favoring surgical resection include:

- Extent of systemic disease.
- Neurologic status of patient.
- Number of cerebral metastases.
- Interval between diagnosis of primary cancer and occurrence of brain metastasis.
- Primary cancer.
- Location of tumor.

Single brain metastasis: Several controlled studies suggest a benefit of surgery combined with whole-brain irradiation for patients with single brain metastasis and stable extracranial disease.

Multiple brain metastases: For patients with multiple brain metastases, the role of surgery generally is limited to:

- Large, symptomatic, or life-threatening lesions.
- Tissue diagnosis in unknown primary.
- Differentiation of metastasis from primary brain tumor like meningioma.

The value of resection of multiple brain metastases with therapeutic intent has not been established.

Radiation Therapy

- Considered primary therapy for patients with brain metastasis.
- Whole-brain irradiation increases median survival to 3 to 6 months.
- Overall response rate, 64% to 85%.
- Cranial nerve deficit improvement, 40%.

Fractionation Schedule

- From 30 to 50 Gy in 1.5- to 4-Gy fractions.
- Most common: 30 Gy in 10 fractions over 2 weeks.
- Patients with good prognosis: more prolonged fractionation like 40 Gy in 2-Gy fractions may reduce long-term morbidity.

Postoperative Radiation Therapy

- A 62% reduction in treatment failure.
- A 30% reduction in risk of death from neurologic causes.

- No improvement of overall survival or duration of functional independence.
- Dosing: 50.4 Gy in 28 fractions.

Late Toxicities

- In patients receiving total dose of greater than 30 Gy, 11% dementia.
- Recommended dosing: 40 to 45 Gy in 1- to 2-Gy fractions.

Reirradiation

- Radiosurgery for patients with solitary or fewer than three metastases.
- Whole or partial brain irradiation for patients not eligible for radiosurgery/chemotherapy.
- Clinical response, 42% to 75%.
- Median survival, 3.5 to 5 months.
- Dosing schedules vary without established consensus.

Radiosurgery

Indications

- Young patient.
- Good performance status.
- Limited extracranial disease.
- One to two small lesions.
- Recurrent brain metastasis after whole-brain irradiation.

Adverse Prognostic Factors

- Poor performance status.
- Progressive systemic disease.
- Infratentorial location.
- Large tumor size.
- More than two lesions.

Interstitial Brachytherapy

For postsurgical treatment of residual tumor, may be indicated for metastases too large for radiosurgery.

Chemotherapy

In selected malignancies, brain metastases may show responses to systemic treatment of the underlying cancer.

Breast Cancer

Regimens including cyclophosphamide/5-fluorouracil/cisplatin (CFP), cyclophosphamide/methotrexate/5-fluorouracil (CMF), doxorubicin (Adriamycin)/cyclophosphamide (AC) have been used, generally directed at the systemic cancer. Responses are noted in 50% to 70% of cases. There appears to be a survival advantage for responders.

TABLE 16. *Prognosis*

	Median survival (mo)
Untreated brain metastasis	1
Addition of steroids	2
With whole-brain irradiation	3–6
Single metastasis, limited extracranial disease, surgery and whole-brain radiation	10–16

Small-cell Lung Cancer

Experience exists with regimens including etoposide and platinating agents. Overall response rates for primary brain metastasis approach 76%. Responses at CNS relapse decrease to 43%.

Prognostic Factors

- Karnofsky PS more than 70.
- Age <65 years.
- Controlled primary disease.
- No extracranial metastasis.

Median survival ranges from 2.3 to 7.1 months depending on the presence of good prognostic indicators (Table 16).

SELECTED REFERENCES

1. Ahmed Rasheed BK, Wiltshire RN, Bigner SH, et al. Molecular pathogenesis of malignant gliomas. *Curr Opin Oncol* 1999;11:162–167.
2. Avgeropoulos NG, Batchelor TT. New treatment strategies for malignant gliomas. *Oncologist* 1999;4:209–224.
3. Black PM. Meningiomas. *Neurosurgery* 1993;31:643–657.
4. DeVita VT Jr, Hellman S, Rosenberg SA, eds. *Cancer: principles and practice of oncology.* 5th ed. Philadelphia: Lippincott-Raven, 1997.
5. Davey P. Brain metastases. *Curr Probl Cancer* 1999;23:59–98.
6. Haskell CM, ed. *Cancer treatment.* 4th ed. Philadelphia: WB Saunders, 1995.
7. Hoffman HJ. Brain stem gliomas. *Clin Neurosurg* 1997;44:549–558.
8. Kyritsis AP, Yung WKA, Bruner JB, et al. The treatment of anaplastic oligodendrogliomas and mixed gliomas. *Neurosurgery* 1993;32:365–370.
9. Levin VA, Silver P, Hannigan J, et al. Superiority of post-radiotherapy adjuvant chemotherapy with CCNU, procarbazine, and vincristine (PCV) over BCNU for anaplastic astrocytoma: NCOG 6G61 final report. *Int J Radiat Oncol Biol Phys* 1990;18:321–324.
10. Maldjian JA, Patel RS. Cerebral neoplasms in adults. *Semin Roentgenol* 1999;34:102–122.
11. Newton HB, Turowski RC, Stroup TJ. Clinical presentation, diagnosis, and pharmacotherapy of patients with primary brain tumors. *Ann Pharmacother* 1999;33:816–832.
12. Packer RJ. Brain tumors in children. *Arch Neurol* 1999;56:421–425.
13. Packer RJ, Goldwein J, Nicholson HS, et al. Treatment of children with medulloblastomas with reduced-dose craniospinal radiation therapy and adjuvant chemotherapy: a Children's Cancer Group study. *J Clin Oncol* 1999;17:2127–2136.
14. Pech IV, Peterson K, Cairncross JG. Chemotherapy for brain tumors. *Oncology* 1998;12:537–547.
15. Pizzo PA, Poplack DG, eds. *Principles and practice of pediatric oncology.* 3rd ed. Philadelphia: Lippincott-Raven, 1997.
16. Schiffer D. Classification and biology of astrocytic gliomas. *Forum* 1998;8:244–255.
17. Perez CA, Brady LW, eds. *Principles and practice of radiation oncology.* 3rd ed. Philadelphia: Lippincott-Raven, 1998.

18. Schild SE, Haddock MG, Scheithauer BW, et al. Nongerminomatous germ cell tumors of the brain. *Int J Radiat Oncol Biol Phys* 1996;36:557–563.
19. Sanford RA, Gajjar A. Ependymomas. *Clin Neurosurg* 1997;44:559–570.
20. Tomlinson FH, Kurtin PJ, Suman VJ, et al. Primary intracerebral malignant lymphoma: a clinico-pathologic study of 89 patients. *J Neurosurg* 1995;82:558–566.
21. Wen PY, Loeffler JS. Management of brain metastases. *Oncology* 1999;13:941–961.
22. Shaw EG, Daumas-Duport C, Scheithauer BW, et al. Radiation therapy in the management of low-grade supratentorial astrocytomas. *J Neurosurg* 1989;70:853–861.

34

Endocrine Tumors

Jame Abraham and Tito Fojo

Medicine Branch, DCS, National Cancer Institute, National Institutes of Health, Bethesda, Maryland

Endocrine tumors are relatively uncommon. They are often difficult to diagnose and treat effectively. As per American Cancer Society (ACS) data, 20,200 new endocrine cancers will be diagnosed in 2000, and 2,100 patients will die of the disease.

In this chapter we discuss:

1. Thyroid cancer.
2. Cancer of the parathyroid gland.
3. Adrenocortical cancer.
4. Pheochromocytoma.
5. Pancreatic endocrine tumors (PET).
6. Carcinoid tumors.
7. Multiple endocrine neoplasia (MEN).

Epidemiology is outlined in Table 1.

THYROID CANCER

Cancer of the thyroid gland is rare. Papillary carcinoma of the thyroid is the most common form of thyroid cancer. It is one of the least aggressive cancers in humans, but anaplastic thyroid carcinoma is one of the most aggressive cancers in human beings.

Epidemiology

About 18,400 cases of thyroid carcinoma will have been diagnosed in the United States in 2000, and the estimated number of deaths is 1,200. Incidence of thyroid cancer is twice as high in women as in men. Over the past 20 years, incidence of thyroid carcinoma increased by 21%, whereas the mortality decreased by 23%. Peak incidence is in the third and fourth decades.

In solitary and multinodular goiter, the prevalence of thyroid cancer is 10% to 15%.

Pathogenesis

Oncogenes

- Rearrangements of the tyrosine kinase domains of the *RET* and *TRK* genes with the amino terminal sequence of an unlinked gene are found in some papillary carcinomas.
- *RET* rearrangements are found in 3% to 33% of the papillary carcinomas unassociated with irradiation and in 60% to 80% of those occurring after radiation.

TABLE 1. *Incidence and proportion of all endocrine cancers*

Type	Number	% of total
All endocrine cancers		
Thyroid	13,900	87
Endocrine pancreas	800	5
Adrenal	550	3.4
Thymus	425	2.6
Pineal gland	128	0.8
Pituitary gland	77	0.5
Parathyroid	65	0.4
Carotid body or paraganglia	33	0.2

From references 1 and 3, with permission.

Radiation

- External radiation administered in childhood for benign conditions of the head and neck increases the risk for papillary carcinoma.
- Latency period is at least 5 years, and risk is maximal at about 20 years and then decreases gradually.
- High incidence of malignancy is reported at a dose of 200 to 1,000 rads, and at greater than 2,000 rads, the risk is low.
- The risk is not increased in patients given iodine-131 for diagnostic or therapeutic purposes.

Other Factors

- Where iodine intake is adequate, well differentiated carcinomas account for more than 80% of all thyroid carcinomas, with papillary histology being more frequent (60–80% of cases).
- High incidence of medullary thyroid carcinoma is seen in MEN-II.

Pathology

Clinical features (Table 2)

- Usually presents as an asymptomatic thyroid nodule.
- Can present as a dominant nodule in a multinodular goiter.

TABLE 2. *Pathology of thyroid cancer*

Well Differentiated
   Papillary
   Follicular
Moderately Differentiated
   Papillary variants
      Tall cell
      Columnar
      Diffuse sclerosis
   Hurthle cell carcinoma
Poorly differentiated/undifferentiated
   Anaplastic thyroid carcinoma
Medullary thyroid carcinoma
Lymphoma
Sarcoma and others

- Bilateral discrete nodules suggest familial medullary thyroid carcinoma (especially in a setting of MEN).
- Anaplastic carcinoma may present as a fixed or rapidly enlarging tumor with symptoms of hoarseness, dysphagia, stridor, or neck pain.
- Metastatic disease:
  - Occurs in 4% of papillary carcinomas.
  - From 16% to 33% of follicular carcinomas.
  - Sites of metastatic disease are lung, lymph nodes, bone, contralateral thyroid lobe, and adjacent cervical structures.

Diagnostic Workup

History and physical examination.

- Women develop nodules more frequently than men.
- Risk of malignancy:
  - Men have a higher risk for malignancy.
  - Overall risk for malignancy is 5% to 10%.
  - Risk with history of thyroid radiation is 35%.
- High-risk lesions:
  - Solitary nodule/dominant nodule/change in nodule.
  - Rapid increase in size.
  - Pain.
  - Hoarseness.
  - Horner's syndrome.
  - Dyspnea.
  - Dysphagia.

Fine-needle aspiration (FNA)

- The single most important study is the evaluation of a thyroid nodule.
- Accuracy of cytologic diagnosis from FNA is between 70–97%.
- Any thyroid nodule more than 1.5 cm should be evaluated with an FNA.
- If the lesion is solid, cytology results can be:
  - Benign.
  - Malignant or suggestive.
  - Indeterminate.
- Complete further evaluation as per the algorithm (Fig. 1).

Radiologic studies

- **Ultrasound scan:**
  - To differentiate cystic from solid.
  - To diagnose multinodular goiter and to identify the dominant lesion.
- **Thyroid scans** with radioiodine are used to differentiate "cold" nodule (that does not take up radioiodine) from "hot" nodule (that concentrates radioiodine).
  - Of the cold nodules, 10% are malignant.
  - It is not necessary to operate on all cold nodules.
  - Hot nodules essentially excludes malignancy.

Laboratory tests

- **Calcitonin:**
  - It is used as a tumor marker in medullary carcinoma of the thyroid.

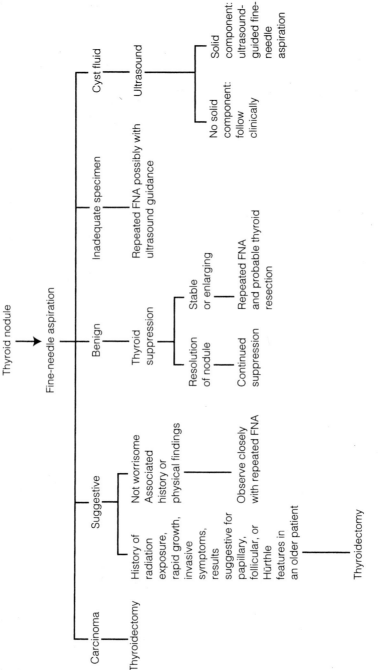

FIG. 1. Algorithm for evaluation of solitary thyroid nodule.

- It is a specific product of thyroid C cells (parafollicular cells).
- In medullary carcinoma, calcitonin level is always elevated.
- **Carcinoembryonic antigen (CEA)** is elevated in medullary and anaplastic thyroid carcinoma.
- Other tests like serum thyroxine and thyroid-stimulating hormone (TSH) may not be helpful in distinguishing benign process from thyroid carcinoma.

Genetic testing: RET proto-oncogene.

- Germline mutations in the *RET* proto-oncogene cause familial non-MEN medullary thyroid carcinoma, MEN-IIA and MEN-IIB.
- DNA analysis of peripheral blood is a highly reliable method for identifying the presence of *RET* mutation.

Staging of Thyroid Cancer

See Table 3.

Papillary Carcinoma of the Thyroid

This is the most common type of thyroid carcinoma. Since iodine supplementation started in endemic areas, the incidence of papillary carcinoma has increased compared with that of follicular thyroid carcinoma.

- Papillary carcinoma is one of the least aggressive human cancers and has the best prognosis.
- It invades the lymphatics and causes metastatic spread to the regional lymph nodes and microscopic metastatic lesions in the gland.
- Some rare variants of papillary carcinoma are more aggressive:
  - Tall-cell variant.
  - Columnar variant.
  - Diffuse sclerosis variant.

Follicular Carcinoma

Constitutes 5% to 10% of the thyroid malignancies. Since the initiation of iodine prophylaxis, follicular carcinoma is diagnosed less frequently. Metastatic spread is through vascular invasion rather than lymphatic spread, and lymph node involvement is rare. It has a slightly worse prognosis than papillary thyroid carcinoma.

Prognostic Factors of Well-differentiated Thyroid Carcinoma

The overall survival rate at 10 years for middle-aged adults with thyroid carcinoma is about 80% to 95%. From 5% to 20% of the patients will have local or regional recurrences, and 10% to 15% will have distant metastatic disease.

The prognostic indicators for recurrent disease and death are the patient's age at the time of diagnosis, histologic subtype, and extent of the tumor (Table 4).

Treatment of Well-Differentiated Thyroid Carcinoma

Surgery.
Iodine-131.
Chemotherapy.
External radiation.
Thyroxine treatment.

TABLE 3. *Definition of TNM and Stage Grouping (AJCC)*

Primary tumor (T)

TX	Primary tumor cannot be assessed
T0	No evidence of primary tumor
T1	Tumor ≤1 cm in greatest dimension limited to the thyroid
T2	Tumor >1 cm but ≤4 cm in greatest dimension limited to the thyroid
T3	Tumor >4 cm in greatest dimension limited to the throid
T4	Tumor of any size extending beyond the thyroid capsule

Regional lymph nodes (N): the cervical and upper mediastinal lymph nodes

NX	Regional lymph nodes cannot be assessed	
N0	No regional lymph node metastasis	
N1	Regional lymph node metastasis	
	N1a	Metastasis in ipsilateral cervical lymph node(s)
	N1b	Metastasis in bilateral, midline, or contralateral cervical or mediastinal lymph node(s)

Distant metastasis (M)

MX	Distant metastasis cannot be assessed
M0	No distant metastasis
M1	Distant metastasis

Stage grouping: Separate stage groupings are recommended for papillary, follicular, medullary, or undifferentiated (anaplastic)

Papillary or follicular

	Under 45 years	45 years and older
Stage I	Any T, any N, M0	T1, N0, M0
Stage II	Any T, any N, M1	T2, N0, M0
Stage III		T3, N0, M0
		T4, N0, M0
		Any T, N1, M0
Stage IV		Any T, any N, M1

Medullary

Stage I	T1	N0	M0
Stage II	T2	N0	M0
	T3	N0	M0
	T4	N0	M0
Stage III	Any T	N1	M0
Stage IV	Any T	N1	M1

Undifferentiated (anaplastic): All cases are stage IV

Stage IV	Any T	Any N	Any M

All categories may be subdivided: (a) solitary tumor, (b) multifocal tumor (the largest determines the classification).

Surgery

- If lesion is less than 1.5 cm, lobectomy is appropriate.
- **Lobectomy:** contralateral lobe is not dissected, only examined for abnormalities.
- **Subtotal thyroidectomy:**
  - Leaves 2 to 4 g of the thyroid tissue of the upper part of the contralateral thyroid.
  - Preserves the recurrent laryngeal nerve and the blood supply to the upper parathyroid glands.
- **Near-total thyroidectomy:**
  - Leaves a much smaller portion of the thyroid tissue near the ligament of Berry.
  - Preserves the recurrent laryngeal nerve, but not the blood supply for the parathyroid glands.
- **Total thyroidectomy:**
  - Removes all thyroid tissue.
  - Can cause permanent hypocalcemia.

TABLE 4. *Schema for categorizing patients with well-differentiated thyroid cancer prognostic risk categories*

AMES: age, metastases, extent of primary cancer, tumor size
  Low risk/high risk
    Age: males <41 yr, females <51 yr/males >40 yr, females >50 yr
    Metastases: no distant metastases/distant metastases
    Extent: intrathyroidal papillary or follicular with minor capsule invasion/extrathyroidal
      papillary or follicular with major invasion
    Size: <5 cm/>5 cm
  Low-risk patients are (1) any low-risk age group without metastases or (2) high-risk age
    group without metastases and with low-risk extent and size
  High-risk patients are (1) any patient with metastases or (2) high-risk age group with either
    high-risk extent or size
DAMES: AMES system modified by tumor cell DNA content measured by flow cytometry
  Low-risk AMES + euploid = low risk
  Low-risk AMES + aneuploid = intermediate risk
  High-risk AMES + aneuploid = high risk
AGES: age, tumor grade, tumor extent, tumor size
  Prognostic score (PS) = 0.05 × age in years (except patients <40 y = 0), +1 (grade 2) or +3
    (grade 3 or 4), +1 (if extrathyroidal) or +3 (if distant metastases), +0.2 × tumor size in cm
    (maximum diameter)
  PS range: 0–11.65, median 2.6
  Risk categories: 0–3.99, 4–4.99, 5–5.99, >6
MACIS: metastasis, age, completeness of resection, invasion, size
  PS = 3.1 (age <39 yr) or 0.08 × age (if age >40), +0.3 × tumor size in cm, +1
    (if incompletely resected), +1 (if locally invasive), +3 (if distant metastases)
  PS risk categories: 0–5.99, 6–6.99, 7–7.99, >8

- The choice of surgery is a controversial topic.
- Prognostic factors (Table 4) can guide the surgeon in his decision making.

Iodine-131

Iodine-131 is used in papillary or follicular thyroid carcinoma for:

- Ablation of the normal residual thyroid tissue after thyroid surgery, thereby increasing the sensitivity of subsequent iodine-131 total body scanning and measurement of serum thyroglobulin for the presence of recurrent disease.
- Treatment of microscopic occult thyroid cancer in the neck or in the metastatic sites.
- No randomized study in the treatment of patients with well-differentiated thyroid cancer.
- Radioiodine treatment decreases cancer-related death, tumor recurrence, and development of distant metastases.
- The dose varies from 30 to 150 mCi.
- See Table 5 for indications for iodine-131 treatment after surgery.
- See Figure 2 for the recommended follow up of patient after total thyroid ablation.

Complications of Iodine-131 Treatment

- Sialadenitis.
- Nausea.
- Transient marrow suppression.
- Transient testicular dysfunction.
- Dose-dependent development of leukemia.

TABLE 5. *Indications for ablative treatment with iodine-131*
after surgery in patients with thyroid cancer

No indication
 Low risk of cancer-specific mortality and low risk of relapse
Indication
 Distant metastases
 Incomplete excision of tumor
 Complete excision of tumor but high risk of mortality associated with thyroid carcinoma
 Complete excision of tumor but high risk of relapse due to age (<16 or >45 yr), histologic
  subtype (tall cell, columnar cell, or diffuse sclerosing papillary variants; widely invasive or
  poorly differentiated follicular subtypes; Hürthle cell carcinomas), or extent of tumor (large
  tumor mass, extension beyond the thyroid capsule, or lymph node metastases)
 Elevated serum thyroglobulin concentration >3 mo after surgery

Chemotherapy

Chemotherapy has only a limited role. Doxorubicin has a response rate of 30% to 45%, and other single agents like VP-16, carboplatin, and cisplatin have response rates of 20% to 30%.

External Radiation

External-beam radiation therapy has only a limited role. It is indicated in patients with incomplete surgical resection and in tumors that do not take up iodine-131.

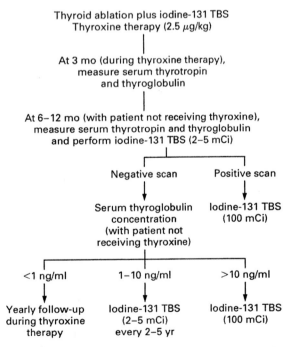

FIG. 2. Recommended follow-up of patients after total thyroid ablation, on the basis of serum thyroglobulin (assessment and iodine – 131Total Body Scanning (TBS) (from Ref.11).

Thyroxine Treatment

- The growth of the thyroid tumor cells is controlled by thyrotropin, and the inhibition of thyrotropin secretion with thyroxine improves the recurrence and survival rates.
- Thyroxine in the form of levothyroxine sodium should be given to all patients with thyroid carcinoma, whatever the extent of the surgery and other treatment.
- In patients without evidence of disease, keep the TSH level at below the normal range (0.5–5 mU/mL).
- In patients with disease, keep the TSH below 0.1 mU/mL.

Follow-up of Patients with Well-Differentiated Thyroid Carcinoma

The goals of follow-up after initial therapy are to maintain adequate thyroxine therapy and the detection of recurrent or persistent disease.

- Clinical examination for recurrent nodes in thyroid bed.
- Ultrasonography in patients with suggestive clinical findings and high risk.
- Serum thyroglobulin.

Thyroglobulin

- It is an important tumor marker in the follow-up of thyroid cancer (Fig. 2).
- After thyroidectomy and radioablation, it should be in the athyreotic range (undetectable).
- If there are detectable thyroglobulin levels after suppressive therapy, it is indicative of persistent or recurrent thyroid cancer.
  - Thyroxine can suppress thyroglobulin secretion and mask recurrent disease.
  - Test is more sensitive in the setting of thyroid hormone–suppressive therapy discontinuation and frank hypothyroidism.
- It may be more sensitive than whole-body scan in detecting cancer.

Medullary Thyroid Carcinoma

Incidence of medullary thyroid carcinoma is 5% to 9%. It arises from the parafollicular C cells, which produce calcitonin (which lowers serum calcium). Serum calcitonin is one of the most sensitive tumor markers in oncology. Medullary carcinoma is not associated with radiation exposure. It occurs with familial syndromes (most prominent clinical diagnosis in MEN-IIA and -IIB).

Diagnosis

- In sporadic cases, it can show symptoms of a mass in the thyroid.
- Advanced cases may have hoarseness, dysphagia, or cough.
- Patients with high levels of calcitonin may have secretory diarrhea.
- Most important tool in screening, diagnosis, and follow-up after the treatment is the basal and stimulated serum calcitonin.

Treatment

- Chemotherapy and external-beam radiation are ineffective.
- Total thyroidectomy with central nodal dissection is the treatment of choice.

Anaplastic Thyroid Cancer

- Form 1% to 3% of all thyroid cancer.

- Presents with rapidly growing mass, with invasion of trachea, larynx (stridor), recurrent laryngeal nerve (hoarseness), or esophagus (dysphagia).
- It is a very aggressive tumor with a median survival of 3 to 4 months.
- Most patients die of aggressive locoregional disease with upper airway obstruction or respiratory failure.
- Patients usually have prior or concurrent diagnosis of well-differentiated thyroid cancer or benign thyroid disease.

Treatment

- Options are limited and prognosis is extremely poor.
- **Surgery:** If technically possible, patients should be considered for aggressive local resection.
- **Radiation treatment:** After surgery, they should be considered for radiation therapy. Response rates are low.
- **Chemotherapy:** Doxorubicin is the single most effective agent.

CANCER OF THE PARATHYROID GLAND

Neoplasm of the parathyroid gland is a common endocrine problem, but parathyroid carcinoma is rare. Unlike other endocrine tumors, which become hypofunctional, parathyroid carcinoma is usually hyperfunctional. It presents with symptoms of hyperparathyroidism and accounts for 0.2% of hyperparathyroidism (Table 6). Serum parathyroid hormone (PTH) is an excellent tumor marker.

Clinical Features

Because all parathyroid carcinomas are hyperfunctional and produce unregulated high levels of PTH, they present with signs and symptoms of hormonal excess.

Treatment of Parathyroid Carcinoma

- Aggressive surgery with *en bloc* resection of recurrent laryngeal nerve, if necessary, is the only treatment option.
- Treatment of local recurrence is also surgical resection.

Metastatic Disease

- Nonsurgical treatment options are limited.
- Metastatic disease should also be considered for resection, especially in bone and lungs.

Radiation Therapy

- Should be used as a last resort.
- Response rate is very low.

Chemotherapy

- Has only a limited role.
- Agents used are dacarbazine, 5-fluorouracil (5-FU), and cyclophosphamide.

TABLE 6. *Comparison of the various causes of primary hyperparathyroidism*

Cause	Frequency (%)	Etiologic factors	Gender distribution	Age (yr)	Pathology	
					Gross	Microscopic
Adenoma	83–85	Radiation exposure	F > M (2–3:1)	55–61	Single enlarged soft red–brown gland	Nests of parathyroid chief cells; decreased cytoplasmic fat; possible rim at normal tissue
Hyperplasia	13	Familial in MEN 1 and MEN 2	M = F	25–40	Asymmetric enlargement with red–brown color of 4+ glands	Similar to adenomas Minimal intercellular fat
Carcinoma	<1	Familial Radiation exposure	M = F	45–50	Single large firm white/gray mass frequently invading thyroid or scrap muscle	Trabecular arrangement of tumor cells divided by fibrous bands. Mitotic figures present. Possible capsular, vascular, or adjacent structure invasion

Management of Hypercalcemia (see Chapter 39)

- Surgery if possible.
- Aggressive hydration and diuresis.
- Bisphosphonates are the medical treatment of choice.
- Other agents used with poor results are plicamycin and calcitonin.

ADRENAL CORTICAL CANCER

Adrenal cortical cancer (ACC) is a rare tumor with an incidence of 1 to 2 per million. ACC is more common in women, and functional tumors are seen more often in women. May occur in MEN-I patients. Usually seen in fourth/fifth decades. Adenomas of the adrenal gland are a common finding in routine CT scans. It is not easy to differentiate an adenoma from a carcinoma of the adrenal gland (Table 7).

Clinical Features

- Of the adrenocortical neoplasms, 50% have features of hormone hypersecretion.
- Cushing's syndrome.
- Virilizing or feminizing syndrome.
- Hyperaldosteronism.
- The combination of hirsutism, acne, amenorrhea, and rapidly progressing Cushing's syndrome in a young female is a typical presentation.

Diagnosis

- Made clinically and a pathologic diagnosis is difficult.
- Any patient in whom adrenocortical cancer is suspected, a computed tomography (CT) scan or magnetic resonance imaging (MRI) is indicated.
- Malignancy is diagnosed by the size (>5 cm) of the primary tumor or by evidence of metastatic disease.

Staging is addressed in Tables 8 and 9.

Treatment

Surgery

- Surgery is the treatment of choice at presentation.
- Should also be considered at relapse.
- Repeated surgical resections of the metastatic lesions have been shown to prolong survival in ACC.

TABLE 7. *Adrenal cortical carcinoma versus adenoma*

	Adenoma	Carcinoma
Size	<5 cm	>5 cm
Weight	<100 g	100–500 g
Nuclei	Normal	Polymorphic/hyperchromatic
Nucleoli	Normal	Large
Mitoses	Few	>20/hpf
Vascular invasion	Rare	Common
Lymphatic invasion	Rare	Common
Necrosis	Rare	Abundant
Fibrosis	Rare	Common

TABLE 8. *Staging of adrenocortical cancer*

Stage	Criteria
1	Tumor <5 cm
	Negative nodes
	No local invasion
	No metastases
2	Tumor >5 cm
	Negative nodes
	No local invasion
	No metastases
3	Positive nodes or local invasion
4	Positive nodes and local invasion or distant metastases

TABLE 9. *Sites of spread in stage 4 adrenocortical cancers*

Organ	Percentage
Lung	45
Liver	42
Lymph nodes	24
Bone	15
Pancreas	12
Spleen	6
Diaphragm	12
Miscellaneous (brain, peritoneum, skin, palate)	12

Chemotherapy

- **Mitotane (o,p-DDD)** is the only conventional treatment.
- Can improve excess hormone production without affecting the tumor size.
- Usual starting dose is 2 to 6 g/day (can be given as twice a day).
- Dose should be increased to achieve a therapeutic serum level of 15 mg/L.
- At higher doses, it has significant gastrointestinal toxicities and neurotoxicity.
- Retrospective studies report a response rate around 18% to 30% with mitotane.
- No impact on survival was documented with mitotane.

Other chemotherapy agents:

- Cisplatin, VP-16, and doxorubicin (Adriamycin) are used in combination with or without mitotane.
- Response rate is around 18% to 30%.
- Advantage over mitotane is not clear.

Radiation Therapy

- Has only a limited role.
- Mainly used for palliation.

PHEOCHROMOCYTOMA

These are rare tumors arising from the chromaffin cells in the adrenal medulla (90%) and elsewhere (10%). Most of the tumors are not malignant (10–40%). Extraadrenal tumors are

TABLE 10. *Clinical features*

Mild labile hypertension to malignant hypertension
Myocardial infarction
Cerebrovascular accident
Classic pattern of paroxysmal hypertension occurs in 30%–50% of cases
Spells of paroxysmal headache
Pallor or flushing
Tremor
Apprehension
Palpitation
Hypertension
Diaphoresis

TABLE 11. *Benign versus malignant*

	Benign	Malignant
Weight	<200 g	>500 g
Mitoses	Few	Many
Ploidy	Diploid	Aneuploid
Necrosis	Some	More
Metastases	Never	Frequent
Neuropeptide Y	Yes	±

usually cancerous. Of the pheochromocytomas, 10% occur with endocrine and nonendocrine inherited disorders like MEN-IIA, MEN-IIB (nonmalignant), and as part of Von Hippel–Lindau disease and von Recklinghausen's disease (Tables 10 and 11).

Malignant Pheochromocytoma

Approximately 10% of pheochromocytomas are malignant. Pathologic analysis is not always helpful. Clinical features including metastases are more important in making the diagnosis. Males have greater incidence of developing malignant pheochromocytoma.

Development of metastases can occur up to 30 years after surgery. After surgical resection, lifetime follow-up with [131I]MIBG (metaiodobenzylguanidine) scan or catecholamines is recommended.

Diagnosis

Catecholamines

- Diagnosis of pheochromocytoma is based on measuring catecholamines and metabolites in the urine.
- Best study is 24-hour urine assay for catecholamines, metanephrine, and vanillylmandelic acid (VMA). VMA and norepinephrine have a sensitivity of 97%. VMA has a specificity of 91%.

Localization Studies

CT and MRI are widely used and have comparable sensitivity.

TABLE 12. *Chemotherapy regimen*

CVD
Cyclophosphamide 750 mg/m² i.v. on day 1
Vincristine, 1.4 mg/m² i.v. on day 1
Dacarbazine, 600 mg/m² i.v. on day 1 and 2
Repeat every 21 days

Nuclear medicine scanning ([^{131}I]MIBG scan).

- MIBG is similar to norepinephrine.
- Taken up and concentrated in functional adrenergic tissue.
- High sensitivity and specificity.
- It can be false-positive in neuroblastoma and medullary thyroid carcinoma.
- Bone scan is better than MIBG for bone involvement.

Management

Surgery (Fig. 3):

- Surgical resection is the mainstay of treatment.
- Should be considered for primary, metastatic, and recurrent disease.
- Hypertension should be managed appropriately before and during the surgery.

Radiation therapy:

- Used for bony and soft-tissue metastases.
- Has only limited utility.

Medical management:

- [^{131}I]MIBG has a response rate of 40%.
- None of these responses is durable.

Chemotherapy:

- In one study from the National Cancer Institute (NCI), 14 patients who were treated with CVD (cyclophosphamide, vincristine, dacarbazine) had an overall response rate of about 80%. The median duration of response was 22 months (Table 12).
- Occasional hypertensive crisis can occur after chemotherapy.

PANCREATIC ENDOCRINE TUMORS

Pancreatic endocrine tumors (PETs) are neuroendocrine neoplasms. They include tumors of alpha cells (glucagonomas), beta cells (insulinomas), and delta cells (Zollinger–Ellison tumors or gastrinomas). PETs are classified as APUDomas (amine precursor uptake and decarboxylation). The percentage of tumors of the endocrine pancreas that are malignant ranges from 10% for insulinomas to 50% for glucagonomas, and at least 65% for Zollinger–Ellison and diarrheogenic tumors. Malignancy is definitely established only by the presence of metastases.

Gastrinoma

Patients with gastrinoma can present with features of increased basal gastric acid secretion due to hypergastrinemia, which causes trophic changes in gastric mucosa.

- From 70% to 90% of gastrinoma occur in pancreatic head and duodenum.
- Frequently multiple and extrapancreatic.
- Of gastrinomas, 20% are "familial," and 57% of MEN-I patients develop gastrinomas.
- Slightly more common in males.
- Diagnosis is made by fasting hypergastrinemia and elevated basal acid output (BAO).
- Alternatively, if pH of gastric contents is more than 2.5, gastrinoma can be excluded.

Clinical Features and Diagnosis

- Gastrinomas are usually recognized because of Zollinger-Ellison Syndrome (ZES).
- Abdominal pain.
- Diarrhea.
- Esophageal symptoms.
- Peptic ulcer with diarrhea.
- Peptic ulcer in unusual location.
- Recurrent or refractory peptic ulcer.
- Family history of peptic ulcer.

Localization

A number of different techniques can be used in localizing the tumor.

- SRS (somatostatin-receptor scintigraphy).
- MRI, CT, and abdominal ultrasound scans can be useful.
- EUS (endoscopic ultrasound).
- Selective abdominal angiography.
- PVS (portal venous sampling).
- Intraarterial secretin.
- IOUS (intraoperative ultrasound).

Treatment of Gastrinomas

With advances in medical treatment, the indications for surgical treatment of gastric acid hypersecretion are few. The malignant behavior of the tumor is the principal determinant of survival.

Medical Treatment of Gastric Acid Hypersecretion

- Histamine H_2 antagonists including ranitidine, cimetidine, and famotidine.
- Substituted benzimidazoles including omeprazole and lansoprazole.
- Anticholinergic agents including probanthine and isopropamide.

Evaluation of Medical Treatment

- Relief of symptoms is an insufficient guide.
- The treatment should cause a decrease in acid output to 10 mEq/hour.
- May require high-dose therapy with frequent reevaluation.

Surgery

- All patients with ZES should be considered for surgical resection.
- Surgical resection can improve survival.
- Indications for surgery in patients with MEN-I are not well defined.

Unproven Therapy

- Chemotherapy.
- Hepatic embolization.
- Somatostatin analogues.
- α-Interferon.
- Liver transplantation.

Insulinoma

Insulinomas are more common in women and are infrequently malignant (5–10%). Documentation of metastases is the only definitive way to diagnose malignant disease. It is usually confined to the pancreas. Metastases are not always secretory. It is usually a solitary tumor, but if multiple, consider MEN-I.

Clinical Features

- Whipple's triad consists of:
  - Hypoglycemia associated with blood glucose less than 50 mg/dL and immediate relief with ingestion of glucose.
  - Neuroglycopenic symptoms include confusion (51%), visual changes (59%), altered consciousness (38%), weakness (32%), and seizures (23%).
  - Adrenergic symptoms include sweating (43%) and tremulousness (23%).

Diagnosis

- Documentation of hypoglycemia during neuroglycopenic episodes.
- Diagnosis of insulinoma can be made by documenting "organic hypoglycemia" (<40 mg/dL) after overnight or prolonged fast. In healthy individuals, usually blood glucose level does not decrease below 70 mg/dL.
- Inappropriately elevated insulin levels after overnight fast.
- In more than 55% of patients, the test may have to be repeated after 72-hour fasting and measuring serum glucose and insulin level at 2- to 4-hour intervals.

Treatment

Surgery

Surgery is indicated in all patients, even in those with metastatic disease. Of all insulinomas, 80% to 90% are benign lesions, and they are completely cured with surgical resection.

Medical Therapy

The best nonsurgical therapy is dietary management. Many patients begin small, frequent meals before seeking medical attention. Slowly absorbed foods such as bread, rice, potatoes, and cornstarch are recommended.

The most effective medications used to control hyperinsulinemia are diazoxide and octreotide. Other medications are verapamil, phenytoin, glucocorticoids, and glucagon.

Less Frequent Pancreatic Endocrine Tumors

- VIPomas.
- Glucagonomas.
- Somatostatinomas.
- GRFomas.

CARCINOID TUMORS

These rare neuroendocrine tumors are derived from the diffuse neuroendocrine system, made up of peptide- and amine-producing cells with different hormonal profiles depending on the site of origin. They have distinct clinical features; diagnosis can be made clinically. Prognosis is excellent even with metastatic spread, so they are managed symptomatically.

• The incidence of carcinoid syndrome is 1.5/100,000.
• Primary carcinoids are classified according to their presumed derivation from different embryonic divisions of the gut.
• Commonest site is the appendix, followed by the rectum.

Clinical Features

• Diarrhea due to GI hypermotility, usually after a meal.
• Flushing is the commonest symptom, often triggered by alcohol or emotional stress.
• Abdominal pain.
• Bronchospasm.
• Valvular heart disease.
• Rarely features of pellagra (diarrhea, dermatitis, and dementia).

Pathology

• Pathologists cannot differentiate malignant from benign carcinoid based on histology.
• Unequivocal diagnosis of malignancy is determined only if there is lymph node invasion or distant metastatic disease.
• Symptoms of carcinoid syndrome are due to the secretory products such as serotonin.

Laboratory Findings

• Measurement of serotonin or its metabolites in the urine.
• Urinary 5-hydroxy indoleacetic acid (5-HIAA) is the commonest test.

Management of carcinoid tumors

Medical treatment (Fig. 4):

• Diarrhea can be effectively treated with octreotide, a somatostatin analogue.
• Symptomatic improvement in 70% of patients.
• From 50% to 70% of patients have more than 50% reduction in urinary 5-HIAA secretion.
• Dose of octreotide is 100 to 600 mcgm/day subcutaneously in two to four divided doses.
• Dose should be titrated according to symptoms.

Surgery:

• Surgical resection of the all-neoplastic tissue is the preferred therapy.
• Until octreotide was introduced, surgical resection was used for palliation in recurrent disease.

Radiation:

These tumors are responsive to higher doses of external radiation, with a response rate of 40% to 50%.

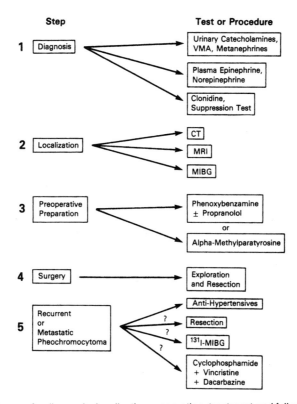

FIG. 3. Flow diagram for diagnosis, localization preparation, treatment and follow-up of a patient with a pheochromocytoma.

Chemotherapy:

- Generally chemotherapy resistant.
- α-Interferon has a biochemical response rate of 50% and a symptomatic response rate of 70%.

MULTIPLE ENDOCRINE NEOPLASIA

Multiple endocrine neoplasias (MEN) are characterized by the occurrence of tumors involving two or more endocrine glands within a single patient.

MEN-I is Wermer's syndrome, and MEN-II is Sipple's syndrome.

MENs are uncommon, but because they are inherited as autosomal dominant traits, they have important implications for other family members. First-degree relatives have about a 50% risk of developing disease (Fig. 4).

MEN-I

1. Parathyroid hyperplasia.
2. Pancreatic endocrine tumors, benign and malignant.
3. Pituitary adenoma.

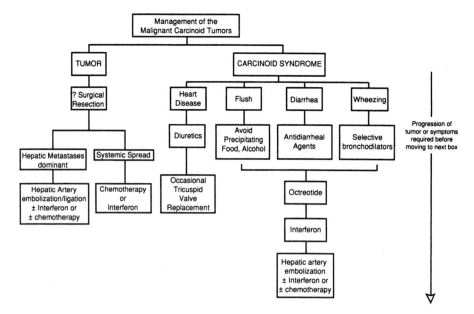

FIG. 4. Management of malignant carcinoid tumors (from Ref. 1, with permission).

4. Benign adrenocortical tumors.
5. Benign thyroid tumors.
6. Carcinoids.
7. Lipomas.

Clinical Features

 1. Hypercalcemia.
 2. Nephrolithiasis.
 3. Peptic ulcer disease.
 4. Hypoglycemia.
 5. Headache.
 6. Visual loss.
 7. Hypopituitarism.
 8. Acromegaly.
 9. Galactorrhea/amenorrhea.
10. Cushing's syndrome.

For treatment, see Table 13.

MEN-II

See Table 14 and Fig. 5.

TABLE 13. *MEN 1: Treatment options*

Disease	Intervention	Comment
Hyperparathyroidism	Remove 3.5 to 4 glands	Complication rate high
	Autograft if needed	
Pancreatic tumors		
ZES/gastrinomas	Surgical resection	Low success rate
	Medical management	Low success rate
Hypoglycemia/insulinoma	Medical management	Low success rate
Watery diarrhea/VIPoma	Medical management	Low success rate
Pituitary tumors		
Prolactinomas		
Others	Bromocriptine	Variable success
	Resect transphenoidal	Variable success

TABLE 14. *MEN 2*

MEN 2A	MEN 2B
1. Medullary thyroid carcinoma	1. Medullary thyroid carcinoma
2. Pheochromocytoma	2. Pheochromocytoma
3. Parathyroid adenomas or hyperplasia	3. Diffuse neuronal hypertrophy with mucosal and gastrointestinal ganglioneuromatosis

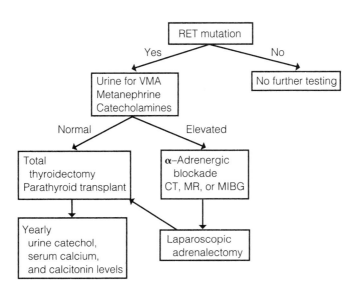

FIG. 5. Suggested diagram for treatment of individuals from kindreds of MEN 2a (from Ref. 1, with permission).

REFERENCES

1. Norton JA. Adrenal tumors. In: DeVita VT Jr, Hellman S, Rosenberg SA, eds. *Cancer: principles and practice of oncology*. 5th ed. Philadelphia: Lippincott-Raven, 1997:1659–1677.
2. Icard P, Chapuis Y, Andreassian B, et al. Adrenocortical carcinoma in surgically treated patients: a retrospective study on 156 cases by the French Association of Endocrine Surgery. *Surgery* 1992;112: 972–979.
3. Luton JP, Cerdas S, Billaud L, et al. Clinical features of adrenocortical carcinoma, prognostic factors, and the effect of mitotane therapy. *N Engl J Med* 1990;322:1195–1201.
4. Hundahl SA, Fleming ID, Fremgen AM, et al. A National Cancer Data Base report on 53,856 cases of thyroid carcinoma treated in the U.S., 1985-1995. *Cancer* 1998;83:2638–2648.
5. Grant CS, Hay ID, Gough IR, et al. Local recurrence in papillary thyroid carcinoma: is extent of surgical resection important? *Surgery* 1998;104:954–962.
6. Sanders LE, Cady B. Differentiated thyroid cancer: reexamination of risk groups and outcome of treatment. *Arch Surg* 1998;133:419–425.
7. Mazzaferri EL. Treating differentiated thyroid carcinoma: where do we draw the line? *Mayo Clin Proc* 1991;66:105–111.
8. Lairmore TC, Ball DW, Baylin SB, et al. Management of pheochromocytomas in patients with multiple endocrine neoplasia type 2 syndromes. *Ann Surg* 1993;217:595–603.
9. Neumann HP, Berger DP, Sigmund G, et al. Pheochromocytomas, multiple endocrine neoplasia type 2, and Von Hippel-Lindau disease. *N Engl J Med* 1993;329:1531–1538.
10. Sclafani LM, Woodruff JM, Brennan MF. Extraadrenal retroperitoneal paragangliomas: natural history and response to treatment. *Surgery* 1990;108:1124–1129.
11. Schlumberger MJ. Papillary and follicular thyroid carcinoma. *N Eng J Med* 1998;338:297–308.

SECTION 11

Supportive Care

35

Transfusion Medicine

Kenneth B. Johnson and Brian P. Monahan

*Division of Hematology and Medical Oncology, Department of Medicine,
Uniformed Services University of the Health Sciences, National Naval
Medical Center, Bethesda, Maryland*

With the intensive nature of chemotherapeutic regimens in use today and increased implementation of bone marrow transplantation, transfusion of blood products plays an important role supporting patients through the expected period of pancytopenia. The clinician must consider appropriate use of the many blood components available, indications for blood-product irradiation, washing, and leukocyte reduction by filtration, and management of potential adverse effects.

Understanding the principles of transfusion medicine begins with knowledge of the different components obtained from blood donation. The process of blood donation, screening of donors, the required pretransfusion testing of donor blood for infectious diseases, and compatibility testing are not reviewed here, but are essential checkpoints along the way to ensure the safety of the patient when the indication for transfusion arises. Figure 1 illustrates the different components that are derived from a single unit of donated blood.

BLOOD COMPONENTS

Whole blood

- Approximately 450 to 500 mL which contains red blood cells (RBCs), plasma, white blood cells (WBCs), platelets, and anticoagulant.
- No routine indication to transfuse whole blood in the oncology patient.

Packed RBCs

- Final volume of packed RBCs is approximately 350 mL.
- The anticipated response in a 70kg recipient to one unit of packed RBCs is an increase in the hemoglobin of 1 g/dL or the hematocrit of 3%.
- Recent data suggest that a transfusion threshold of 7.0 to 8.0 g/dL is safe in the asymptomatic patient with anemia (1).
- In patients with symptomatic cardiac or pulmonary disease with anemia, the hemoglobin should be maintained at a level that results in control of presenting symptoms.

Irradiated RBCs

- From 25 to 30 Gy will inhibit lymphocyte proliferation without affecting the functional properties of all other cell types (2).

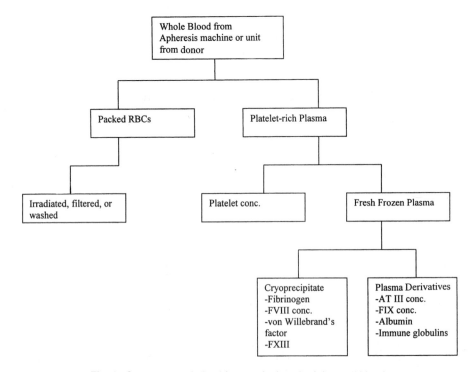

Fig. 1. Components derived from a single unit of donated blood.

- Irradiation is indicated to prevent the almost universally fatal complication of transfusion-associated graft-versus-host disease (TA-GVHD).
- Those at greatest risk for TA-GVHD include patients with congenital immunodeficiencies, patients who are immunocompromised because of allogeneic or autologous bone marrow transplantation, and patients receiving transfusions from haploidentical individuals (i.e., siblings, parents, and children). Other patients at risk include those who have undergone solid organ transplantation and are receiving immunosuppressive medication, and those with Hodgkin's disease, leukemia, and lymphoma.
- If there is an indication for irradiated RBCs, then all cellular blood products should be irradiated before transfusion.
- Acellular products such as fresh-frozen plasma, cryoprecipitate, and clotting factor concentrates do not require irradiation (2).
- Leukocyte reduction through filtration is not an acceptable substitute.

Washed RBCs

- Isotonic saline solution is used to wash RBCs to remove plasma proteins.
- Used to prevent recurrent febrile nonhemolytic reactions and severe allergic reactions caused by transfused donor plasma proteins. Most commonly, this involves immunoglobulin A (IgA)-deficient recipients who have preformed antibody to IgA (3).
- The practice of using washed RBCs to prevent febrile nonhemolytic transfusion reactions has been made obsolete by leukocyte reduction filters.

Leukocyte-reduced RBCs

- Contaminating WBCs, transfused along with packed RBCs, are responsible for several potential complications: febrile nonhemolytic transfusion reactions, platelet alloimmunization, and transmission of some infectious diseases [e.g., cytomegalovirus (CMV)].
- Current leukocyte filters remove 99.9% of WBCs from one unit of RBCs, leaving approximately 5 million WBCs (4).
- The reduction in contaminating leukocytes transfused is sufficient to significantly reduce febrile reactions, platelet alloimmunization, and CMV transmission (4–6).
- If there is an indication for leukocyte-reduced RBCs, then filtration should be used with all cellular blood products.

Platelets

- Obtained from a single-donor apheresis procedure or pooled from multiple random donors.
- The potential advantages of single-donor platelet transfusion include reduction in the risk of infectious disease transmission by reducing donor exposure, and delayed development of platelet alloimmunization and refractoriness.
- Maintaining a platelet count greater than 5,000 to 10,000/μL appears to be sufficient to prevent spontaneous hemorrhage in afebrile patients without serious concurrent infection and in the absence of coagulopathy.
- In patients with fever, concurrent infection, or coagulopathy, a platelet count of 20,000/μL or greater should be maintained.
- If invasive procedures are required, the platelet count should be maintained above 50,000/μL.
- Indications for irradiated, washed, and leukocyte-reduced platelets are the same as noted earlier for RBCs.

Fresh Frozen Plasma

- Contains all the coagulation factors and fibrinogen reduced to a volume of 200 to 250 mL.
- The usual recipient dose is 10 to 15 mL/kg.
- The effects are transient, as the half-lives of the transfused clotting factors are short.
- Uses include treatment of patients with deficiency of multiple coagulation factors such as disseminated intravascular coagulation (DIC), reversal of warfarin effects, and in patients requiring massive transfusion. In general, 2 units of fresh frozen plasma are given with every 10 units of packed RBCs in massively transfused patients. Another use includes replacement therapy in patients with thrombotic thrombocytopenic purpura undergoing plasma exchange.

Cryoprecipitate

- Contains fibrinogen, factor VIII, von Willebrand's factor, factor XIII, and fibronectin in approximately 50 mL.
- The typical recipient dose is 10 units of cryoprecipitate.
- It is indicated primarily as a source of fibrinogen in defining states such as DIC. H is also used for factor XIII deficiency.

COMPLICATIONS OF BLOOD TRANSFUSION

Approximately 20% of transfusions result in some adverse reaction, with about 0.5% considered serious (13). All blood products transfused in the United States are tested for human immunodeficiency virus (HIV) 1 and 2, human T-cell leukemia virus (HTLV) I and II, hepati-

TABLE 1. *List of potential transfusion-transmitted diseases*

Viruses: HIV 1 and 2, HTLV I and II, CMV, hepatitis A, B, C, D, E, and G, parvo B-19, human herpes virus 6 and 8
Parasites: *Plasmodium, Trypanosoma, Babesia, Toxoplasma*
Bacteria: *Yersinia, Serratia, Pseudomonas, Enterobacter, Staphylococcus, Bacillus, Streptococcus, Klebsiella*
Other organisms: *Treponema,* prion associated with Creutzfeldt–Jakob disease

tis B and C, and syphilis. The infectious risks are not limited to the infectious agents screened for. Table 1 is a list of possible transfusion-transmitted diseases.

The best strategy for the management of these potential transmitted infectious diseases is prevention. Donor counseling and screening blood products for different pathogens before transfusion have made blood products safer, even in developing countries (7).

Transfusion-related Sepsis

• Fever, chills, and/or rigor usually occur within 30 minutes of initiation of the transfusion. Nausea, vomiting, and hypotension may follow.
• Life-threatening complications such as DIC, renal failure, and congestive heart failure are potential sequelae.
• If bacterial contamination is suspected with any blood product transfusion, the transfusion is immediately stopped, and the product is sent for culture and Gram stain. Supportive care is of utmost importance in these patients. In addition, the patient's blood is cultured, and empiric broad-spectrum antibiotics are started (8).

Listed in Table 2 are the noninfectious complications associated with transfusion of blood products. They can be divided into acute and delayed processes.

Acute Hemolytic Transfusion Reaction (AHTR)

• Most commonly due to clerical errors, resulting in intravascular hemolysis from ABO incompatibility (9).
• Signs and symptoms, attributed to systemic complement activation and RBC lysis, include fever, chills, back pain, nausea, flushing, dyspnea, oliguria, and hypotension. DIC and death can follow.
• Positive direct agglutination test (DAT), hemoglobinemia, low haptoglobin, indirect hyperbilirubinemia, and schistocytes or spherocytes on examination of the peripheral blood smear are seen.

TABLE 2. *Acute and delayed noninfectious complications of blood transfusions*

Acute	Acute hemolytic transfusion reaction
	Febrile nonhemolytic transfusion reaction
	Anaphylaxis
	Urticaria
	Transfusion-related acute lung injury
	Circulatory overload
Delayed	Delayed hemolytic transfusion reaction
	Transfusion-associated graft-vs-host disease
	Posttransfusion purpura

- Management includes immediate termination of the transfusion along with supportive measures to maintain blood pressure and urine output.

Febrile Nonhemolytic Transfusion Reaction

- Common transfusion reaction with an incidence of 0.5% to 1% attributed to cytokines from WBCs present in the transfused blood products and preformed recipient antibodies reacting against donor leukocytes (9).
- Management includes excluding an acute hemolytic reaction. Pretreatment with an antipyretic and use of leukocyte-filtered blood products will prevent most febrile nonhemolytic transfusion reactions.

Anaphylaxis

- Classically associated with IgA-deficient patients who have anti-IgA antibodies, signs and symptoms of flushing, dyspnea, wheezing, cyanosis, and circulatory collapse that are clinically apparent immediately upon initiation of the transfusion (10).
- Treatment includes administration of epinephrine and other supportive measures. Preventive measures include washing of blood products or use of blood products from IgA-deficient donors (10).

Urticaria

- Most common transfusion reaction, with mild reactions occurring at a rate of 1% to 3%.
- Caused by hypersensitivity to transfused donor plasma proteins (9).
- Urticaria and pruritus commonly occur, notably without fever.
- The transfusion may be continued, along with administration of antihistamines. This is the only circumstance when a patient can be treated with an antihistamine and have the transfusion resumed. Pretreatment with antihistamines will minimize recurrent urticarial reactions.

Transfusion-related Acute Lung Injury

- Rare, life-threatening complication occurring within 4 hours of the transfusion because of infusion of donor leukocyte agglutinating antibodies.
- It occurs with a frequency of approximately 1 in 5,000 transfusions (11).
- Donor antileukocyte antibodies activate the complement cascade, with subsequent sequestration of recipient neutrophils in the pulmonary microvasculature.
- Clinically indistinguishable from noncardiogenic pulmonary edema. With supportive care and short-term mechanical ventilation, improvement occurs within 48 to 96 hours, thus differentiating this entity from noncardiogenic pulmonary edema. Diagnosis is often retrospective, with demonstration of lymphocytotoxic, human leukocyte antigen (HLA), or granulocyte-specific antibodies present in the donor or recipient serum (11).

Circulatory Overload

- Acute pulmonary edema may occur in patients with underlying cardiac or pulmonary disease.
- Management is supportive, with the judicious use of diuretics.

Delayed Hemolytic Transfusion Reaction (DHTR)

- A delayed hemolytic reaction can occur 1 to 7 days after a transfusion.
- Less dramatic than AHTR, it is characterized by low-grade fever and jaundice. The most common manifestation is a decreasing hemoglobin after transfusion.

- Laboratory findings include elevated indirect bilirubin and lactate dehydrogenase (LDH), and a positive DAT. These reactions occur in multiparous women or previously transfused patients.
- An amnestic response from exposure to one of the minor RBC antigens such as Rh, Kidd, Kell, or Duffy is the usual cause of DHTR (9).
- Treatment is usually not necessary, as a DHTR is often self-limited. However, rare cases of a severe delayed hemolytic reaction will require general supportive measures. A high index of suspicion is required for accurate diagnosis.

Transfusion-associated Graft-versus-Host Disease

- Rare but almost universally fatal transfusion complication due to immunocompetent lymphocytes in the donor blood reacting against histoincompatible recipient target tissues.
- The target tissue is predominantly the bone marrow, with lesser involvement of the skin, liver, and gastrointestinal tract (9).
- Symptoms manifest 3 to 30 days after transfusion.
- Bone marrow aplasia with resultant sepsis is often the cause of death with TA-GVHD.
- The only effective treatment is prevention, with the use of prophylactic irradiation of cellular blood products in patients at risk (see section on irradiation of blood products).

Posttransfusion Purpura (PTP)

- Rare transfusion reaction characterized by the development of severe thrombocytopenia 5 to 14 days after receiving blood products (12).
- Other causes of thrombocytopenia may coexist; therefore a high clinical suspicion is needed.
- The pathogenesis of PTP involves a PL^{A1}-negative recipient receiving PL^{A1}-positive platelets contaminating a red cell transfusion and then developing severe thrombocytopenia by a poorly understood immune complex–mediated accelerated platelet clearance.
- Although the syndrome is self-limited, significant morbidity and mortality can occur because of severe thrombocytopenia.
- Treatment is aimed at decreasing the period of thrombocytopenia with intravenous immunoglobulin, steroids, or plasmapheresis. Platelet transfusions are seldom effective.

REFERENCES

1. Goodnough LT, Brecher ME, Kanter MH, et al. Transfusion medicine. *N Engl J Med* 1999;340: 438–446.
2. Przepiorka D, LeParc GF, Stovall MA, et al. Use of irradiated blood components. *Am J Clin Pathol* 1996;106:6–11.
3. Hoffman R, Benz EJ, Shattil SJ, et al. eds. *Hematology: basic principles and practice.* 2nd ed. New York: Churchill Livingstone, 1995.
4. Miller JP, Mintz PD. The use of leukocyte-reduced blood components. *Hematol Oncol Clin North Am* 1995;9:69–82.
5. Bowden RA, Slichter SJ, Sayers M, et al. A comparison of filtered leukocyte-reduced and cytomegalovirus (CMV) seronegative blood products for the prevention of transfusion-associated CMV infection after marrow transplant. *Blood* 1995;86:3598–3603.
6. Slichter S, Gernsheimer T, Townsend-McCall D, et al. Leukocyte reduction and ultraviolet B irradiation of platelets to prevent alloimmunization and refractoriness to platelet transfusions. *N Engl J Med* 1997;337:1861–1869.
7. Moor AC, Dubbelman TM, VanSteveninck J, et al. Transfusion-transmitted diseases: risks, prevention and perspectives. *Eur J Haematol* 1999;62:1–18.
8. Krishnan LG, Brecher ME. Transfusion-transmitted bacterial infection. *Hematol Oncol Clin North Am* 1995;9:167–185.

9. Winkelstein A, Kiss JE. Immunohematologic disorders. *JAMA* 1997;278:1982–1992.
10. Jeter EK, Spivey MA. Noninfectious complications of blood transfusion. *Hematol Oncol Clin North Am* 1995;9:187–201.
11. Popovsky MA. Case 40-1998 of the Massachusetts General Hospital. *N Engl J Med* 1998;339:2005–2012.
12. McCrae KR, Herman JH. Post-transfusion purpura: two unusual cases and a literature review. *Am J Hematol* 1996;52:205–211.
13. Walker RH. Special report: transfusion risks. *Am J Clin Pathol* 1987;88:374.

36

Hematopoietic Growth Factors

Kevin Knopf and Frederic Kaye

*Medicine Branch, DCS, National Cancer Institute, National Institutes of Health,
Bethesda, Maryland*

Hematologic toxicity from chemotherapy is the most frequent serious side effect encountered in clinical practice. Reduction in all three cell lineages (white blood cells, red blood cells, and platelets) can lead to complications such as fever that complicates neutropenia and requires patient hospitalization, severe anemia, and thrombocytopenia that may necessitate transfusion.

All three cell lines arise from differentiation of totipotent hematopoietic stem cells; the fully differentiated cells are mature leukocytes, erythrocytes, or platelets (the breakdown product of megakaryoctes). Hematopoietic growth factors are regulatory molecules for all three cell lines. Several have been identified, synthesized, and approved for use in clinical practice to mitigate hematologic toxicity from chemotherapy. Recommendations in this chapter come primarily from the American Society of Clinical Oncology (ASCO) evidence-based clinical practice guidelines (1–3).

In many clinical situations, hematopoietic growth factor use is both judicious (4) and cost-effective (5,6). New agents continue to be sought, developed, and evaluated in clinical trials.

MYELOID GROWTH FACTORS: G-CSF AND GM-CSF

Currently two myeloid growth factors have been approved for clinical use by the United States Food and Drug Administration (FDA). They are filgrastim [granulocyte colony-stimulating factor (G-CSF; Neupogen; Amgen, Inc., Thousand Oaks, CA, U.S.A.)] and sargramostim [(granulocyte macrophage colony-stimulating factor (GM-CSF, Leukine; Immunex Corporation, Seattle, WA, U.S.A.)]. Whereas G-CSF is specific for the production of neutrophils, GM-CSF stimulates the production of monocytes and eosinophils in addition to neutrophils. There is no firm clinical evidence to indicate that either agent produces a clinical benefit that is greater than the other drug. Although the use of exogenous myeloid growth factor decreases the duration of absolute neutropenia, the depth of the neutropenic nadir is unchanged by their use.

Indications

Primary Prophylaxis

As primary prophylaxis after a first cycle of chemotherapy, myeloid growth factors are reserved for patients with a greater than 40% probability of experiencing febrile neutropenia.

This includes patients receiving high-dose chemotherapy regimens. Their use may be exceptionally warranted in patients thought to be at higher risk for chemotherapy-induced infectious complications due to (a) preexisting neutropenia due to disease, (b) extensive prior chemotherapy, (c) previous irradiation to areas containing large amounts of bone marrow, (d) a history of febrile neutropenia during prior myelosuppressive treatments that are similarly or less dose intensive, or (e) conditions that potentially increase a risk for a serious infection (e.g., poor performance status, decreased immune function, open wounds, preexisting active tissue infections).

Secondary Prophylaxis

In patients who have had an episode of febrile neutropenia during prior courses of chemotherapy, myeloid growth factors have been shown to decrease the probability of fever after repeated myelosuppressive treatment courses. Myeloid growth factor support also may be considered if prolonged neutropenia causes excessive dose reductions or, in the absence of febrile events, delays administering planned chemotherapy. However, when there is no clinical experience to indicate that dose reduction compromises a therapeutic response, dose reduction should be considered a viable alternative to myeloid growth factor use.

Treatment of Neutropenic Patients

Treatment of afebrile neutropenic patients is not recommended. Growth factors may be considered along with antibiotics in some febrile neutropenic patients who have prognostic factors considered predictive of clinical deterioration (e.g., pneumonia, sepsis syndrome, fungal infection).

Transplantation and Peripheral Blood Stem Cell Mobilization

Myeloid growth factors are useful for mobilizing peripheral blood stem cells (PBSCs). Myeloid growth factors use can be routinely recommended after autologous PBSC transplantation and autologous or allogeneic bone marrow transplantation to speed hematopoietic recovery or as an aid to engraftment.

Leukemias and Myelodysplastic Syndrome

Myeloid growth factors can be given after completion of induction chemotherapy for acute myelogenous leukemia (AML) in patients age 55 years or older. Despite concerns that myeloid growth factors might actually induce growth of the underlying leukemia, clinical studies have not shown any detrimental effect from their use in this setting. Data on the use of growth factors in leukemic patients younger than 55 years are limited.

In myelodysplastic syndrome (MDS), there are no data regarding the safety of long-term use of myeloid growth factors; however, intermittent use may be considered in patients with MDS who have severe disease-related neutropenia and recurrent infections.

ERYTHROCYTIC GROWTH FACTOR: EPOETIN

Indication: Anemia in Cancer Patients

Erythropoietin is specific for erythrocyte differentiation (Table 1). Anemia in cancer is multifactorial and often related to decreased endogenous erythropoietin (EPO) production. Patient selection is important in EPO treatment to ensure cost-effectiveness before initiating supportive treatment with epoetin alfa (EPO; Procrit, Ortho Biotech Inc. Raritan, NJ; Epogen: Amgen, Inc. Thousand Oaks, CA, U.S.A.). Patients at greatest risk for transfusion are those

TABLE 1. *Summary of growth factor indications and prescribing information*

Drug	Indications	Dosage, route of administration, and schedule	Adverse effects
Filgrastim	Primary and secondary prophylaxis after chemotherapy After induction chemotherapy for AML in elderly patients Refractory neutropenic fever during neutropenia Peripheral blood stem cell mobilization and transplantation Autologous and allogeneic bone marrow transplantation Treatment of myelodysplastic syndrome	Filgrastim, 5 μg/kg per day s.c. or i.v. (doses may rounded to nearest vial size) Filgrastim, 10 μg/kg per day s.c. or i.v. for PBSC mobilization or after BMT Start 24–72 h after chemotherapy Discontinue when ANC recovers to 10 × 10^3/μL after neutrophil nadir has passed (occasionally earlier), and discontinue ≥24 h before next chemotherapy cycle. Rounding doses (±10%) to the nearest vial size reduces cost without compromising clinical benefit	Bone pain Often in lower back or pelvis Can be treated with analgesics as needed Rare side effects Sweet's syndrome Cutaneous vasculitis Recrudescent psoriasis Laboratory changes Increases in serum LDH, uric acid, and alkaline phosphatase Occasionally a modest decrease in platelet counts
Sargramostim	As for filgrastim	Sargramostim, 250 μg/m^2 per day s.c. or i.v. (may round dose to nearest vial size) Start 24–72 h after chemotherapy Discontinue when ANC recovers to 10 × 10^3/μL after neutrophil nadir has passed occasionally earlier), and discontinue ≥24 h before next chemotherapy cycle	Bone pain Constitutional symptoms Fever, chills, headache, myalgias (associated with high doses and i.v. route) Rare side effects Diarrhea Flushing Dyspnea Edema Anorexia Laboratory changes: Increases in serum LDH, uric acid, and alkaline phosphatase Decreases in cholesterol, albumin, and occasionally platelet counts
Epoetin alfa	Anemia in cancer patients	Epoetin alfa, 150 Units/kg s.c. 3 times weekly, may increase dose to epoetin alfa, 300 Units/kg s.c.3 times weekly after 2–4 weeks if inadequate response occurs at a lower dosage Give iron supplements to maximize response	Fever Diarrhea Edema Rare side effects Hypertension (BP should be monitored when starting treatment and after dosage increases) Seizures in patients with underlying CNS disease and hypertension Edema, usually mild and self-limited, but may require diuretics if pulmonary edema or increase in pleural effusions Tachycardia, usually mild and self-limited Atrial arrhythmias (10%)
Oprelvekin	To prevent severe thrombocytopenia and decrease the need for platelet transfusions in patients with nonmyeloid cancers who are at high risk of developing chemotherapy-induced thrombocytopenia	Oprelvekin, 50 μg/kg s.c. daily Start 6–24 h after completing chemotherapy Discontinue when the platelet count recovers to 50 × 10^3/μL after platelet nadir has passed	Due to increased fluid retention Monitor and use diuretics as needed Dilutional anemia, due to fluid retention

CNS, central nervous system; BP, blood pressure; LDH, lactate dehydrogenase; BMT, bone marrow transplant; PBSC, peripheral blood stem cell; AML, acute myelogenous leukemia; ANC, absolute neutrophil count.

who have anemia before commencing antineoplastic treatment and who experience a decrease in hemoglobin more than 2 g/dL after the first cycle of chemotherapy. Predictors of response include (7–9):

- Serum erythropoietin concentrations less than 100 mUnits/mL plus an increase in hemoglobin concentration of 0.5 g/dL after a 2-week trial of epoetin, 150 Units/kg (patient body weight) given subcutaneously 3 times weekly.
- Serum ferritin concentration less than 400 ng/mL after 2 weeks of epoetin.
- Response to epoetin is unlikely in patients whose hemoglobin increases less than 0.5 g/dL and reticulocyte counts increase less than $40 \times 10^3/\mu L$ after 2 to 4 weeks of treatment.
- Patients with chronic cancer-related anemia and an observed-to-expected (O/E) serum erythropoietin ratio less than 0.9 (a serum erythropoietin concentration of 50 mUnits/mL).

In summary, serum erythropoietin concentrations at baseline and a change in erythropoietin concentrations after a brief trial of epoetin have been shown to correlate with response to epoetin treatment; however, their predictive accuracy is approximately 75%. Because ASCO has not yet established guidelines for EPO use, the decision to use epoetin requires an empiric approach and obligates patients to complete a therapeutic trial of up to 4 weeks' duration before clinicians can assess whether they are among the subset of individuals who will benefit from continued treatment.

PLATELET GROWTH FACTOR: INTERLEUKIN-11

Thrombocytopenia can be a life-threatening consequence of antineoplastic treatments that requires clinicians to monitor patients' platelet counts, and, when necessary to prevent or mitigate hemorrhagic complications, to provide platelet transfusions. Patients at high risk of bleeding or experiencing delays in receiving planned chemotherapy include those with poor bone marrow reserve or a previous history of bleeding, those receiving regimens highly toxic to the bone marrow, and patients with a potential bleeding site (e.g., necrotic tumor) (10).

Although several thrombopoietic agents are in clinical development, oprelvekin (Neumega; Genetics Institute, Inc., Cambridge, MA, U.S.A.) is the only thrombocytopoietic agent that has received FDA approval for clinical use. Oprelvekin is a product of recombinant DNA technology and is nearly homologous with native interleukin-11 (IL-11), lacking only an amino-terminal proline residue. Oprelvekin promotes proliferation of hematopoietic stem cells, induces maturation of megakaryocytes, and clinically, has been shown to shorten the duration of thrombocytopenia and reduce the need for platelet transfusions in patients who developed platelet counts less than $20 \times 10^3/\mu L$ after prior antineoplastic treatments (11).

Fortunately, iatrogenic thrombocytopenia that requires platelet transfusion or causes major bleeding is relatively uncommon, although it tends to increase with cumulative cycles of chemotherapy that are toxic to hematopoietic progenitor cells. At present, neither ASCO nor the National Comprehensive Cancer Network (NCCN) has published formal guidelines for using thrombopoietic growth factors, although they are under development. The results of clinical trials and economic analyses with this class of agents will aid in determining optimal clinical use.

REFERENCES

1. American Society of Clinical Oncology. Recommendations for the use of hematopoietic colony-stimulating factors: evidence-based clinical practice guidelines. *J Clin Oncol* 1994;12:2471–2508.
2. American Society of Clinical Oncology. Update of recommendations for the use of hematopoietic colony-stimulating factors: evidence-based clinical practice guidelines. *J Clin Oncol* 1996;14:1957–1960.
3. Bennett CL, Smith TJ, Weeks JC, et al. Use of hematopoietic colony-stimulating factors: the American Society of Clinical Oncology survey. *J Clin Oncol* 1996;14:2511–2520.

4. Croockewit AJ, Bronchud MH, Aapro MS, et al. A European perspective on haematopoietic growth factors in haemato-oncology: report of an expert meeting of the EORTC. *Eur J Cancer* 1997;33: 1732–1746.

5. Lyman GH, Balducci L. A cost analysis of hematopoietic colony-stimulating factors. *Oncology* 1995; 9S:85–91.

6. Schulman KA, Dorsainvil D, Yabroff KR, et al. Prospective economic evaluation accompanying a trial of GM-CSF/IL-3 in patients undergoing autologous bone marrow transplantation for Hodgkin's and non-Hodgkin's lymphoma. *Bone Marrow Transplant* 1998;21:607–614.

7. Henry D, Abels R, Larholt K. Prediction of response to recombinant human erythropoietin (r-HuEPO/epoetin-a) therapy in cancer patients [Letter]. *Blood* 1995;85:1676–1678. Comment on: *Blood* 1994;84:1056–1063.

8. Cazzola M, Messinger D, Battistel V, et al. Recombinant human erythropoietin in the anemia associated with multiple myeloma or non-Hodgkin's lymphoma: dose finding and identification of predictors of response. *Blood* 1995;86:4446–4453.

9. Ludwig H, Fritz E, Leitgeb C, et al. Prediction of response to erythropoietin treatment in chronic anemia of cancer [see comments]. *Blood* 1994;84:1056–1063.

10. Rubenstein EB, Elting L. Incorporating new modalities into practice guidelines: platelet growth factors. *Oncology* 1998;12:381–386.

11. Tepler I, Elias S, Smith JW II, et al. A randomized placebo-controlled trial of recombinant human IL-11 in cancer patients with severe thrombocytopenia due to chemotherapy. *Blood* 1996;87:3607–3614.

37

Infectious Complications in Oncology

Rebecca Thomas and Alison G. Freifeld

Medicine Branch, Division of Clinical Sciences, National Cancer Institute,
National Institutes of Health, Bethesda, Maryland

Infectious morbidity and mortality in cancer patients stem from the underlying malignancy, intensive immunosuppressive treatment regimens, or both. As cancer treatment options expand and intensify, the risk of infectious complications increases. Therefore an oncologist must be familiar with factors contributing to these infections and treatment options currently available.

FEVER IN THE NONNEUTROPENIC CANCER PATIENT

- Fever may be due to infection, medication, blood products, graft-versus-host disease, allergy, or tumor.
- Patients require routine evaluation including history, physical examination, blood and urine cultures, and chest radiograph.
- Empiric coverage with a broad-spectrum agent such as intravenous ceftriaxone is prudent in patients with indwelling venous catheters until blood culture results are available.
- Empiric vancomycin is not recommended for fever without localizing signs, even if an indwelling venous catheter is in place, unless there is a very high incidence of methicillin-resistant *Staphylococcus aureus* in the health care setting. Empiric coverage for coagulase-negative staphylococci is unnecessary because of the low virulence of these organisms.
- Vancomycin is indicated if coagulase-negative staphylococcus is isolated or there is a catheter tunnel infection.

FEVER IN THE NEUTROPENIC CANCER PATIENT

Febrile neutropenic patients require immediate evaluation and prompt initiation of empiric antibiotics.

Definition

- Fever: one oral temperature greater than 38.3°C or two oral temperatures greater than 38°C measured an hour apart.
- Neutropenia: an absolute neutrophil count (ANC) less than 500/mm^3, or ANC between 500/mm^3 and 1,000/mm^3, with a predicted decline to less than 500/mL within 48 hours.
- It is important to remember that in the absence of white cells:
  - Signs and symptoms of invasive infections may be absent.
  - Infections can invade and spread quickly.
  - Fever may be the only manifestation of a potentially life-threatening infection.

Pathogens

- From 60% to 70% of fevers during neutropenia have no identifiable etiology (i.e., fever of unknown origin).
- Bacteremia is seen in 10% to 20% of patients with fever and neutropenia. Gram-positive bacteremia predominates (70%), especially due to coagulase-negative staphylococcus and *S. aureus.* Gram-negative bacteremia (30%) is usually due to *Escherichia coli, Klebsiella* sp., *Enterobacter* sp., and rarely, *Pseudomonas aeruginosa.*
- Common sites of local infection include the respiratory tract, sinuses, skin, soft tissue, venous catheter entry/exit sites, urinary tract, and gastrointestinal tract.

Evaluation

- History and physical (with a focus on potential sites of infections) should take no longer than 60 minutes to complete, and then administer first antibiotic dose.
- Laboratory evaluation:
  - Complete blood count (check for degree of neutropenia).
  - Chemistries (check for hepatic and renal function).
  - Blood cultures (including through all catheter lumens).
  - Chest radiograph.
  - Urine analysis and culture.
  - Any accessible sites of possible infection should be sampled for culture and Gram stain.
- After initial survey, the patient is categorized as either high or low risk, based on the cancer type, chemotherapy regimen, the presence or absence of medical comorbidity, and the expected duration of neutropenia (see Table 1). Patients in the low-risk category may be candidates for oral empiric antibiotic therapy.

Empiric Antibiotic Therapy

Broad-spectrum empiric antibiotic therapy must be started promptly at the onset of fever and neutropenia. Survival is greater than 90% when patients are treated with appropriate empiric therapy. Several options are available for empiric therapy:

- **Combination therapy.** Two or more antibiotics have been traditionally used to provide antibacterial synergy as well as rapid and intense bactericidal activity against gram-negative organisms in serum.

TABLE 1. *Risk stratification of patients with fever and neutropenia*

Low risk	High risk
Neutropenia anticipated to last <7 days	Neutropenia anticipated to last >7 days
Solid tumor or maintenance chemotherapy for leukemia	Leukemia induction or bone marrow transplantation
Absence of comorbid medical conditions (see list in adjacent column)	Comorbid medical condition present: Hypotension Dehydration Uncontrolled pain Altered mental status Respiratory compromise Acute abdominal pain New neurologic changes Bleeding
Fever of undetermined origin or mild infection (cellulitis, urinary tract infection) on initial examination	Pneumonia, typhlitis, or other serious documented infection on initial examination

- Effective antibiotic combinations include semisynthetic antipseudomonal penicillin (e.g., ticarcillin, piperacillin) plus an aminoglycoside, with or without an antistaphylococcal agent such as cephalothin or vancomycin.
- Drawbacks include complexity of administering multiple drugs, expense, and toxicity, particularly when aminoglycosides are given.
- Vancomycin is no longer considered a necessary component of the empiric regimen. This drug should be used in a very limited fashion.
- **Monotherapy.** Monotherapy with certain broad-spectrum bactericidal activity has been shown to be as effective as combination antibiotic regimens for empiric therapy of fever and neutropenia in a number of clinical trials, as long as appropriate modifications of therapy are made during the course of treatment. Antibiotics proven effective include (doses for adults with normal renal function):
  - Ceftazidime, 30 mg/kg i.v. every 8 hours (maximal daily dose, 6,000 mg).
  - Imipenem, 12.5 mg/kg i.v. every 6 hours (maximal daily dose, 50 mg/kg or 4,000 mg, whichever is less). Administer doses of 500 mg or less over 20 to 30 minutes; doses greater than 500 mg over 40 to 60 minutes. Slow the infusion rate if nausea occurs.
  - Meropenem, 1,000 mg i.v. every 8 hours.
  - Cefepime, 2,000 mg i.v. every 8 hours.
- **Oral therapy.** Sequential intravenous/oral or oral therapies may be acceptable for initial empiric therapy in low-risk febrile neutropenic patients (Table 1). Oral regimens that have proven useful:
  - Ciprofloxacin, 750 mg p.o. every 12 hours, plus amoxicillin/clavulanate, 500 mg (amoxicillin component) p.o. every 8 hours.
  - Most patients should be maintained as inpatients. Outpatient management is acceptable for selected stable low-risk patients. These patients should be seen in clinic daily and instructed to call or come in to clinic for new or worsening symptoms or persistent high fevers.
- Modifications to therapy are often necessary during the course of neutropenia, regardless of the specific empiric antibiotic regimen that is initially used. Specific modifications are dictated by clinical changes or by specific microbiologic isolates (Table 2).

TABLE 2. *Modifications of initial empiric therapy for fever and neutropenia*

Clinical event	Possible modification of therapy
Breakthrough bacteremia	Gram-positive isolate: add vancomycin until antibiotic sensitivities available, then switch accordingly. Gram-negative isolate: switch to noncross-resistant antibiotic regimen (e.g., from third-generation cephalosporin to aminoglycoside plus carbapenem or fluoroquinolone
Diarrhea	Add oral metronidazole, send *C. difficile* toxin assay
Severe oral mucositis or necrotizing gingivitis	Add antianaerobic agent such as metronidazole or clindamycin
Esophagitis	Trial of oral or i.v. fluconazole or i.v. amphotericin B and/or i.v. acyclovir
Pneumonia: diffuse or interstitial	Trial of trimethoprim–sulfamethoxazole plus macrolide (e.g., erythromycin, azithromycin, clarithromycin)
Pneumonia: new infiltrate in neutropenic patients	If ANC rising, watch and wait. If ANC is not recovering, perform biopsy to establish diagnosis. If cannot perform biopsy, add amphotericin B empirically
Perianal tenderness	Already on broad-spectrum antibiotics, add anaerobic agent. If not on antibiotics, begin broad-spectrum therapy with anaerobic coverage
Persistent or recurrent fever and neutropenia after 5–7 days of broad-spectrum antibiotics	Add antifungal therapy: amphotericin B, liposomal amphotericin B

- **Empiric antifungal therapy.** An antifungal agent (e.g., amphotericin B, liposomal amphotericin, or fluconazole) should be added empirically for neutropenic patients with persistent or recurrent fever after 5 to 7 days of broad-spectrum antibiotic therapy.
  - Amphotericin B deoxycholate, 0.5 mg/kg/day i.v.
  - Liposomal amphotericin B (Ambisome), 3 to 5 mg/kg/day i.v.
  - Fluconazole, 400 mg/day i.v. or p.o. has been compared with amphotericin B in small studies, with promising results for empiric use.

SPECIFIC INFECTIONS

Gram-positive Bacteremia

- Gram-positive organisms account for nearly 70% of all bacteremias in cancer patients.
- Coagulase-negative staphylococci are most common and are often catheter-related.
- *Staphylococcus aureus* also causes catheter-related infections, and is the most common cause of catheter tunnel infections. High fever, sepsis syndrome, and metastatic lesions in lung, kidney, and skin may occur with *S. aureus* bacteremia.
- Enterococci (*E. faecalis, E. faecium*) often cause bacteremia in very debilitated patients who have been taking prolonged courses of antibiotics. Vancomycin-resistant enterococci (VRE) and other antibiotic-resistance patterns (as seen with aminoglycoside, β-lactam) are increasingly common. Management of VRE is difficult: Synercid (quinupristin/dalfopristin) or linezolid may be useful; chloramphenicol, doxycycline, high-dose ampicillin, and gentamicin (if sensitive) may also be active. *In vitro* antibiotic susceptibility testing is critical to choosing appropriate antibiotics.
- α-Streptococcal bacteremia during neutropenia may cause a sepsis syndrome and adult respiratory distress syndrome in 10% of patients. Risk factors for α-streptococcal sepsis are severe mucositis, fluoroquinolone prophylaxis, and recent therapy with cytarabine. Vancomycin therapy is used until antibiotic susceptibilities are known.
- Vancomycin use should be limited. It is rarely required empirically and should be reserved for specific infections known or thought to be gram-positive in origin.
- Specific therapy of gram-positive bacteria may safely be delayed in most cases of fever and neutropenia until organism identification and sensitivity results are available, particularly for the low-virulence coagulase-negative staphylococci.
- However, it may be prudent to use empiric vancomycin in hospitals with a high incidence of methicillin-resistant *S. aureus.*
- Vancomycin prophylaxis of indwelling catheters is very strongly discouraged.
- Treat simple gram-positive bloodstream infections for 10 days or until neutropenia resolves (whichever is longer); 6 weeks for endovascular infections or other deep sites of infection.

Gram-negative Bacteremia

- *Escherichia coli, Klebsiella,* and *Enterobacter* sp. are currently the predominant gram-negative pathogens in neutropenic patients. Gram-negative organisms account for 30% or fewer of bacteremias in neutropenic cancer patients.
- *Pseudomonas aeruginosa,* once the most frequent cause of sepsis in cancer patients, is now uncommon.
- Non-aeruginosa gram-negative pseudomonads, including *Stenotrophomonas (Xanthomonas) maltophilia* and *Burkholderia (Pseudomonas) cepacia* appear to be increasing in frequency. These organisms are often intrinsically resistant to the β-lactam antibiotics and should be treated with trimethoprim–sulfamethoxasole initially.
- *Citrobacter, Serratia,* and *Enterobacter* sp. contain inducible β-lactamases, and these organisms may quickly become resistant to β-lactam antibiotics during the course of treatment. Addition of an aminoglycoside or a switch to carbapenem is prudent.

- Treat simple gram-negative bloodstream infections for 14 days or until neutropenia resolves (whichever is longer); 6 weeks for endovascular infections.

Intraluminal Indwelling Venous Catheter Infections

- More than 80% of coagulase-negative *Staphylococcus* catheter infections do not require catheter removal and can be treated with i.v. antibiotics rotated through all catheter lumens for 10 days. *S. aureus* venous catheter-related bloodstream infections also may be successfully treated in this way, as long as there is no evidence of sepsis syndrome or metastatic foci of infection.
- Gram-negative catheter-related infections may require catheter removal, especially if sepsis syndrome is present. If fever is the only clinical manifestation of catheter infection, many gram-negative infections can be treated by rotated antibiotics through all catheter lumens for 14 days.
- If initial blood cultures are positive, repeated catheter and peripheral cultures should be obtained 48 hours after the start of antibiotics. Persistent positive blood cultures after 48 hours of antibiotic therapy is an indication for line removal (see Figs. 1 and 2).
- There is no role for oral antibiotics in the management of intraluminal venous catheter infections if the catheter remains *in situ*. The entire course of therapy must be given intravenously.
- Line removal is generally recommended if there is evidence of fungal, *Corynebacterium jekeium,* or *Bacillus* sp. intraluminal catheter infection. Staphylococcus aureus or gran-negative line infections often require line removal.

Catheter-site Infections

- Localized exit-site infection is characterized by erythema, tenderness, and/or purulent discharge within 2 cm of where the catheter penetrates the skin.
- Tunnel infection should be suspected if there is erythema, tenderness, and/or induration extending more than 2 cm out from the exit site, along the subcutaneous track of the tunneled catheter.
- Swab culture of exit-site discharge and blood cultures from all catheter lumens and peripheral sites should be obtained.
- *Staphylococcus aureus* is the most common cause of catheter-exit site and tunnel infections; coagulase-negative staphylococcus infections occur less often.
- Gram-negative bacteria, rapidly growing mycobacteria (e.g., *M. fortuitum* and *M. chelonei*), *Candida* sp., *Corynebacterium jekeium,* and *Bacillus* sp. occasionally cause catheter-site infections, and catheter removal is generally required for these organisms. Mycobacterial site infections require surgical debridement, in addition to catheter removal.
- In most cases of bacterial catheter-site infections, the catheter can be treated without removal. Appropriate antibiotics for gram-positive bacteria are recommended for 10 to 14 days, and for at least 14 days for gram-negative bacteria. If improvement is dramatic after several days, initial intravenous antibiotics may be switched to an oral regimen as long as blood cultures through the catheter have always been negative. Antibiotics should always be continued throughout any neutropenic periods.

Cellulitis and Skin Lesion

- Necrotic lesions, single or scattered, may represent pyoderma gangrenosa, often due to systemic *Pseudomonas* or *Candida* infections.

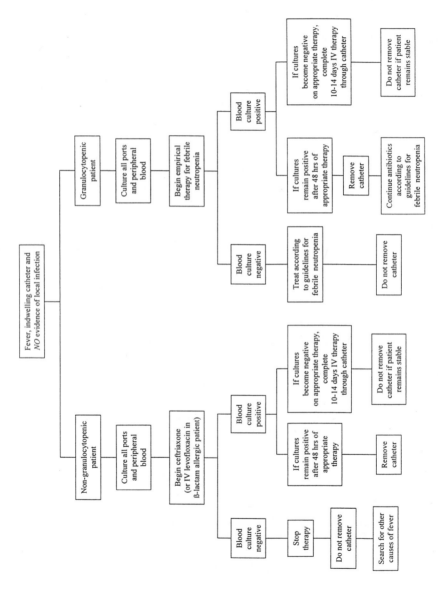

FIG 1. Fever, indwelling catheter, and no evidence of local infection.

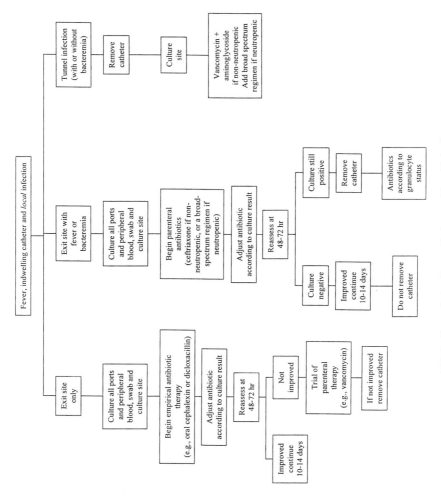

FIG 2. Fever, indwelling catheter, and local infection.

- Pustular lesions may be due to *S. aureus* or *Candida* bloodstream infections. It is important to remember, however, that neutropenic patients may not produce pus, and these lesions may appear as small, erythematous papules.
- Vesicular lesions are likely due to *Herpes simplex* or *Varicella zoster.*
- Mild HSV: Acyclovir, 400 mg p.o. or i.v., five doses daily for 7 days, or famciclovir, 500 mg p.o. every 12 hours for 7 days.
- Moderate-to-severe HSV: Acyclovir, 5 mg/kg (250 mg/m^2) i.v. every 8 hours for 7 to 14 days. Ensure good intravenous hydration to avoid nephrotoxicity.
- Varicella zoster: Acyclovir, 10 to 12 mg/kg (500 mg/m^2) i.v. every 8 hours for 7 days. Ensure good intravenous hydration to avoid nephrotoxicity. Acyclovir, 800 mg p.o., five doses daily, or famciclovir, 500 mg p.o. every 8 hours for 7 days, may be used in mild, localized zoster in a less immunocompromised patient. If progression, switch to i.v. acyclovir.
- Perform a biopsy or aspirate representative lesions by dermatology consultant, perform blood cultures, and perform computed tomography (CT) scan if there is evidence of soft tissue crepitus. The base of vesicular lesions should be scraped for immunofluorescence testing for herpes viruses (HSV or VZV).
- Streptococcal cellulitis of the upper extremity may occur after axillary node dissection for breast cancer. There is no evidence to support penicillin prophylaxis for recurrent cellulitis in this setting.
- Perirectal tenderness may signify cellulitis. Usual pathogens are gram-negative aerobes, anaerobes, and enterococci. A carbapenem (e.g., Imipenem/Cilastatin, Meropenem) provides good initial coverage. For fluctuence at perirectal site, progression of soft-tissue infection, or ongoing sepsis, surgical incision and drainage are generally indicated.

Sinusitis

- Sinus tenderness, headache, and chronic cough suggest sinusitis. Tumor obstruction of the sinus can promote recurrent infections.
- In addition to the usual pathogens (*Streptococcus pneumoniae, H. influenzae,* and *Moraxella catarrhalis*), sinusitis in immunocompromised hosts may involve gram-negative aerobes, *P. aeruginosa,* and anaerobic bacteria.
- Patients with prolonged neutropenia are at high risk for fungal sinus infections (e.g., *Aspergillus* and agents of mucormycosis). Note that fungal sinus infections are often accompanied by pulmonary and/or cerebral fungal disease, so CT scans of these sites are required.
- If sinusitis is a result of local tumor mass obstruction or damage secondary to radiotherapy, surgical opening of the sinus or an "antral window" may be beneficial for drainage.

Treatment

- **Nonneutropenic host:** 10 days of an oral regimen such as amoxicillin/clavulanate, 875 mg (amoxicillin component) p.o. every 12 hours, clarithromycin, 500 mg p.o. b.i.d., or cefuroxime, 250 mg p.o. b.i.d. Severe or recurrent sinusitis requires 21 days of therapy.
- **Neutropenic patients** require broad-spectrum antibiotics, including an antibiotic active against *P. aeruginosa* (carbapenem, third-generation cephalosporin).
- *Aspergillus* infections: amphotericin B deoxycholate, 1 to 1.5 mg/kg/day i.v., or liposomal amphotericin B (Ambisome), 5 mg/kg/day i.v. If intolerant or refractory to other amphotericin formulations, then amphotericin B lipid complex (Abelcet) or amphotericin B cholesteryl (Amphotec) may be used.
- If sinusitis does not improve within 72 hours after starting empiric antibiotics in a neutropenic host, CT scan and aspiration or biopsy of the sinus should be performed to look for fungal infection. CT evidence of bony erosion suggests fungal invasion and requires immediate biopsy and initiation of amphotericin B deoxycholate, 1 to 1.5 mg/kg/day.

Mucositis

- Pain and shallow ulcerations of tongue and buccal mucosa; usually are secondary to chemotherapy but may be superinfected with oral pathogens such as α-hemolytic streptococci, oral anaerobes, *Candida* sp., and *Herpes simplex* virus (HSV).
- Examine mouth for characteristic white plaques (often *Candida*) or ulcers (often HSV) or erythema along gum line (marginal gingivitis due to anaerobes).
- Swab white plaques for Gram's stain to look for characteristic budding yeast forms of *Candida*. Swab ulcers for culture in viral media to look for HSV.

Treatment

- Mouth-cleansing salts and solutions should be initiated before onset of chemotherapy-induced mucositis.
- **Candidiasis:** Clotrimazole, 10 mg troche, dissolved slowly in the mouth 5 times daily for mild to moderate oral thrush. Oral fluconazole with a loading dose of 200 mg p.o. or i.v., and then 100 mg daily for 10 to 14 days, or amphotericin B, 0.3 mg/kg i.v. daily for 7 days, for more extensive cases of oral or esophageal candidiasis.
- **HSV:** Acyclovir, 5 mg/kg (250 mg/m^2) i.v. every 8 hours for 7 days, or acyclovir, 400 mg p.o., five doses daily for 14 to 21 days, or famciclovir, 500 mg p.o. b.i.d. for 7 days.
- Marginal gingivitis: add metronidazole, 7.5 mg/kg every 6 hours i.v.

Esophagitis

- Sore throat, odynophagia, and substernal discomfort often are due to cytotoxic chemotherapy, but may be related to infections.
- *Herpes simplex* and *Candida albicans* are the most common pathogens. *Cytomegalovirus* occurs occasionally in severely immunocompromised patients (acute leukemia, allogeneic marrow transplant). Bacterial pathogens (e.g., *S. aureus*) rarely cause esophagitis.
- Endoscopic biopsy and culture are required for definitive diagnosis. However, endoscopy is not recommended during neutropenia, and empiric therapy must be instituted as described later.

Treatment

- Fluconazole, 100 to 200 mg i.v. or p.o. daily should be initiated empirically, and endoscopic biopsy performed as soon as possible if patient is not neutropenic.
- If esophagitis persists or worsens, a trial of low-dose amphotericin B, 0.3 mg/kg i.v. daily
- Acyclovir, 5 mg/kg (250 mg/m^2) i.v. every 8 hours should be initiated empirically if there is not prompt response to antifungal therapy or if HSV esophagitis is strongly suspected.

Diarrhea

- Moderate diarrhea is defined as four or more stools a day.
- *Clostridium difficile* is the most common pathogen causing diarrhea in cancer patients. *Salmonella, Shigella, Aeromonas,* toxigenic or invasive *E. coli, Campylobacter, Giardia,* and other parasites and viruses such as Norwalk virus are less frequent pathogens. Chemotherapy and other drugs also commonly cause diarrhea in cancer patients.
- Fever and generalized crampy abdominal pain are common in cases of *C. difficile* and those due to invasive pathogens such as *E. coli, Salmonella,* and *Shigella.* Bloody diarrhea may also occur.
- Evaluate by sending stool for *C. difficile* toxin assay, and culture for bacterial pathogens. If these do not yield an etiology, three stool samples for ova and parasite examination are recommended.

Treatment

- *C. difficile:* metronidazole, 500 mg p.o. t.i.d. for 10 to 14 days. Vancomycin, 125 mg p.o. q.i.d. should be used only in cases in which metronidazole has failed; it is not recommended for routine use. Intravenous metronidazole may be used in patients who are unable to tolerate oral, but i.v. vancomycin is not effective.
- Although bacterial diarrheas (e.g., *Campylobacter, Salmonella, Shigella, Aeromonas*) are often self-limited and do not require antibiotic treatment in the normal host, they should be treated with antibiotics in cancer patients to prevent bacteremic complications. Specific therapy should be directed to individual pathogens (infectious diseases consultation).
- Correct signs of dehydration.
- Antimotility agents should be avoided in patients with fever or bloody stools.

Typhlitis

- Acute or subacute right lower quadrant abdominal pain, rebound tenderness, fever, bloody diarrhea during neutropenia ("neutropenic enterocolitis" or "cecitis" are synonyms for typhlitis).
- CT scan shows focal bowel wall thickening around the cecum, ascites, inflammation of the pericolic fat, and pneumatosis intestinalis.
- Pathogens: mixed infections usually, although *Clostridium* sp. (especially *septicum*) and *P. aeruginosa* predominate. *Clostridium difficile* may play a role.
- Treatment consists of broad-spectrum antibiotics including metronidazole to cover *C. difficile,* bowel rest, and supportive care. If bleeding is intractable or positive blood cultures persist, consider surgical intervention.

Pulmonary Infiltrates

Pathogens are shown in Table 3 and management algorithm is shown in Fig. 3. Some of the common causes of pneumonia are discussed below.

Bacterial Pneumonias

- Gram-negative organisms (e.g., *Klebsiella* sp., *E. coli, P. aeruginosa*) predominate in neutropenic patients.
- Community-acquired pathogens (e.g., *H. influenzae, S. pneumoniae*) may cause severe pneumonia in immunocompromised cancer patients, even if they are not neutropenic.
- Sputum culture (routine, *Legionella* sp, mycobacteria, respiratory viruses) Gram's stain, acid-fast/modified acid-fast stains, fungal wet mount.
- Bronchoscopy should be performed in neutropenic patients or in those who do not respond promptly to empiric antibiotics.
- Empiric coverage with third-generation cephalosporin, possibly with the addition of a macrolide to cover *Legionella.* If highly resistant *S. pneumoniae* is suspected (community-acquired pneumonia), then vancomycin may be added until antibiotic susceptibilities are known, although intermediately resistant strains will respond to cephalosporins in general.
- Tuberculosis and *Nocardia* should be considered in patients with new pulmonary infiltrates that appear during immunosuppressive therapy and are unresponsive to routine antibiotic therapy.

Cytomegalovirus Pneumonia

- CMV disease typically occurs 30 to 90 days after allogeneic marrow transplant, although late CMV pneumonia can occur after prophylaxis is discontinued (after 180 days). Autologous transplant patients have less than 10% incidence of CMV pneumonitis.

TABLE 3. *Differential diagnosis of pneumonia in cancer patients*

	Localized infiltrate	Diffuse infiltrate
Non-neutropenic patients		
Bacteria	*Streptococcus pneumoniae, Moraxella, Legionella, Mycobacterium, Mycoplasma*	*Mycobacteria, Nocardia, Legionella, Mycoplasma, Chlamydia*
Fungi	*Cryptococcus, Histoplasma, Coccidioides*	*Aspergillus, Candida, Zygomycetes, Cryptococcus, Histoplasma*
Viruses	RSV, adenovirus, influenza	RSV, adenovirus, HSV, VZV, CMV, influenza
Protozoa		*Pneumocystis carinii, Toxoplasma gondii*
Other	Radiation pneumonitis	Radiation pneumonitis
Neutropenic patients		
Bacteria	Any gram-positive or gram-negative organism, *Mycobacterium, Nocardia*	*Mycobacteria, Nocardia, Legionella, Mycoplasma, Chlamydia*
Fungi	*Aspergillus, Candida, Zygomycetes, Cryptococcus, Histoplasma*	*Candida, Cryptococcus, Histoplasma*
Virus	RSV, adenovirus, influenza	RSV, adenovirus, HSV, VZV, CMV, influenza
Protozoa		*Pneumocystis carinii, Toxoplasma gondii*
Other	Radiation pneumonitis	Radiation pneumonitis

RSV, respiratory syncytial virus; HSV, herpes simplex virus; VZV, varicella zoster virus; CMV, cytomegalovirus.

- Rapid onset of fever, dry cough, dyspnea, and oxygen desaturation.
- Diffuse interstitial infiltrates (idiopathic interstitial pneumonia and other viral infections have similar presentation).
- Bronchoscopy for lavage and biopsy must be performed promptly to diagnose CMV either by cytology or by pathology (the "gold standard"). Positive CMV culture from bronchoalveolar lavage is not diagnostic because it may simply represent shedding of reactivated virus rather than actual invasive disease.
- Initiate broad-spectrum β-lactam plus aminoglycoside until bronchoscopy results are available.
- Combination therapy with intravenous immunoglobulin plus ganciclovir appears to provide the best therapeutic outcome for CMV pneumonia. Nonetheless, mortality usually exceeds 50%.
- Other viral pneumonias in immunocompromised cancer or transplant patients: respiratory syncytial virus, adenovirus, influenza, *Varicella zoster virus* (VZV). Usually present as diffuse interstitial infiltrates and require aggressive evaluation with bronchoscopy and virus cultures. VZV pneumonia is treated with high-dose acyclovir ($\geq$12 mg/kg i.v. every 8 hours). Treatment of other viral pneumonia is experimental, and outcome is often poor.

Fungal Pneumonia

- Usually in patients with prolonged granulocytopenia and fever despite 5 to 7 days of broad-spectrum antibiotics. Pleuritic chest pain, bloody sputum, or mild nasal stuffiness are clinical clues to sinopulmonary fungal disease.

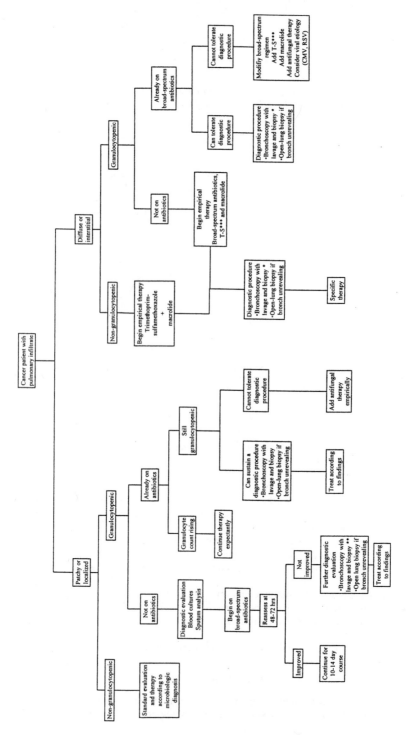

FIG 3. Cancer patient with pulmonary infiltrate.

- Rapidly progressive nodular, alveolar, or cavitary infiltrates. Pulmonary infarction may result from fungal invasion of blood vessels. Uncontrolled hemoptysis can be fatal.
- *Aspergillus* sp. are most common pathogens. *Mucor* sp. and *Pseudallescheria boydii* are less common.
- Demonstration of fungal elements in tissue obtained by bronchoscopic or open-lung biopsy is essential for diagnosis. Positive culture of sputum or lavage fluid will not distinguish between fungal colonization and invasive disease, although they are suggestive of invasion if positive in a high-risk patient.
- *Aspergillus* and similar pathogens also typically invade paranasal sinuses and central nervous system, so CT scan evaluation of these areas is important.
- High-dose amphotericin B deoxycholate at 1 to 1.5 mg/kg/day i.v. must be initiated early. Liposomal preparations are indicated if failure or intolerance of routine amphotericin B is encountered. Surgical debridement of sinus disease should be performed.
- Mortality is high unless granulocyte recovery is imminent and high-dose amphotericin B is started early.

Pneumocystis *Pneumonia*

Rapid onset of dyspnea and fevers is typical in cancer patients, in contrast to the insidious onset in those with acquired immunodeficiency syndrome (AIDS).

- Most common in patients with lymphoproliferative cancers or after marrow transplant, but can occur during a variety of cancer therapies. Steroid and cytotoxic therapies are predisposing factors.
- Diffuse interstitial infiltrates predominate, although radiographic manifestations are variable. In early disease, chest radiograph may be normal, have very subtle infiltrates, or have localized patchy infiltrates.
- Induced sputum for diagnostic stains for *Pneumocystis* (fluorescent monoclonal antibody against *Pneumocystis carinii* is most sensitive and specific). Bronchoalveolar lavage for same stains if induced sputum is unrevealing.
- Treatment: Trimethoprim–sulfamethoxazole (cotrimoxazole) 5 mg (trimethoprim)/kg i.v. every 6 to 8 hours for 21 days. Alternatives in sulfonamide-allergic patients include pentamidine isethionate, 4 mg/kg/day slow i.v. infusion over 1 to 2 hours for 21 days or atovaquone, 750 mg p.o. with food b.i.d. for 21 days.
- Clinical data in AIDS patients recommend the addition of a prednisone taper over 3 weeks in acutely ill patients with *pneumocystis carinii* pneumonia (PCP). This may be extrapolated to include cancer patients, although there are no data addressing this practice.

PREVENTION OF INFECTION

Antibiotic Prophylaxis

- Antimicrobial agents such as trimethoprim–sulfamethoxazole and fluoroquinolones have been used to decrease the incidence of gram-negative bacterial infections. However, gram-negative infections are less common in most cancer patients now.
- Widespread use of prophylactic antibiotics contributes to antibiotic resistance among pathogens, so benefits may be attenuated. Therefore antibiotic prophylaxis should not be used routinely in oncology patients.
- Prophylaxis should be used only in patients who are considered high risk for serious gram-negative infections (e.g., patients receiving intensive therapy for acute leukemia or allogeneic bone marrow transplantation).

Antiviral

Herpes Simplex Virus

- Acyclovir prophylaxis will effectively suppress almost all symptomatic HSV recurrences in seropositive patients who are undergoing bone marrow transplantation or highly immuno-suppressive chemotherapy. Risk of developing acyclovir resistance is low.
- Acyclovir is typically given beginning 1 week before until 4 weeks after transplant, corresponding with the period of highest recurrence risk.
- Acyclovir, 250 mg/m^2 i.v. every 8 hours, or acyclovir, 200 to 400 mg p.o. b.i.d. to t.i.d. are effective, with the higher dosing schemes being appropriate for higher levels of immuno-suppression (allogeneic marrow transplant).

Varicella Zoster Virus

- Immunocompromised patients who are seronegative for VZV should be isolated from those with active (noncrusted) zoster or varicella.
- Significant exposure (e.g., prolonged face-to-face contact or sharing living quarters) between a seronegative patient and persons with active VZV should receive varicella-zoster immune globulin (VZIG) within 96 hours after exposure: 125 units/10 kg of body weight by deep i.m. injection. Inject not more than 125 units (2.5 mL)/injection site; minimal dose, 125 units; maximal dose, 625 units.
- Exposed seronegative patients should be isolated for 21 days (the "incubation period" of VZV) from other seronegatives.

Cytomegalovirus

- Intravenous immunoglobulin can decrease the incidence of CMV infection (replication and shedding of virus without clinical manifestations) in marrow transplant recipients, but no consistent prophylactic benefit against CMV disease (pneumonitis, colitis) has been demonstrated.
- Prophylactic high-dose acyclovir, 500 mg/m^2 i.v. every 8 hours, decreases the occurrence of CMV disease and significantly lowers patient mortality in allogeneic marrow transplant recipients.
- Ganciclovir given prophylactically to all allogeneic marrow transplant recipients can reduce the incidence of invasive CMV, but myelosuppressive toxicity limits its utility.
- Preemptive ganciclovir therapy:
  - Candidates for preemptive ganciclovir include patients with evidence of active CMV replication after marrow engraftment such as (a) positive CMV pp65 antigenemia test (unfortunately, there is no current standardization of antigenemia test performance or interpretation); (b) positive CMV culture from blood, urine, or sputum; (c) polymerase chain reaction (PCR)-positive CMV blood test (no standardization).
  - Ganciclovir, 5 mg/kg i.v. every 12 hours for 1 week, and then ganciclovir, 5 mg/kg/day i.v. for the first 100 days after transplantation is a common preemptive protocol.
  - Markedly decreases mortality in bone marrow transplant recipients who have evidence of active CMV replication.

Pneumocystis carinii *Pneumonia*

- The use of PCP prophylaxis depends on the patient's underlying disease, intensity of therapy, and history. Patients who routinely receive prophylaxis:
  - Diagnosis of lymphoma.
  - Initial 3 to 6 months after allogeneic or autologous marrow transplant.

- History of an episode of PCP.
- Trimethoprim (TMP)–sulfamethoxazole (SMZ), 160 mg TMP/800 mg SMZ p.o. 3 times per week, is as effective as and less toxic than daily therapy. In sulfonamide-allergic patients, other options include dapsone, atovaquone, or aerosolized pentamidine.

Antifungal

- Most prophylactic regimens are aimed at reducing invasive infections of *Candida.*
- Fluconazole, 400 mg p.o. daily, may prevent disseminated candidiasis in allogeneic marrow patients and others undergoing intensive cytotoxic chemotherapy, but it does not reduce the incidence of *Aspergillus* infection.
- Widespread use of fluconazole prophylaxis has led to increased incidence of fluconazole-resistant infections (e.g., *Candida tropicalis, C. parapsilosis, C. glabrata, C. krusei.* These species may be more difficult to treat than *C. albicans.*
- The decision to use prophylactic antifungal therapy should be dependent on the institution, cytotoxic therapy, and patient.

SUGGESTED READING

1. Hughes WT, Armstrong D, Bodey GP, et al. 1997 guidelines for the use of antimicrobial agents in neutropenic patients with unexplained fever. *Clin Infect Dis* 1997;25:551–573.
2. NCCN. NCCN practice guidelines for fever and neutropenia. *Oncology* 1999;13:197–257.
3. Pizzo PA. Management of fever in patients with cancer and treatment-induced neutropenia. *N Engl J Med* 1993;328:1323–1332.
4. Talcott JA, Whalen A, Clark J, et al. Antibiotic therapy for low-risk cancer patients with fever and neutropenia: a pilot study of 30 patients based on a validated prediction rule. *J Clin Oncol* 1994;12: 107–114.
5. Malik IA, Khan WA, Karim M, et al. Feasibility of outpatient management of fever in cancer patients with low-risk neutropenia: results of a prospective randomized trial. *Am J Med* 1995;98:224–231.
6. Freifeld A, Marchigiani D, Walsh T, et al. A double-blind comparison of empirical oral and intravenous antibiotic therapy for low-risk febrile patients with neutropenia during cancer chemotherapy. *N Engl J Med* 1999;341:305–311.
7. Raad I. Intravascular-catheter-related infections. *Lancet* 1998;351:893–898.
8. Goodrich JM, Mori M, Gleaves CA, et al. Early treatment with ganciclovir to prevent cytomegalovirus disease after allogeneic bone marrow transplantation. *N Engl J Med* 1991;325:1601–1607.
9. Viscoli C, Castagnola E, Van Lint MT, et al. Fluconazole versus amphotericin B as empirical antifungal therapy of unexplained fever in granulocytopenic cancer patients: a pragmatic, multicentre, prospective and randomised clinical trial. *Eur J Cancer* 1996;32:814–820.
10. De Pauw BE, Meis JF. Progress in fighting systemic fungal infections in haematological neoplasia. *Support Care Cancer* 1998;6:31–38.
11. Noskin GA. Prevention of infection in immunocompromised hosts. *Cancer Treat Res* 1998;96: 223–246.
12. Reusser P. Current concepts and challenges in the prevention and treatment of viral infections in immunocompromised cancer patients. *Support Care Cancer* 1998;6:39–45.
13. Whimbey E, Champlin RE, Couch RB, et al. Community respiratory virus infections among hospitalized adult bone marrow transplant recipients. *Clin Infect Dis* 1996;22:778–782.
14. Roy V, Weisdorf D. Mycobacterial infections following bone marrow transplantation: a 20 year retrospective review. *Bone Marrow Transplant* 1997;19:467–470.

38

General Principles of
Cancer Pain Management

Richard A. Messmann and *David R. Kohler

*Medicine Branch, Division of Clinical Sciences,
National Cancer Institute, National Institutes of Health, and
National Institutes of Health Clinical Center Pharmacy Department, Bethesda, Maryland

Inappropriate or inadequate pain management is a significant problem that results in suffering and decreased quality of life for cancer patients. This chapter is designed to help clinicians focus on the three major components of any comprehensive pain-management plan: initial patient assessment followed by analgesic therapy and reassessment. The chapter is not intended to be an exhaustive review of pain management, but it may act as a helpful guide to facilitate an understanding of pain assessment and control.

INITIAL PATIENT ASSESSMENT

The initial assessment of any cancer patient in pain should include a comprehensive history with documentation of the following items:

- The primary cancer diagnosis: this may help define the etiology of the painful stimuli (e.g., prostate cancer and bone pain).
- Any current or prior treatment of pain: is the patient opiate naïve? This may affect dosing considerations. Identify the type(s) of analgesics in use by the patient as well as the administration route (is delivery optimized?), dose (sufficient for analgesia?), schedule (appropriate regularly scheduled "around-the-clock" coverage? Is the dosing interval consistent with the duration of action of the prescribed drug?), and change in effectiveness of current regimen (is tolerance developing?).
- Location of pain.
- Date of onset: is this an acute or chronic problem?
- Quality of pain: characterization may help to elucidate the etiology of pain. Is the pain cramping, burning, aching, dull, sharp?
- Character of pain: waxing/waning? Aggravating/alleviating factors. Constant versus intermittent?
- Intensity/severity of pain: use a visual analogue scale (VAS)/numeric scale (Fig. 1) to quantify and document the intensity of pain. Believe the patient's subjective interpretation of the level of pain. Chronic cancer pain may not be accompanied by sympathetic stimulation, normally manifested as tachypnea or tachycardia, in spite of the presence of severe pain.
- Psychosocial evaluation (any concomitant major stresses?).
- Document these baseline findings in the patient's chart to facilitate future management.
- Document pertinent medical history.

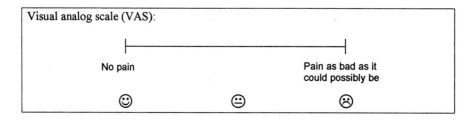

Visual analog scale (VAS):

No pain   Pain as bad as it
                           could possibly be

Simple descriptive pain intensity scale:

No   Mild   Moderate Severe   Very   Worst
Pain   Pain   Pain   Pain   Severe   Possible Pain
                                   Pain

FIG 1. Pain intensity scales: (Top) Visual Analogue Scale (VAS). (Bottom) Simple descriptive pain intensity scale.

Complete a thorough physical examination: Characterize the physical examination manifestations of pain, such as atrophy, muscle weakness, trigger points, etc.

Obtain appropriate laboratory/imaging studies.

Therapy

The five principles of general pain management, modified from the World Health Organization (WHO) report see references) are as follows:

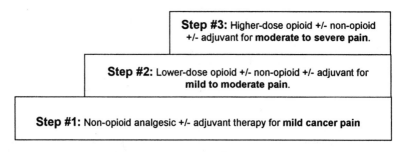

Step #3: Higher-dose opioid +/- non-opioid +/- adjuvant for **moderate to severe pain.**

Step #2: Lower-dose opioid +/- non-opioid +/- adjuvant for **mild to moderate pain.**

Step #1: Non-opioid analgesic +/- adjuvant therapy for **mild cancer pain**

Reproduced (and modified) by permission of WHO, from Cancer Pain Relief, 2nd ed. Geneva, World Health Organization, 1996.

FIG 2. Three-step World Health Organization (WHO) analgesic ladder. Step 1: Nonopioid analgesic ± adjuvant therapy for mild cancer pain. Reproduced (and modified) from *Cancer pain relief.* 2nd ed. Geneva: World Health Organization, 1996, with permission.

TABLE 1. *Selected nonopioid analgesics*

Generic drug name	Usual dose and administration schedule	Maximum daily dose[a]	Comments
Aspirin	325–650 mg p.o. every 4–6 h	Usually ≤4000 mg daily Therapeutic salicylate concentration range, 150–300 μg/mL.	Analgesic, antiinflammatory, and antipyretic. Irreversibly inhibits platelet aggregation. Irritating to GI mucosa; may cause GI bleeding. May trigger allergic reactions in atopic patients
Acetaminophen (APAP)	325–650 mg p.o. every 4–6 h, or 975–1,000 mg p.o. every 4–6 h	Limit total daily APAP dose to ≤4,000 mg	Analgesic and antipyretic. May be hepatotoxic at high doses and in chronic alcohol users
Ibuprofen	200–400 mg p.o. every 4–6 h	Limit total daily ibuprofen dose to ≤3,200 mg	See NSAIDs general statement (below)[b]
Naproxen	Naproxen immediate release: 250–500 mg p.o. every 12 h Naproxen delayed release, 375–500 mg p.o. every 12 h Naproxen controlled release: 750–1,000 mg p.o. once daily Naproxen sodium: 275–550 mg p.o. every 12 h	Limit total daily dose to ≤4,000 mg naproxen ≤1,375 mg naproxen sodium	See NSAIDs general statement (below).
Ketorolac	Parenterally Age <65 yr: 30 mg i.m./i.v. every 6 h Age ≥65 yr, renal impairment, or body weight <55 kg: 15 mg i.m./i.v. every 6 h	Limit total daily ketorolac dose to ≤40 mg orally, ≤120 mg i.v/i.m. For patients aged ≥65 yr, renal impairment, or body weight <55 kg, the total daily dose should not exceed 60 mg.	See NSAIDs general statement (below). Duration of use by all routes of administration should not exceed 5 consecutive days. Doses and treatment duration greater than recommended and shorter dosing intervals increase the potential for adverse effects.
Tramadol	50–100 mg p.o. every 4–6 h In renal impairment (GFR <30 mL/min), recommended tramadol dosage is 50–100 mg p.o. every 12 h. In patients with cirrhosis, recommended dosage is tramadol, 50 mg p.o. every 12 h.	Limit total daily tramadol dose to ≤400 mg. For patients aged ≥75 yr, maximal daily tramadol dose should not exceed 300 mg. In renal impairment (GFR, <30 mL/min) maximal daily tramadol dose should not exceed 200 mg.	Potential adverse effects in drug accumulation and overdose include respiratory depression and seizure.

[a]In the absence of concomitant diseases and other contraindications.

[b]NSAIDs' analgesic, antiinflammatory, and antipyretic effects vary among compounds. Consider alternative NSAID if one agent is ineffective. Potency and duration of inhibitory effect on platelet aggregation varies among compounds, but is reversible. NSAIDs are irritating to GI mucosa; may cause GI erosion and bleeding. NSAIDs may trigger allergic reactions in atopic patients. NSAIDs may produce dermatitis. NSAIDs decrease renal blood flow and may exacerbate renal insufficiency.

GI, gastrointestinal; GFR, glomerular filtration rate; p.o., orally; i.m., intramuscularly; i.v., intravenously; NSAIDS, nonsteroidal anti-inflammatory drugs.

TABLE 2. *Selected adjuvant therapy*

Modality	Comments	Considerations
TCA antidepressants	Relieves neuropathic pain and post-herpetic neuralgia. Analgesic effects start at lower doses than required for antidepressant effect	Use associated with anticholinergic effects such as dry mouth, urinary retention, orthostatic hypotension, and conduction abnormalities
Benzodiazepines/ anxiolytics	Decreases anxiety, as a sedative or muscle relaxant	Prolonged use may affect REM sleep
Steroids	Decreases inflammatory component (i.e., nerve-root compression). May potentiate analgesia, provide euphoria, increase appetite. Particularly useful in managing neuropathic pain	Prolonged use associated with a variety of side effects including weight gain and adrenal insufficiency. Increases risk of GI bleeding, especially when used with NSAIDs

GI, gastrointestinal; NSAIDS, nonsteroidal antiinflamatory drugs.

1. Dose "by mouth" whenever possible (for patient convenience and to avoid painful i.m. injections).
2. Basal analgesic administration should be based on a fixed schedule around the clock (ATC) and not on an "as needed" (prn) basis. Rationally designed, regularly scheduled ATC dosing avoids the peak-and-trough effect of prn dosing in which high serum levels correlate with adverse effects like nausea, pruritus, or somnolence, and low levels correspond to periods of suboptimal analgesia. Patients should not be required to rely on prn analgesics to cover basal pain-control requirements. Always order prn analgesics, however, for breakthrough pain control.
3. Dose by the WHO three-step ladder (Fig. 2).
   • Step 1: For mild pain, nonopioid analgesics (Table 1) with or without adjuvant therapy (Table 2), at recommended dose and frequency.
   • Step 2: For moderate pain, add a weak opioid analgesic (Table 3) to the nonopioid, or alternatively, use a narcotic analgesic combination (Table 4) with or without adjuvant therapy.
   • Step 3: For severe pain, substitute a strong opioid analgesic (Table 3) for the weak opioid, in addition to the nonopioid, with or without adjuvant therapy (Table 2). Note: The initial point of entry into the WHO analgesic ladder should correspond to the patient's level of pain. For example, patients with mild pain may start at step 1, whereas patients experiencing severe pain would start at step 3 to attain prompt analgesia.
4. A comprehensive analgesic regimen requires therapeutic customization to the patient's needs, including careful dose titration and reassessment to eliminate cancer pain and the appropriate management of opioid-related side effects (Table 5). Once the pain "type" is identified and characterized (e.g., bone, visceral, neuropathic; see Table 6), initiate an appropriate regimen of analgesics by the appropriate route (Table 7).
5. Consider the need for adjuvant therapies (Table 2) including the use of antidepressants (to enhance analgesia or to treat depression/insomnia/loss of appetite). Depression often accompanies chronic pain, and tricyclic antidepressants at low doses augment analgesia, whereas full-dose selective serotonin reuptake inhibitors (SSRIs) improve sleep and appetite and elevate mood. Use pain-management consultants (e.g., anesthesia pain management service).

TABLE 3. *Selected opioid analgesics*

Generic (proprietary) drug names	Equianalgesic doses[a,b] Parenteral	Oral	Duration of action	Comments
Alfentanil (Alfenta)	0.4–0.8 mg (i.m.)	—	—	High potency. Primarily used for anesthesia induction and maintenance
Codeine	120 mg	200 mg	4–6 h	Very low potency; high emetic potential. Excellent anti-tussive activity at less-than-analgesic doses (~15 mg)
Fentanyl[c] [Sublimaze (injection); Duragesic (transdermal patches); Oralet (lozenges); Actiq (lozenge on a stick)]	0.1 mg[c]	—	1–2 h	Available formulations include injectable solution, patches for transdermal drug delivery, and lozenges for transmucosal delivery. Caution: transdermal patches deliver fentanyl continuously.
Hydromorphone (Dilaudid)	1.5–2 mg	7.5 mg	3–5 h	Low emetic potential. Solid and liquid oral formulations, rectal suppositories, and injectable formulations available
Levorphanol (Levo-Dromoran)	2 mg	4 mg	6–8 h	Very low emetic potential
Meperidine	100 mg	300 mg	2–4 h	Primary metabolite is a neuroexcitatory compound, normeperidine, which is eliminated more slowly than meperidine and may produce muscle tremors, fasciculations, or seizures in patients with renal insufficiency.
Methadone[c] (Dolophine)	10 mg	10 mg	4–8 h†	Accumulates with repeated use
Morphine	10 mg	30–60 mg	4–6 h	Immediate- and sustained-release oral formulations available
Oxycodone	—	20 mg	4–6 h	Immediate- and sustained-release oral formulations available
Oxymorphone (Numorphan)	1–1.5 mg (injection) 5–10 mg (per rectum)	—	3–6 h	Injectable and rectal suppository formulations available
Propoxyphene (Darvon)	—	130 mg	3–6 h	Low potency. Often used in combination with aspirin or acetaminophen
Sufentanil (Sufenta)	0.01–0.04 mg	—	—	High potency. Primarily used for anesthesia induction and maintenance

[a]Equianalgesic doses are approximately equal to 10 mg parenterally administered morphine sulfate.
[b]Generally, elderly patients are much more sensitive to opioid pharmacologic effects.
[c]Duration of action increases with repeated or prolonged use.
i.m., intramuscularly.

TABLE 4. Selected opioid analgesic combinations

Generic (proprietary) drug names	Drug content	Usual dose and administration schedule		Comments
Acetaminophen (APAP) with codeine (Tylenol with codeine #2, #3, or #4; many others)	APAP w/codeine #2 — APAP 300 mg APAP w/codeine #3 — 300 mg APAP w/codeine #4 — 300 mg	Codeine 15 mg 30 mg 60 mg	300–600 mg APAP + 15–60 mg codeine p.o every 4–6 h	Limit patient's daily APAP use to ≤4,000 mg
Acetaminophen + hydrocodone	APAP 500–750 mg Hydrocodene 2.5–5 mg		5–10 mg hydrocodone p.o. every 4–6 h	Limit patient's daily APAP use to ≤4,000 mg
Acetaminophen + propoxyphene (Darvocet-N 50, Darvocet-N 100, Wygesic)	APAP Darvocet-N 50 — 325 mg Darvocet-N 100 — 650 mg Wygesic — 650 mg	Propoxyphene 50 mg 100 mg 65 mg	50–100 mg propoxyphene p.o. every 4–6 h	Limit patient's daily APAP use to ≤4,000 mg
Acetaminophen + oxycodone (Percocet, Roxicet, Tylox, Roxicet 5/500, Roxilox)	Percocet, Roxicet: APAP 325 mg Tylox, Roxicet 5/500, Roxilox: 500 mg	Oxycodone 5 mg 5 mg	5–10 mg oxycodone p.o. every 4–6 h	Limit patient's daily APAP use to ≤4,000 mg
Aspirin + oxycodone (Percodan)	Percodan Aspirin 325 mg	Oxycodone ~5 mg	5–10 mg oxycodone p.o. every 4–6 h	Gastrointestinal mucosal integrity and platelet aggregation may be adversely affected by aspirin

[a] Propoxyphene napsylate.
[b] Propoxyphene hydrochloride.
p.o., orally

TABLE 5. *Management of opioid-induced adverse effects*

Reaction	Comments	Therapeutic alternatives and suggestions
Constipation	Very common. Requires aggressive vigilance and therapy. Always order a bowel regimen for any patient on regularly scheduled opioids	Bowel regimen: Senna 2 tabs p.o. hs (up to maximum of 8 tabs/day) + 100 mg docusate sodium p.o. hs (titrate to effect) ± bisacodyl. Obstipation: consider lactulose, milk of magnesia, etc., prn disimpaction
Nausea	Tolerance often develops in 3–5 days	Hydrate patient. Relieve constipation. Decrease opioid dose with increased frequency to avoid high serum peaks. Consider antiemetics, anxiolytics, and anticholinergic agents such as prochlorperazine, metoclopramide, lorazepam, meclizine, or Transderm Scop → scopolamine patch
Pruritus	Morphine releases histamine; consider using fentanyl or oxymorphone	Consider using diphenhydramine, hydroxyzine, or cyproheptadine
Sedation	Patients may develop a varying degree of tolerance over several days	Decrease opioid dose with increased frequency to avoid high serum peaks. Consider using stimulants like caffeine, 100–200 mg p.o. q 3–4 h, or methylphenidate, 5–10 mg p.o. at breakfast; repeat at lunch
Respiratory depression	Rarely a significant problem. Patients develop rapid tolerance	May simply require physical stimulation. If severe/emergency use, 0.4 mg naloxone/10 ml NS as a 0.5-ml i.v. push q2 min, titrating to effect. Use with caution; may precipitate acute pain, withdrawal, and/or seizures

TABLE 6. *Treatment of cancer pain by etiology*

Type of pain	Characteristics	Suggested treatment options
Bone	Aching, dull	NSAIDs, opioids, strontium, pamidronate, plicamycin, samarium, lexidronam, calcitonin
Soft tissue infiltration/nerve compression/spinal cord compression		Corticosteroids (dexamethasone, prednisone), radiation therapy, neurolytic procedures
Neuropathic	Burning, tingling	Tricyclic antidepressants, opioids, anticonvulsants
Neuralgic	Lancinating (sharp, shooting)	Opioids, anticonvulsants (carbamazepine, clonazepam, phenytoin, gabapentin), antidepressants. Herpetic neuralgia; sympathetic or epidural blocks
Somatic	Deep, dull	See below. Chest wall pain: consider intrapleural analgesia, or intercostal nerve block
Visceral	Complaint depends on site of disease: If pleural or pericardial, worse with deep breathing, sharp. If organ-based, cramping, gnawing	Three-step ladder ± adjuvant therapy. Versus mucositis, consider opioids, topical anesthetics, PCA, oral rinses

PCA, patient-controlled analgesia; NSAIDS, nonsteroidal antiinflammatory drugs.

TABLE 7. Selected routes of analgesic administration

Route	Advantages	Comments
Oral	Facilitates long-term administration. Tablet/capsule or liquid formulations	Preferred route whenever possible
Intramuscular	None	Painful administration, slower onset than i.v. route. Variable time to peak effect
Subcutaneous	Steady serum levels without peak/trough effect when used to administer continuous infusion of medication	As with i.v. and transdermal routes, subcutaneous route is ideal for certain infusional techniques
Intravenous	Rapid onset to peak effect and ease of titration	May require repeated i.v. boluses for titration to analgesic effect, followed by maintenance dosing
Sublingual	Circumvents first-pass hepatic metabolism. Fast onset	Facilitates ease-of-use for liquid preparations (Roxanol, etc.)
Rectal	As an alternative to oral administration of drug	Not often considered
Transdermal	Convenient for nonfluctuating analgesic or basal requirements or for long-term administration	Slow onset (≈48 hs to steady-state levels). Difficult to titrate during changing analgesic requirements
Epidural or intrathecal	Can utilize opioid or local anesthetics or both in combination	Optimally requires "pain service" consult. Respiratory depression if dermatome levels too high
Injection techniques	Trigger-point injections and nerve blocks	Optimally requires "pain service" consult
Neurosurgery	Neuroablative techniques	Requires "pain service" or neurosurgical consult

GENERAL CONSIDERATIONS REGARDING THERAPY

Use short-acting opioid analgesics (i.e., shorter acting i.v./p.o. morphine sulfate vs. long-acting MS Contin-uous) until the patient has attained adequate pain control. Short-acting analgesics may offer advantages over longer-acting formulations in the initial management of acute cancer pain, including (a) ease of dose adjustment and (b) rapid onset of analgesic effect. After attaining effective analgesia, total daily-dose requirements can be determined, facilitating conversion to long-acting formulations.

Be aware that there is wide interpatient variability in the amount of analgesics required to obtain pain control.

Consider relaxation exercises for cancer patients: slow breathing, touch, massage therapy, and positive visualization to enhance well-being and analgesia.

Avoid using meperidine (Demerol), which is metabolized to normeperidine, a metabolite with neuroexcitatory (seizure-producing) effects. Risk of toxicity is increased after prolonged administration (more than 48 hours) and in patients with renal insufficiency.

Avoid using mixed opioid agonist/antagonists, like pentazocine or butorphanol, which may cause dysphoria, confusion, and hallucinations.

Consider using patient-controlled analgesia (PCA), which administers small intravenous or epidural doses of opioids on demand. Often used for treatment of acute varying or postoperative cancer pain, this modality affords a high degree of patient satisfaction and safety. Frequent evaluation to determine analgesic effect, and the need for dose modification, suggests that PCA may be best used through formal consultation of in-house anesthesia or multimodality "pain-management teams." Programmable PCA pumps often allow basal or maintenance rates of opioid infusion, in addition to bolus dose amounts and "lockout" time intervals. Maintenance PCA orders can be initiated after bolus opioid dosing achieves adequate analgesic effect.

PATIENT REASSESSMENT

Pain management is a dynamic process that requires frequent reassessment to determine the effectiveness of therapy and to facilitate dose adjustment. Disease progression often requires increasing doses of analgesics, whereas opioid tolerance is often manifested as decreased duration of analgesia.

The appropriate management of opioid-related side effects (Table 5), like constipation or pruritus, is of paramount importance because their mismanagement often acts as a barrier that precludes administration of adequate analgesia. Optimization of patient management requires that the clinician be proactive in managing opioid-related side effects, and in assessing and reassessing cancer pain.

REFERENCES AND SUGGESTED READINGS

1. American Pain Society. *Principles of analgesic use in the treatment of acute pain and cancer pain.* 3rd ed. Skokie, IL: American Pain Society, 1992.
2. Abraham J. *A physician's guide to pain and symptom management in cancer patients.* Baltimore: Johns Hopkins University, 2000.
3. Arbit E. *Management of cancer-related pain.* Mount Kisco, NY: Futura Publishing, 1993.
4. Brisman R. *Neurosurgical and medical management of pain: trigeminal neuralgia, chronic pain, and cancer pain.* Boston: Kluwer Academic Publishers, 1989.
5. Brooks PM, Day RO. Nonsteroidal antiinflammatory drugs: differences and similarities [published erratum appears in *N Engl J Med* 1991;325:747] [see comments]. *N Engl J Med* 1991;324:1716–1725.
6. Cleeland CS, Gonin R, Hatfield AK, et al. Pain and its treatment in outpatients with metastatic cancer [see comments]. *N Engl J Med* 1994;330:592–596.

7. Djulbegovia B, Sullivan DM. *Decision making in oncology: evidence-based management.* New York: Churchill Livingstone, 1997.
8. Epps RP, Stewart SC. *American Medical Women's Association: guide to cancer and pain management.* New York: Dell Publishing, 1996.
9. Kaiko RF, Foley KM, Grabinski PY, et al. Central nervous system excitatory effects of meperidine in cancer patients. *Ann Neurol* 1983;13:180–185.
10. Kanner R. *Diagnosis and management of pain in patients with cancer.* Basel: Karger, 1988.
11. Magni G. The use of antidepressants in the treatment of chronic pain: a review of the current evidence. *Drugs* 1991;42:730–748.
12. McGuire DB, Yarbro CH. *Cancer pain management.* Orlando: Grune & Stratton, 1987.
13. McGuire DB, Yarbro CH, Ferrell B. *Cancer pain management.* 2nd ed. Boston: Jones & Bartlett, 1995.
14. Mellick LB, Mellick GA. Successful treatment of reflex sympathetic dystrophy with gabapentin [Letter]. *Am J Emerg Med* 1995;13:96.
15. Parris WCV. *Cancer pain management: principles and practice.* Boston: Butterworth-Heinemann, 1997.
16. Schug SA, Zech D, Dorr U. Cancer pain management according to WHO analgesic guidelines. *J Pain Symptom Manage* 1990;5:27–32.
17. Agency for Health Care Policy and Research. *Management of cancer pain guideline panel.* Rockville, MD: U.S. Dept. of Health and Human Services, Public Health Service Agency for Health Care Policy and Research, 1994.
18. Ventafridda V, Tamburini M, Caraceni A, et al. A validation study of the WHO method for cancer pain relief. *Cancer* 1987;59:850–856.
19. Waller A, Caroline NL. *Handbook of palliative care in cancer.* Boston: Butterworth-Heinemann, 1996.
20. Watson CP. Antidepressant drugs as adjuvant analgesics. *J Pain Symptom Manage* 1994;9:392–405.

39

Oncologic Emergencies and Paraneoplastic Syndromes

Richard A. Messmann and *Brian P. Monahan

*Medicine Branch, Division of Clinical Sciences, National Cancer Institute, National Institutes of Health, and *Division of Hematology and Medical Oncology, Department of Medicine, Uniformed Services University of the Health Sciences, National Naval Medical Center, Bethesda, Maryland*

SPINAL CORD COMPRESSION

- Spinal cord compression (SCC) is a true oncologic emergency.
- Delay in evaluation/treatment can result in permanent bowel and bladder dysfunction or paralysis.
- The majority of cord compression cases involve tumor or collapsed bone fragments in the epidural space; few cases are subdural; and intramedullary metastasis is very rare.

Etiology of SCC

- Metastatic tumors from primary breast, lung, and prostate cancer; lymphoma, multiple myeloma; renal and gastrointestinal tumors (1).
- SCC infrequently is the first sign of cancer.

Clinical Signs and Symptoms of SCC

- Back or radicular pain.
- Muscle weakness.
- Acute or slowly evolving changes in bowel or bladder function.
- Sensory loss or autonomic dysfunction.

  Any of these clinical signs should initiate a prompt clinical evaluation for SCC (2,3).

Diagnosis of SCC

A thorough neurologic and physical examination (4), including:
- Gentle percussion of the spinal column.
- Evaluation for motor or sensory weakness.
- Passive neck flexion.
- Straight-leg raising.
- Rectal examination (to evaluate sphincter tone).
- Pinprick testing from toe to head to establish if a "sensory level" is present.

- Clinical suspicion of SCC should prompt initiation of steroid therapy (see Treatment, below) (5).
- Most SCC occurs at the level of the thoracic spine, and with lesser frequency, at the lumbar and cervical spinal areas (1).

The choice of diagnostic imaging should be suggested by the results of the neurologic examination. Magnetic resonance imaging (MRI) with gadolinium contrast is the standard for diagnosis because of its high sensitivity and specificity for detecting SCC (2,4,5). The entire neuraxis is readily imaged such that the superior and inferior extent of the compression can be used to target radiotherapy.

Some limitations include limited availability in some communities, inability of the patient to lie absolutely still and supine for 30 to 60 minutes of imaging, and issues that preclude MRI (e.g., history of metallic vertebral stabilization surgery, prior pacemaker/automatic implantable cardioverter defibrillator (AICD) placement, or certain other implanted devices).

Conventional radiographs are readily obtained and inexpensive:
- Radiographs exploit the finding that almost all SCC begins as vertebral bone metastases that lead to subsequent fracture and cord compression by bone and tumor.
- The value of conventional radiographs is limited to verifying a diagnostic impression of SCC, assessing surgical options, and evaluating spinal stability.
- They do not exclude the diagnosis of SCC if "normal" and are insufficient to plan radiotherapy.
- Computed tomography (CT) scan of the spinal region combined with i.v. and intrathecal radiocontrast.
- Provides an excellent assessment of the epidural space and surrounding soft tissue and is useful in diagnosis and therapy planning.
- Generally more available than MRI and is an acceptable imaging modality when MRI is not possible.
- Technical limitations include the need for lumbar puncture to administer radiocontrast, as well as a requirement that the ordering physician identify the expected spinal region to be imaged. The procedure is impractical for the entire neuraxis and may require supplemental studies to exclude a more superior level of compression.

Management of SCC

Symptomatic patients with **abnormal** neurologic examination:

- Receive steroid therapy at once, as detailed below.
- The majority of patients with SCC have abnormal conventional radiograph findings that will aid prompt confirmation of the diagnosis.
- Proceed to MRI to define the proximal and distal extent of the compression to facilitate the therapeutic plan.

Symptomatic patients with **normal** neurologic examination:

- Conventional radiographs of the spine followed by MRI if the conventional radiograph is abnormal (as earlier), or if clinical progression occurs, or if symptom complex fails to resolve. Note that a very small percentage of intradural tumor metastasis will be visible only to MRI.

Additionally, any abnormal findings should prompt initiation of steroid therapy. Myelography (often assisted by simultaneous CT scan) may be useful if an MRI is not available.

Treatment of SCC

- Once SCC is suspected, begin treatment with a "loading" dose of dexamethasone, 10 mg by i.v. infusion. Six hours after the loading dose, and every 6 hours thereafter, administer dexamethasone, 4 mg by i.v. infusion (5,6).

- An alternative treatment strategy includes an initial bolus dose of dexamethasone, 100 mg by i.v. infusion, followed 6 hours later by dexamethasone, 4 mg by i.v. infusion every 6 hours; however, this regimen is associated with additional toxicities related to high-dose steroid administration (7) and no improvement has been seen versus low-dose therapy with respect to neurologic improvement.
- Radiation oncology and/or surgical consultation(s) are required, and further therapy is decided by degree of spinal stability.
  - Radiotherapy is used to treat radiosensitive tumors in individuals with stable vertebral bodies and nonsurgical candidates with unstable spinal columns.
  - Radiosensitive tumors include breast and prostate tumors, lymphoma, multiple myeloma, and neuroblastoma, among others.
  - Radiotherapy candidates may also include patients with multiple areas of compression, or those with slowly evolving SCC.
  - May require surgical intervention (with or without radiation therapy), as would patients who are surgical candidates with unstable spinal columns.
- Additional surgical candidates include those patients with relapsed compression at a site of prior irradiation and patients with progression of deficits during radiation therapy. Selected patients with chemosensitive tumors may benefit from chemotherapy in addition to either radiation or surgical intervention (6,8).
- Chemotherapy may be an appropriate first-line therapy for chemosensitive tumors (lymphoma, myeloma, germ cell tumors, breast and prostate cancer) and in adults who are not candidates for radiation or surgery. The reader is directed to a number of references for specific details (2,9–16).

SUPERIOR VENA CAVA SYNDROME

- Superior vena cava syndrome (SVCS) is a common occurrence in cancer patients and may occur as a manifestation of either primary or metastatic tumor, or as a thrombosis associated with central venous access devices.
- Superior vena caval obstruction can result in life-threatening cerebral edema ($\uparrow$ intracranial pressure) or laryngeal edema (airway compromise).

Etiology of SVCS

It is most often due to extrinsic compression of the SVC by (intrathoracic) tumor in the setting of (1,4):

- Lung cancer, especially right-sided bronchogenic carcinoma.
- Non-Hodgkin's lymphoma, especially diffuse large cell or lymphoblastic lymphoma in the anterior mediastinum.
- Metastatic disease to the mediastinum, from primary:
  - Breast cancer.
  - Testicular cancer.
  - Gastrointestinal (GI) cancers.
- Primary tumors:
  - Sarcomas (e.g., malignant fibrous histiocytoma).
  - Melanomas.

It may also have an infectious etiology: tuberculosis, syphilis, histoplasmosis.
Other causes include:

- Central line thrombus and other iatrogenic causes.
- Idiopathic fibrosing mediastinitis.
- Congestive heart failure (CHF).
- Goiter.

Clinical Signs and Symptoms of SVCS

- Clinical evolution may occur acutely or gradually.
- Physical examination findings may include neck or chest wall superficial venous distention, facial and periorbital edema, cyanosis, facial plethora, mental status changes, lethargy, or edema of the upper extremities.
- SVCS symptoms include dyspnea, orthopnea, facial swelling, complaint of head "fullness," cough, arm swelling, chest pain, dysphagia, hoarseness, and positional worsening of symptoms (5).

Diagnosis of SVCS

- A thorough physical examination may be sufficient to establish the diagnosis of SVCS (17).
- Noninvasive imaging that may facilitate the diagnosis of SVCS includes:
  - Contrast-enhanced CT or MRI.
  - Chest radiograph may show mediastinal widening.
  - Doppler ultrasound examination of the jugular or subclavian vein may help differentiate thrombus from extrinsic obstruction.
  - Radiocontrast or other injections into veins of the affected extremity are not recommended because of extravasation risk and delayed central circulation entry.

Treatment of SVCS

- Options depend on the underlying etiology and the pace of symptom progression (17,18).
- Emergent radiation therapy is required when respiratory compromise (e.g., stridor) or central nervous system (CNS) symptoms are present.
- Nonemergent treatment end points are symptom relief and treatment of the malignant/infectious/other process causing the SVCS.
- If SVCS is a presenting symptom (i.e., no history of cancer), and if time allows (i.e., no respiratory distress or changing neurologic status), obtain tissue to establish a diagnosis before treatment.
- Diagnostic strategies may be limited by the patient's inability to lie supine (worsened SVCS symptoms). The majority of malignancies causing SVCS can be identified without major thoracic surgical procedures by using thoracentesis, bronchoscopy, lymph node biopsy, and bone marrow biopsy, or by analyzing sputum cytology. Limited thoracotomy and mediastinoscopy may be required in some cases.
- Conservative treatment includes elevation of the head of the bed, supplemental O_2, and bed rest.
- Emergent treatment of malignancy or treatment once the histologic diagnosis is established, may include:
  - Radiation therapy (especially if non–small-cell lung cancer (NSCLC))
  - Chemotherapy (lymphoma or germ cell tumor).
  - Chemotherapy and radiation therapy for limited-disease small-cell lung cancer.
  - Anticoagulant or thrombolytic therapy (for caval thrombosis and in catheter-associated thrombosis).
  - In cases of SVCS due to catheter-associated thrombosis, removal of the catheter with a brief period of anticoagulation remains an option. Alternatively, the catheter can often be retained (if functional) and the patient treated indefinitely with therapeutic-dose warfarin.
  - Surgery (especially in the setting of refractory disease or nonmalignant causes).
  - Intraluminal stenting (4,5,19).
  - Adjunct medical therapy with steroids can be used but is seldom helpful. Hydrocortisone, 100 to 500 mg i.v., followed by lower doses of hydrocortisone every 6 to 8 hours.

HYPERCALCEMIA

Etiology of Hypercalcemia

Hypercalcemia most often occurs in the setting of the following cancers:

- Non–small-cell lung cancer: squamous cell/bulky disease.
- Breast: adenocarcinoma/during hormonal therapy.
- Genitourinary tumors: renal, small-cell ovarian.
- Multiple myeloma.
- Head and neck tumors.
- Lymphoma: older Hodgkin's patients with bulky disease/intermediate or high-grade non-Hodgkin's lymphoma (NHL)/adult T-cell.
- Leukemias and unknown primary neoplasms (1,4).
- Patients with solid tumor metastasis to the bone comprise a large percentage of cancer patients with hypercalcemia (small-cell lung and prostate cancers are seldom associated).

Clinical Signs and Symptoms of Hypercalcemia

- May be general: dehydration, weakness, fatigue, pruritus.
- May involve many organ systems including CNS (hyporeflexia, mental status changes, seizure, coma, proximal myopathy); GI/genitourinary (GI: weight loss, nausea/vomiting, constipation, ileus, polyuria, polydipsia, azotemia, dyspepsia, pancreatitis).
- Cardiac: bradycardia, short-QT interval, wide T wave, prolonged PR interval, arrhythmias, arrest.

Diagnosis of Hypercalcemia

- It may be difficult to distinguish between hypercalcemia as a paraneoplastic syndrome and the hypercalcemia that results from metastatic disease to the bone.
  - Hypercalcemia of malignancy: serum iPTH is low or undetectable; serum PTH-related peptide (PTH-RP) levels are elevated while both 1,25-dihydroxyvitamin D and inorganic phosphate levels are low or normal. Serum PTH-RP has a high prevalence in malignancy-related hypercalcemia, which results from osteoclastic bone resorption and increased renal resorption of calcium.
  - Osteolytic hypercalcemia is seen in the setting of multiple myeloma, NSCLC, and breast cancer.
  - Calcitriol-mediated hypercalcemia is seen in relation to Hodgkin's and non-Hodgkin's lymphomas.
- In general terms, the degree of hypercalcemia can be characterized as follows: *Mild hypercalcemia* is characterized by serum calcium above normal limits but less than 12 mg/dL, whereas *moderate hypercalcemia* ranges from 12 to 13.5 mg/dL, and *severe hypercalcemia* occurs at levels greater than 13.5 mg/dL, although patients with chronic hypercalcemia may tolerate levels well in excess of 14 mg/dL without any apparent symptoms. The reader is cautioned, therefore, that the clinical manifestations and severity of hypercalcemia do not necessarily correlate with the absolute serum level of hypercalcemia, but may be more directly related to the speed with which hypercalcemia develops (1).
- Albumin and certain serum proteins bind serum calcium and may distort "true" serum calcium levels, for example, in cases of myeloma, in which dramatic elevations in serum calcium simply reflect elevated concentrations of serum calcium-binding proteins as opposed to severe hypercalcemia. Approximation of the "corrected" serum calcium level can be calculated by using one of several formulas that account for serum albumin levels, for example (13):

- Formulae for corrected serum calcium:

$$(mg/dL) = serum\ Ca_{(measured)} + 0.8 \times [4.0 - serum\ albumin\ (g/dL)] \quad [1]$$

$$(mEq/L) = serum\ Ca_{(measured)} + 0.4 \times [4.0 - serum\ albumin\ (g/dL)] \quad [2]$$

$$(mmol/L) = serum\ Ca_{(measured)} + 0.2 \times [4.0 - serum\ albumin\ (g/dL)] \quad [3]$$

Treatment of Hypercalcemia

- Any symptomatic patient with hypercalcemia, regardless of absolute serum calcium level, should be treated for correction of the hypercalcemia (20,21). Outpatient therapy includes observation during fluid rehydration and pharmacologic correction of the hypercalcemia. Corticosteroid administration inhibits osteoclastic bone resorption and is useful in patients with tumors responsive to this steroid effect. These tumors include lymphoma, leukemia, myeloma (prednisone, 40–100 mg/day) and breast cancers (prednisone, 15–30 mg/day) during hormonal therapy (4,22–24). The hypocalcemic effect of corticosteroid administration is inconsistent, however, in steroid-resistant tumor types, and caution is advised (4). Symptomatic patients with severely elevated calcium levels often require profound fluid volume replacement, which makes outpatient therapy impractical and unsafe.
- The most effective treatment of hypercalcemia requires effective therapy directed at the underlying malignancy (i.e., the source of the hypercalcemia). Unfortunately, hypercalcemia most often occurs in advanced states of disease and in patients who have progressed through available standard chemotherapy. In patients with solid tumor primary cancers, survival is often less than 6 months.

Practical and General Management of Hypercalcemia

- Initiate therapy by increasing urinary calcium excretion through vigorous hydration and decreasing bone resorption through osteoclast inhibition (see later).
- Assess the fluid and hemodynamic status by evaluating blood pressure/pulse/orthostatics/urine volume/appropriate laboratory values of the patient (4,21). Hypercalcemic patients are often severely dehydrated (i.e., they need many liters) and require immediate administration of isotonic saline (300–400 mL/h over 3–4 hours) to increase renal blood flow and calcium excretion. Small doses of furosemide may be used when the patient's volume status has first been restored.
- During treatment, patients require frequent monitoring of clinical status and metabolic laboratory testing because forced diuresis may be complicated by hypomagnesemia, hypokalemia, fluid overload, or subsequent pulmonary edema.

Once rehydration is complete and urinary output is optimized, assess the need for bisphosphonate administration. These pyrophosphate analogues interfere with osteoclast function, and thus inhibit calcium release.

- Intravenous pamidronate (60 or 90 mg in 1 L NS, infused over 2–4 hours) is effective (60–75%) and indicated for moderate to severe hypercalcemia (25,26). Bisphosphonate administration is well tolerated except for occasional i.v. site irritation and fever during infusion. Its onset of action occurs within 24 to 48 hours; maximal effect may not be achieved until 72 hours after treatment.
- An additional and perhaps more effective intervention for hypercalcemia includes the use of gallium nitrate (not the radioisotope), which also inhibits bone resorption (4).
  - Gallium nitrate intravenous administration (100–200 mg/m^2/day over 24 hours for up to 5 days) in rehydrated nonoliguric (target urine output, 1,500–2,000 mL/day) patients is highly effective (70–90%) in the treatment of hypercalcemia. Care should be taken to discontinue gallium nitrate use once normocalcemia is achieved, but to maintain close metabolic monitoring, because maximal drug effect occurs days after cessation of administra-

tion. Avoid the concomitant use of nephrotoxic drugs when using gallium nitrate. Hypercalcemic patients who do not respond to pamidronate may benefit from subsequent gallium nitrate administration. Conversely, gallium nitrate nonresponders may benefit from pamidronate (1,4).

- Calcitonin has a rapid onset of action (within 4 hours) and is often useful in severe and symptomatic hypercalcemia until more slowly acting agents become effective (e.g., pamidronate and gallium nitrate). Salmon calcitonin is initially given at 4 units/kg (body weight) s.c. or i.m. every 12 hours. If response is not satisfactory after 1 to 2 days, the dosage may be increased to 8 units/kg s.c./i.m. every 12 hours. If response is still not adequate after a 1- to 2-day trial at the higher dosage, the dosing interval should be decreased to 8 units/kg s.c./i.m. every 6 hours. Although many patients initially will respond to calcitonin, tachyphylaxis often develops rapidly, which renders patients refractory to its hypocalcemic effect (20–27).
- Plicamycin (mithramycin) also has a rapid onset of hypocalcemic activity (<12 hours), with a duration of response from 3 to 7 days. Its hypocalcemic effect is attributed to a direct cytotoxic effect on osteoclasts. Single doses of plicamycin, 0.025 mg/kg (body weight) in 150 to 250 mL 0.9% sodium chloride injection or 5% dextrose injection, USP, by i.v. infusion over 30 to 60 minutes, are usually well tolerated. The duration of hypocalcemic response with plicamycin is typically 3 to 7 days; however, it is essential to note that a maximal hypocalcemic effect may not be achieved until 48 hours after treatment. Consequently, repeated doses should not be given more frequently than every 48 hours to avoid producing hypocalcemia. Greater dosages and shorter treatment intervals also increase the risk of plicamycin-induced hepatic and renal toxicities, hemorrhagic diathesis, and thrombocytopenia (4,29).

TUMOR LYSIS SYNDROME

Etiology of Tumor Lysis Syndrome

- The administration of antitumor agents can lead to cell death, with subsequent release of intracellular contents.
- Tumor lysis syndrome (TLS) occurs when cellular disruption results in life-threatening lactic acidosis, with concomitant hyperuricemia, hyperkalemia, hyperphosphatemia, and hypocalcemia (4). The patient rapidly develops renal failure or has renal insufficiency at presentation.

Clinical Setting, Signs, and Symptoms of TLS

- TLS usually occurs in bulky disease treated with cytotoxic agents directed at rapidly proliferating tumors (1).
- TLS most often occurs during treatment of leukemia or high-grade lymphomas but also may occur during the treatment of other solid tumors (30).
- Cardiac arrhythmias may result from the severe hyperkalemia or hypocalcemia that accompanies TLS.
- Hypocalcemia can result in tetany, whereas hyperphosphatemia and hyperuricemia can result in acute renal failure.

Prevention and Treatment of TLS

- The pretreatment identification of individuals at risk, along with 24 to 48 hours of prehydration, use of pretherapy allopurinol, and vigilant metabolic monitoring (q 3–4 hour laboratory tests) after institution of therapy, are the hallmarks of TLS prevention and management (30,31). Elevated lactate dehydrogenase (LDH), uric acid, or creatinine at presentation identify a particularly high-risk patient.

- Corrective measures should be directed toward any metabolic abnormalities that occur after starting cytotoxic therapy, and particular care should be given to appropriate monitoring [e.g., continuous or serial electrocardiograms (ECGs)] and early interventions during correction of hyperkalemia, intensive care unit (ICU) admission for severe hemodynamic instability, and hemodialysis when faced with worsening or severely compromised renal function (4).
- The correction of metabolic abnormalities during TLS is similar to general ICU patient management with specific interventions for the following conditions.

Hyperphosphatemia

- If mild to moderate: restrict dietary phosphate to 0.6 to 0.9 g/day or add aluminum hydroxide, 300 to 600 mg (e.g., Amphojel, 5–10 mL or one to two tablets) p.o. t.i.d before meals.
- If severe: volume expansion with 1,000 to 3,000 mL 0.9% sodium chloride injection over 1 to 2 hours. Consider hemodialysis.

Hypocalcemia

- If symptomatic and after correction of hyperphosphatemia: calcium chloride, 10% (270 mg calcium/10 mL vial) with 5 to 10 mL given i.v. slowly over 10 minutes, or diluted in 100 mL of D5W and infused over 20 minutes. Repeat as often as q 20 minutes, while symptomatic *OR*
- Calcium gluconate, 10% solution, 20 mL given i.v. over 10 to 15 minutes, followed by infusion of 60 mL of calcium gluconate in 500 mL of D5W at 1 mg/kg/hour, with continued monitoring of serum calcium q 4 to 6 hours and prn correction of hypomagnesemia.
- Primary management of the hyperphosphatemia is critical to minimize metastatic deposition of insoluble calcium phosphate. Hemodialysis is almost always required by this time.

Hyperkalemia

- Confirm that the elevation is genuine.
  1. If nonemergent, withhold potassium and initiate administration of cation exchange resins.
  2. If emergent (cardiac toxicity, paralysis, or levels greater than 6.5 to 7 mEq/L), consider glucose and insulin, calcium administration, or nebulized β-agonist and prepare for hemodialysis (32,33).
- Measures to reduce serum potassium:
  1. Calcium gluconate, 10% solution, 10 to 30 mL i.v. over 2 to 5 minutes (onset, 0–5 minutes, 1 hour duration), *OR*
  2. Regular insulin (onset, 15–60 minutes, 4–6-hour duration) 10 to 20 U in 500 mL of dextrose 10% in water i.v. over 1 hour, *OR*
  3. Regular insulin, 10 U i.v. push with 1 ampule 50% glucose i.v. over 5 minutes.
  4. Adrenergic β2-antagonist such as nebulized albuterol, 10 to 20 mg in 4 mL normal saline, inhaled over 10 minutes (onset, 15–30 minutes, duration of 2–4 hours). Adrenergic β2-antagonists induce hypokalemia by stimulating transport of potassium into skeletal muscle.
  5. Kayexalate orally, 15 to 50 g in 50 to 100 mL of 20% sorbitol solution, repeated q 3 to 4 hours prn up to 5 times per day. Rectally, 50 g in 20% sorbitol. Each modality has an approximate duration of 1 to 3 hours.
- Minimize administration of drugs that can cause or potentiate hyperkalemia [nonsteroidal antiinflammatory drugs (NSAIDs), β-blockers, angiotensin-converting enzyme (ACE) inhibitors, potassium-sparing diuretics].

Hyperuricemia and Renal Failure

- Hyperuricemic acute renal failure may be avoided by (a) prechemotherapy identification of patients at risk for developing TLS, and (b) administration of allopurinol at doses of 600 to 900 mg qd, starting several days before chemotherapy, with tapering doses to maintain uric acid levels of less than 7 mg/dL. Hyperuricemic acute renal failure is usually refractory to conservative intervention (hydration, diuretics, etc.), and patients require hemodialysis for supportive therapy and renal recovery.

REFERENCES

1. Abeloff MD. *Clinical oncology,* 2nd ed. New York: Churchill Livingstone, 1999.
2. Boogerd W, van der Sande JJ. Diagnosis and treatment of spinal cord compression in malignant disease. *Cancer Treat Rev* 1993;19:129–150.
3. Talcott JA, Stomper PC, Drislane FW, et al. Assessing suspected spinal cord compression: a multidisciplinary outcomes analysis of 342 episodes. *Support Care Cancer* 1999;7:31–38.
4. DeVita VT, Hellman S, Rosenberg SA. *Cancer: principles and practice of oncology,* 5th ed. Philadelphia: Lippincott-Raven, 1997.
5. Djulbegovic B, Sullivan DM. *Decision making in oncology: evidence-based management.* New York: Churchill Livingstone, 1997.
6. Loblaw DA, Laperriere NJ. Emergency treatment of malignant extradural spinal cord compression: an evidence-based guideline. *J Clin Oncol* 1998;16:1613–1624.
7. Vecht CJ, Haaxma-Reiche H, van Putten WL, et al. Initial bolus of conventional versus high-dose dexamethasone in metastatic spinal cord compression. *Neurology* 1989;39:1255–1257.
8. Byrne TN. Spinal cord compression from epidural metastases. *N Engl J Med* 1992;327:614–619.
9. Burch PA, Grossman SA. Treatment of epidural cord compressions from Hodgkin's disease with chemotherapy: a report of two cases and a review of the literature. *Am J Med* 1988;84:555–558.
10. Clarke PR, Saunders M. Steroid-induced remission in spinal canal reticulum cell sarcoma: report of two cases. *J Neurosurg* 1975;42:346–348.
11. Cooper K, Bajorin D, Shapiro W, et al. Decompression of epidural metastases from germ cell tumors with chemotherapy. *J Neurooncol* 1990;8:275–280.
12. Friedman HM, Sheetz S, Levine HL, et al. Combination chemotherapy and radiation therapy: the medical management of epidural spinal cord compression from testicular cancer. *Arch Intern Med* 1986;146:509–512.
13. Payne RB, Carver ME, Morgan DB. Interpretation of serum total calcium: effects of adjustment for albumin concentration on frequency of abnormal values and on detection of change in the individual. *J Clin Pathol* 1979;32:56–60.
14. Sanderson IR, Pritchard J, Marsh HT. Chemotherapy as the initial treatment of spinal cord compression due to disseminated neuroblastoma. *J Neurosurg* 1989;70:688–690.
15. Sinoff CL, Blumsohn A. Spinal cord compression in myelomatosis: response to chemotherapy alone. *Eur J Cancer Clin Oncol* 1989;25:197–200.
16. Sasagawa I, Gotoh H, Miyabayashi H, et al. Hormonal treatment of symptomatic spinal cord compression in advanced prostatic cancer. *Int Urol Nephrol* 1991;23:351–356.
17. Ostler PJ, Clarke DP, Watkinson AF, et al. Superior vena cava obstruction: a modern management strategy. *Clin Oncol* 1997;9:83–89.
18. Patel V, Igwebe T, Mast H, et al. Superior vena cava syndrome: current concepts of management. *N Engl J Med* 1995;92:245–248.
19. Greenberg S, Kosinski R, Daniels J. Treatment of superior vena cava thrombosis with recombinant tissue type plasminogen activator. *Chest* 1991;99:1298–1301.
20. Chisholm MA, Mulloy AL, Taylor AT. Acute management of cancer-related hypercalcemia. *Ann Pharmacother* 1996;30:507–513.
21. Bilezikian JP. Management of acute hypercalcemia. *N Engl J Med* 1992;326:1196–1203.
22. Raisz LG, Trummel CL, Wener JA, et al. Effect of glucocorticoids on bone resorption in tissue culture. *Endocrinology* 1972;90:961–967.
23. Percival RC, Yates AJ, Gray RE, et al. Role of glucocorticoids in management of malignant hypercalcaemia. *Br Med J* 1984;289:287.

24. Kristensen B, Ejlertsen B, Holmegaard SN, et al. Prednisolone in the treatment of severe malignant hypercalcaemia in metastatic breast cancer: a randomized study. *J Intern Med* 1992;232:237–245.
25. Gucalp R, Theriault R, Gill I, et al. Treatment of cancer-associated hypercalcemia: double-blind comparison of rapid and slow intravenous infusion regimens of pamidronate disodium and saline alone. *Arch Intern Med* 1994;154:1935–1944.
26. Ralston SH, Gallacher SJ, Patel U, et al. Comparison of three intravenous bisphosphonates in cancer-associated hypercalcaemia. *Lancet* 1989;2:1180–1182.
27. Chan FK, Koberle LM, Thys-Jacobs S, et al. Differential diagnosis, causes, and management of hypercalcemia. *Curr Probl Surg* 1997;34:445–523.
28. Kiang DT, Loken MK, Kennedy BJ. Mechanism of the hypocalcemic effect of mithramycin. *J Clin Endocrinol Metab* 1979;48:341–344.
29. Green L, Donehower RC. Hepatic toxicity of low doses of mithramycin in hypercalcemia. *Cancer Treat Rep* 1984;68:1379–1381.
30. Fleming DR, Doukas MA. Acute tumor lysis syndrome in hematologic malignancies. *Leuk Lymphoma* 1992;8:315–318.
31. Jones DP, Mahmoud H, Chesney RW. Tumor lysis syndrome: pathogenesis and management. *Pediatr Nephrol* 1995;9:206–212.
32. Fluid and electrolyte disorders. In: Tierney LM, McPhee SJ, Papadakis MA, eds. *Current medical diagnosis and treatment*, 38th ed. Stamford, CT: Appleton & Lange, 1999:847.
33. Cogan MG. *Fluid and electrolytes: physiology and pathophysiology*, 1st ed. Norwalk, CT: Appleton & Lange, 1991.

40

Psychopharmacologic Management in Oncology

June Cai and Donald L. Rosenstein

National Institute of Mental Health, National Institutes of Health, Bethesda, Maryland

Psychiatric syndromes, predominantly depression and anxiety, occur commonly in cancer patients and, if misdiagnosed or poorly managed, can have a profoundly negative impact on optimal oncologic care. The comprehensive psychiatric care of cancer patients includes psychosocial, behavioral, and psychoeducational interventions as well as pharmacologic and psychotherapeutic treatment. The focus of this chapter is on the psychopharmacologic management of the major psychiatric syndromes encountered in the oncology setting.

CONSIDERATIONS BEFORE PRESCRIBING PSYCHOPHARMACOLOGIC AGENTS

1. Psychiatric symptoms are often manifestations of an underlying medical disorder or complication (Table 1). For example, specific malignancies (e.g., lung, breast, gastrointestinal, renal, and prostate cancers) are particularly prone to metastasize to the central nervous system (CNS). Additionally, any cancer at an advanced stage can result in structural or metabolic CNS insults that precipitate psychiatric symptoms. For those patients whose psychiatric symptoms fail to respond to psychopharmacologic treatment, CNS involvement should be reconsidered, even in malignancies that do not commonly metastasize to the brain, such as ovarian cancer.
2. Medically ill patients are particularly susceptible to CNS adverse effects of medications. For example, corticosteroids, interferon-α, dopamine-blocking antiemetics, and isotretinoin commonly produce mood, cognitive, and behavioral symptoms (Table 2). In these patients, it is often more prudent to lower the dose or discontinue the use of a currently prescribed medication than to introduce yet another agent that might exacerbate a psychiatric syndrome. In any event, when prescribing psychopharmacologic agents in patients with cancer, it is important to start low and go slow to avoid adverse CNS effects.
3. Polypharmacy often is unavoidable in oncology patients; however, most clinically significant interactions with psychotropic agents are predictable and can be avoided by choosing alternative agents or making dose adjustments. The use of monoamine oxidase inhibitors (MAOIs) with meperidine (Demerol) or selective serotonin reuptake inhibitors (SSRIs) is life threatening. [Up-to-date drug-interaction tables can be found at the Georgetown University Medical Center Division of Clinical Pharmacology website at http;//www.Drug-Interactions.com].

TABLE 1. *Medical conditions in oncology associated with anxiety and depression*

Neoplasms	Cardiovascular
Brain tumors	Ischemic heart disease
Insulinoma	Arrhythmias
Lymphoma	Congestive heart failure
Small-cell carcinoma	
Pancreatic cancer	Metabolic
Leukemia	Electrolyte disturbances
	Uremia
Endocrinologic	Vitamin B_{12} or folate deficiency
Cushing's syndrome	
Adrenal insufficiency	Others
Hypopituitarism	Substance abuse and withdrawal
Pheochromocytoma	Pain (uncontrolled)
Thyroid dysfunction	Hematologic (e.g., anemia)

TABLE 2. *Psychiatric symptoms associated with selected medications used in oncology*

	Chemotherapy agents		Other medications	
Depression	Cyproterone	Corticosteroids	Metoclopramide	Methyldopa
	Decarbazine	Vinblastine	Anticonvulsants	Barbiturates
	Interferon-α	Interleukin-1	Antimicrobials[a]	β-Blockers
	Asparaginase	Methotrexate	Bromocriptine	Isotretinoin
	Procarbazine	Tamoxifen	Opioid and nonopioid analgesics	
	Hexamethylmelamine	Vincristine		
Anxiety	Decarbazine	Flutamide	Anticholinergics	Analgesics
	Hexamethylmelamine	Interferon-α	Antimicrobials[a]	Corticosteroids
	Levamisole	Vinblastine	Thyroid hormone	Antiemetics
	Procarbazine		Bronchodilators	
Delirium	Aminoglutethimide	Bleomycin	Analgesics (especially meperidine)	
	Carmustine	Cisplatin	Corticosteroids	
	Cyclophosphamide	Corticosteroids	Anticholinergics	
	Vinblastine	Vincristine	Anticonvulsants	
	Fluorouracil	Fludarabine	Sedative–hypnotics	
	Hexamethylmelamine	Interferon-α	Ergotamines	
	Interleukin-1	Ifosfamide	Cimetidine	
	Methotrexate	Mitotane	Antiemetics	
	Procarbazine	Tamoxifen	Antimicrobials[a]	
	Cytarabine			

[a]Amphotericin B, isoniazid, acyclovir, metronidazole.

4. Inadequate pain control frequently elicits symptoms of anxiety, irritability, or depression. Therefore it is essential to have pain well controlled so that the appropriate psychiatric diagnosis and treatment can proceed (see Chapter 38).

COMMON PSYCHIATRIC SYNDROMES IN THE ONCOLOGY SETTING

1. Adjustment disorder: This is a time-limited, maladaptive reaction to a specific stressor that typically involves symptoms of depression, anxiety, or behavioral changes and impairs psychosocial functioning. The diagnostic criteria for an adjustment disorder include the onset of symptoms within 3 months of the stressor but symptom duration of no more than 6 months. The differential diagnosis includes the following disorders:

TABLE 3. *Symptoms of major depression*

Sleep disturbance	Impaired concentration and memory
Loss of interest or pleasure (anhedonia)	Change in appetite or weight
Feelings of guilt or worthlessness	Psychomotor retardation or agitation
Fatigue or loss of energy	Suicidality

Mnemonic: sig e caps.

- Bereavement.
- Posttraumatic stress disorder.
- Other mood and anxiety disorders.

Management: The initial treatment approach consists of crisis intervention and brief psychotherapy. Time-limited symptom management with medications may be indicated.

2. Major depression: Major depression is defined by the presence of a depressed mood and a majority of the following symptoms lasting at least 2 weeks (Table 3).

In cancer patients, psychological symptoms such as guilt and anhedonia are more helpful in diagnosing depression than are neurovegetative symptoms that may be due to cancer or its treatment. Particular attention should be paid to symptoms of hopelessness, helplessness, and suicidal ideation, because patients with cancer have twice the risk of suicide compared with the general population. Having cancer at certain sites [oral pharyngeal, lung, gastrointestinal (GI) tract, urogenital, breast] is associated with an even greater risk of suicide (Table 4).

Differential diagnosis of major depression:
- Adjustment disorder.
- Dysthymic disorder.
- Delirium.
- Dementia.
- Substance abuse.
- Bipolar disorder.
- Bereavement.
- Mood disorder due to a medical disorder or medication (see Tables 1 and 2).

Management: Treatment modalities include pharmacotherapy (Table 5), psychotherapy, and electroconvulsive therapy (ECT). The selection of an antidepressant should be based on a number of considerations such as prior treatment response, an optimal match between the patient's target symptoms and the side-effect profile of the antidepressant (e.g., using a sedating agent for the patient with anxiety and insomnia), and the potential for drug interactions.

3. Anxiety disorders: Many medical conditions seen in the oncology setting, such as heart failure, respiratory compromise, seizure disorders, pheochromocytoma, and chemotherapy-induced ovarian failure, may cause anxiety. Additional conditions that may cause both

TABLE 4. *Risk factors for suicide in cancer patients*

Historical considerations	Clinical descriptors
Prior suicide attempts	Elderly male
Family history of suicide	Recent loss and poor social support
Prior psychiatric illness	Current depression, substance abuse
History of substance abuse	Advanced cancer, pain, poor prognosis
Impulsive behavior	Delirium, psychosis, illogical thoughts

TABLE 5. *Commonly used antidepressants in cancer patients*

Generic names (brand names)	Dosage range (mg)	Important adverse effects and comments
Selective serotonin reuptake inhibitors (SSRIs)		
fluoxetine (Prozac)	10–60	Sexual dysfunction, diarrhea, weight changes, insomnia, agitation, anxiety, hyponatremia, night sweats
sertraline (Zoloft)	25–200	Sedation, weight gain, GI symptoms, sexual dysfunction, hyponatremia
paroxetine (Paxil)	10–60	Sexual dysfunction, sedation, akathisia, anticholinergic effects, hyponatremia
citalopram (Celexa)	20–60	Nausea, dry mouth, somnolence, ejaculation disorder. Weak inhibition of P450 isoenzymes
fluvoxamine (Luvox)	50–300	Night sweats, sexual dysfunction, potent inhibitor of CYP-1A2 and -3A3/4
Novel antidepressants		
venlafaxine (Effexor)	18.75–300	GI distress, sexual dysfunction, sedation, anticholinergic effects, hypertension at dose >225 mg
nefazodone (Serzone)	25–450	Sedation, GI upset, headache, weight gain, potent inhibitor of CYP-3A3/4, lack of sexual dysfunction
mirtazapine (Remeron)	7.5–45	Sedation, dry mouth, increased appetite and weight gain, constipation, asthenia, dizziness
bupropion (Wellbutrin)	75–300	GI distress, tremor, excitement, seizure at high dose or with brain tumors
trazodone (Desyrel)	25–200	Sedation, anticholinergic effects, orthostatic hypotension, priapism. Useful for anxiety and insomnia at low doses
CNS stimulants		
methylphenidate (Ritalin)	2.5–30	Insomnia, agitation, GI distress, headache, tics, rebound depression
dextroamphetamine (Dexedrine)	2.5–30	Insomnia, agitation, confusion, delusion, psychosis, tics, rebound depression
pemoline (Cylert)	18.75–150	Insomnia/drowsiness, dizziness, seizures, hallucinations, dyskinetic movements, GI upset, irritability
Tricyclic antidepressants		
amitriptyline (Elavil)	25–150	Dry mouth, sedation, weight gain, ECG changes, orthostatic hypotension, anticholinergic effects
desipramine (Norpramin)	25–150	Dry mouth, tachycardia, ECG changes
nortriptyline (Pamelor)	25–100	Tremor, confusion, anticholinergic effects

GI, gastrointestinal; CNS, central nervous system; ECG, electrocardiogram.

anxiety and depression are listed in Table 1. Similarly, anxiety is an adverse effect of numerous medications (Table 2). Of particular note, dopamine-blocking antiemetics such as metoclopramide (Reglan), prochlorperazine (Compazine), and promethazine (Phenergan) frequently cause akathisia, an adverse effect characterized by subjective restlessness and increased motor activity, which is commonly misdiagnosed as anxiety.

The differential diagnosis of anxiety disorders in the oncology setting includes:
- Exacerbation of medical illness.
- Agitated depression.
- Adverse effects of medications.
- Substance abuse.
- Adjustment disorder.
- Delirium.

Management of anxiety: In addition to behavioral therapy and psychotherapy, benzodiazepines (BZDs) are the medications most frequently used for the short-term treatment of anxiety (Table 6). For anxiety that persists beyond a few weeks, treatment with an antidepressant (Table 5) is indicated. Additionally, low-dose atypical antipsychotics are often useful for severe and persistent anxiety or for conditions such as anxiety secondary to steroids and delirium (Table 7).

The following issues associated with benzodiazepine use require attention:
- BZDs are the treatment of choice for delirium due to alcohol or sedative–hypnotic withdrawal, but typically worsen other types of delirium.
- In patients with hepatic failure, lorazepam or oxazepam is the preferred BZD.
- BZDs may result in "disinhibition," especially in delirium, substance abuse, organic disorders, and preexisting personality disorders.
- The abrupt discontinuation of BZDs with short half-lives [e.g., alprazolam (Xanax), triazolam (Halcion)] can cause rebound anxiety and precipitate a withdrawal syndrome.

4. Delirium: Delirium is an acute confusional state characterized by a fluctuating course of cognitive impairment, perceptual disturbances, mood changes, delusions, and sleep–wake cycle disruption. Patients can have a hyperactive (agitated) or hypoactive ("quiet") delirium. Virtually any psychiatric symptom can be a manifestation of delirium, among which anxiety and/or labile mood are common presentations often misdiagnosed as "depression." Delirium is a syndrome caused by the pathophysiology of the underlying medical condition or drug intoxication or withdrawal. In general, it reflects global brain dysfunction and is a medical emergency. Electroencephalogram (EEG) reveals widespread slow waves in most cases, except for drug withdrawal. Elderly patients and patients with existing brain pathology are more prone to delirium (i.e., so-called "sundowning"). Delirium in terminally ill patients is prevalent and often underdiagnosed. The differential diagnosis includes:
- Dementia.
- Affective disorders with psychosis (mania or depression).
- Psychotic disorders.

TABLE 6. *Preferred benzodiazepines in the oncology setting*

	Lorazepam (Ativan)	Clonazepam (Klonopin)
Dose equivalency	1 mg	0.25 mg
Dose range	0.5–2 mg p.o., sublingual, i.m. or i.v. routes, every 1–6 h (maximum daily dose, 8 mg)	0.25–1 mg p.o. route only, every 12 h
Advantages	Rapid onset of action	Less frequent dosing than with lorazepam

p.o., orally; i.m., intramuscularly; i.v., intravenously.

TABLE 7. *Commonly used neuroleptics in the oncology setting*

	Initial dose	Administration routes and schedules	Maximum daily dose	Important adverse effects
haloperidol (Haldol)	0.5–5 mg	p.o., s.c., i.m., or i.v., every 2–12 h	20 mg	EPS, hypotension, elevated prolactin
chlorpromazine (Thorazine)	12.5–50 mg	p.o., i.m., or i.v., every 4–12 h	300 mg	Decreased seizure threshold, EPS, hypotension
risperidone (Risperdal)	0.25–3 mg	p.o., every 12 h	6 mg	Hypotension, sedation, increased (serum?) prolactin
olanzapine (Zyprexa)	2.5–10 mg	p.o., every 12–24 h	20 mg	Sedation, anticholinergic effects

EPS, extrapyramidal symptoms; p.o., orally; s.c., subcutaneously; i.m., intramuscularly; i.v., intravenously.

- Medication effects (Table 2) or substance abuse.

Management: The first steps in the management of delirium are the identification and treatment of precipitating factors and the discontinuation of nonessential medications. Haloperidol (Haldol) continues to be the treatment of choice for delirium in most cases (Table 7). Delirium secondary to BZD or sedative–hypnotic withdrawal should be treated with BZDs.

SUMMARY

Psychiatric syndromes are frequently misdiagnosed and poorly treated in cancer patients. Before initiating psychopharmacologic treatments, underlying medical disorders and medication adverse effects must be addressed and potential drug interactions anticipated. Psychiatric symptoms should then be treated promptly and aggressively. Consultation from a psychiatrist is indicated when a patient (a) has a complex psychiatric history and is taking multiple psychotropic medications; (b) exhibits depressive symptoms associated with extreme guilt, anxiety, and/or suicidal thoughts; (c) is confused, disorganized, agitated, or violent; and (d) rejects treatment and/or seeks physician-assisted suicide.

SUGGESTED READINGS

1. Holland J, ed. *Psycho-oncology*. Oxford University Press, 1998.
2. Goldman LS, Wise TN, Brody DS, eds. *Psychiatry for primary care physicians*. Washington, D.C.: American Psychiatric Press, 1997.
3. Fawzy I, Greenburg D. *Oncology*. In: Rundell JR, Wise MG, eds. Textbook of Consultation-liasion psychiatry. Washington, D.C.: The American Psychiatric Press, Inc., 1995.
4. Psychiatric aspects of excellent end-of-life care: a position statement of the academy of psychosomatic medicine. 1998 (Website: http://www.apm.org/eol-care.html)
5. Caring for the dying: identification and promotion of physician competency. American Board of Internal Medicine, 1998.
6. Lipsett DR, Payne EC, Cassem NH, et al. On death and dying: discussion. *Geriatr Psychiatry* 1974;7:108–120.
7. Wise TN. The physician and his patient with cancer. *Primary Care* 1974;1:407–415.
8. Colye N, Adelhardt J, Foley K, et al. Character of terminal illness in the advanced cancer patient: pain and other symptoms during the last four weeks of life. *J Pain Sympt Manage* 1990;5.
9. Goldberg RJ. Psychiatric aspects of cancer. *Adv Psychosom Med* 1988.
10. *Diagnostic and statistical manual IV* (DSM-IV). Washington, D.C.: American Psychiatric Press, 1996.

41

Management of Emesis in Oncology

David R. Kohler

Oncology Clinical Pharmacy Specialist, National Institutes of Health Clinical Center Pharmacy Department, Bethesda, Maryland

TYPES OF TREATMENT-RELATED EMETIC SYMPTOMS

Radiation- and chemotherapy-associated emetic symptoms are categorized as acute, delayed, or anticipatory (see Fig. 1) (1).

Acute-phase symptoms have been correlated with serotonin (5-HT) release from entero-chromaffin cells. Emetic signals are propagated at local 5-HT_3 receptors, and transmitted along afferent vagus nerve fibers, and activate a diffuse series of effector nuclei in the medulla

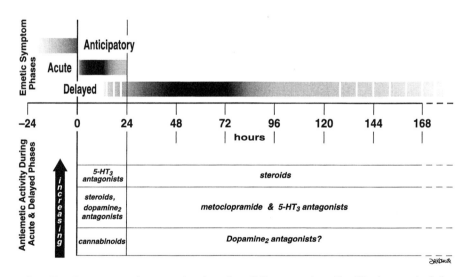

FIG 1. Emetic symptom phases and antiemetic activity comparison. Top: The temporal relation between the time of exposure to emetogenic treatment [hour zero (0)] and the emetic symptom phases. For each phase, a shaded bar indicates generally the periods during which nausea and emesis occur; symptom incidence corresponds with color intensity. Bottom: The most highly active drug categories are ranked by their relative effectiveness during the acute and delayed emetic phases.

TABLE 1. *Antineoplastic drugs implicated in causing delayed emesis*

Carboplatin ≥300 mg/m^2 (± other cytotoxic agents)
Cisplatin ≥50 mg/m^2
Cyclophosphamide ≥600 mg/m^2
Cyclophosphamide ± other cytotoxic agents
Cyclophosphamide + anthracycline combinations
Doxorubicin ≥50 mg/m^2

oblongata (the so-called "vomiting center"), which integrates afferent emetic signals and subsequently activates and coordinates motor nuclei that produce the physiologic changes associated with vomiting.

Although a physiologic basis for delayed symptoms has remained elusive, it appears not to be related to serotonin. Delayed-phase symptoms have been associated with numerous chemotherapy regimens (see Table 1). Symptoms may occur as early as 16 to 18 hours after emetogenic treatment, with a period of greatest incidence between 24 and 96 hours after treatment. Delayed-phase symptom severity and duration often correlate with drug dosage (2,3).

Delayed emesis may occur in patients who do not experience symptoms acutely, but the incidence characteristically is decreased in patients who achieve complete control during the acute phase. Although the severity of emesis typically is less during the delayed phase than that which occurs acutely, nausea severity reportedly is similar during both phases.

Anticipatory emetic symptoms are an aversive conditioned response that develops after repeated antineoplastic treatments that are characterized by poor emetic control. Consequently, complete control throughout antineoplastic treatment remains the best preventive strategy against developing anticipatory symptoms. Although anxiolytic amnestic drugs are helpful in preventing anticipatory symptoms from developing, behavior-modification and cognitive-distraction techniques become the primary interventional modalities after symptoms occur. After anticipatory symptoms develop, the role for medical intervention during subsequent emetogenic treatment is limited to preventing conditioned stimulus reinforcement, which may exacerbate anticipatory symptoms.

EMETIC (EMETOGENIC) POTENTIAL

The potential for producing emesis and the patterns in which symptoms manifest vary among antineoplastic medications and radiation therapy techniques. Generally, acute emetic symptoms begin within 1 to 3 hours after commencing chemotherapy administration (see Table 2).

Symptoms characteristically occur with greatest incidence during a 2- to 6-hour period after treatment, and may persist or intermittently recur for 12 hours or longer after treatment; however, there are some notable exceptions. The onset of emesis after mechlorethamine (nitrogen mustard) is often exaggeratedly described as occurring "on the tip of the needle" or coincident with treatment. In fact, symptoms characteristically occur within 30 to 60 minutes after administration. In contrast, both cyclophosphamide and carboplatin characteristically exhibit 8 to 18 hours latency between treatment and the onset of emesis.

Among antineoplastic drugs, dosage is the factor that most often affects emetogenic potential and the duration for which symptoms occur. The number of emetogenic drugs administered in combination, administration schedule, treatment duration, and route of drug administration also are mitigating factors. Emetic potential often is a function of treatment duration; it may be decreased or eliminated by attenuating drug delivery over hours or days (e.g., continuous infusional therapies), but often is increased by rapid administration (e.g., i.v. push or bolus), by brief intervals between repeated doses, and when emetogenic treatment is given repeatedly, one or more times per day for two or more consecutive days.

TABLE 2. *Time to onset and duration of emesis*

Drug name	Time to onset (h)	Duration (h)
Aldesleukin	0–6	—
Altretamine	3–6	—
Asparaginase	1–3	—
Bleomycin	3–6	—
Carboplatin	6–8	>24
Carmustine	2–6	4–24
Chlorambucil	48–72	—
Cisplatin	1–6	24 to >48
Cyclophosphamide	6–18	6 to >24
Cytarabine	6–12	3–5
Dacarbazine	1–5	1–24
Dactinomycin	2–6	12–24
Daunorubicin	2–6	24
Doxorubicin	4–6	6 to >24
Etoposide	3–8	6–12
Fluorouracil	3–6	3–4
Hydroxyurea	6–12	—
Ifosfamide	1–6	6–12
Irinotecan	2–6	6–12
Lomustine	2–6	4–12
Mechlorethamine	0.5–2	1–24
Melphalan	6–12	—
Mercaptopurine	4–8	—
Methotrexate	4–12	3–12
Mitomycin	1–6	3–12
Mitotane	Long latency	Persistent
Paclitaxel	3–8	3–8
Pentostatin	Long latency	Persistent, >24
Plicamycin	4–6	12–24
Procarbazine	24–27	Variable
Streptozocin	1–4	12–24
Teniposide	3–8	6–12
Thioguanine	4–8	—
Thiotepa	6–12	Variable
Vinblastine	4–8	—
Vincristine	4–8	—
Vinorelbine	4–8	—

Adapted from references 4 and 5, with permission.

For ionizing radiation, emetic potential correlates directly with the amount of radiation administered per dose and the dose rate. Large treatment volumes and fields including the upper abdomen, the upper hemithorax, and the whole body are prominent risk factors for severe emesis. Generally, emetic risk is increased when radiation and chemotherapy are administered concomitantly.

PATIENT RISK FACTORS THAT AFFECT EMETIC CONTROL

It is generally more difficult to prevent and control emesis in:

- Female than in male patients, particularly among women with a history of persistent or severe emetic symptoms during pregnancy.
- Children and young adults than in older patients.

- Patients with a history of incomplete antiemetic control during prior treatments, whether acutely, during the delayed phase, or during both periods.

Patients in the latter category are at greatest risk for poor antiemetic control during subsequent treatments (6).

Decreased performance status and a predisposition to motion sickness also have been associated with poor emetic control. In contrast, patients who have chronically consumed alcoholic beverages (generally, ≥100 g ethanol/day for several years) are more likely to have complete emetic control than are "non-drinkers," even if they are not still using alcohol.

For a minority of patients who receive treatment-appropriate antiemetic prophylaxis, effective emetic control is beyond the scope of evidence-based guidelines and requires a rational empiric approach. Unfortunately, empiric interventions predispose to a risk of overtreatment that may adversely affect patients' safety and unjustifiably increase treatment costs. In comparison, undertreatment is equally unsatisfactory, as it places patients at risk for emesis and debilitating morbidity that may adversely affect their safety, comfort, and quality of life, and complicate their care.

PRIMARY ANTIEMETIC PROPHYLAXIS

To prevent emetic symptoms during each antineoplastic treatment, treatment-appropriate antiemetic prophylaxis should begin before emetogenic treatment commences, and antiemetics should be given on a fixed schedule. Unscheduled medications require patients to recognize prodromes or develop symptoms before an antiemetic is administered. It is essential that patients are not left to rely on unscheduled antiemetics; however, it is also rational to provide a supply of antiemetic medications that patients can self-administer for symptoms that surmount primary prophylaxis.

TREATMENT FOR BREAKTHROUGH SYMPTOMS

Up to 50% of patients receiving highly emetogenic therapy may experience symptoms that surmount (i.e., "breakthrough") primary antiemetic prophylaxis. Gastrointestinal motility and drug absorption from the gut may be impaired around times when emetic symptoms occur, thus potentially compromising an orally administered drug's beneficial effect. In addition, some patients may be too ill to swallow and retain oral medications. For ambulatory outpatients, rectal suppositories are a practical alternative; however, before relying on a rectally administered drug, clinicians should ascertain whether their patient finds that route of administration acceptable. Clinicians also should avoid prescribing sustained-release drug products to treat acute breakthrough symptoms. Although sustained-release formulations are very useful for maintaining emetic control, breakthrough symptoms require a rapidly acting intervention for which sustained-release drug products are ill suited.

ANTIEMETIC COMBINATIONS

Antiemetics in combination can be more effective than single agents. The rationale for combining antiemetic agents is to:

- Improve neurotransmitter receptor blockade by targeting multiple receptor types.
- Lessen the adverse effects associated with a patient's malignant disease (e.g., anxiety), antineoplastic treatment (e.g., diarrhea), and other antiemetic agents (e.g., sedation, extrapyramidal effects), which consequently improves their overall comfort and ability to tolerate treatment.
- Develop simple antiemetic strategies suitable for outpatients that decrease the duration of hospitalization and the amount of time spent in an ambulatory care setting.

Numerous studies have demonstrated that acute phase emetic control is significantly improved when 5-HT$_3$ receptor antagonists and glucocorticoids are combined. Likewise, delayed-phase control is improved when glucocorticoids are combined with either metoclopramide or 5-HT$_3$ antagonists and perhaps with D$_2$-receptor antagonists.

PLANNING ANTIEMETIC PROPHYLAXIS

Planning effective antiemetic prophylaxis for chemotherapy entails evaluating each agent's emetic potential; characteristic severity, onset, and duration; and how those factors may be affected by drug dosage, schedule, and route of administration. Recently an expert panel developed a method for categorizing the emetic potential of drugs (see Table 3) and a companion algorithm with which one may predict the cumulative emetic potential of drug combinations (see Table 4) (7–11).

The guidelines for selecting treatment-appropriate antiemetic prophylaxis and treatment described in Fig. 2 integrate evidence-based guidelines recommended by leading professional oncology organizations [National Comprehensive Cancer Network (NCCN), American Society of Clinical Oncology (ASCO)], and the consensus of experts in oncology practice (11–14).

In Fig. 2, primary prophylaxis is indicated for all patients whose treatment has a cumulative emetic potential of 2 or more [i.e., a level at which more than 30% of persons receiving similar chemotherapy would be predicted to experience emetic symptoms (derived from Tables 2 and 3)]. Like the NCCN and ASCO guidelines, prophylaxis and treatment are based on an assessment of emetic risk; they generally are limited in application to adult patients and may not be appropriate in all clinical situations. Decisions to follow the recommendations must be based on professional judgment, individual patient circumstances, and available resources.

ANTIEMETIC OPTIONS

Serotonin (5-HT$_3$) receptor antagonists

- Dolasetron, granisetron, and ondansetron are equally effective at maximally effective dosages.
- Must exceed a "threshold" dosage to achieve optimal antiemetic responses.
  - Doses greater than a maximally effective dose do not improve antiemetic control.
  - Additional doses administered within the first 24 hours after emetogenic treatment have not been shown to improve emetic control.
- Are more effective and safer to use than other types of antiemetics.
- Are convenient to use because they have excellent oral bioavailability and a long duration of action.
- Provide equivalent antiemetic protection after either oral or parenteral administration.
- Activity against delayed-phase symptoms is similar to that of less expensive alternatives such as metoclopramide.
- Adverse-effects profiles are similar among agents and include:
  - Headache.
  - Diarrhea.
  - Constipation.
  - Transiently increased hepatic transaminase concentrations.
  - Transient ECG changes ± decreased cardiac rate.

Glucocorticoids (Steroids)

- Effective as single agents against mildly to moderately emetogenic acute-phase symptoms (emetic potential level 2 or less).

TABLE 3. *Emetic potential as a function of drug, dosage, and route of administration*

Emetic potential		Incidence of emesis[a]
Level 5 (very high)	Carmustine (>250 mg/m^2) Cisplatin (>50 mg/m^2) Cyclophosphamide (>1,500 mg/m^2) Dacarbazine Mechlorethamine Pentostatin Streptozocin	>90%
Level 4 (high)	Carboplatin Carmustine (≤250 mg/m^2) Cisplatin (<50 mg/m^2) Cyclophosphamide (>750–1,500 mg/m^2) Cytarabine (>1,000 mg/m^2) Dactinomycin (>1.5 mg/m^2) Doxorubicin (>60 mg/m^2) Irinotecan Lomustine Methotrexate (>1,000 mg/m^2) Mitoxantrone (>15 mg/m^2) Procarbazine (oral)	60%–90%
Level 3 (moderate)	Aldesleukin Altretamine Cyclophosphamide (≤750 mg/m^2) Cyclophosphamide (oral, for multiple consecutive days) Dactinomycin (≤1.5 mg/m^2) Daunorubicin Doxorubicin (20–60 mg/m^2) Epirubicin (≤90 mg/m^2) Idarubicin Ifosfamide Methotrexate (250–1,000 mg/m^2) Mitoxantrone (<15 mg/m^2)	30%–60%
Level 2 (low)	Asparaginase Cytarabine (<1,000 mg/m^2) Docetaxel Doxorubicin (<20 mg/m^2) Doxorubicin, liposomal Etoposide Fluorouracil (≤1,000 mg/m^2) Gemcitabine Methotrexate (>50–<250 mg/m^2) Mitomycin Pacilitaxel Teniposide Thiotepa Topotecan	10%–30%
Level 1 (very low)	Bleomycin Busulfan Chlorambucil (oral) Cladribine Estramustine Fludarabine Hydroxyurea Melphalan (oral) Mercaptopurine Methotrexate (≤50 mg/m^2) Thioguanine (oral) Vinblastine Vincristine Vinorelbine	<10%

Drugs are arranged alphabetically within the emetic potential levels. All drugs are administered by the intravenous route unless noted otherwise.

[a]The incidence of emesis among patients who received the drug without antiemetic protection.

TABLE 4. Algorithm for estimating the emetogenic potential of combination chemotherapy regimens

1. Identify the most emetogenic agent in a drug combination to determine the BASE SCORE.
2. FOR ANY NUMBER OF LEVEL 2 agents in the combination, ADD ONE to the BASE SCORE
3. FOR EACH LEVEL 3 or LEVEL 4 agent, ADD ONE to the BASE SCORE.
4. The sum of all amounts added to the BASE SCORE produces a CUMULATIVE EMETOGENICITY score for the drug combination.

Chemotherapy regimen[a]	Emetogenic level by drug	Cumulative emetogenicity SCORE	Predicted frequency of emesis
CMF			
Cyclophosphamide, 600 mg/m^2 i.v. on day 1	**3** (base score)	3 + 1 = 4	60–90%
Methotrexate, 40 mg/m^2 i.v. on day 1	1		
Fluorouracil, 600 mg/m^2 i.v. on day 1	2 (add 1)		
• Cycle repeats every 21 days			
CAF			
Cyclophosphamide, 500 mg/m^2 i.v. on day 1	**3** (base score)	3 + 1 + 1 = 5	>90%
doxorubicin, 50 mg/m^2 i.v. on day 1	**3** (add 1)		
fluorouracil, 500 mg/m^2 i.v. on day 1	2 (add 1)		
• Cycle repeats every 21 days			
CHOP			
Cyclophosphamide, 750 mg/m^2 i.v. on day 1	**3** (base score)	3 + 1 = 4	60–90%
Doxorubicin, 50 mg/m^2 i.v. on day 1	**3** (add 1)		
Vincristine, 1.4 mg/m^2 i.v. on day 1	1		
Prednisone, 100 mg orally days 1–5	Not applicable		
• Cycle repeats every 21 days			
ABVD			
Doxorubicin, 25 mg/m^2/d i.v. on days 1 and 14	3 (add 1)	5 + 1 = 6 (day 1)	>90% (day 1)
Bleomycin, 10 Units/m^2/d i.v. on days 1 and 14	1	5 (days 2–5)	>90% (days 2–5)
Vinblastine, 6 mg/m^2/d i.v. on days 1 and 14	1	3 (day 14)	>30–60% (day 14)
Dacarbazine 150 mg/m^2/d i.v. on days 1–5	**5** (base score)		
• Cycle repeats every 28 days			

[a]The most emetogenic agents in a combination appear in bold-faced type. I.v., intravenously.

Emetic Potential

Acute Phase - Primary Prophylaxis*,†,‡

Treatment for Breakthrough Symptoms*,‡,**

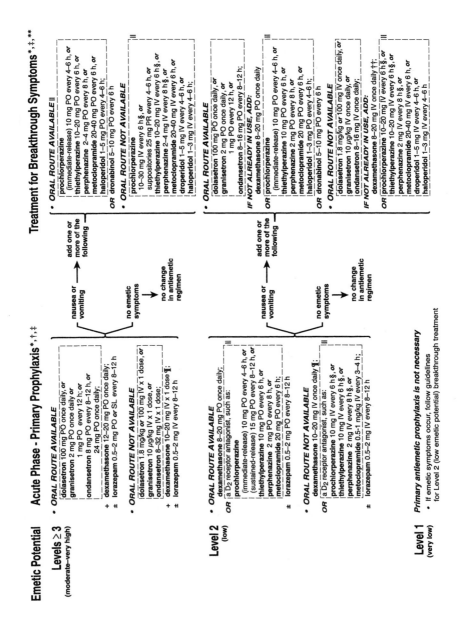

Levels ≥ 3
(moderate–very high)

- *ORAL ROUTE AVAILABLE*
  - dolasetron 100 mg PO once daily, *or*
  - granisetron 2 mg PO once daily or
    1 mg PO every 12 h; *or*
  - ondansetron 8 mg PO every 8-12 h, *or*
    24 mg PO once daily;
  - + dexamethasone 12–20 mg PO once daily;
  - ‡ lorazepam 0.5–2 mg PO or SL every 8–12 h ‖

- *ORAL ROUTE NOT AVAILABLE*
  - dolasetron 1.8 mg/kg or 100 mg IV x 1 dose, *or*
  - granisetron 10 µg/kg IV x 1 dose, *or*
  - ondansetron 8–32 mg IV x 1 dose;
  - + dexamethasone 10–20 mg IV x 1 dose ¶;
  - ‡ lorazepam 0.5–2 mg IV every 8–12 h ‖

nausea or vomiting → add one or more of the following

no emetic symptoms → no change in antiemetic regimen

- *ORAL ROUTE AVAILABLE* ‖
  - prochlorperazine
    (immediate-release) 10 mg PO every 4–6 h, *or*
  - thiethylperazine 10–20 mg PO every 6 h, *or*
  - perphenazine 2–4 mg PO every 8 h, *or*
  - metoclopramide 20–40 mg PO every 6 h, *or*
  - haloperidol 1–5 mg PO every 4–6 h;
  - *OR* dronabinol 5–10 mg PO every 6 h

- *ORAL ROUTE NOT AVAILABLE*
  - prochlorperazine
    10–30 mg IV every 6 h §, *or*
    suppositories 25 mg PR every 4–6 h, *or*
  - thiethylperazine 10–20 mg IV every 6 h §, *or*
  - perphenazine 2–4 mg IV every 8 h §, *or*
  - metoclopramide 20–40 mg IV every 6 h, *or*
  - droperidol 1–5 mg IV every 4–6 h, *or*
  - haloperidol 1–3 mg IV every 4–6 h;

Level 2
(low)

- *ORAL ROUTE AVAILABLE*
  - dexamethasone 8–20 mg PO once daily;
  - *OR* a D₂ receptor antagonist, such as:
  - prochlorperazine
    (sustained-release) 15 mg PO every 8–12 h, *or*
  - thiethylperazine 10 mg PO every 6 h, *or*
  - perphenazine 2 mg PO every 8 h, *or*
  - metoclopramide 20 mg PO every 6 h;
  - ‡ lorazepam 0.5–2 mg PO every 8–12 h ‖

- *ORAL ROUTE NOT AVAILABLE*
  - dexamethasone 10–20 mg IV once daily ¶;
  - *OR* a D₂ receptor antagonist, such as:
  - prochlorperazine 10 mg IV every 6 h §, *or*
  - thiethylperazine 10 mg IV every 6 h §, *or*
  - perphenazine 2 mg IV every 8 h §, *or*
  - metoclopramide 0.5–1 mg/kg IV every 3–4 h;
  - ‡ lorazepam 0.5–2 mg IV every 8–12 h ‖

nausea or vomiting → add one or more of the following

no emetic symptoms → no change in antiemetic regimen

- *ORAL ROUTE AVAILABLE*
  - dolasetron 100 mg PO once daily, *or*
  - granisetron 2 mg PO once daily, *or*
    1 mg PO every 12 h; *or*
  - ondansetron 8–16 mg PO every 8–12 h;
  - *IF NOT ALREADY IN USE, ADD:*
    dexamethasone 8–20 mg PO once daily
  - *OR* prochlorperazine
    (immediate-release) 10 mg PO every 4–6 h, *or*
  - thiethylperazine 10 mg PO every 6 h, *or*
  - perphenazine 2 mg PO every 8 h, *or*
  - metoclopramide 20 mg PO every 6 h, *or*
  - haloperidol 1–3 mg PO every 4–6 h;
  - *OR* dronabinol 5–10 mg PO every 6 h

- *ORAL ROUTE NOT AVAILABLE*
  - dolasetron 1.8 mg/kg or 100 mg IV once daily, *or*
  - granisetron 10 µg/kg IV once daily, *or*
  - ondansetron 8–16 mg IV once daily;
  - *IF NOT ALREADY IN USE, ADD:*
    dexamethasone 8–20 mg IV once daily ††;
  - *OR* prochlorperazine 10–20 mg IV every 6 h §, *or*
  - thiethylperazine 10–20 mg IV every 6 h §, *or*
  - perphenazine 2 mg IV every 8 h §, *or*
  - metoclopramide 20–40 mg IV every 6 h, *or*
  - droperidol 1–5 mg IV every 4–6 h, *or*
  - haloperidol 1–3 mg IV every 4–6 h

Level 1
(very low)

Primary antiemetic prophylaxis is not necessary

- If emetic symptoms occur, follow guidelines for Level 2 (low emetic potential) breakthrough treatment

Delayed Phase Prophylaxis *, ††

dexamethasone 8 mg PO every 12 h
- for 4 or 5 doses total, followed by

dexamethasone 4 mg PO every 12 h for 2 d
- 4 doses total;

or **dexamethasone** 4–8 mg PO every 8–12 h for 3 d

± **metoclopramide** 10–40 mg or 0.5 mg/kg PO
- every 6 h *or*

granisetron 2 mg PO once daily *or*
granisetron 1 mg PO every 12 h *or*
ondansetron 8 mg PO every 8 h *or* } = for 2–4 d

prochlorperazine sustained-release 15 mg PO
- every 8–12 h

± **lorazepam** 0.5–2 mg PO every 8–12 h
± **diphenhydramine** 25–50 mg PO every 6 h

Prophylaxis During Second and Subsequent Treatments

Control achieved during previous cycle	*Intervention*
No emetic symptoms	No change in initial antiemetic regimen
Nausea without emesis	Include in prophylaxis any rescue medications used during the previous cycle. All antiemetics should be given as scheduled medications
Emetic symptoms controlled by rescue ('breakthrough') medications	
Uncontrolled emetic symptoms	Implement fluid and electrolyte support. Consider: alternative primary agents, adding additional secondary agents, adding non-pharmacologic interventions, *or* an alternative antineoplastic treatment

Prophylaxis for Radiation Therapy *

Type of Radiation Therapy (RT)	*Primary Prophylaxis*	*Treatment for Breakthrough Symptoms **
Fields that include the abdomen, hemibody, mantle, craniospinal, and cranium (radiosurgery)	**granisetron** 2 mg PO once daily *or* **ondansetron** 8 mg PO every 8 h • each day RT is given	Apply chemotherapy breakthrough guidelines for emetic potential ≥3 ± **dexamethasone**
RT + Chemotherapy	Give antiemetic prophylaxis appropriate for the chemotherapy in use	
Total Body Irradiation	**granisetron** 2 mg PO *or* 10 μg/kg IV once daily *or* **ondansetron** 8 mg PO *or* IV every 8–12 h • start prophylaxis before TBI begins • repeat antiemetic prophylaxis before each TBI dose fraction • continue for ≥24 h after TBI is completed	**ondansetron** 8 mg PO *or* IV every 8-12 h • repeat each day RT is given
RT to other sites	None necessary	

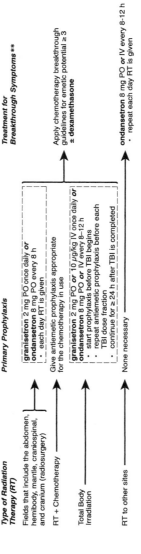

Prophylaxis for Anticipatory Symptoms *

Prevention
- complete protection against emetic symptoms during each treatment

Behavior modification and relaxation techniques
- distraction
- desensitization
- biofeedback
- relaxation
- guided imagery
- hypnosis

Pharmacotherapy
[**lorazepam** 0.5–2 mg PO *or* sublingually *or* **alprazolam** 0.5–1 mg PO]
- in the morning, before treatment
- ± an additional dose the night before treatment

- Are the most active agents against delayed-phase symptoms: dexamethasone and methyl-prednisolone are especially useful in combination with 5-HT$_3$- and D$_2$-receptor antagonists.
- Parenteral and oral doses are equivalent.
- Prophylaxis and treatment are empirically based; safety and efficacy comparisons are lacking.
- Single doses are as effective as multiple-dose schedules.
- Optimal dosages and schedules have yet to be determined.
  - Dexamethasone doses vary from 2 to 40 mg.
  - No evidence that dexamethasone doses greater than 20 mg improve antiemetic response.

Incidence of adverse effects after single doses is:
  - Usually very low.
  - Limited to "activating" psychogenic effects such as insomnia and sleep disturbances that may be minimized by administering steroids early during a patient's waking cycle.
- Adrenocortical suppression is not a problem when steroids are used for brief periods.
- Limited use for short durations may cause hyperglycemia: Glycemic control may be problematic in patients with incipient or frank diabetes.

Metoclopramide

- A weak competitive 5-HT$_3$-receptor antagonist at high dosages; activity is not superior to that of other 5-HT$_3$ antagonists against acute symptoms.
- Activity is at least equivalent to that of ondansetron against delayed-phase symptoms: metoclopramide, 20 to 40 mg (or 0.5 mg/kg) orally or i.v. 2 to 4 times daily.
- Adverse-effect profile is similar to that of other potent D$_2$ antagonists.
  - Dose-related sedation.
  - Extrapyramidal reactions.
- Gastrointestinal prokinetic effects may be useful for patients who have concomitant gastrointestinal motility disorders or gastroesophageal reflux disease.

Dopaminergic (D$_2$)-Receptor Antagonists

- Includes clinically useful phenothiazines.
  - Prochlorperazine.
  - Thiethylperazine.

←————————————————————————————————————

FIG 2. Algorithms for antiemetic prophylaxis and treatment. IV (intravenous administration); PO (oral administration); PR (rectal insertion); SL (sublingual administration). *Medications are not listed in order of preference. Pharmacologically similar alternatives are bounded by broken lines. [†]Oral prophylaxis should begin 1 hour before commencing cytotoxic treatment. Intravenous prophylaxis may be given within minutes before emetogenic treatment. [‡]Antiemetic prophylaxis should be repeated each day emetogenic treatment is administered. [§]When administered IV, phenothiazines should be given over 30 minutes to prevent hypotension. [‖]Generally, regimens containing D$_2$-receptor antagonists and metoclopramide doses ≥20 mg should include primary prophylaxis with anticholinergic agents against acute dystonic extrapyramidal reactions. For prophylaxis, diphenhydramine, 25 to 50 mg p.o. or IV every 6 hours, is often used; benztropine and trihexyphenidyl are alternatives. Parenteral administration is preferred for treating extrapyramidal symptoms. [¶]When administered IV, dexamethasone should be given as a short infusion over 10 to 15 minutes to prevent uncomfortable sensations of warmth. [**]Medications used for "breakthrough" symptoms are not alternatives to primary prophylaxis, but should be added to a patient's antiemetic regimen. [††]Delayed-phase prophylaxis may begin 12 to 24 hours after emetogenic treatment began.

- Perphenazine.
- Includes clinically useful butyrophenones.
  - Droperidol.
  - Haloperidol.
- Overall, antiemetic activity varies directly with D_2-receptor antagonism.
- Optimal dosages and schedules have not been established.
- A direct correlation between dose and antiemetic response has been demonstrated for prochlorperazine.
- Adverse-effect incidence also correlates with D_2-antagonist dose and the frequency of administration.
  - Sedation.
  - Extrapyramidal reactions (EPRs).
  - Anticholinergic effects.
- At present, only meager data support combinations of D_2-receptor antagonists with 5-HT_3 antagonists ± steroids for acute-phase symptoms and combinations with steroids, metoclopramide, or lorazepam for delayed-phase symptoms.

Benzodiazepines

- Important adjuncts to antiemetics for their anxiolytic and amnestic effects.
- Clinically useful for mitigating EPRs associated with D_2 antagonists and metoclopramide.
- Many clinically useful agents are available in oral, injectable, or both formulations. Lorazepam and alprazolam tablets are rapidly absorbed after sublingual administration.
- Primary liability is dose-related sedation.
- Pharmacodynamic effects are exaggerated in elderly patients.

Cannabinoids

- Dronabinol is an oral formulation of Δ^9-tetrahydrocannabinol (THC).
  - Empirically, dronabinol, 2.5 to 10 mg orally every 6 to 8 hours.
  - Antiemetic activity is similar to that of prochlorperazine (at low doses).
  - Produces a greater incidence of adverse effects than phenothiazines at dronabinol doses and schedules that produce comparable antiemetic effects.
- Antiemetic benefit may be achieved without producing psychotropic effects.
- Dose-related side effects occur throughout the range of clinically useful doses.
- Regulated as (Schedule II) controlled substances in the United states.
- Potential for misuse.
- Adverse effect profile includes:
  - Sedation.
  - Confusion.
  - Dizziness.
  - Recent memory impairment.
  - Euphoria or dysphoria.
  - Ataxia.
  - Dry mouth.
  - Orthostatic hypotension ± an increased heart rate.

REFERENCES

1. Kris MG, Gralla RJ, Clark RA, et al. Incidence, course, and severity of delayed nausea and vomiting following the administration of high-dose cisplatin. *J Clin Oncol* 1985;3:1379–1384.
2. Morrow GR, Hickok JT, Burish TG, et al. Frequency and clinical implications of delayed nausea and delayed emesis. *Am J Clin Oncol* 1996;19:199–203.

3. Kris MG, Roila F, De Mulder PHM, et al. Delayed emesis following anticancer chemotherapy. *Support Care Cancer* 1998;6:228–232.
4. Borison HL, McCarthy LE. Neuropharmacology of chemotherapy-induced emesis. *Drugs* 1983;25 (suppl 1):8–17.
5. Aapro M. Methodological issues in antiemetic studies. *Invest New Drugs* 1993;11:243–253.
6. Italian Group for Antiemetic Research. Cisplatin-induced delayed emesis: pattern and prognostic factors during three subsequent cycles. *Ann Oncol* 1994;5:585–589.
7. Lindley CM, Bernard S, Fields SM. Incidence and duration of chemotherapy-induced nausea and vomiting in the outpatient oncology population. *J Clin Oncol* 1989;7:1142–1149.
8. Hesketh PJ, Kris MG, Grunberg SM, et al. Proposal for classifying the acute emetogenicity of cancer chemotherapy. *J Clin Oncol* 1997;15:103–109.
9. Hesketh PJ, Gralla RJ, du Bois A, et al. Methodology of antiemetic trials: response assessment, evaluation of new agents and definition of chemotherapy emetogenicity. *Support Care Cancer* 1998;6:221–227.
10. Gralla RJ. Antiemetic therapy. *Semin Oncol* 1998;25:577–583.
11. ASHP. Therapeutic guidelines on the pharmacologic management of nausea and vomiting in adult and pediatric patients receiving chemotherapy or radiation therapy or undergoing surgery [see comments]. *Am J Health Syst Pharm* 1999;56:729–764. Comment in: *Am J Health Syst Pharm* 1999;56:728.
12. NCCN. Antiemesis practice guidelines. *Oncology (Huntingt)* 1997;11(suppl 11A):57–89.
13. Gandara DR, Roila F, Warr D, et al. Consensus proposal for 5HT$_3$ antagonists in the prevention of acute emesis related to highly emetogenic chemotherapy: dose, schedule, and route of administration. *Support Care Cancer* 1998;6:237–243.
14. Gralla RJ, Osoba D, Kris MG, et al. Recommendations for the use of antiemetics: evidence-based, clinical practice guidelines. *J Clin Oncol* 1999;17:2971–2994.

42

Malnutrition in Oncology Patients

Marnie Dobbin

Nutrition Department, National Institutes of Health, Bethesda, Maryland

Incidence: more than 40% of oncology patients develop signs of malnutrition during treatment.

Impact: malnourished patients have

- Impaired responses to treatment (1,2).
- Incur higher costs for their care.
- Have increased rates of mortality and morbidity (2).
- As many as 20% of oncology patients die of nutritional complications rather than of their primary diagnosis (3).

To minimize malnutrition: Nutritional deterioration in oncology patients is not inevitable and can be minimized dramatically with appropriate screening and timely intervention.

IDENTIFYING NUTRITIONAL RISK

For nutrition interventions to be effective, patients at risk for malnutrition must be identified before irreversible deficits occur.

Parameters most useful in identifying patients at nutritional risk include (see Fig. 1):

- Weight change.
- Functional status.
- Symptom status.
- Changes in food intake.
- Changes in body composition.
- Visceral protein markers.

Simple, validated tools have been developed to allow the timely identification of patients at risk.

- The Subjective Global Assessment (SGA) form developed by Dr. Jeejeebhoy et al. (1987) has been adapted for use with oncology patients by Dr. Faith Ottery [Contact Ottery & Associates Inc., phone, 215-351-4050].
- This patient-generated tool (PG-SGA) helps identify patients at nutritional risk and may improve patient satisfaction, as attention to a patient's nutritional health is a major concern for patients and their families.

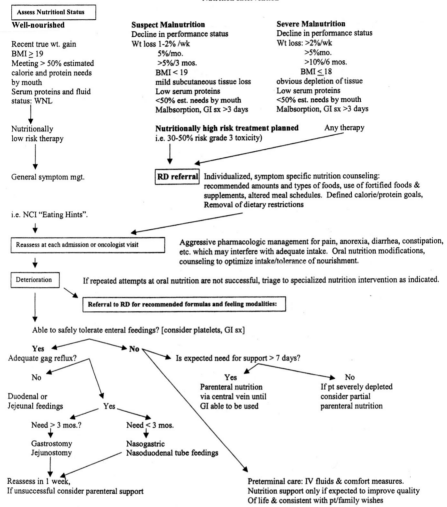

Nutrition Intervention

Assess Nutritionl Status

Well-nourished	Suspect Malnutrition	Severe Malnutrition
	Decline in performance status	Decline in performance status
Recent true wt. gain	Wt loss 1-2% /wk	Wt loss: >2%/wk
BMI ≥ 19	5%/mo.	>5%mo.
Meeting > 50% estimated	>5%/3 mos.	>10%/6 mos.
calorie and protein needs	BMI < 19	BMI ≤ 18
by mouth	mild subcutaneous tissue loss	obvious depletion of tissue
Serum proteins and fluid	Low serum proteins	Low serum proteins
status: WNL	<50% est. needs by mouth	<50% est. needs by mouth
	Malbsorption, GI sx >3 days	Malbsorption, GI sx >3 days

Nutritionally low risk therapy

Nutritionally high risk treatment planned i.e. 30-50% risk grade 3 toxicity)   Any therapy

General symptom mgt.

RD referral   Individualized, symptom specific nutrition counseling: recommended amounts and types of foods, use of fortified foods & supplements, altered meal schedules. Defined calorie/protein goals, Removal of dietary restrictions

i.e. NCI "Eating Hints".

Reassess at each admission or oncologist visit   Aggressive pharmacologic management for pain, anorexia, diarrhea, constipation, etc. which may interfere with adequate intake. Oral nutrition modifications, counseling to optimize intake/tolerance of nourishment.

Deterioration   If repeated attempts at oral nutrition are not successful, triage to specialized nutrition intervention as indicated.

Referral to RD for recommended formulas and feeling modalities:

Able to safely tolerate enteral feedings? [consider platelets, GI sx]

Yes   No

Adequate gag reflux?   Is expected need for support > 7 days?

No   Yes   No

Duodenal or   Parenteral nutrition   If pt severely depleted
Jejeunal feedings   Yes   via central vein until   consider partial
                                    GI able to be used   parenteral nutrition

Need > 3 mos.?   Need < 3 mos.

Gastrostomy   Nasogastric
Jejunostomy   Nasoduodenal tube feedings

Reassess in 1 week,   Preterminal care: IV fluids & comfort measures.
If unsuccessful consider parenteral support   Nutrition support only if expected to improve quality
                                                      Of life & consistent with pt/family wishes

FIG. 1. Parameters most useful in identifying patients at nutritional risk. RD, registered dietician; BMI, body mass index; GI, gastrointestinal.

EFFECTIVE NUTRITION INTERVENTION

Continual reassessment, pharmacologic management, and nutrition counseling can reduce the need for costly, risky nutrition support options.

Identifying Risk

When nutritional risk is identified early, with realistic nutrition interventions implemented in a timely manner, there can be:

• Improvement in quality of life and nutritional status.
• Weight maintenance.

Nutrition counseling by registered dietitians (R.D.) is associated with improvement in quality of life, improvement in nutritional parameters, and the success of oral nutrition intervention for oncology patients (Table 1).

Effective nutrition intervention by an R.D. may include:

• Modifications of foods and feeding schedules.
• Fortification of foods with modular nutrition products.
• Supplementation with meal-replacement products.
• Eating is highly individualized and complex, affected by such factors as food aversions/associations, cultural influences, and family dynamics.
• Nutrition recommendations must be tailored to the individual's needs, incorporating input from the patient and family to be successful.
• Providing nutrition samples and written information alone is not associated with nutritional success.
• Self-imposed diets and the use of dietary supplements should be evaluated by an R.D. for possible risks and the potential to confound results of protocols (see Table 2).

NUTRITION SUPPORT

Controversies

Although tumor growth is stimulated by a number of nutrients, limitation of the nutrients preferred by tumors can lead to detriments in the host.

• Maintenance of good nutritional status does not appear to have deleterious effects on tumor growth.

TABLE 1. *Simple food/oral nutrition supplement recommendations*

Neutropenia: emphasize food-borne illness prevention (well-washed produce is not contraindicated)
Early satiety: calorically dense foods/nutrition products (*e.g., Scandi and Polycose*)
Poor appetite/fatigue: to ↓ dependence on appetite >5 scheduled feedings/day, reliance on nutritious liquids (quenching thirst) without need for appetite
Nausea: ↓ fat foods/supplements (*Biocare, Boost, Resource drink*)
Malabsortion: semielemental palatable products (*Propeptide oral formulation*)
Diarrhea: ↓ lactose, ↓ fat, ↓ insoluble fiber, ↑ soluble fiber (*Benefiber and Ensure light*)
Fat malabsorption: ↓ fat diet and MCT–oil fortified foods/products (*e.g., Lipisorb*)
Aversion to canned "milkshake-type" products: fortification of preferred foods (*e.g.*, soups) with modular kcal or protein supplements (*Polycose, Promod*)

Refer to R.D., for comparable products at your facility. Brand names provided as examples only–does not imply endorsement.

TABLE 2. *Quick nutrition reference for adult oncology patients*

Estimated requirements
 Kilocalories: 20 kcals/kg (actual wt) for obese
 25–30 kcals/kg for sedentary
 35 kcals/kg for hypermetabolic pt or malabsorption
 Fluid: 1 cc/kcal; 35 ml/kg; 1,500 m/m^2 body surface
 1,500 ml/kg for first 20 kg, plus 25 ml/kg for the remaining wt
 Protein: 1.2 g/kg. Weekly 24-hr urine for UUN to assess adequacy 0.8 g pro/kg = RDA and
  is appropriate for nondialyzed renal insufficiency
BMI (body mass index): Wt (kg)/Ht(m^2) BMI 19–25, healthy wt range
Nutrient limitations for nutrition support:
 Dextrose (parenteral nutrition via central-line TPN):
  Maximal glucose oxidation rate ~4–6 mg/kg/min (TPN)
  Initial dextrose concentration: 10–15%; final, 20–25% [peripheral parenteral nutrition
   (PPN)]: final dextrose conc., 10%
 Lipids to provide 30% of total kcals usually (up to 60% Tkcals for PPN)
Diets and supplements that pose a risk: Gerson's diet, strict macrobiotic diet;
 Chapparal, P'au D'arco, Mistletoe, DHEA; Vit A >5,000 IU/d, B$_6$ >200 mg/d, chromium
  >200 µg/d
 Vit D >1,600 IU/d, Fe >15 mg/d (unless Fe deficiency clear), Zn >25 mg/d. Vit C >250 mg/d
  may alter renal excretion of chemotherapy. Any single antioxidant taken in excess (e.g., β-
  carotene) may cause a pro-oxidant state or malabsorption of other antioxidants (Vit E
  <800 IU/day has not been found to be harmful in Vit K–sufficient adults not taking
  anticoagulants).

- In more than 200 Hodgkin's disease (HD) patients, malnourished patients had greater rates of tumor growth (demonstrated by incorporation of [^{3}H]thymidine-labeling index in the tumor tissue) than well-nourished patients (6).

Enteral Nutrition

The superiority of enteral nutrition over parenteral has been reviewed in many references (7).
- If the gut works, it should be used.
- To be successful, enteral nutrition should be implemented as soon as the need arises.
- Surgeons may approve feeding within 4 hours of placement of gastrostomy tubes and immediately after jejunostomy placement (as bowel sounds are not needed).
- Prophylactic placement of gastrointestinal (GI) tubes can significantly reduce the amount of weight loss during radiotherapy and decrease the number of admissions due to dehydration, weight loss, or other complications of mucositis (8).
- Reviews of nutrition-support practices indicate that parenteral nutrition is often instituted when safer, more physiologic enteral nutrition support could have been provided (7,9).

Parenteral Nutrition

- Total parenteral nutrition (TPN) can be beneficial to cancer patients when response to treatment is good but the associated nutritional morbidity high, and the GI tract is unavailable to nutrition support.
- The use of perioperative TPN should be limited to patients who are severely malnourished, with surgery expected to prevent oral intake for more than 10 days after surgery (8,10) (see Table 2).

- Feeding is synonymous with caring by many family members. Provision of nominal supportive care for preterminal patients can reduce family tension and may reduce readmissions due to hydration and electrolyte maintenance problems.
- Data indicate that there can be improved quality of life and functional status for selected preterminal patients receiving parenteral nutrition. The risks and benefits of nutrition support must be addressed individually and evaluated with patient and family input.

REFERENCES

1. Aker SN. Oral feedings in the cancer patient. *Cancer* 1979;43(suppl):2103–2107.
2. Ottery FD. Nutritional oncology: a proactive, integrated approach to the cancer patient. In: Chernoff R, ed. *Nutrition support theory and therapeutics*. New York: Chapman & Hall, 1997:395–409.
3. Ambrus J, Ambrus CM, Mink IB, et al. Causes of death in cancer patients. *J Med Clin Exp Ther* 1975; 6:61–64.
4. Ottery FD. Supportive nutrition to prevent cachexia and improve quality of life. *Semin Oncol* 1995; 22(2 suppl 3):98–111.
5. Osoba D. Current applications of health-related quality of life assessment in oncology. *Support Care Cancer* 1997;5:100–104.
6. Bozzetti FEA. Relationship between nutritional status and tumor growth in humans. *Tumori* 1995; 81:1–6.
7. Mercadante S. Parenteral versus enteral nutrition in cancer patients: indications and practice. *Support Care Cancer* 1998;6:85–93.
8. Lee JH, Machtay M, Unger LD, et al. Prophylactic gastrostomy tubes in patients undergoing intensive irradiation for cancer of the head and neck. *Arch Otolaryngol Head Neck Surg* 1998;124: 871–875.
9. Bowman LEA. Algorithm for nutritional support: experience of the metabolic and infusion support service of St. Jude Children's research hospital. *Int J Cancer* 1998;11:76–80.
10. Kelly CJ, Daly JM. Perioperative care of the oncology patient. *World J Surg* 1993;17:199–206.

43

Rehabilitation of the Cancer Patient

Usha Chaudhry and Jay P. Shah

Rehabilitation Medicine Department, National Institutes of Health, Bethesda, Maryland

Cancer is a chronic and complex disease with distinct and predictable phases that present opportunities for rehabilitation intervention (see Fig. 1). Disability is a major problem for patients undergoing cancer treatments. It is a result of local and distant effects of tumor as well as treatment sequelae. Treatment and prevention of disability require a comprehensive and multidisciplinary approach and frequently span several life stages.

The cancer rehabilitation team is committed to helping the patient achieve his or her functional goals through all phases of the disease and its treatments. Cancer patients frequently require rehabilitation for the following general problems: pain, decreased mobility and self-care, fatigue, and weakness. There may also be problems more specific to tumor type, size, location, and proximity to other critical structures (bone, nerve, vessels). These include dysphagia, lymphedema, cognitive impairment, neuropathy, and bony metastatic disease. The rehabilitation professions can make significant contributions in these situations.

As Fig. 1 indicates, rehabilitation is a dynamic process that can and should begin as soon after the diagnosis as possible and continue for the duration of the illness and its treatments. Physiatrists are often introduced into staging and treatment decision making to assess the functional aspects of potential treatment options at each phase of illness. This may have a significant impact on the patient's abilities and quality of life.

The physiatrist is a physician who specializes in rehabilitation medicine and is uniquely qualified to evaluate the impact of disease/injury on the patient's physical status, abilities, vocational, avocational, and psychological background, family/societal roles, and aspirations. The physiatrist formulates a problem list and appropriate treatment plan to optimize their functional abilities in each of these domains. The ultimate goal of cancer rehabilitation is optimal function.

There are important problems and rehabilitation interventions in Fig. 1 that merit further discussion: pain (see Chapter 38), lymphedema, bony metastatic disease, peripheral neuropathy, and deficits in strength, range of motion (ROM), and endurance.

LYMPHEDEMA

Any patient with a diagnosis of cancer who has undergone lymphadenectomy and/or radiation therapy has the potential to develop lymphedema. For example, lymphedema occurs in patients with breast cancer, prostate cancer, ovarian cancer, renal cell carcinoma, post-ILP (isolated limb perfusion), and IL-2 (interleukin 2) treatments for patients with melanoma, renal cell carcinoma, and soft tissue sarcoma. Risk factors for lymphedema include extent of surgery, receipt of axillary radiation, obesity, and possible surgical intervention. Prevention of lymphedema depends on two factors: (a) not interfering with lymph outflow, by not constricting the arm and by protecting from infection, scarring, and burns; and (b) limiting capillary

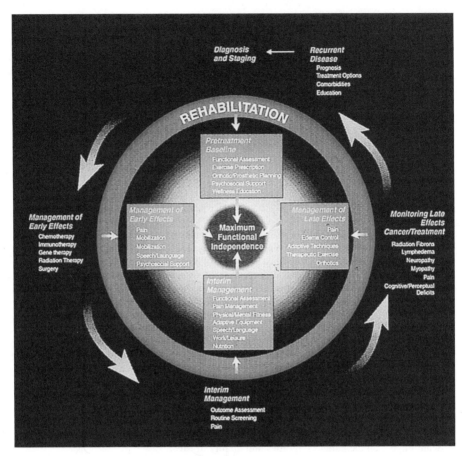

FIG 1. Rehabilitation cycle.

filtration by using compression garments when exercising and avoiding vasodilation through heat exposure (sun, sauna, and steam).

Best results are obtained with early detection, diagnosis, and intervention. Helpful treatments include elevation of the extremity; compression therapy with bandages, garments, and pneumatic pumps; benzopyrone (acts by increasing the hydraulic resistance of the capillary membrane and by exerting a proteolytic effect in lymphedema); manual lymph-drainage massage; and patient education on how to protect the limb at risk for developing lymphedema.

BONY METASTATIC DISEASE

Bony metastatic disease can occur with most types of cancers but is especially common in tumors of the breast, lung, prostate, kidney, thyroid, and hematologic system (myeloma, lymphoma, and leukemia). Immediate attention is required to prevent pathologic fracture or spinal cord compression. Locations particularly at risk for pathologic fracture include the femur, thoracolumbar junction, proximal humerus, pelvis, ribs, and skull. Symptoms may include pain, instability with risk of pathologic fracture, and, in the case of spine or skull metastasis, compromise of adjacent neurologic structures.

Assessment of fracture risk depends on the size, location, and type of metastatic lesion (lytic or blastic). Fracture risk (see Fig. 2) increases for lesions greater than 2.5 cm in the lower and 3.0 cm in the upper extremities; involvement of more than 50% of the bony cortex; intramedullary lesions more than 50% cross-sectional diameter; and involvement of length of cortex more than cross-sectional diameter of bone.

Lytic lesions are more likely to fracture than are blastic lesions and typically occur in tumors of the breast, lung, kidney, and thyroid; gastrointestinal tumors; neuroblastoma; melanoma; and lymphoma.

Plain radiographs are obtained to evaluate bony stability of the long bones. In the spine, flexion–extension films also should be obtained, although lesions less than 1 cm require computed tomography (CT) or magnetic resonance imaging (MRI). When an unstable lesion is suspected, surgical referral should be initiated and the patient should be non–weight bearing on the affected extremity. Although bony metastasis is a finding of progressive malignancy,

FEMORAL LESIONS AT RISK
FOR FRACTURE

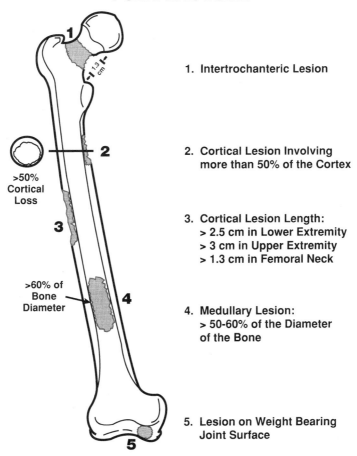

1. Intertrochanteric Lesion

2. Cortical Lesion Involving more than 50% of the Cortex

3. Cortical Lesion Length:
   > 2.5 cm in Lower Extremity
   > 3 cm in Upper Extremity
   > 1.3 cm in Femoral Neck

4. Medullary Lesion:
   > 50-60% of the Diameter of the Bone

5. Lesion on Weight Bearing Joint Surface

FIG 2. Femoral lesions at risk for fracture.

SPINAL COLUMNS
THREE COLUMN SPINE CONCEPT

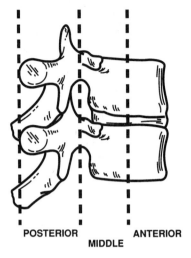

POSTERIOR   ANTERIOR
MIDDLE

ANTERIOR -
    Anterior Longitudinal Ligament
    Anterior Wall of the Vertebral Body
    Anterior Part of the Annulus Fibrosus

MIDDLE -
    Posterior Longitudinal Ligament
    Posterior Wall of the Vertebral Body
    Posterior Part of the Annulus Fibrosus

POSTERIOR -
    Supraspinous Ligament
    Interspinous Ligament
    Facet Capsule
    Ligamentum Flavum

FIG 3. Three-column spine concept.

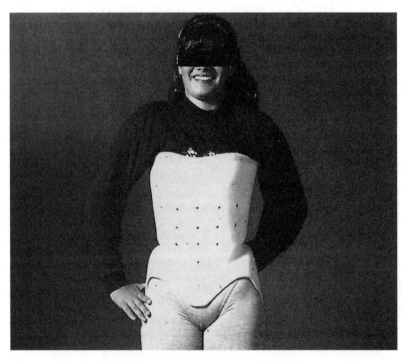

FIG 4. a: Thoracolumbar orthosis (aka clamshell brace), front view.

usually without hope of cure, patients may survive for a period of years, especially with breast, prostate, and thyroid malignancies.

After assessing the severity of the lesion, the physiatrist will recommend mobility precautions that may range from complete non–weight bearing of an affected limb to no precautions whatsoever. Bed rest is to be avoided because additional functional loss will occur, and hypercalcemia and thromboembolic disease may complicate the course.

In cases of spinal metastasis, the three-column model of Denis (Fig. 3) is often used, with the spine considered to have anterior, middle, and posterior columns (see figure for description). If two or more of these columns are involved, or the middle column alone is involved, the lesion is considered unstable. Jewett bracing or a custom-molded thoracolumbosacral orthosis (TLSO; Fig. 4) can be used in cases of anterior or middle column involvement. However, patients are often resistant to spinal orthotics because of poor skin tolerance, perceived

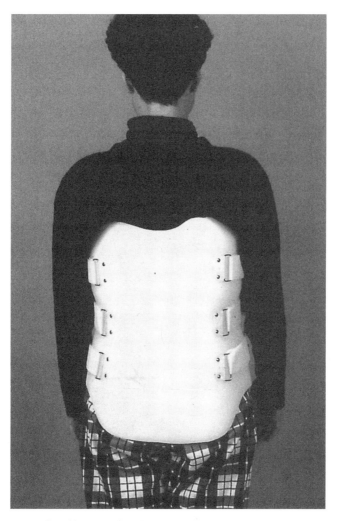

FIG 4. *(Continued)* **b:** Thoracolumbar orthosis, rear view.

discomfort, and lack of a clear end point. In such cases, a thoracolumbar corset is recommended to provide limited support and pain relief. Its use in combination with a gait aid such as a walker will minimize torque across the spine.

For lesions involving the cervical spine, a Philadelphia collar (Fig. 5), sternal/occipital/mandibular immobilizer (SOMI) or even a halo orthotic can be used, depending on the severity of the findings.

Activity recommendations should focus on exercises that increase strength and stamina while minimizing bony impact. Examples include isometric strengthening, isotonic nonresistive exercise, and aerobic exercise such as swimming, riding a stationary bicycle, or walking. Patient education should focus on attention to proper body mechanics such as avoiding sud-

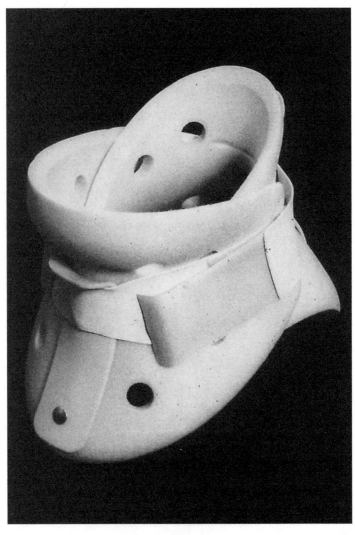

FIG 5. Philadelphia collar.

den spine or limb torsions, and on fall-prevention strategies given the possible influence of medication on balance and blood pressure.

PERIPHERAL NEUROPATHY

Chemotherapy is the most common cause of peripheral neuropathy in patients with cancer. It can also be caused by remote effects of tumor, such as lung, breast, and colon cancers, among others. Common findings include pain, paresthesias, numbness, and unsteady gait.

Treatment includes medication, such as carbamazepine, quinidine, or tricyclic agents to treat pain or cramping, and therapy for the underlying malignancy. The physiatrist can recommend appropriate nonconstrictive footwear to minimize the likelihood of ulceration resulting from poor sensory feedback. Other measures include exercise to maintain strength and

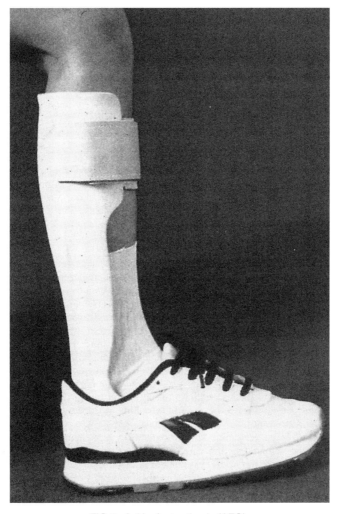

FIG 6. Ankle–foot orthosis (AFO).

range of motion, appropriate prescription of orthotics (Fig. 6), assistive and adaptive devices, and energy-conservation strategies.

STRENGTH, ROM, AND ENDURANCE DEFICITS

Strength, range of motion (ROM), and endurance deficits in cancer patients may be caused by the cancer itself, prolonged periods of bed rest, local cast use, chemotherapy, steroids, radiation, and surgical treatments. The use of therapeutic exercise programs to maintain ROM and increase strength and endurance is appropriate.

Strength deficits may be caused by a variety of factors including disuse, local casts, inactivity, poor nutrition, steroid myopathy, peripheral neuropathy, plexopathy, surgical excision of muscle and nerves and malignancies associated with polymyositis.

ROM deficits may result from local compression of a nerve plexus or peripheral nerves, tumor invasion of soft tissue or bone, prolonged bed rest, inactivity, casting procedures, and high-dose radiation therapy around joints.

Deconditioning always follows prolonged bed rest or inactivity, with frequent concomitant orthostatic intolerance, ataxia, diminution in heart rate and stroke volume, and increased pulse rate. Furthermore, the cancer itself can decrease static muscle and dynamic cardiorespiratory endurance.

Cancer patients may have increased metabolic needs and impaired protein-sparing mechanisms. These problems, combined with inactivity, decreased caloric intake, and administration of chemotherapeutic agents and anabolic steroids may result in varying degrees of loss of lean body mass and decreased muscle endurance. Therefore any method that spares protein breakdown and enhances incorporation of nutrient protein into lean muscle should be beneficial for cancer patients.

There is a scientific basis for exercise in cancer patients. Muscle tension is widely believed to enhance protein synthesis, thereby preventing muscle atrophy and increasing muscle mass in cancer patients. Moderate exercise increases the efficacy of dietary protein utilization. In normal individuals, various forms of exercise (isometric, isotonic, isokinetic) have been shown to increase muscle strength. Furthermore, aerobic exercise increases cardiorespiratory fitness, work capacity, and functional ability, and leads to a decrease in mortality rate and diminution of disease risk factors (hyperlipidemia, elevated blood pressure, obesity), as well as risk of coronary artery disease.

Professionals who work with large numbers of cancer patients believe that therapeutic exercise increases their strength, endurance, well-being, and functional levels. When prescribing therapeutic exercise, one must determine the exercise goals with consideration of the stage of cancer. During the early stages of cancer, goals may be clearly preventive and restorative in nature. The restorative group may include patients with complete cure or in remission.

If functional deficits already exist when the patient is first evaluated, or if they occur during treatment, restorative goals are obvious, and ROM and stretching may be needed. Preventive therapies, such as ROM exercises, should be given during all the cancer-treatment periods. When the patient is confined to bed, isometric and isotonic exercise with a Theraband™ (an elastic rubber band in different colors for different amounts of resistance used for mild resistive exercises) tied to the bed is useful for the upper and lower extremities. Isometric exercises for the lower extremities can be done by installing a bedboard (piece of plywood) for hamstrings and gastrocnemius.

Endurance exercises are very important for patients with preventive and restorative goals. However, before they are initiated, a careful and ongoing review of the patient's electrocardiogram (ECG), chest film, cardiovascular examination, electrolyte balance, hydration, hematocrit/hemoglobin (Hct/Hb), and current medications must be done.

Moderate exercise is thought to be beneficial for patients with cancer. However, one needs to consider hematologic, cardiac, pulmonary, and skeletal factors when establishing exercise precautions.

We gratefully acknowledge the editorial assistance of Jeanne E. Hicks, M.D.

REFERENCES

1. Gerber LH, Vargo M. Rehabilitation for patients with cancer diagnoses. In: Delisa JA, Gans BM, eds. *Rehabilitation medicine: principles and practice.* 3rd ed. Philadelphia: Lippincott-Raven, 1998:1293.
2. Denis F. Spinal instability as defined by the three-column spine concept in acute spinal trauma. *Clin Orthop* 1984;189:65–76.
3. Gerber LH. Rehabilitation management for women with breast cancer: maximizing functional outcomes. In: Harris JR, Lippman MG, Morow M, et al., eds. *Disease of the breast.* Philadelphia: Lippincott–Raven, 1996:939–947.
4. Given CW, Given BA, Stommel M. The impact of age, treatment and symptoms on the physical and mental and mental health of cancer patients: a longitudinal perspective. *Cancer* 1994;74(suppl 7): 2128–2138.
5. Hicks JE. Exercise for cancer patients. In: Basmajian JV, Wolf SL, eds. *Therapeutic exercise.* Baltimore: Williams & Wilkins, 1990:351–369.

44

Clinical Trials

Helgi Van de Velde and *Louise Grochow

*Janssen Pharmaceutica N.V., Beerse, Belgium, and *Investigational Drug Branch,
Cancer Therapy and Evaluation Program, National Cancer Institute,
National Institutes of Health, Bethesda, Maryland*

AIMS OF THIS CHAPTER

- Describe the different steps in the cancer drug–development process to help the reader understand the clinical trial reports published in the literature.
- Provide practical suggestions on how to obtain further information on currently available clinical trials or on compounds currently in development.

PHASE I TRIAL

- **Phase I trial:** the initial clinical test of a new agent or of a new combination of agents in humans. Patients are treated at predefined escalating dose levels.
- **Objectives:** Principal objective is to define a safe dose and schedule suitable for later efficacy testing. Additional objectives of most phase I studies are the gathering of pharmacokinetic data and the preliminary assessment of the effect of the agent (tumor responses, pharmacologic effect on drug target).
- **Patient characteristics:**
  - With any type of cancer for which no effective therapeutic options are known.
  - Adequate major organ function and good performance status are required in initial trials.
  - Generally, a relatively small number of patients (20 to 40) are enrolled. Patients are treated in small cohorts (one to six, depending on the study design) per dose level.
- **Starting dose:** chosen as a low drug dose that was nontoxic in non–tumor-bearing animals. A typical starting dose is 1/10 of the equivalent dose in mg/m^2 of the LD_{10} (dose lethal to 10% of animals) of a rodent species, unless that dose was found to be severely toxic to a nonrodent species. If this dose is found safe in the first patient cohort, the next cohort will be treated at the next dose level.
- **Dose-escalation schemes:** typically consist of a rapid escalation of lower, presumably more tolerable, doses and a slower escalation as the dose increases and/or side effects become apparent.
  - Most conventional escalation scheme is the *modified Fibonacci scheme,* in which the second dose is double the starting dose, the third dose is 67% greater than the second, the fourth dose is 50% greater than the third, and each subsequent step is 33% greater than the preceding dose.
  - Alternative *accelerated titration* schemes have been designed to limit the number of patients treated at the lower (presumably inactive) dose levels (1).

TABLE 1. *Data bases of cancer trials*

PDQ Clinical Trials Database	NCI's comprehensive database of currently open cancer clinical trials worldwide (*contains separate user-friendly search forms for health professionals and for patients*)	cancernet.nci.nih.gov/pdq.htm
Cancer Trials	NCI's clinical trials information resource (*contains background reading on clinical trials and research news*)	cancertrials.nci.nih.gov
NCI CTC 2.0	NCI Common Toxicity Criteria version 2.0 (*commonly used grading system of treatment-induced toxicities*)	ctep.info.nih.gov/CTC3/ctc.htm
CANCERLIT	Major cancer-related bibliographic data base (*particularly useful for clinical trial abstracts presented at conferences and not readily available in other data bases*)	cnetdb.nci.nih.gov/cancerlit.shtml
MedWatch	FDA Medical Products Reporting Program (*program to report serious drug-related adverse events in the context of postmarketing surveillance*)	www.fda.gov/medwatch
Cooperative groups		
CALGB	Cancer And Leukemia Group B	www-calgb.uchicago.edu
ECOG	Eastern Cooperative Oncology Group	ecog.dfci.harvard.edu
NCCTG	North Central Cancer Treatment Group	ncctg.mayo.edu
NSABP	National Surgical Adjuvant Breast and Bowel Project	www.nsabp.pitt.edu
POG	Pediatric Oncology Group	www.pog.ufl.edu
RTOG	Radiation Therapy Oncology Group	www.rtog.org
SWOG	Southwest Oncology Group	www.swog.saci.org
EORTC	European Organization for Research and Treatment of Cancer	www.eortc.be
NCIC-CTG	National Cancer Institute of Canada Clinical Trials Group	www.ctg.queensu.ca

Some study designs permit the patient cohorts to be subsequently re-treated at a higher dose level (*intrapatient dose escalation*).
- End of dose escalation:
  - For drugs in which toxicity is anticipated: escalation continues until a *maximal tolerated dose* (MTD) is defined. This MTD is the dose level below the dose for which *dose-limiting toxicity* (DLT) is observed in a predefined number of patients. A dose for further phase II studies is chosen based on this MTD (usually 80% of the MTD). Toxicities are graded according to predefined criteria (e.g., NCI CTC 2.0, Table 1).
  - For agents in which little or no toxicity is anticipated: dose escalation can be stopped based on measurements of immunologic or other host responses (biologically effective dose) or based on practical limitations (e.g., maximal possible volume that can be locally administered).

PHASE II TRIAL

- **Objectives:** to obtain an estimate of the response rate of a tumor type to a new agent or combination of agents administered in a dose schedule as determined in phase I. Additional objective is the gathering of more safety data, especially the identification of unusual or chronic toxicities that may not be identified in small phase I studies.
- **Patients:**
  - Trials are tumor-type specific (or may be specific for same molecular target).
  - Most trials will require patients to have *measurable* primary tumors or metastases (whose dimensions can be defined with reasonable accuracy) in order to assess tumor response. This is in contrast to *evaluable* disease, in which dimensions cannot be precisely determined (e.g., bone metastases on bone scan, pleural effusions, lymphangitic pulmonary metastases).
  - Usually 25 to 50 patients per tumor type. Trials often have a two-stage design allowing early termination of the study if a predefined response rate of interest is not achieved after the first stage. For example, if the minimal response rate of interest is 20%, there is a 95% chance that one or more responses will be observed in 14 consecutive cases. If no responses are seen in these 14 patients, the trial may end there. To minimize the number of patients treated with ineffective agents in phase II trials, alternative two-stage designs have been evaluated (2).
- **Assessment of response:** most commonly used response categories are complete response, partial response, progression, or stable disease. Definitions of these response categories depend on whether lesions are measured in two dimensions (WHO criteria, 1979) or only in their largest dimension (RECIST criteria, 1999; Table 2) (3). Although an appropriate end point, tumor response should not automatically be assumed to reflect patient benefit.
- ***Randomized phase II study:*** two therapeutic approaches are comparatively studied in a preliminary fashion to identify the one that is least likely to be found useful in a subsequent phase III study.

PHASE III TRIAL

- **Objective:** to compare a new agent or combination of agents (*test arm*) quantitatively with a treatment of proven efficacy or with placebo (*control arm*). The study can be designed to demonstrate *superiority* over the control arm or *therapeutic equivalence* between the two arms.
- **Patients:**
  - Trials are tumor specific.
  - Often, large sample sizes of 100 to 3,000 patients or more are required, and accrual may take 2 to 5 years or more. For example, 2,105 patients were included in NSABP-B06 (total mastectomy vs. lumpectomy with or without irradiation in breast cancer), whereas only

TABLE 2. *Response categories*

Response category	WHO criteria	RECIST criteria
Complete response (CR)	Disappearance of all known disease sites without development of new sites for ≥1 mo	Disappearance of all lesions
Partial response (PR)	At least 50% decrease in sum of products of the bidimensional measurements of all lesions with no new lesions appearing for ≥1 mo	At least 30% decrease in sum of longest diameter (LD) of target lesions with no lesions appearing for ≥1 mo
Stable disease (SD)	No significant change in tumor size	Neither sufficient shrinkage to qualify for PR nor sufficient increase to qualify for PD, taking as references the smallest sum of LD of target lesions
Progressive disease (PD)	At least 25% increase in same sum of products or appearance of any new lesion	At least 20% increase in sum of LD of target lesions, taking as references the smallest sum LD recorded since treatment started or appearance of any new lesion

121 patients were required in INT-R8501 (radiation vs. radiation plus chemotherapy in esophageal cancer). Because of the large sample size, phase III trials are nearly always multiinstitutional and are often coordinated by *cooperative oncology groups* (Table 1).
- Each arm of the study should be composed of comparable groups of patients. *Randomization:* patients are randomly (presumably without any bias) assigned to one of the treatment arms at the moment of study entry. *Stratification* for major prognostic factors is an additional way of reducing imbalance.
- Phase III trials often have multiple end points. These end points should address the clinical benefit to patients.
  - Primary end point is the parameter predicted to be most informative for the value of the new approach, and the trial sample size (the minimal number of patients in the study) is calculated such that the difference between the two treatment groups for this end point is statistically significant. Most common primary end points in phase III: overall survival, disease-free survival, or time to progression, although in palliative settings, quality of life can be an equally valid end point of patient benefit.
  - Limited data on other, secondary end points also are collected.

PHASE IV TRIAL

- Phase IV trials: large-scale postmarketing safety studies.
- **Objective:** detection of rare but serious side effects when a new treatment is applied to a large population.
- **Rationale:** Regulatory approval and marketing of a new treatment is usually based on the experience with a relatively small number of patients treated for relatively short periods in the phase I to III trials. When such treatment is applied to a large population, there is a possibility of encountering uncommon serious side effects.
- Serious adverse events associated with the use of a new drug and encountered outside of a phase IV trial should be reported by the individual physician through the FDA MedWatch program (Table 1).

PRACTICAL SUGGESTIONS

Table 1 provides a list of useful internet websites related to clinical trials in oncology.
- *PDQ Clinical Trials database* provides detailed information on trials currently open in particular diseases. It can be searched by phase of study, disease site, drug name, and geographic location or institution.
- *CancerLit* allows access to clinical trial abstracts that are presented at conferences but are not yet available as manuscripts.
- *CancerTrials* provides research news and background reading on clinical trials in oncology.
- *NCI CTC 2.0* is a commonly used grading system to grade treatment-related toxicities.
- *FDA MedWatch* program allows reporting of serious drug-related adverse events for compounds approved for off-study use.
- Description of predicted toxicities of experimental compounds should be available in the study protocol, which is often available through the institution's website. If not, it can be obtained through the pharmacy of the institution participating in the study.

REFERENCES

1. Simon R, Freidlin B, Rubinstein L, et al. Accelerated titration designs for phase I clinical trials in oncology. *J Natl Cancer Inst* 1997;89:1138–1147.
2. Simon R. Optimal two-stage designs for phase II clinical trials. *Control Clin Trials* 1989;10:1–10.
3. James K, Eisenhauer E, Christian M, et al. Measuring response in solid tumors: unidimensional versus bidimensional measurement. *J Natl Cancer Inst* 1999;91:523–528.
4. Leventhal BG, Wittes RE. *Research methods in clinical oncology.* New York: Raven Press, 1988:246.
5. Schilsky RL, Milano GA, Ratain MJ. Principles of antineoplastic drug development and pharmacology. In: Cheson BD, ed. *Basic and clinical oncology.* Vol 9. New York: Marcel Dekker, 1996:741.
6. Teicher BA. Anticancer drug development guide: preclinical screening, clinical trials, and approval. In: Teicher BA, ed. *Cancer drug discovery and development.* Vol 2. Totowa, NJ: Humana Press, 1997:311.

45

End-of-Life Care

Jane Carter

Nursing Department, Clinical Center, National Institutes of Health,
Bethesda, Maryland

When disease reaches its terminal stage, the goal of treatment ceases to be a cure or an extension of life. Rather, there is an awareness of the futility of further treatment, and focus of care shifts to one of palliation of symptoms and relief of suffering to enhance the quality of remaining life for both patient and family. Such care can be given by a hospice agency in the patient's home or by the oncologic team in a hospice or acute care setting. The key to what is called a "good death" in the hospice movement is a holistic approach that embraces care in four dimensions: physical, emotional, spiritual, and social.

COMMUNICATION

Patients will often know intuitively when a transition is reached. They may not voice awareness of the shift, especially if they sense an unwillingness of physicians, nurses, or family members to explore their thoughts and feelings. Open and honest communications between the physician and patient as death approaches help to ease the patient's fears, relieve anxiety, and prepare the patient for death (1).

THE "GOOD DEATH"

Patients' end-of-life needs are multifaceted, but it is only control of the physical symptoms that is uniquely medical (2) and consists of:

- The need to have adequate relief of pain.
- The need to have ongoing assessment and prompt relief of discomfort from distressing symptoms.
- The need to be cared for by physicians and nurses who have a positive attitude toward palliative care.
- The need to be allowed a measure of control over decisions and respect for their stated wishes as put forth in advance directives, to have the quality of life they choose.
- The need to have a trusting relationship with their physician that permits open, truthful communication (3).

PALLIATIVE CARE MEASURES

"Skilled physical symptom control is the linchpin of good hospice and palliative care...without which the many psychological, social and spiritual needs of the patient and family cannot be met" (4).

Pain

In the early days of the contemporary hospice movement in the late 1960s, founder Dr. Cicely Saunders identified the failure of medicine to control cancer pain. Pain continues to be the most important, feared, and undertreated symptom in end-stage cancer patients. It has many dimensions and is often described as "total pain" (5).

- The key to effective pain control is constant assessment and modification until relief is obtained, using the World Health Organization three-step analgesic ladder.
- Morphine is the strong opioid of choice and should be titrated to a level that provides relief.
- The appropriate dose is the amount of opioid that controls pain with the fewest side effects (6).

Other Symptoms

Other symptoms that arise in the course of dying should be addressed as they occur, keeping in mind the underlying principle of promoting comfort (care) rather than prolonging life (cure). Optimal interventions for all symptoms will be ones that have minimal negative impact on quality of life. The practitioner who keeps this in mind at each decision point will avoid making decisions that unnecessarily burden the dying patient. Symptoms should be assessed and treated quickly. Accordingly, certain practices appropriate within the traditional medical model of caring for a hospitalized patient become contraindicated, such as extensive testing and diagnostic procedures; monitoring of vital signs; gathering of blood and other body fluids for laboratory analysis; and medications that are not specifically ordered to enhance comfort.

Medications

As long as the oral route of administration is viable, it should be used. When swallowing is no longer possible, or if the gastrointestinal (GI) absorption is in question, an alternative route should be attempted, such as transdermal, sublingual, subcutaneous, or rectal/vaginal. Administration of sedatives and other essential drugs can be given intravenously only if such access is readily available. The goal is to use the least-invasive means possible to provide the maximal benefit.

Hydration and Nutrition

This is one of the most provocative areas of terminal care, in which personal values and religious beliefs may conflict with accepted medical knowledge. A natural stage in dying occurs when the patient ceases to eat or drink. Although appetite has diminished gradually over many days or even weeks, as death approaches, the patient may refuse all food and oral fluids. It is at this point that physicians, sometimes at the urging of well-meaning family members, will consider ordering intravenous hydration and/or insertion of a tube for enteral nutrition. Terminal patients do not need invasive nutritional support. It will not prolong life or reverse weight loss or weakness, or make the person feel stronger (4). Feeding tubes and intravenous lines have the effect of increasing the emotional distance between the patient and family. Hunger is rarely a source of discomfort. Some literature suggests that reduced food intake can produce a euphoric-like feeling such as one experienced by a healthy person who is fasting.

Similarly, hydration by artificial means exacerbates discomfort and should be used only when the patient complains of thirst and is unable to drink. Dehydration in the terminal phase decreases pulmonary secretions that increase dyspnea; decreases urine output, which minimizes incontinence; and minimizes the possibility of vomiting.

Altered Mental Status and Terminal Restlessness

"Nearing death" experiences can be observed with a remarkable similarity among dying patients in which the person in the final minutes or hours before death appears to be "seeing" into another dimension beyond earthly life (7). This usually is brief and transitory just before the patient lapses into the final unconsciousness. Should the patient become physically agitated and distressed to the point of attempting to climb out of bed, or if agitation is prolonged and causing dyspnea, adequate sedation should be given to ease the anguish. It is important at this point that careful discussion takes place with family members for them to understand that this agitation is a terminal event, part of the illness, probably due to profound hypoxia, requiring sedation, and is not emotional distress or a sign of lack of readiness to die (4).

Family Needs as Death Approaches

Families will need close contact and communication with the physician and nurses as death approaches. Practitioners must guide families through this difficult time with empathy and the wisdom of experience. Each death experience will be unique, as the individuals' coping strategies and experiences with death and their attachment to the dying person will affect their response. It is incumbent on the professional at the bedside to meet them at whatever level they are experiencing the death.

The most frequently asked question, "How long will it be?" can best be answered by a simple explanation of the significance of signs as they appear: changes in breathing, changes of skin color, weakening of pulses, and such. Simple explanations can guide the family in deciding when it is time to come together for the last time to say goodbye if they so desire.

REFERENCES

1. Kubler-Ross, E. *On death and dying.* New York: Macmillan, 1969.
2. Byock I. *Dying well.* New York: Riverhead Books, 1997.
3. Nuland SB. *How we die.* New York: Knopf, 1994.
4. Kaye P. *Notes on symptom control in hospice and palliative care.* Essex, CT: Education Institute, 1992.
5. Rossman P. *Hospice.* New York: Fawcett Columbine, 1979.
6. U.S. Department of Health and Human Services. *Management of cancer pain: adults.* Rockville, MD: Agency for Health Care Policy and Research, AHCPR Publication No. 94-0593, 1994.

SECTION 12

Common Therapeutic Procedures

46

Central Venous Access Devices for Cancer Patients

Deborah C. Gutierrez and Peter Q. Eichacker

Vascular Access Device Service, Critical Care Medicine Department,
Warren Magnuson Clinical Center, National Institutes of Health, Bethesda, Maryland

Treatment for patients with cancer frequently requires placement of a vascular access device (VAD) for administration of either chemotherapy, total parenteral nutrition, analgesics, antibiotics or for frequent blood sampling. In some cases, vascular access may only require a peripheral intravenous (i.v.) catheter (i.e., the tip of the catheter remains within the peripheral circulation). With increasing frequency, however, there is need for access to the central venous circulation with a central VAD [i.e. the tip of the catheter is positioned in a large central vessel such as the superior vena cava (SVC)]. A VAD that is inserted into a peripheral vein but is long enough for tip positioning in a central vessel is termed a peripherally inserted central venous catheter (PICC). Indications for a central VAD are shown in Table 1.

Several different types of central VADs are available for use in patients with cancer (1–6). Individual circumstances will determine which type of VAD is best for a particular patient. Placing and maintaining any central VAD is more complex, however, than a simple peripheral i.v. catheter. It is very important that the potential infectious and mechanical complications with central VADs be recognized and minimized.

CLASSIFICATION AND APPLICATION OF DIFFERENT CENTRAL VADS

Classification of central VADs is based in large part on characteristics of each catheter's composition (e.g., polyurethane or silicone) and location (i.e., central or peripheral) and method of insertion (i.e., percutaneous, tunneled, or implanted). These characteristics are associated with both advantages and disadvantages, which are outlined in Table 2. A percutaneous catheter is inserted directly from the skin into the vessel. When tunneled, part of a catheter is placed in the subcutaneous tissue between the sites of insertion at the skin (usually midway between the nipple and sternum on the anterior chest) and vein (subclavian or internal jugular). A Dacron cuff positioned several inches above the exit site promotes fibrous ingrowth, better securing the tunneled catheter and possibly decreasing bacterial colonization of the catheter below the cuff. Implanted VADs have a stainless-steel, titanium, or plastic port at their proximal end, which includes a Silastic self-sealing septum. Once the catheter is inserted, the port is placed in a subcutaneous pocket that is sutured closed. The Silastic septum of the port can be accessed by a needle introduced through the skin and septum, into the port chamber itself. This is frequently done with a Huber needle, which was designed with a side hole to minimize damage (coring) to the Silastic septum. Port housings are designed to provide minimal distortion artifact on magnetic resonance imaging (MRI) or computed tomographic (CT) scans.

TABLE 1. *Indications for central venous access devices*

- Administration of a sclerosing agent
- Inadequate peripheral access
- Venous access required for >3 days
- Administration of total parenteral nutrition
- Need for frequent blood sampling

The characteristics outlined in Table 2 determine in large part the applicability of a catheter for a particular patient. Polyurethane percutaneous catheters, although relatively easy to place at either central or peripheral sites, are generally not applicable for long-term use, given their greater risk of infection and vascular trauma. Tunneled and implanted Silastic catheters, however, although more difficult to place, may be associated with lower risk of infection and vascular injury and can be used over longer periods. The ease of care and limited restrictions associated with implanted catheters make their use most desirable in patients who will require frequent catheter use over very prolonged periods. The optimal duration of use for percutaneous or Silastic catheters located centrally or peripherally has not been adequately defined. With careful care and prompt removal when clinically indicated, these catheters may be maintained in some patients for several months.

Other characteristics of central VADs may make one more applicable for an individual patient than another. For example, catheters located centrally are usually larger gauge (4 to 12 Fr) than those placed peripherally (2 to 6 Fr) and permit higher flow rates and easier blood drawing. Larger-gauge catheters can also be constructed with more lumens. Although most central VADs are open at the peripheral tip, the Groshong catheter (Bard Access Systems, Salt Lake City, UT, U.S.A.) has a closed end with a three-way slit valve to reduce potential backflow of blood into the catheter. Figure 1 shows an algorithm for determining the type of

TABLE 2. *Advantages and disadvantages of different catheter compositions, locations, and methods of insertion*

Type	Advantages	Disadvantages
Composition		
Polyurethane	• Durable • Easy to position	• Increased vascular injury
Silicone	• Decreased vascular injury	• Easily broken • More difficult to position
Location of insertion		
Peripheral (basilic or cephalic veins)	• Limited central insertion complication • Insertion by nurse	• Migration with movement • Mechanical phlebitis • Maximum of two lumens
Central insertion (internal jugular or subclavian veins)	• Limited tip migration • More than two lumens possible	• Insertion by physician • Greater central insertion complications
Method of insertion		
Percutaneous	• Bedside placement • Easy to remove	• Increased risk of infection • Activity restrictions • Frequent maintenance
Tunneled	• Decreased risk of infection • Easy to remove	• Radiologist or surgeon insertion • Activity restrictions • Frequent maintenance
Implanted	• Decreased risk of infection • No activity restrictions • Infrequent maintenance	• Insertion by surgeon • Maximum of two lumens • Removal by surgeon

Vascular Access Device (VAD) Decision Algorithm

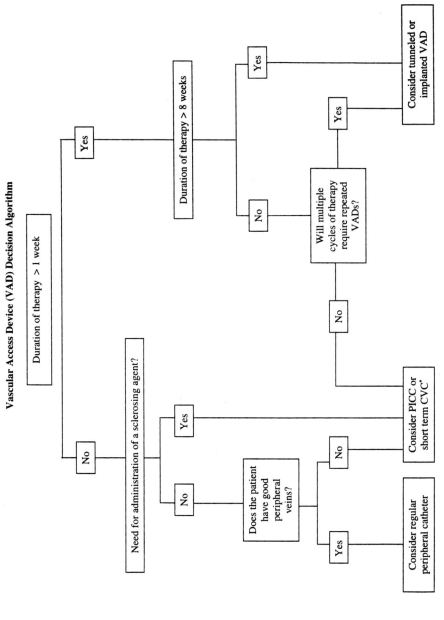

Fig. 1. Algorithm for determining the appropriate type of catheter.

TABLE 3. *Examples of frequently inserted VADs at the NIH Warren G. Magnuson Clinical Center*

Catheter type and manufacturer	Composition	Size	Lumens	Typical duration of insertion
Nontunneled CVC[a]				
Arrow	Polyurethane	4, 5, 7, or 8 FR	3	3–30 days
		12 FR[c]	2	2–10 days
Bard Hohn	Silicone	5 FR	2	6–8 wks
Gesco Per-Q-Cath	Silicone	5 FR	2	6–8 wks
Quinton Mahurkar	Silicone	11.5 FR[c]	2	2–10 days
PICC[b]				
Arrow	Polyurethane	4 FR	1	4–8 wks
		5 FR	2	
Bard Groshong	Silicone	4 FR	1	
		5 FR	2	
Tunneled CVC				
Bard Hickman	Silicone	7 FR	2	≤1 yr
		10 FR	2	
		10 FR	3	
Bard Groshong	Silicone	9.5 FR	2	
Implanted ports				
Bard MRI	Silicone	9.6 FR	1	≤2 yr

[a]Centrally inserted central venous catheter.
[b]Peripherally inserted CVC.
[c]Used for dialysis or apheresis.

catheter most appropriate for a particular patient. Table 3 shows examples of different catheter types frequently used at the NIH Warren G. Magnuson Clinical Center.

COMPLICATIONS WITH INSERTION

Insertion of every central VAD, whether at the bedside, in radiology or in surgery, has the risk of mechanical or infectious complications (1–3,5,6). Mechanical complications generally arise when catheter placement results in injury to either central vascular structures (e.g., venous or arterial perforation) or the lungs (e.g., pneumo-, hemo-, or hydrothorax). These types of complications or their sequelae can be reduced by ensuring first, that abnormalities of anatomy related to previous therapy (e.g., surgery, radiation, or earlier VADs) or disease (e.g., tumor) are recognized before VAD placement; second, that the patient's coagulation profile has been optimized (i.e., platelets more than 50,000/mL and prothrombin and partial thromboplastin times corrected); and third, that careful attention is given to identification of complications that may only be apparent several hours after VAD placement (e.g., pneumo-, hemo-, or hydrothorax). In some patients in whom complete correction of the coagulation profile is not possible, a procedure may still be done while the appropriate replacement products are infused through an additional catheter. Because of the difficulties associated with compressing subclavian vascular structures, percutaneous or tunneled catheter insertions should generally not be performed at this site unless an adequate coagulation profile can be achieved. Infectious complications at insertion can be reduced by ensuring that operators use strict sterile technique and barrier precautions.

CARE AND MAINTENANCE

Once inserted, care and maintenance of all central VADs includes regular flushing with a saline and heparin solution and changing of dressings (i.e., gauze or transparent) and catheter injection caps. No clear standard has been established with respect to the volume, dose, and frequency of heparin flushing, the type, frequency, or cleansing agent for dressing changes, or the frequency of cap changes. However, general guidelines do exist, and successful maintenance of a central VAD is the result of an established care routine (7–9). Most central VADs are flushed daily with a quantity of saline (5–10 mL) and heparin (1–5 mL of a 10 to 1,000 U/mL) solution equivalent to 2 times the volume of the catheter and any additional infusion devices in series with the catheter. Implanted VADs are flushed monthly with saline and heparin when not accessed. Groshong catheters are flushed weekly with saline only or after each use. Gauze and transparent dressings are changed every 48 hours or 3 to 7 days, respectively. Catheter caps are changed after wiping with cleansing solution at least every 7 days or whenever they are damaged or have residual blood. Povidine–iodine (10%) and alcohol (70–92%) are the most frequently recommended cleansing solutions, although chlorhexidine and hydrogen peroxide can be used.

Whenever accessing a central VAD, precautions must be taken to prevent entry of air into the catheter and circulation (i.e., air embolus). The central VAD should be clamped between the point of access and the patient. If a catheter does have to remain open for short periods, such as during initial wire removal at insertion, the patient should be in the Trendelenberg position.

COMPLICATIONS AFTER INSERTION

Maintaining a central VAD for any period of time is associated with the risk of infection, thrombotic or nonthrombotic catheter obstruction, vascular injury, or failure of the VAD itself. These complications may occur at any time.

The reported incidence of infection related to central VADs ranges from 3% to 60% but is usually less than 10% (1–5,9–12). This incidence may be higher in cancer patients with neutropenia related to therapy or disease. Infections with central VADs occur locally (i.e., exit site, tunnel or pocket infections) or systemically [i.e., catheter-related bloodstream infections (CR-BSI)]. Definitions developed by the Centers for Disease Control (CDC) are shown in Table 4 (9). Different types of infections with VADs will be managed differently (1,3–6,10–12,14). Exit-site infections, most frequently related to *Staphylococcus epidermidis,* can be initially treated with local wound care and oral antibiotics without removing the catheter. However, exit-site infections resulting in bacteremia may require catheter removal, especially with *Staphylococcus aureus.* Tunnel or pocket infections are most frequently related to *S. epidermidis* or *aureus* and almost always require systemic antibiotic treatment and catheter removal, with surgical drainage of the infected site. Definitive diagnosis of CR-BSI, while not always possible, requires that the same pathogen be cultured in blood drawn from both the central VAD and another site. Documented or suspected CR-BSI should always be treated with systemic antibiotics. These infections, most frequently related to *S. epidermidis* and *aureus,* may also be due to either the gram-negative bacteria or fungal species to which immunosuppressed cancer patients are susceptible. Institution of empiric antibiotic coverage in such patients must take these other organisms into account. CR-BSI can sometimes be treated with systemic antibiotics alone, but evidence of worsening infection or the presence of *S. aureus* or candidal infection should cause prompt catheter removal. Some central VADs are impregnated with antimicrobial agents [chlorhexidine and silver sulfadiazine (Arrowguard Blue; Arrow International, Reading, PA, U.S.A.) or minocycline and rifampin (Cook Spectrum; Cook Critical Care, Bloomington, IN, U.S.A.)] or have an attached antimicrobial cuff [silver ion (Vita Cuff; Vitaphore, CA, U.S.A.)]. The overall effectiveness of such agents in preventing infection over the lifetime of a central VAD continues to be studied (13–18). At present, data supports the use of antiseptic impregnated catheters. The effectiveness of antimicrobial cuffs is not clear.

Obstruction of a VAD can be related to thrombotic or nonthrombotic causes (10,19–22). Thrombotic obstructions can be classified as those present within (intraluminal) or around the outside of (fibrin sheath) the catheter itself and those in association with the vessel wall (mural thrombus). A catheter may sometimes become encased in a mural thrombus. Non-thrombotic obstruction of a central VAD can be due to malpositioning of a catheter tip against a vessel wall, catheter kinking, luminal occlusion due to drug precipitation, or fracture of the catheter. These types of obstruction may require either repositioning or removal of the catheter. When diagnosing the cause of an obstruction, it is helpful to first determine whether the obstruction interferes with withdrawal, infusion, or both. An algorithm to aid in the diagnosis and treatment of catheter obstruction is shown in Figure 2.

Vascular injury resulting in actual perforation of a vessel wall is not common with the flexible central VADs now in use. Nevertheless, catheter tips should not be positioned perpendicular to an adjacent vessel such as in the innominate vein at its junction with the SVC. Given the smaller diameter of the basilic and cephalic veins, mechanical phlebitis can sometimes

TABLE 4. *CDC catheter infection definitions*

Exit-site infection	Erythema, tenderness, induration and/or purulence within 2 cm of the skin at the catheter exit site
Tunnel infection	Erythema, tenderness, and induration in the tissues overlying the catheter and >2 cm from the exit site
Pocket infection	Erythema and necrosis of the skin over the reservoir of a totally implanted device or purulent exudate in the subcutaneous pocket containing the reservoir
CR-BSI	Isolation of the same organism from a semiquantitative or quantitative culture of a catheter segment and from the blood, preferably peripherally drawn, from a patient with accompanying clinical symptoms and no other source of infection

CR-BSI, catheter-related bloodstream infection; CDC, Centers for Disease Control.

Occluded Catheter Algorithm

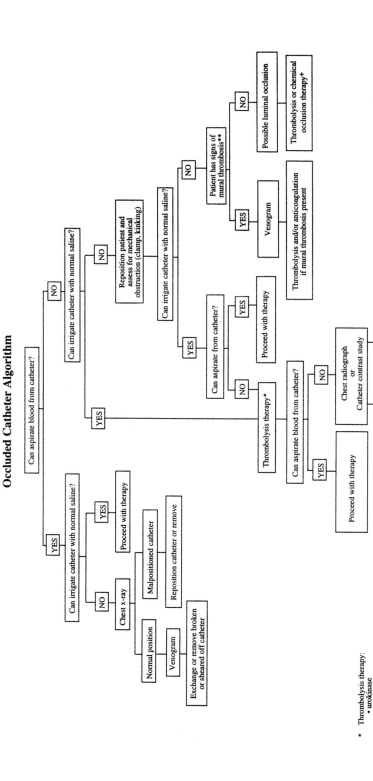

FIG. 2. Algorithm to aid in the diagnosis and treatment of catheter obstruction.

* Thrombolysis therapy:
  • urokinase
  • streptokinase
  • rtPA
** Jugular vein distention, evidence of collateral circulation, unilateral arm swelling
+ Chemical occlusion therapy:
  • Alcohol for lipid precipitates
  • 0.1N HCl for nonlipid precipitates

occur after PICC insertion. This usually manifests itself within 1 to 7 days of insertion with erythema, tenderness, induration, and a palpable venous cord along the vessel tract. Treatment is with moist heat, arm elevation, mild range-of-motion exercises, and an antiinflammatory agent. Mechanical phlebitis should respond to treatment within 24 to 48 hours. If such a response is not noted, the catheter should be removed, local treatment continued, and consideration given to a course of antibiotic therapy.

With use, VADs may themselves fail. In percutaneous catheters, the sutures or anchoring device may loosen, and the catheter may be pulled out partially or completely. Any catheter that has been partially pulled out should not be readvanced. If a chest radiograph does not show the catheter tip in the SVC, the catheter should be removed. The external parts of a catheter that are frequently manipulated may break. Some catheters have repair kits available from the manufacturers and can be safely repaired. If no repair kits are available, the catheter should be removed. In rare instances, an internal part of a VAD may break and embolize. This problem, which may be recognized only at the time the catheter is removed, should be discussed immediately with interventional radiology.

CENTRAL VAD REMOVAL

VADs which are neither tunneled or implanted can be removed at the bedside. Whenever resistance is encountered during removal, care should be taken not to sever the catheter. A radiograph or fluoroscopy should be used to determine whether the catheter has become kinked or knotted. In some cases, especially with PICC VADs, thrombosis may develop, which prevents catheter removal. After prolonged VAD placement, especially with centrally placed polyurethane catheters, a fistula may develop large enough to permit air entry after catheter removal. After VAD removal, the site should be dressed to prevent this occurrence.

Tunneled Silastic catheters can also be removed at the bedside. However, if a tunneled catheter has a cuff (or cuffs) associated with it, resultant adhesions may necessitate incision and dissection for catheter removal. Implanted catheters require surgical removal.

REFERENCES

1. Alexander HR. Vascular access and specialized techniques of drug delivery. In: DeVita VT Jr, Hellman S, Rosenberg SA, eds. *Cancer: principles and practice of oncology.* 5th ed. Philadelphia: Lippincott-Raven, 1997:725–734.
2. Lucas AB, Steinhaus EP, Torosian MH. Long term venous access catheters and implanted ports. In: Alexander HR, ed. *Vascular access in the cancer patient, devices, insertion techniques, maintenance, and prevention and management of complications.* Philadelphia: JB Lippincott, 1994:3–35.
3. Garcia JP, Osteen RT. Vascular access for cancer therapy. In: Macdonald JS, Haller DG, Mayer RJ, eds. *Manual of oncologic therapeutics.* 3rd ed. Philadelphia: JB Lippincott, 1995:67–70.
4. Lucas AB. A critical review of venous access devices: the nursing perspective. In: Hubbard SM, Green PE, Knobf MT, eds. *Current issues in cancer nursing practice.* Philadelphia: JB Lippincott, 1991:1–10.
5. Raaf J. Vascular access, catheter technology and infusion pumps. In: Moosa AR, Schimpff SC, Robson MC, eds. *Comprehensive textbook of oncology.* Vol 1. 2nd ed. Baltimore: Williams & Wilkins, 1991:583–589.
6. Shoemaker WC. Intravascular access and long-term catheter maintenance. In: Ayres SM, Grenvik A, Holbrook PR, et al., eds. *Textbook of critical care.* 3rd ed. Philadelphia: WB Saunders, 1995: 234–252.
7. Intravenous Nursing Society. Standards of practice supplement. *J Intraven Nurs* 1998:21:1S.
8. Oncology Nursing Society. *Access device guidelines module: catheters: recommendations for nursing education and practice.* Pittsburgh: Oncology Nursing Press, 1995.
9. Center for Prevention and Disease Control. Guidelines for prevention of intravascular infections: Atlanta, GA. *Am J Infection Control* 1996:24:262–293.
10. Hoch JR. Management of complications of long-term venous access. *Semin Vasc Surg* 1997;10: 135–143.

11. Groeger JS, Lucas AB, Thaler HT, et al. Infectious morbidity associated with long-term use of venous access devices in patients with cancer. *Ann Intern Med* 1993;119:1168–1174.

12. Lucas AB, Steinhaus EP, Torosian MH. Types of catheter related infections. In: Alexander HR, ed. *Vascular access in the cancer patient, devices, insertion techniques, maintenance, and prevention and management of complications.* Philadelphia: JB Lippincott, 1994:113–127.

13. Groeger JS, Lucas AB, Coit D, et al. A prospective, randomized evaluation of the effect of silver impregnated subcutaneous cuffs for preventing tunneled chronic venous access catheter infections in cancer patients. *Ann Surg* 1993;218:206–210.

14. Toltzis P, Goldmann DA. Current issues in central venous catheter infection. *Annu Rev Med* 1990; 41:169–176.

15. Maki DG, Cobb L, Garman JK, et al. An attachable silver-impregnated cuff for the prevention of infection with central venous catheters: a prospective randomized multicenter trial. *Am J Med* 1988; 85:307–314.

16. Darouiche RO, Raad II, Heard SO, et al. A comparison of two antimicrobial-impregnated central venous catheters. *N Engl J Med* 1999;340:1–8.

17. Maki DG, Stolz SM, Wheeler S, et al. Prevention of central venous catheter-related bloodstream infection by use of an antiseptic-impregnated catheter. *Ann Intern Med* 1997;127:257–266.

18. Raad II, Darouiche R, Dupuis J, et al. Central venous catheters coated with minocycline and rifampin for the prevention of catheter-related colonization and bloodstream infections. *Ann Intern Med* 1997; 127:267–274.

19. Rumsey K, Richardson D. Management of infection and occlusion associated with vascular access devices. *Semin Oncol Nurs* 1995;11:174–183.

20. Williams E. Catheter-related thrombosis. *Clin Cardiol* 1990;13:34–36.

21. Lucas AB, Steinhaus EP, Torosian MH. Catheter occlusion and persistent withdrawal occlusion. In: Alexander HR, ed. *Vascular access in the cancer patient, devices, insertion techniques, maintenance, and prevention and management of complications.* Philadelphia: JB Lippincott, 1994:91–107.

22. Reed T, Phillips D. Management of central venous catheter occlusions and repairs. *J Intraven Nurs* 1996;19:289–294.

47

Procedures in Medical Oncology

Suzanne G. Demko and Jennifer Loud

Medicine Branch, DCS, National Cancer Institute, National Institutes of Health, Bethesda, Maryland

As in other subspecialties, procedures performed in an oncology setting can serve the dual purposes of diagnosis and treatment. This chapter outlines those medical oncology procedures commonly performed and briefly discusses any special considerations or techniques that may assist you in performing these procedures rapidly, with confidence, and with an eye toward patient comfort and education.

INFORMED CONSENT

Unless a procedure is being performed as part of a research or treatment protocol that a patient has signed previously, informed consent, or a legally sufficient substitute, must be obtained before every procedure.

ANESTHESIA

Local anesthesia should be used for all procedures, and premedication with a narcotic and benzodiazepine [we prefer fentanyl and midazolam (Versed)] should be considered for certain patients and procedures. Lidocaine, 1% mixed in a 3:1 or 5:1 ratio with $NaHCO_3$, will ensure proper anesthetic effect and will also virtually eliminate the usual sting of lidocaine.

INSTRUMENTATION

Most offices and hospitals are equipped with sterile trays or self-contained disposable kits that are specific to each procedure. Where additional instruments are needed, based on operator preference or other considerations, they may be added.

PROCEDURES

Bone Marrow Aspirate/Bone Marrow Biopsy

Indications

Diagnostic: analysis of abnormality in blood cell production; staging purposes in hematologic and nonhematologic malignancies

Contraindications

• Few: Severe thrombocytopenia (<20,000), may give platelet transfusion before procedure).
• Sternal biopsy.
• Sternal aspirate: patients with thoracic aortic aneurysms, patients with lytic bone disease of ribs or sternum, patients taking heparin. Heparin should be discontinued before procedure and resumed after hemostasis is achieved.

Anatomy

• Sternal aspiration.
• Patient is in supine position without elevation of head.
• Landmarks:
    1. Sternal angle of Louis.
    2. Lateral borders of the sternum in the second intercostal space.
• Posterior superior iliac spine aspiration and biopsy (Fig. 1).
• Patient is in prone or lateral decubitus position for posterior superior iliac spine aspiration/biopsy or supine for anterior iliac crest position (patients with history of radiation to pelvis or extremely obese patients).

Procedure

• Sternal aspirate.
    1. Once landmarks have been identified, the area is cleaned and draped with a fenestrated drape, using sterile technique.

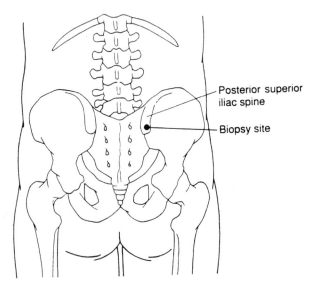

FIG. 1. Biopsy site in the posterior superior iliac spine. The needle should be directed toward the anterior superior iliac spine. From Chestnut MS, Dewar TN, Locksley RM, et al. Bone marrow aspiration & biopsy. In: Chestnut MS, Dewer TN, Locksley RM, eds. *Office & bedside procedures.* Norwalk, CT: Appleton & Lange, 1992:381, with permission.

2. The skin, subcutaneous tissues, and periosteum in the area to be aspirated are infiltrated with lidocaine, 1%, for anesthesia. "Sounding" of the surface of the bone can be done with the infiltration needle to approximate the distance from the skin to the periosteum.
3. A 16-gauge sternal aspiration needle with guard is used to prevent penetration of the posterior table of the sternum. Adjustment of the needle guard is based on approximation of distance from skin to periosteum.
4. A 2-mm, superficial skin incision is made with a surgical blade, in the midsternum, laterally at the second intercostal space.
5. Aspirate needle with guard is introduced using gentle, corkscrew-type pressure to advance the needle, until fixed in bone. Remove obturator, attach a 10- to 12-mL syringe, and aspirate. Pain will accompany the aspiration, which cannot be prevented and will last only seconds.

One milliliter of aspirate is obtained. Greater than 1 mL will be diluted by peripheral blood. Spicules of bone marrow will be present unless significant fibrosis is present or the marrow is packed with leukemia or other malignancy.

If no specimen is obtained, replace the obturator and carefully advance the needle 2 to 3 mm. Repeat the aspiration process. Smears are then prepared for evaluation.

- Posterior Superior Iliac Spine Aspiration and Biopsy

In general, an 11-gauge Jamshidi-type needle is most frequently used to obtain biopsy specimens. Under special circumstances (for example, spongy bone marrow, or easily compressed marrow), a larger-gauge needle (8 g) may be used to obtain an adequate biopsy specimen.

The patient may be positioned prone; however, the lateral decubitus position may also be used for better identification of anatomic sites or for patient comfort. For all but the most obese patient, these positions may be used to obtain aspirate and biopsy. For extremely obese patients or for those who have had radiation to the pelvis, the anterior iliac crest may be used for sampling.

1. Once the site has been prepared and anesthetized, the needle is advanced into the cortex of the bone until it is fixed. Aspiration is then attempted, and if unsuccessful, the needle is advanced slightly, and aspiration is attempted again.
2. Once the aspirate is obtained, the needle, without the obturator in place, is advanced to obtain the biopsy specimen, using a twisting motion. A 1.5- to 2-cm specimen is recommended. To ensure that the specimen is collected when the needle is removed, the needle is first rotated briskly in one direction and then the other, and then "rocked" gently by exerting pressure perpendicular to the shaft of the needle in four directions with the needle capped. The needle is then gently removed while rotating in a corkscrew manner. The specimen is removed from the needle by pushing it up through the hub with a stylet provided for this purpose, with care to avoid needle stick while removing the specimen.

Aftercare

- A pressure dressing is placed over the site, and external pressure is applied for 5 to 10 minutes. Direct pressure is the preferred method to avoid prolonged bleeding and hematoma formation. The pressure dressing should remain in place for 24 hours. The patient may remove the pressure dressing and shower after 24 hours; however, the patient should avoid immersion in water for 1 week after the procedure to avoid infection.

Complications

- Infection and hematoma formation are the most common complications after bone marrow biopsy and aspiration, and can be minimized using careful technique during and after the procedure.

Documentation

• Procedure note.

LUMBAR PUNCTURE
Indications

• Diagnostic [analysis of cerebrospinal fluid (CSF) to assess adequacy of treatment].
• CSF pressure measurement to assess adequacy of treatment.

Contraindications

• Increased intracranial pressure.
• Coagulopathy.
• Infectious process near the planned access site.

Anatomy

• The conus medullaris rarely ends below L-3 (L-1 to L-2 in adults, L-2 to L-3 in children), and interspaces above this should be avoided (Fig. 2).
• The L-4 spinous process lies in the center of the supracristal plane (a line drawn between the posterior and superior iliac crests).
• There are eight layers from the skin to the subarachnoid space; they are skin, supraspinous ligament, interspinous ligament, ligamentum flava, epidural space, dura, subarachnoid membrane, and subarachnoid space.

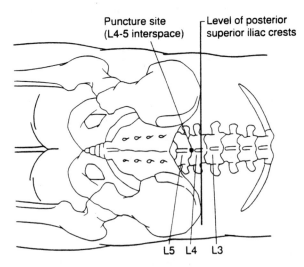

Puncture site
(L4-5 interspace)

Level of posterior
superior iliac crests

L5   L4   L3

FIG. 2. Anatomy of the lumbar spine. From Chestnut MS, Dewar TN, Locksley RM, et al. Lumbar puncture. In: Chestnut MS, Dewer TN, Locksley RM, eds. *Office & bedside procedures.* Norwalk, CT: Appleton & Lange, 1992:391, with permission.

Procedure

1. Explain the procedure to the patient with assurance that you will explain what you are about to do before you do it.
2. Position in lateral decubitus position at edge of table or bed with knees pulled upward and head flexed downward toward chest (Fig. 3). If the spinal column appears to be mis-aligned, place a pillow beneath the patient to assure proper alignment. The seated position may be substituted if the patient is obese or has difficulty remaining in the lateral decubitus position for any reason.
3. Assess your anatomic landmarks and identify the interspace to be used for the procedure.
4. Using sterile technique, prep the area and one interspace above or below it with povidone–iodine solution. Drape the patient, establishing a sterile field.
5. Using 1% lidocaine/bicarb mixture, anesthetize the skin and deeper tissues, being careful to avoid giving epidural or spinal anesthesia.
6. Insert the spinal needle, bevel upward, into the anesthetized skin and into the spinous ligament, keeping the needle parallel to the bed or table. Immediately change the angle of the needle to 30 to 45 degrees, directing the needle cephalad. Begin to advance the needle in small increments through the layers and remove the stylet to check for cerebrospinal fluid (CSF) before each new advance of the needle. With practice, you may be able to identify the "pop" through the dura into the subarachnoid space, but even an experienced operator would be wise to check for CSF before each advance of the needle.
7. Confirming the presence of CSF, attach a manometer to measure opening pressure. Collect appropriate samples of CSF. Samples are to be sent in the following order: tube 1, cultures; tube 2, chemistries (especially glucose and protein); tube 3, cell count and differential; tube 4, cytopathology or other special studies (flow cytometry, cytogenetics, etc.).
8. Withdraw the needle, observe the site for CSF leak or hemorrhage, and place an appropriate bandage over the site.

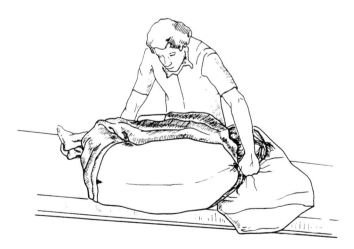

FIG. 3. Lateral decubitus position for lumbar puncture. From Chestnut MS, Dewar TN, Locksley RM, et al. Lumbar puncture. In: Chestnut MS, Dewer TN, Locksley RM, eds. *Office & bedside procedures.* Norwalk, CT: Appleton & Lange, 1992:390, with permission.

9. Reposition the patient to recumbent and ask the patient to remain in this position for 5 to 10 minutes. There appears to be no relation between postprocedure positioning and spinal headache; however, a relationship does exist among needle size, CSF leak, and spinal headache. The patient should be instructed to drink 2 to 3 L of fluid over the next 24 hours, to replenish the CSF removed.

Complications

- Spinal headache can occur in approximately 20% of patients after lumbar puncture. It is a characteristic headache in that it is present and pounding in the occipital region when the patient is upright, and it resolves when the patient lies down. Fluid intake should be encouraged, over-the-counter analgesia should be suggested, and the patient should be instructed to remain recumbent, if possible. Spinal headaches can be quite severe and last for about 1 week; if this is the case, stronger analgesia, caffeine, or a blood patch may be indicated.
- Nerve root trauma can occur, but does so only infrequently. This complication can be avoided by choosing a low interspace as entry site.
- Cerebellar or medullar herniation occurs only rarely in patients who have increased intracranial pressure. If recognized early, this process can be reversed.
- Infections, including meningitis, also can occur.

PARACENTESIS

Indications

- Patients with ascites as a result of tumor metastasis or obstruction often benefit from therapeutic paracentesis. Where the diagnosis is in doubt or to assess diagnostic markers, diagnostic paracentesis can be performed

Contraindications

- There are few situations in which one would hesitate to perform a paracentesis. The complication rate for this procedure is minuscule (about 1%), and the benefit derived by the patient can be quite remarkable. This is especially true of therapeutic paracentesis.
- Even in the event of a coagulopathy, the benefit outweighs the risks for performing this procedure.

Anatomy

- One should identify the area of greatest dullness in the abdomen by percussion. As an alternative, one can have the ascites "marked" by having the patient undergo an ultrasound. Care should be taken to avoid abdominal vasculature and viscera.

Procedure

1. Place the patient in a comfortable supine position on the edge of the bed or table.
2. Identify the area of the abdomen to be accessed (Fig. 4).
3. Prepare the area with povidone–iodine solution, and establish a sterile field by draping the patient.
4. Anesthetize the area with 1% lidocaine/bicarb mixture.

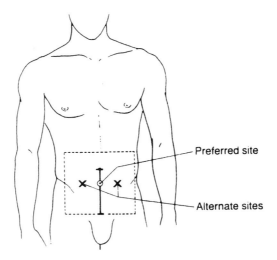

FIG. 4. Sites for diagnostic paracentesis. From Chestnut MS, Dewar TN, Locksley RM, et al. Gastrointestinal procedures. In: Chestnut MS, Dewer TN, Locksley RM, eds. *Office & bedside procedures.* Norwalk, CT: Appleton & Lange, 1992:269, with permission.

5. For diagnostic paracentesis, insert a 22- to 25-gauge needle attached to a sterile syringe into the skin, and pull the skin laterally before advancing the needle into the abdomen. After releasing the tension on the skin, the needle is advanced in the peritoneal cavity, and an appropriate amount of fluid is withdrawn and sent for testing. The skin-retraction method creates a "z" tract into the peritoneal cavity, which minimizes the risk of ascitic leak after the procedure (Fig. 5).

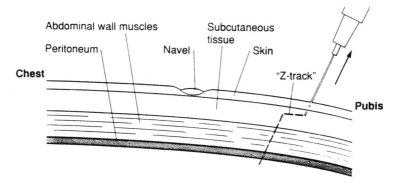

FIG. 5. "Z-tracking" technique for needle insertion into the peritoneal cavity. From Chestnut MS, Dewar TN, Locksley RM, et al. Bone marrow aspiration & biopsy. In: Chestnut MS, Dewer TN, Locksley RM, eds. *Office & bedside procedures.* Norwalk, CT: Appleton & Lange, 1992:381, with permission.

6. For therapeutic paracentesis, the z-tract method also is used with a flexible catheter with multiple ports over a guide needle. When the catheter is in place, the ascites may be evacuated into multiple containers. One must, however, be careful that the patient remain hemodynamically stable during the removal of large amounts of ascites.
7. When the procedure has been completed, the needle or catheter is withdrawn, and a pressure bandage may be placed over the site. The operator should note any bleeding or ascitic leakage before placing the bandage.
8. After a therapeutic paracentesis is performed, the patient should remain in a supine position until all vital signs are stable, and the patient should be assisted when arising from the bed or table for the first time.
9. If the patient becomes orthostatic, standard medical measures should be used to reverse this process, and the patient should be hemodynamically stable before being allowed to leave the area where the procedure was performed.

Complications

- Although choice of an adequate site for paracentesis virtually eliminates complications, the following have been reported: hemorrhage, ascitic leak, infection, perforated abdominal viscus.

THORACENTESIS
Indications

- Removal of pleural fluid for diagnostic or therapeutic purposes.

Contraindications

- Relative: Coagulopathies (correct coagulation abnormality)
- Bullous emphysema due to increased risk of pneumothorax.
- Cardiovascular disease (cardiac arrhythmias).
- Inability of patient to cooperate.
- Cellulitis, if the thoracentesis would require penetrating the inflamed tissue.
- Care must be taken to ascertain the location of the diaphragm before the procedure to avoid accidental injury to the abdominal organs and viscera.
- Chest radiographs should be viewed by the person who is performing the procedure, and if loculation of fluid is suspected, decubitus films and possibly computed tomography or ultrasound may be helpful before thoracentesis is attempted.

Anatomy

- The procedure may be performed with the patient in a sitting position, with arms resting on a pillow, placed on a table. This allows the patient to lean forward 10 to 15 degrees, allowing the intercostal spaces to spread.
- The procedure is performed through the seventh or eighth intercostal space, posterior axillary line. With fluoroscopic, sonographic, or computed tomographic guidance, the procedure may be performed below the fifth rib anteriorly, the seventh rib laterally, and the ninth rib posteriorly. Without such guidance, injury to underlying organs may occur.
Assessment of the size of the pleural effusion with physical examination includes decreased tactile fremitus and dullness to percussion over the pleural effusion. Begin percussion at the top of the chest, listening for the change in the sound of percussion with downward motion. When the change in sound is first noted, compare with the percussion note in the same interspace and location on the opposite side. This is the highest level of the pleural effusion.

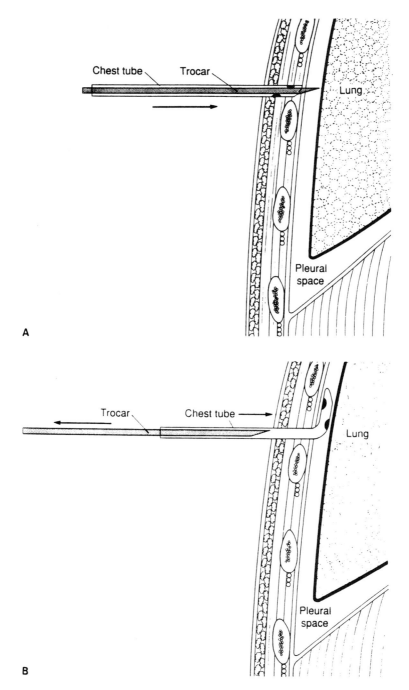

FIG. 6. Trocar technique for inserting a chest tube. **A:** Insertion of chest tube. **B:** Advancement of the chest tube off the trocar into the pleural space. From Chestnut MS, Dewar TN, Locksley RM, et al. Bone marrow aspiration & biopsy. In: *Office & bedside procedures.* Norwalk, CT: Appleton & Lange, 1992:221, with permission.

Procedure

1. With the patient in the proper position, the site is cleaned with antiseptic solution, and local anesthesia is begun. The skin is infiltrated with 1% lidocaine using a 25-gauge needle. Infiltration to the deeper tissues is achieved using a 22-gauge needle, advancing the needle slowly, at a right angle to the chest wall in the center of the intercostal space. The needle is directed into the intercostal space just above the rib to avoid injury to the intercostal nerve and vessels that may run just below the rib. Aspiration is done frequently to ensure that a vessel has not been entered and to determine distance from the skin to the pleural fluid. Once pleural fluid has been obtained, the anesthesia needle is removed, and the depth is noted.
2. A small skin incision may be needed to ease the passage of a larger-gauge thoracentesis needle into the pleural space. Generally, a 16- to 19-gauge needle with its intracath is introduced just to the level of obtaining pleural fluid. If the fluid at this time is bloody or different in appearance from that when identified with the anesthesia needle, vessel injury must be suspected, and the procedure is stopped. If the fluid appears to be the same as previously aspirated, a flexible intracath is then advanced, and the needle withdrawn to avoid puncture of the lung as the fluid is drained. The placement of a flexible intracath with a three-way stopcock allows the removal of large volumes of fluid with lower risk of pneumothorax. (For sampling small amounts of pleural fluid, without the need to drain large amounts of pleural fluid, a 22-gauge needle connected to an air-tight, three-way stopcock will suffice.) Tubing is then attached to the three-way stopcock, and fluid is removed by hand or by vacutainer. Careful monitoring of hemodynamic status must be taken when withdrawing more than 1,000 mL per procedure.
3. A chest radiograph is done after the procedure to determine the amount of fluid that remains and the presence of pneumothorax, and to assess the lung parenchyma. Small pneumothoraces do not need treatment, whereas major pneumothoraces (greater than 50% lung collapse) do (Fig. 6).

Complications

• Pneumothorax.
• Air embolism, rare.
• Infection.

REFERENCES

1. Butler E, Lichtman M, Giler B, et al. *Williams hematology.* 5th ed. New York: McGraw-Hill, 1995.
2. Jashidi K, Swaim WR. Bone marrow biopsy with unaltered architecture: a new biopsy device. *J Lab Clin Med* 1971;77:335.
3. Isselbacher K, et al., *Harison's principles of internal medicine.* 13th ed. 1994.

Appendix

Part One: Anticancer Agents.

Nishaat Saini and *Barry R. Goldspiel

*Pharmacy Department, University College Hospital, London, England; and *Pharmacy Department, NIH Clinical Center, Bethesda, Maryland*

FOOTNOTES AND ABBREVIATIONS

All information obtained from current product labeling as of September 1, 2000.

Single-Agent Dose

Doses listed are those from the package insert and apply when the agent is given alone, unless otherwise noted.

Doses are expressed in accordance with nomenclature guidelines from Kohler DR, Montello MJ, Green L, et al. Standardizing the expression and nomenclature of cancer treatment regimens. *Am J Health Syst Pharm* 1998;55:137–144.

Adverse Reactions

- CNS: central nervous system.
- CV: cardiovascular system.
- DERM: skin and integument system.
- ELECTRO: electrolyte abnormalities.
- ENDO: endocrine system.
- GI: gastrointestinal system.
- GU: genitourinary system.
- HEMAT: hematopoietic system.
- INFUS: infusion-related reactions.
- OCULAR: ocular system.
- PULM: pulmonary system.
- LFTs: liver function tests.
- Cr: serum creatinine.
- CrCl: creatinine clearance.
- N/V Lx: Nausea and vomiting graded according to Hesketh PJ, Kris MG, Grunberg SM, et al. Proposal for classifying the acute emetogenicity of cancer chemotherapy. *J Clin Oncol* 1997;15:103–109, with permission.

Aldesleukin (Proleukin)

Mechanism of Action

Cellular immunity activation.

Food and Drug Administration (FDA)-approved Indications

Metastatic renal cell carcinoma, metastatic melanoma.

FDA-approved Dosage

- 600,000 IU/kg i.v. over 15 minutes every 8 hours for a maximum of 14 doses.
- May be repeated after 9 days of rest for a maximum of 28 doses per course.

Dose Modification Criteria

Withhold or interrupt a dose for toxicity.

Adverse Reactions

CNS: confusion, somnolence, anxiety, dizziness; CV: hypotension, tachycardia, arrhythmia; DERM: rash, pruritis; GI: diarrhea, N/V LS, stomatitis, anorexia; GU: oliguria, acute renal failure; HEMAT: myelosuppression; PULM: dyspnea, pulmonary edema; OTHER: pain, fever, chills, malaise.

Comments

- Restrict use to patients with normal cardiac and pulmonary function.
- Monitor for capillary-leak syndrome.
- Associated with impaired neutrophil function; consider antibiotic prophylaxis for patients with indwelling central lines.

Altretamine (Hexalen)

Mechanism of Action

Unknown, but like an alkylating agent in structure.

FDA-approved Indications

Second-line, palliative treatment of persistent or recurrent ovarian cancer.

FDA-approved Dosage

65 mg/m^2 p.o. q.i.d. (total daily dose, 260 mg/m^2) p.o. for 14 or 21 consecutive days, every 28 days.

Dose Modification Criteria

GI intolerance, myelosuppression.

Adverse Reactions

CNS: peripheral sensory neuropathy, mood disorders, ataxia, dizziness; GI: N/V L3; HEMAT: myelosuppression (WBC, RBC, platelets).

Comments

Monitor for neurologic toxicity.

Anastrazole (Arimidex)

Mechanism of Action

Selective, nonsteroidal aromatase inhibitor.

FDA-approved Indications

First-line: Postmenopausal women with hormone receptor positive or hormone receptor unknown locally advanced or metastatic breast cancer.
Second-line therapy (after tamoxifen) in postmenopausal women with advanced breast cancer.

FDA-approved Dosage

1 mg p.o. daily (no requirement for glucocorticoid or mineralocorticoid replacement).

Dose Modification Criteria

Renal: No; Mild-to-moderate hepatic: no; Severe hepatic: unknown.

Adverse Reactions

CNS: headache, asthenia, pain; CV: flushing; GI: N/V L2, diarrhea, LFT elevations [in patients with liver metastases (mets)]; PULM: dyspnea; OTHER: pain, back pain, vaginal bleeding.

Comments

Patients with estrogen receptor (ER)-negative disease and patients who do not respond to tamoxifen rarely respond to anastrazole.

Asparaginase (Elspar)

Mechanism of Action

Depletes asparagine, an amino acid required by some leukemic cells.

FDA-approved Indications

Acute lymphocytic leukemia (ALL) induction therapy (primarily in combination with other agents).

FDA-approved Dosage

- Consult current literature for doses.
- ALL: Induction in combination with prednisone and vincristine: 1,000 IU/m^2 i.v. every day for 10 days starting day 22 *OR* 6,000 IU/m^2 i.m. every 3 days for nine doses, starting day 4 of induction (day 1 is first day of chemotherapy).

Dose Modification Criteria

None available.

Adverse Reactions

DERM: skin rash; ENDO: dysglycemia; GI: N/V L3, pancreatitis, Inc. SGOT, Bili, PT; GU: prerenal azotemia; OTHER: HEMAT, hypersensitivity, anaphylactic reactions.

Comments

- Contraindicated in patients with active pancreatitis or history of pancreatitis.
- Hypersensitivity and anaphylactic reactions can occur.
- Consult package insert regarding test doses and desensitization schedules.
- i.m. administration preferred over i.v. administration (lower incidence of anaphylaxis).
- i.v. infusions should be over at least 30 minutes.

BCG Live (Intravesical), [TheraCys, Tice(BCG)]

Mechanism of Action

Local inflammatory and immune response.

FDA-approved Indications

Primary and relapsed carcinoma-in-situ of the urinary bladder.

FDA-approved Dosage

(TheraCys; Vial contains $10.5 \pm 8.7 \times 10^8$ colony-forming units/mL when resuspended in diluent provided.)

One vial diluted in 50 ml normal saline (NS) and instill into bladder for 2 hours once weekly for 6 weeks followed by one treatment at 3, 6, 12, 18, and 24 months after initial treatment.

(Tice BCG; Vial contains 1 to 8×10^8 colony-forming units/mL or 50 mg.)

One vial diluted in 50 mL NS and instill into bladder for 2 hours once weekly for 6 weeks followed by once monthly for 6 to 12 months.

Dose Modification Criteria

Withhold on any suspicion of systemic infection.

Adverse Reactions

CNS: malaise, fever, chills; GU: irritative bladder symptoms.

Comments

May complicate tuberculin skin test interpretation.

Bicalutamide (Casodex)

Mechanism of Action

Antiandrogen.

FDA-approved Indications

Palliation of advanced prostate cancer (stage D2) in combination therapy with a luteinizing hormone releasing hormone (LHRH) agonist.

FDA-approved Dosage

50 mg p.o. daily.

Dose Modification Criteria

None available.

Adverse Reactions

ENDO: loss of libido, hot flashes, gynecomastia; GI: N/V, diarrhea, constipation; GU: impotence.

Comments

Monitor LFTs periodically.

Bleomycin (Blenoxane)

Mechanism of Action

Unknown, but may inhibit DNA and RNA synthesis.

FDA-approved Indications

Squamous cell cancers, non-Hodgkin's lymphoma, testicular cancer, Hodgkin's disease, malignant pleural effusions.

FDA-approved Dosage

- A test dose (2 U or less) for the first two doses is recommended in lymphoma patients.
- From 0.25 to 0.50 units/kg (10 to 20 units/m^2) i.v. or i.m. or s.c. weekly or twice weekly.
- Malignant pleural effusions: 60 units as single intrapleural bolus dose.

Dose Modification Criteria

Renal: Yes.

Adverse Reactions

DERM: erythema, rash, hyperpigmentation, alopecia, nail changes, pruritus, stomatitis; PULM: pulmonary fibrosis (increases at cumulative doses greater than 400 units, but can happen at lower total doses), pneumonitis; OTHER: idiosyncratic reaction consisting of hypotension, mental confusion, fever, chills, and wheezing has been reported in 1% of lymphoma patients.

Comments

- Monitor for fine rales as an early indication of pulmonary toxicity.
- Pulmonary toxicity is increased when oxygen is used during surgery.

Busulfan (Myleran); Busulfan Injection (Busulfex)

Mechanism of Action

Alkylating agent.

FDA-approved Indications

- p.o.: CML.
- i.v.: Combination (with cyclophosphamide) before allogeneic hematopoietic progenitor cell transplantation for CML.

FDA-approved Dosage

- p.o.: Induction: 4 to 8 mg daily; maintenance: 1 to 3 mg daily.
- i.v.: Premedicate patients with phenytoin before busulfan administration.
- For nonobese patients, use ideal body weight (IBW) or actual body weight, whichever is lower.
- For obese or severely obese patients, use adjusted IBW. Adjusted IBW (AIBW) should be calculated as follows: AIBW = IBW + 0.25 × (actual weight − IBW).
- 0.8 mg/kg over 2 hours q6h × 16 doses (total course dose, 12.8 mg/kg) with cyclophosphamide.

Dose Modification Criteria

Myelosuppression.

Adverse Reactions

CNS: seizures; DERM: hyperpigmentation; GI: N/V oral L1, i.v. L5; HEMAT: severe myelosuppression; HEPAT: veno-occlusive disease; RESP: pulmonary fibrosis, veno-occlusive disease.

Comments

Phenytoin reduces busulfan plasma area under the curve (AUC) by 15%. Use of other anticonvulsants may result in higher busulfan plasma AUCs, and an increased risk of veno-occlusive disease or seizures. Monitor plasma busulfan exposure if other anticonvulsants are used.

Capecitabine (Xeloda)

Mechanism of Action

Antimetabolite that is anabolized to fluorouracil in tumors.

FDA-approved Indications

Third-line therapy for metastatic breast cancer (after paclitaxel and an anthracycline-containing chemotherapy regimen) or second-line (after paclitaxel) if anthracycline is not indicated.

FDA-approved Dosage

Give 1,250 mg/m^2 p.o. b.i.d. (total daily dose, 2,500 mg/m^2) at the end of a meal for 2 weeks, followed by a 1-week rest period, given as 3-week cycles. See product labeling for a dosing chart.

Dose Modification Criteria

Mild to moderate hepatic (due to liver metastases): No; grade 2 toxicity or higher: Yes.

Adverse Reactions

CNS: fatigue, paresthesia; DERM: hand and foot syndrome, dermatitis; GI: N/V, diarrhea, stomatitis, abdominal pain, anorexia, hyperbilirubinemia; HEMAT: myelosuppression.

Carboplatin (Paraplatin)

Mechanism of Action

Alkylating-like agent producing interstrand DNA cross-links.

FDA-approved Indications

- First-line: Advanced ovarian cancer (in combination with other agents).
- Second-line: Advanced ovarian cancer (including patients who have previously received cisplatin).

FDA-approved Dosage

- With cyclophosphamide: 300 mg/m^2 i.v. × one dose on day 1 q4wk × six cycles.
- Single agent: 360 mg/m^2 i.v. × one dose q4wk.
- Formula dosing may be used as an alternative to body surface area (BSA)-based dosing.
- Total dose in milligrams = (target AUC) × [glomerular filtration rate (GFR) + 25].
- Target AUC: 4 to 6 mg/mL/min; GFR: estimated by ^{51}Cr-EDTA clearance.

Dose Modification Criteria

Myelosuppression: yes; renal: yes.

Adverse Reactions

CNS: neuropathy; GI: N/V L4; ELECTRO: Mg, Na, Ca, K alterations; HEME: thrombocytopenia > leukopenia and anemia; OTHER: anaphylactic reactions.

Comments

Do not confuse with cisplatin for dosing or during preparation.

Carmustine (BiCNU)

Mechanism of Action

Alkylating agent.

FDA-approved Indications

Brain tumors, multiple myeloma, Hodgkin's disease, non-Hodgkin's lymphomas.

FDA-approved Dosage

150 to 200 mg/m^2 i.v. qd × one dose q6wk *OR* 75 to 100 mg/m^2 i.v. qd × 2d every 6 weeks.

Dose Modification Criteria

Myelosuppression: Yes.

Adverse Reactions

GI: N/V ≥ 250 mg/m^2; L5, <250 mg/m^2: L4; HEMAT: myelosuppression (can be delayed); OCULAR: retinal hemorrhages; PULM: pulmonary fibrosis (acute and delayed).

Comments

Risk of pulmonary toxicity increases with cumulative total doses >1,400 mg/m^2 and in patients with a history of lung disease, radiation therapy, or concomitant bleomycin.

Chlorambucil (Leukeran)

Mechanism of Action

Alkylating agent.

FDA-approved Indications

Palliation of CLL, Hodgkin's disease, non-Hodgkin's disease.

FDA-approved Dosage

- Initial and short courses of therapy: 0.1 to 0.2 mg/kg p.o. qd for 3 to 6 weeks as required. Usually the 0.1 mg/kg/d dose is used except for Hodgkin's disease, in which 0.2 mg/kg/d is used.
- Alternate regimen in CLL (intermittent, biweekly, or once monthly pulses). Initial single dose of 0.4 mg/kg p.o. × one dose. Increase dose by 0.1 mg/kg until control of lymphocytosis.
- Maintenance: Not to exceed 0.1 mg/kg/day.

Dose Modification Criteria

Myelosuppression: Yes.

Adverse Reactions

CNS: seizures, confusion, twitching, hallucinations; DERM: rash; GI: N/V L1, increased LFTs; HEMAT: myelosuppression, lymphopenia; PULM: pulmonary fibrosis; OTHER: secondary acute myelomonocytic leukemia (AML) (long-term therapy).

Comments

Separate radiation therapy and chlorambucil by at least 4 weeks.

Cisplatin (Platinol)

Mechanism of Action

Alkylating-like agent producing interstrand DNA cross-links.

FDA-approved Indications

• First-line: Metastatic testicular tumors (in combination with other agents), metastatic ovarian tumors.
• Second-line: Transitional cell advanced bladder cancer.

FDA-approved Dosage

20 mg/m^2 i.v. qd × 5 days q4wk *OR* 75 to 100 mg/m^2 i.v. × one dose (in combo with cyclophosphamide) q4wk *OR* 100 mg/m^2 i.v. × one dose q4wk *OR* 50 to 70 mg/m^2 i.v. × one dose q3 to 4 weeks.

Dose Modification Criteria

Renal: Yes.

Adverse Reactions

CNS: neuropathy, paresthesia, ototoxicity; ELECTRO: Mg, Na, Ca, K alterations; GI: N/V L5, increased SGOT; GU: increased Cr and BUN (cumulative); HEMAT: anemia; OTHER: anaphylactic reactions.

Comments

• Check auditory acuity.
• Vigorous hydration recommended before and after cisplatin administration.
• Use other nephrotoxic agents (e.g., aminoglycosides) concomitantly with caution.
• Exercise precaution to prevent inadvertent cisplatin overdose and confusion with carboplatin.

Cladribine (Leustatin)

Mechanism of Action

Antimetabolite.

FDA-approved Indications

Hairy cell leukemia.

FDA-approved Dosage

- 0.09 mg/kg i.v. qd × 7 days × one course.
- Inadequate data on dosing of patients with renal or hepatic insufficiency.

Dose Modification Criteria

Renal: No data; Hepatic: no data.

Adverse Reactions

CNS: fatigue, headache, peripheral neuropathy; GI: N/V L1; HEMAT: myelosuppression; DERM: rash; OTHER: fever.

Comments

Immunosuppression persists for up to 1 year after cladribine therapy.

Cyclophosphamide (Cytoxan)

Mechanism of Action

Activated by liver to alkylating agent.

FDA-approved Indications

Lymphomas, leukemias, multiple myeloma, mycosis fungoides, neuroblastoma, adenocarcinoma of the ovary, retinoblastoma, breast cancer.

FDA-approved Dosage

- i.v.: Many dosing regimens reported. Consult current literature.
- p.o.: 1 to 5 mg/kg/day.

Dose Modification Criteria

Myelosuppression: Yes.

Adverse Reactions

CNS: syndrome of inappropriate antidiuretic hormone (SIADH); DERM: rash, skin and nail pigmentation, alopecia; GI: N/V >1,500 mg/m^2: L5 >750 mg/m^2: L4, <750 mg/m^2: L3, anorexia, diarrhea; GU: hemorrhagic cystitis, renal tubular necrosis; HEMAT: myelosuppression (leukopenia > thrombocytopenia and anemia); PULM: pulmonary fibrosis.

Comments

Consider using vigorous hydration and mercaptoethane sulfonate (MESNA) therapy with high-dose cyclophosphamide.

Cytarabine (Cytosar and Others)

Mechanism of Action

Antimetabolite.

FDA-approved Indications

In combination with other agents for induction therapy of ANLL, ALL, blast-phase CML, intrathecal prophylaxis and treatment of meningeal leukemia.

FDA-approved Dosage

- Consult current literature for doses in ALL.
- ANLL induction (in combo with other agents): 100 mg/m^2 i.v. over 24 hours × 7 days *OR* 100 mg/m^2 i.v. q12h × 7d.
- Intrathecally: (use preservative-free diluents) 30 mg/m^2 intrathecally q4d until cerebrospinal fluid (CSF) clear, and then one additional dose.

Dose Modification Criteria

Adverse Reactions

CNS: cerebellar dysfunction, somnolence, coma, SIADH; DERM: alopecia; GI: N/V L1 (>1 g/m^2 L4), anorexia, diarrhea, increased LFTs, pancreatitis (in patients who have previously received asparaginase); HEMAT: myelosuppression; OCULAR: conjunctivitis.

Cytarabine Liposomal Injection (DepoCyt)

Mechanism of Action

Antimetabolite.

FDA-approved Indications

Intrathecal treatment of lymphomatous meningitis.

FDA-approved Dosage

- Given only by intrathecal route either via an intraventricular reservoir or directly into the lumbar sac over a period of 1 to 5 minutes.
- Patients should be started on dexamethasone, 4 mg p.o. or i.v. b.i.d.× 5 days beginning on the day of the cytarabine liposomal injection.
- Induction: 50 mg intrathecally q14d × two doses (weeks 1 and 3).
- Consolidation: 50 mg intrathecally q14d × three doses (weeks 5, 7, and 9) followed by an additional dose at week 13.
- Maintenance: 50 mg intrathecally q28d × four doses (weeks 17, 21, 25, 29).

Dose Modification Criteria

Neurotoxicity: Yes.

Adverse Reactions

CNS: Chemical arachnoiditis, headache, confusion, somnolence.

Dacarbazine (DTIC-Dome)

Mechanism of Action

Mechanism unknown.

FDA-approved Indications

Metastatic melanoma, second-line therapy for Hodgkin's disease.

FDA-approved Dosage

- Single agent: 2 to 4.5 mg/kg i.v. qd × 10d; repeat every 4 weeks, *OR* 250 mg/m^2 i.v. qd × 5d; repeat every 3 weeks.
- In combination with other active drugs: 150 mg/m^2 i.v. qd × 5d, repeat every 4 weeks, *OR* 375 mg/m^2 i.v. on day 1, repeat every 15 days.

Dose Modification Criteria

Adverse Reactions

DERM: alopecia; GI: N/V L5, anorexia, diarrhea, increased LFTs, hepatic necrosis; OTHER: pain and burning at infusion, anaphylaxis, fever.

Comments

Vesicant.

Dactinomycin (Cosmegen)

Mechanism of Action

Intercalating agent.

FDA-approved Indications

Wilms' tumor, Ewing's sarcoma, rhabdomyosarcoma, testicular and uterine cancer.

FDA-approved Dosage

- For obese or edematous patients, dose should be based on BSA.
- Not to exceed 15 μg/kg i.v. qd × 5 days *OR* 400 to 600 μg/m² i.v. qd × 5 days, repeated every 3 to 6 weeks.
- Adult: 500 μg i.v. qd × 5 days every 3 weeks.

Dose Modification Criteria

Adverse Reactions

DERM: alopecia, erythema; ELECTRO: hypocalcemia; GI: N/V L5, stomatitis, dysphagia; HEMAT: myelosuppression; OTHER: fever, radiation recall, fatigue, myalgia.

Comments

Vesicant.

Daunorubicin (Cerubidine)

Mechanism of Action

Intercalating agent. Topoisomerase-II inhibition.

FDA-approved Indications

In combination with other agents for remission induction in ANLL (adult) or ALL (children and adults).

FDA-approved Dosage

- ANLL: with cytarabine.
- Age younger than 60: (first course) 45 mg/m^2 i.v. days 1, 2, and 3; (subsequent course) 45 mg/m^2 i.v., days 1 and 2.
- Age $\geq$ 60 years: (first course) 30 mg/m^2 i.v., days 1, 2, and 3; (subsequent course) 30 mg/m^2 i.v., days 1 and 2.
- Adult ALL: (with vincristine, prednisone, L-asparaginase) 45 mg/m^2 i.v., days 1, 2, and 3.

Dose Modification Criteria

Renal: yes; hepatic: yes.

Adverse Reactions

CV: (Risk of cardiotoxicity increases rapidly with total lifetime cumulative doses >400 to 550 mg/m^2 in adults or >300 mg/m^2 in children), congestive heart failure (CHF), arrhythmias; DERM: nail hyperpigmentation, rash, alopecia; GI: N/V L3, mucositis; HEMAT: myelosuppression; OTHER: red-tinged urine, fever, chills.

Comments

Vesicant.

Daunorubicin Citrate Liposomal Injection (Daunoxome)

Mechanism of Action

Intercalating agent. Topoisomerase-II inhibition.

FDA-approved Indications

First line: Advanced human immunodeficiency virus (HIV)-associated Kaposi's sarcoma.

FDA-approved Dosage

40 mg/m^2 i.v. over 60 minutes × one dose q2wk.

Dose Modification Criteria

Hepatic: Yes.

Adverse Reactions

CV: CHF, arrhythmias; DERM: nail, alopecia, hyperpigmentation, rash; GI: N/V L2, mucositis; HEMAT: myelosuppression; INFUS: (Infusion-related reactions usually subside with interruption of the infusion, and generally do not recur if the infusion is then resumed at a slower rate) back pain, flushing, chest tightness; OTHER: red-tinged urine, fever, chills.

Comments

- Do not confuse with nonliposomal forms of daunorubicin.
- Liposomal formulations of the same drug may not be equivalent.
- Evaluate cardiac function by history and physical examination each cycle and determine left ventricular ejection fraction (LVEF) function at total cumulative doses of daunorubicin citrate liposomal injection of 320 mg/m^2 and every 160 mg/m^2 thereafter in anthracycline-naive patients or before daunorubicin citrate liposomal injection therapy and every 160 mg/m^2 thereafter in patients who previously received anthracyclines.

Denileukin diftitox (Ontak)

Mechanism of Action

Fusion protein composed of diphtheria toxin fragments linked to interleukin 2 (IL-2) sequences.

FDA-approved Indications

Treatment of persistent or recurrent cutaneous T-cell lymphoma (CTCL) in patients whose malignant cells express the CD25 component of the IL-2 receptor.

FDA-approved Dosage

- Cells should be tested for CD25 before administration.
- Give 9 or 18 µg/kg i.v. over at least 15 minutes qd × 5d, q21d. Infusion should be stopped or infusion rate should be reduced for infusion-related reactions.

Dose Modification Criteria

Adverse Reactions

CNS: dizziness; CV: vascular leak syndrome, hypotension; DERM: rash, pruritis; GI: N/V L3, anorexia, diarrhea, increased transaminases; HEME: anemia; INFUS: hypotension, back pain, dyspnea, vasodilation, rash, chest pain or tightness, tachycardia, dysphagia, syncope, allergic reactions, or anaphylaxis; PULM: dyspnea, cough; OTHER: acute hypersensitivity reactions, chills, fever, asthenia, hypoalbuminemia.

Docetaxel (Taxotere)

Mechanism of Action

Microtubule assembly stabilization.

FDA-approved Indications

- Locally advanced or metastatic non–small-cell lung cancer (after failure of prior platinum-based chemotherapy).
- Second-line: Locally advanced or metastatic breast cancer.

FDA-approved Dosage

Premedication for hypersensitivity reactions and fluid retention: dexamethasone, 8 mg p.o. b.i.d., for 3 days starting 1 day before docetaxel administration; breast cancer: 60 to 100 mg/m^2 i.v. over 1h every 3 weeks; lung cancer: 75 mg/m^2 i.v. over 1h Q3 weeks..

Dose Modification Criteria

Hepatic: Yes; myelosuppression: yes.

Adverse Reactions

CNS: Fever, asthenia; DERM: alopecia; GI: N/V L2, diarrhea, stomatitis; HEMAT: myelosuppression; OTHER: hypersensitivity reactions, severe fluid retention, myalgia.

Comments

- Use non-DEHP plasticized solution containers and administration sets.

Doxorubicin (Adriamycin and Others)

Mechanism of Action

Intercalating agent. Topoisomerase-II inhibition.

FDA-approved Indications

ALL, ANLL, Wilms' tumor, neuroblastoma, sarcoma, breast, ovarian, bladder, thyroid, bronchiogenic, and gastric cancer, Hodgkin's disease, lymphoma.

FDA-approved Dosage

- Single agent: 60 to 75 mg/m^2 i.v. × one dose repeated every 3 to 4 weeks.
- In combination with other agents: 40 to 60 mg/m^2 i.v. × one dose, repeated every 3 to 4 weeks.

Dose Modification Criteria

Hepatic: Yes; myelosuppression: yes.

Adverse Reactions

CV: (Risk of cardiotoxicity increases rapidly with total lifetime cumulative doses >450 mg/m^2) CHF, arrhythmias; DERM: nail hyperpigmentation, alopecia; GI: N/V >60 mg/m^2: L4, <60 mg/m^2: L3, mucositis; HEMAT: myelosuppression; OTHER: red-tinged urine.

Comments

Vesicant.

Epirubicin (Ellence)

Mechanism of Action

Intercalating agent. Topoisomerase-II inhibition.

FDA-approved Indications

Adjuvant therapy of axillary node–positive breast cancer.

FDA-approved Dosage

- CEF 120: 60 mg/m^2 i.v., days 1, 8, repeated every 28 days for six cycles.
- FEC 100: 100 mg/m^2, day 1, repeated every 21 days for six cycles.

Dose Modification Criteria

Renal: Yes; hepatic: yes; myelosuppression: yes.

Adverse Reactions

CV: (Risk of cardiotoxicity increases rapidly with total lifetime cumulative doses >900 mg/m^2) CHF; DERM: alopecia; GI: N/V (moderate to severe emetogenicity); HEMAT: myelosuppression.

Comments

Vesicant.

Estramustine (Emcyt)

Mechanism of Action

Alkylating agent, estrogen, microtubule instability.

FDA-approved Indications

Palliative treatment of metastatic and/or progressive carcinoma of the prostate.

FDA-approved Dosage

- 4.67 mg/kg p.o. t.i.d. or 3.5 mg/kg p.o. q.i.d. (total daily dose, 14 mg/kg).
- Administer with water, 1 hour before or 2 hours after meals. Avoid calcium-containing beverages.

Dose Modification Criteria

Hepatic: Yes.

Adverse Reactions

CV: Edema, fluid retention, venous thromboembolism; ENDO: hyperglycemia, gynecomastia, impotence; GI: diarrhea, nausea, increased AST or LDH; PULM: dyspnea.

Etoposide (VePesid)

Mechanism of Action

Topoisomerase-II interaction.

FDA-approved Indications

Refractory testicular cancer; first-line therapy for small-cell lung cancer in combination with other agents.

FDA-approved Dosage

- Testicular cancer: 35-50 mg/m^2 i.v. over 30-60 min qd x 4-5 days.
- SCLC: 50-100 mg/m^2 i.v. over 30-60 min qd x 5 days, repeated Q3-4 weeks.

Dose Modification Criteria

Renal: Yes.

Adverse Reactions

CV: tachycardia; DERM: alopecia; GI: N/V L2, mucositis; HEMAT: myelosuppression; INFUS: hypotension (infusion-rate related); PULM: dyspnea; OTHER: anaphylactic reactions, chills, fever.

Etoposide Phosphate (Etophos)

Mechanism of Action

Rapidly and completely converted to etoposide in plasma, leading to topoisomerase-I interaction.

FDA-approved Indications

Refractory testicular cancer; first-line therapy for small-cell lung cancer in combination with other agents.

FDA-approved Dosage

- Testicular cancer: 35–50 mg/m^2 i.v. over 30–60 min qd × 4–5 days.
- SCLC: 50–100 mg/m^2 i.v. over 30–60 min qd × 5 days, repeated Q3–4 weeks.

Dose Modification Criteria

Renal: Yes.

Adverse Reactions

CV: tachycardia; DERM: alopecia; GI: N/V L2, mucositis; HEMAT: myelosuppression; PULM: dyspnea; OTHER: anaphylactic reactions, chills, fever.

Exemestane (Aromisan)

Mechanism of Action

Irreversible steroidal aromatase inactivator.

FDA-approved Indications

Second-line: Advanced breast cancer after tamoxifen failure in postmenopausal women.

FDA-approved Dosage

25 mg p.o. qd after a meal.

Dose Modification Criteria

Renal: No; hepatic: no.

Adverse Reactions

CV: hot flashes; GI: increased LFTs, nausea, increased appetite; HEME: lymphocytopenia; OTHER: fatigue, sweating.

Fludarabine (Fludara)

Mechanism of Action

Antimetabolite.

FDA-approved Indications

Second-line: After alkylating agent therapy in patients with B-cell CLL.

FDA-approved Dosage

25 mg/m^2 i.v. over 30 minutes qd × 5 days, repeated every 28 days.

Dose Modification Criteria

Renal: No data.

Adverse Reactions

GI: N/V L1, anorexia; HEMAT: myelosuppression, hemolytic anemia; NEURO: paresthesia; PULM: pneumonitis; OTHER: myalgia, tumor lysis syndrome, fatigue, associated with life-threatening instances.

Comments

- Watch for hemolytic anemia.
- Pulmonary toxicity is increased in patients who received pentostatin.
- Use only irradiated blood products if transfusions are necessary.

Flutamide (Eulexin)

Mechanism of Action

Antiandrogen.

FDA-approved Indications

Stage D2 metastatic prostate carcinoma (in combination with LHRH agonists) or locally confined stage B2-C (in combination with LHRH agonists and radiation therapy).

FDA-approved Dosage

- Stage D2 metastatic prostate carcinoma: 250 mg p.o. t.i.d. (every 8 hours).
- Stage B2-C prostate cancer: 250 mg p.o. t.i.d. (every 8 hours) beginning 8 weeks before and continuing through radiation.

Adverse Reactions

DERM: Rash; GI: N/V, diarrhea, constipation, increased LFTs (monitor LFTs periodically because of rare associations with cholestatic jaundice, hepatic necrosis, and encephalopathy); GU: impotence; ENDO: loss of libido, hot flashes, gynecomastia.

Comments

Interacts with warfarin; monitor international normalized ratio (INR) closely.

Fluorouracil (Adrucil and Others)

Mechanism of Action

Antimetabolite.

FDA-approved Indications

Palliative management of colon, rectal, breast, stomach, and pancreatic cancer.

FDA-approved Dosage

Consult current literature.

Adverse Reactions

CNS: Acute cerebellar syndrome, nystagmus, headache, visual changes, photophobia; CV: angina, ischemia; DERM: dry skin, photosensitivity, palmar–plantar erythrodysesthesia, alopecia, dermitis, thrombophlebitis; GI: N/V L2, stomatitis, mucositis; HEMAT: myelosuppression; OTHER: anaphylaxis.

Comments

May be given c.i.v. or i.v. push.

Gemcitabine (Gemzar)

Mechanism of Action

Antimetabolite.

FDA-approved Indications

- Second-line: Adenocarcinoma of the pancreas in patients previously treated with fluorouracil.
- First-line (in combination with cisplatin): inoperable, locally advanced (stage IIIa or IIIb) or metastatic (stage IV) non–small-cell lung cancer.

FDA-approved Dosage

- Pancreas cancer: 1,000 mg/m^2 every week for 7 weeks, followed by 1 week of rest from treatment, followed by 1,000 mg/m^2 every week for 3 consecutive weeks of every 4 weeks.
- Lung cancer, 4-week schedule: 1,000 mg/m^2 i.v. over 30 minutes on days 1, 8, and 15 of each 28-day cycle.
- Cisplatin should be administered intravenously at 100 mg/m^2 × one dose on day 1 after the infusion of gemcitabine.
- *OR* 3-week schedule: 1,250 mg/m^2 i.v. over 30 minutes on days 1 and 8 of each 21-day cycle.
- Cisplatin at a dose of 100 mg/m^2 i.v. × one dose after the infusion of gemcitabine on day 1.

Dose Modification Criteria

Myelosuppression: yes; renal: caution; hepatic: caution.

Adverse Reactions

DERM: rash, alopecia; GI: N/V L2, constipation, diarrhea, stomatitis; GU: proteinuria, hematuria; HEMAT: myelosuppression; HEPAT: ↑LFTs and bilirubin; PULM: dyspnea; OTHER: fever, pain.

Comments

Clearance in women and elderly is reduced.

Goserelin Acetate Implant (Zoladex)

Mechanism of Action

LHRH agonist.

FDA-approved Indications

- Stage D2 metastatic prostate carcinoma or locally confined stage B2-C (in combination with flutamide and radiation therapy).
- Palliative treatment of advanced breast cancer in pre- and perimenopausal women.

FDA-approved Dosage

- Stage D2 metastatic prostate carcinoma: 3.6 mg s.c. monthly, *OR* 10.8 mg s.c. q12wk.
- Stage B2-C prostate cancer: start 8 weeks before radiotherapy and continue through radiation, 3.6 mg, followed in 28 days by 10.8 mg s.c.
- Breast cancer: 3.6 mg s.c. q4wk.

Dose Modification Criteria

Renal: no; hepatic: no.

Adverse Reactions

CNS: pain, ENDO: gynecomastia, decreased, hot flashes; GU: erectile dysfunction, lower urinary tract symptoms; OTHER: tumor flare in the first few weeks of therapy.

Comments

Use with caution in patients at risk of developing ureteral obstruction or spinal cord compression.

Hydroxyurea (Hydrea, Droxia)

Mechanism of Action

Inhibits DNA synthesis; radiation sensitizer.

FDA-approved Indications

Melanoma, ovarian cancer, head and neck tumors (not lip) in combination with radiation therapy; CML.

FDA-approved Dosage

- Dose based on actual or ideal body weight, whichever is less: 20 to 30 mg/kg p.o. qd.
- Intermittent therapy: 80 mg/kg p.o. every third day.
- In combination with irradiation: 80 mg/kg p.o. every third day, beginning 7 days before initiation of irradiation and continued indefinitely thereafter, based on adverse effects and response.

Dose Modification Criteria

Myelosuppression: yes; renal: caution; hepatic: caution.

Adverse Reactions

CNS: drowsiness; DERM: rash, facial erythema, alopecia; GI: N/V L1, diarrhea, anorexia, mucositis, constipation; HEMAT: myelosuppression (leukopenia, anemia > thrombocytopenia).

Comments

- Capsule contents may be emptied into glass of water and taken immediately (some inert particles may float on surface).
- Patients should be counseled about proper handling precautions if they open the capsules.

Idarubicin (Idamycin)

Mechanism of Action

Intercalating agent. Topoisomerase-II inhibition.

FDA-approved Indications

In combination with other agents for AML (FAB M1 to M7).

FDA-approved Dosage

AML induction in combination with cytarabine: 12 mg/m^2 slow i.v. (over 10 to 15 minutes) daily for 3 days.

Dose Modification Criteria

Renal: yes; hepatic: yes; mucositis: yes.

Adverse Reactions

CNS: seizures; CV: CHF, arrhythmia; DERM: alopecia; GI: N/V L3, mucositis; HEMAT: myelosuppression.

Comments

• Vesicant.
• Myocardial toxicity is increased in patients with prior anthracycline therapy or heart disease.

Ifosfamide (Ifex)

Mechanism of Action

Alkylating agent.

FDA-approved Indications

Third-line therapy (in combination with other agents) for germ cell testicular cancer.

FDA-approved Dosage

1.2 g/m^2 i.v. daily for 5 days, repeated every 3 weeks. Give MESNA 20% (wt/wt; 240 mg/m^2 per dose for a 1.2 g/m^2 ifosfamide dose) at time of ifosfamide, and then 4 and 8 hours after ifosfamide.

Dose Modification Criteria

Renal: unknown; hepatic: unknown; myelosuppression: yes.

Adverse Reactions

CNS: somnolence, confusion, dizziness, hallucinations; DERM: alopecia; GI: N/V L3, increased LFTs; GU: hemorrhagic cystitis; HEMAT: myelosuppression.

Comments

Ensure adequate hydration. Administer MESNA concurrently.

Interferon α2a (Roferon-A)

Mechanism of Action

Cell-proliferation suppression, macrophage phagocytic activity enhancement, lymphocyte cytotoxicity enhancement.

FDA-approved Indications

Hairy cell leukemia, acquired immunodeficiency syndrome (AIDS)-related Kaposi's sarcoma, CML (Ph-positive).

FDA-approved Dosage

- Hairy cell leukemia: Induction: 3 million IU i.m. or s.c. daily for 16 to 24 weeks. Maintenance: 3 million IU s.c. or i.m. 3 times a week.
- AIDS-related Kaposi's sarcoma: Induction: 36 million IU i.m. or s.c. daily for 10 to 12 weeks. Maintenance: 36 million IU 3 times a week.
- CML: 9 million IU i.m. or s.c. daily. Initial tolerance may be improved over first week by giving 3 MIU daily × 3d, then 6 MIU daily × 3d, then increased to target dose q 9 MIU daily.
- Continue treatment until disease progression or severe toxicity.

Dose Modification Criteria

Serious adverse events: yes.

Adverse Reactions

CNS: dizziness, depression, suicidal ideation; DERM: skin rash; GI: diarrhea, N/V, anorexia, taste alteration, abdominal pain; HEMAT: myelosuppression; PULM: dyspnea; OTHER: fatigue, malaise, fever, chills, myalgia.

Comments

- Patients with a preexisting psychiatric condition, especially depression, should not be treated.
- Use with caution in patients with pulmonary disease, coagulopathies, cardiac disorders.

Interferon α-2b (Intron A)

Mechanism of Action

Cell-proliferation suppression, macrophage phagocytic activity enhancement, lymphocyte cytotoxicity enhancement.

FDA-approved Indications

Hairy cell leukemia in patients older than 18 years, malignant melanoma in patients older than 18 years, AIDS-related Kaposi's sarcoma, follicular lymphoma.

FDA-approved Dosage

- Hairy cell leukemia: 2 million IU/m^2 i.m. or s.c. 3 times a week for up to 6 months.
- Malignant melanoma: induction: 20 million IU/m^2 i.v. for 5 consecutive days per week for 4 weeks. Maintenance: 10 million IU/m^2 s.c. 3 times per week for 48 weeks.
- Kaposi's sarcoma: 30 million IU/m^2 s.c. or i.m. 3 times a week.
- Follicular lymphoma: (in combination with an anthracycline-containing chemotherapy regimen): 5 million IU s.c. 3 times a week for up to 18 months.

Dose Modification Criteria

Serious adverse events: yes.

Adverse Reactions

CNS: dizziness, depression, suicidal ideation; DERM: skin rash; GI: diarrhea, N/V, anorexia, taste alteration, abdominal pain; HEMAT: myelosuppression; PULM: dyspnea; OTHER: fatigue, malaise, fever, chills, myalgia.

Comments

- Patients with a preexisting psychiatric condition, especially depression, should not be treated.
- Use with caution in patients with pulmonary disease, coagulopathies, cardiac disorders.

Irinotecan (Camptosar)

Mechanism of Action

Topoisomerase-I inhibitor.

FDA-approved Indications

- First-line (in combination with fluorouracil and leucovorin): metastatic colon or rectal cancer.
- Second-line: metastatic colon carcinoma (after fluorouracil-based therapy).

FDA-approved Dosage

- First-line: (see product labeling for fluorouracil/leucovorin dosing).
- Regimen 1: 125 mg/m^2 i.v. over 90 minutes every week (days 1, 8, 15, 22) followed by 2 weeks of rest. Repeat every 6 weeks.
- Regimen 2: 180 mg/m^2 i.v. over 90 minutes every 2 weeks (days 1, 15, 29).
- Second-line: 125 mg/m^2 i.v. over 90 minutes weekly for 4 weeks (days 1, 8, 15, 22) followed by 2 weeks rest. Repeat every 6 weeks; *OR* 350 mg/m^2 i.v. over 90 min Q3 weeks.

Dose Modification Criteria

Hepatic: yes; Pelvic/abdominal irradiation: yes; myelosuppression: yes.

Adverse Reactions

CNS: insomnia, dizziness; CV: vasodilation; DERM: alopecia, sweating, rash; GI: N/V L4, diarrhea (early and late), anorexia, flatulence; HEMAT: myelosuppression; PULM: dyspnea, coughing, rhinitis; OTHER: asthenia, fevers.

Comments

Can induce both early (within 24 hours of administration) and late forms of diarrhea. Treat early form with atropine. Treat late diarrhea aggressively with high-dose loperamide.

Letrozole (Femara)

Mechanism of Action

Selective, nonsteroidal aromatase inhibitor.

FDA-approved Indications

Second-line (after antiestrogen therapy): advanced breast cancer in postmenopausal women.

FDA-approved Dosage

2.5 mg p.o. daily.

Dose Modification Criteria

Renal: no (CrCl ≥ 10 mL/min); hepatic: no (mild), unknown (severe).

Adverse Reactions

CNS: headache; GI: nausea, L1, constipation, diarrhea; OTHER: hot flashes, myalgia.

Leuprolide (Lupron, Lupron Depot, Lupron Depot-3 Month, Lupron Depot-4 Month)

Mechanism of Action

LHRH agonist.

FDA-approved Indications

Palliative treatment of advanced prostate cancer.

FDA-approved Dosage

Lupron: 1 mg s.c. daily; Lupron Depot: 7.5 mg i.m. monthly; Lupron Depot-3 month: 22.5 mg i.m. every 3 months; Lupron Depot-4 months: 30 mg i.m. every 4 months.

Adverse Reactions

CNS: pain; CV: edema, ECG changes; ENDO: hot flashes, sweats; GU: testicular atrophy; OTHER: asthenia, injection-site reactions, tumor flare, bone pain.

Comments

Because of different release characteristics, a fractional dose of the 3-month or 4-month lupron depot formulation is not equivalent to the same dose of the monthly formulation and should not be given.

Levimasole (Ergamisol)

Mechanism of Action

Mechanism unknown. May be an immunomodulator.

FDA-approved Indications

Adjuvant treatment in combination with 5-FU after surgical resection in patients with Dukes' stage C colon cancer.

FDA-approved Dosage

Give fluorouracil concomitantly 50 mg every 8 hours for 3 days (starting 7 to 30 days after surgery), and then 50 mg every 8 hours for 3 days every 2 weeks.

Dose Modification Criteria

Hepatic: yes; myelosuppression: yes.

Adverse Reactions

CNS: encephalopathy syndrome; DERM: dermatitis; Heme: agranulocytosis; OTHER: dysguesia.

Comments

Monitor for agranulocytosis. Disulfiram reaction possible. Monitor phenytoin levels when given concomitantly. Interacts with warfarin; monitor INRs carefully.

Liposomal Doxorubicin (Doxil)

Mechanism of Action

Intercalating agent. Topoisomerase-II inhibition.

FDA-approved Indications

- AIDS-related Kaposi's sarcoma.
- Second-line: metastatic ovarian carcinoma (after both paclitaxel- and platinum-based chemotherapy regimens).

FDA-approved Dosage

- AIDS-related Kaposi's sarcoma: 20 mg/m^2 i.v. repeated every 3 weeks.
- Ovarian carcinoma: 50 mg/m^2 i.v. repeated every 4 weeks.
- Infusion should start at an initial rate of 1 mg/min to minimize the risk of infusion reactions. If no infusion-related adverse events are observed, the rate of infusion can be increased to complete administration of the drug over 1 hour.

Dose Modification Criteria

Palmar–plantar erythrodysesthesia: yes; myelosuppression: yes; stomatitis: yes; hepatic

Adverse Reactions

CV: (Risk of cardiotoxicity increases rapidly with total lifetime cumulative doses >450 to 550 mg/m^2), CHF, arrhythmias; DERM: palmar–plantar erythrodysesthesia, alopecia; GI: N/V L3; HEMAT: myelosuppression; INFUS: flushing, shortness of breath, facial swelling, headache, chills, back pain, tightness in chest or throat, and/or hypotension; OTHER: red-tinged urine.

Comments

- Do not confuse with nonliposomal forms of doxorubicin.
- Liposomal formulations of the same drug may not be equivalent.
- Irritant.
- Mix only with D5W.
- Do not use inline filters.

Lomustine, CCNU (CeeNU)
Mechanism of Action

Alkylating agent.

FDA-approved Indications

Primary and metastatic brain tumors; second-line (in combination with other agents) for Hodgkin's disease.

FDA-approved Dosage

Give 100 to 130 mg/m^2 as a single oral dose every 6 weeks.

Dose Modification Criteria

Myelosuppression: yes.

Adverse Reactions

GI: N/V >71 mg: L5, <60 mg: L4, increased LFTs; GU: increased BUN, Cr; HEMAT: severe delayed myelosuppression, cumulative myelosuppression; PULM: (cumulative and usually occurs after 6 months of therapy or a cumulative lifetime dose of 1,100 mg/m^2, although it has been reported with total lifetime doses as low as 600 mg), fibrosis, infiltrate.

Comments

- A single dose is given every 6 weeks.
- Monitor blood counts at least weekly for 6 weeks after a dose.

Mechlorethamine (Mustargen)

Mechanism of Action

Alkylating agent.

FDA-approved Indications

Bronchogenic carcinoma, CLL, CML, Hodgkin's lymphoma, lymphosarcoma, malignant effusions, mycosis fungoides.

FDA-approved Dosage

- Give 0.4 mg/kg ideal dry body weight i.v. single dose per course *OR* 0.2 mg/kg i.v. qd × 2d q3 to 6 weeks.
- MOPP regimen: 6 mg/m^2 i.v. days 1 and 8 of 28-day cycle.

Dose Modification Criteria

Myelosuppression: yes.

Adverse Reactions

CNS: vertigo, tinnitus, diminished hearing; DERM: alopecia, phlebitis; GI: N/V L1, metallic taste in mouth, diarrhea; HEMAT: bone marrow depression; OTHER: hyperuricemia, secondary malignancies, infertility, azospermia.

Comments

Vesicant.

Megestrol (Megace and Others)

Mechanism of Action

Progestational agent.

FDA-approved Indications

Palliative therapy of breast cancer and endometrial cancer.

FDA-approved Dosage

- Breast cancer: 40 mg p.o. q.i.d. (total daily dose, 160 mg/day).
- Endometrial cancer: 10 mg p.o. q.i.d. to 80 mg p.o. q.i.d. (total daily dose, 40 to 320 mg/day).

Adverse Reactions

CNS: mood changes; CV: deep vein thrombosis; DERM: alopecia; ENDO: Cushing-like syndrome, hyperglycemia, glucose intolerance, weight gain, hot flashes; GU: vaginal bleeding; OTHER: carpal tunnel syndrome, tumor flare.

Melphalan (Alkeran); Melphalan Injection

Mechanism of Action

Alkylating agent.

FDA-approved Indications

Palliative therapy of multiple myeloma and nonresectable ovarian cancer.

FDA-approved Dosage

- Myeloma: 6 mg p.o. qd × 2 to 3 weeks. Wait up to 4 weeks for count recovery, and then 2 mg p.o. qd to achieve mild myelosuppression.
- i.v. (if oral therapy not appropriate): 16 mg/m² i.v. over 15 to 20 minutes q2wk × four doses, and then q4wk.
- Ovarian cancer: 0.2 mg/kg p.o. qd × 5 days q4 to 5 weeks.

Dose Modification Criteria

Renal: yes; myelosuppression: yes.

Adverse Reactions

CNS: depression; DERM: HEMAT: marrow suppression; GI: mild anorexia, N/V L1; vasculitis, alopecia; PUL: pulmonary toxicity; OTHER: hypersensitivity (injection), infertility.

Comments

Vesicant.

Mercaptopurine (Purinethol)

Mechanism of Action

Antimetabolite.

FDA-approved Indications

Remission induction and maintenance therapy of acute lymphatic leukemia, ALL; AML; acute myelomonocytic leukemia.

FDA-approved Dosage

- Induction: 2.5 mg/kg (to nearest 25 mg) p.o. qd as a single dose, and then adjust according to blood counts.
- Maintenance: 1.5 to 2.5 mg/kg p.o. qd as a single dose.

Adverse Reactions

GI: anorexia, N/V L1, stomatitis, hepatotoxicity; HEMAT: bone marrow suppression.

Comments

- Usually there is complete cross-resistance with thioguanine.
- Oral mercaptopurine dose should be reduced to 25% to 33% of usual daily dose in patients receiving allopurinol concomitantly.

Methotrexate

Mechanism of Action

Antimetabolite.

FDA-approved Indications

Gestational tumors (choriosarcoma, chorioadenoma destruens, hydatidiform mole) and trophoblastic neoplasms, acute leukemia (induction, maintenance), prophylaxis, treatment, and in combination with other agents for maintenance therapy of meningeal leukemia in ALL, Burkitt's lymphoma, mycosis fungoides, breast, epidermoid head or neck, and lung cancers, non-Hodgkin's lymphoma, lymphosarcoma, high-dose in combination with leucovorin rescue for patients with nonmetastatic osteosarcoma.

FDA-approved Dosage

- Consult current literature for i.v. doses.
- Intrathecally: younger than 1 year: 6 mg intrathecally; 1 to younger than 2 years: 8 mg intrathecally; 3 to younger than 3 years: 10 mg intrathecally; older than 3 years: 12 mg intrathecally.
- Nonmetastatic osteosarcoma: 12 g/m^2 i.v. over 4 hours × one dose (with leucovorin, 15 mg p.o. q6h × 10 days starting 24 hours after beginning of methotrexate infusion) given weekly (weeks 4, 5, 6, 7 after surgery), and then weeks 11, 12, 15, 16, 29, 30, 44, 45. Leucovorin doses should be adjusted based on methotrexate concentrations.

Dose Modification Criteria

Renal: yes.

Adverse Reactions

DERM: alopecia, uticaria, telangiectasia, acne, photosensitivity; GI: N/V <50 mg/m^2 L1, <50 to <250 mg/m^2 L2, 250 to <1,000 mg/m^2 L3, > 1,000 mg/m^2 L4, stomatitis, ulceration, diarrhea, increased LFTs; GU: renal failure, cystitis; HEMAT: bone marrow suppression; PULM: interstitial pneumonitis; OTHER: fever, malaise, chills.

Comments

- Clearance reduced in patients with impaired renal function or third spaces (e.g., ascites, pleural effusions).
- Nonsteroidal antiinflammatory drugs and acidic drugs inhibit methotrexate clearance.
- Use vigorous hydration and alkalinization with high-dose therapy.

Mitomycin-C (Mutamycin)

Mechanism of Action

Induces DNA cross-links.

FDA-approved Indications

Second-line: palliative therapy of gastric cancer or pancreatic cancer.

FDA-approved Dosage

Give 20 mg/m^2 i.v. q6 to 8 weeks.

Dose Modification Criteria

- Renal: yes.
- Myelosuppression: yes.

Adverse Reactions

CV: congestive heart failure (patients with prior doxorubicin exposure); DERM: alopecia, pruritus; GI: anorexia, N/V L2, stomatitis, diarrhea; GU: increased Cr; HEMAT: bone marrow depression (cumulative); PULM: nonproductive cough, dyspnea; OTHER: fever, hemolytic uremic syndrome, malaise, weakness.

Comments

Vesicant.

Mitotane (Lysodren)

Mechanism of Action

Adrenal cytotoxic agent.

FDA-approved Indications

Inoperable, functional, and nonfunctional adrenal cortical carcinoma.

FDA-approved Dosage

Initial dose, 2 to 6 g p.o. qd in three to four divided doses increased to 8 to 10 g/day until excessive toxicity. Maximal tolerated dose varies from 2 to 16 g p.o. daily; usual dose range is 8 to 10 g p.o. daily.

Adverse Reactions

CNS: vertigo, depression, lethargy, somnolence, dizziness; DERM: skin toxicity, transient skin rashes; GI: anorexia, N/V L4, diarrhea; OTHER: adrenal insufficiency.

Comments

Institute adrenal insufficiency precautions.

Mitoxantrone (Novantrone)

Mechanism of Action

Interacts with DNA. Intercalating agent. Topoisomerase-II inhibition.

FDA-approved Indications

First-line: (in combination with other agents) ANLL (myelogenous, promyelocytic, mono-cytic, erythroid) in adults;

Treatment of pain in patients with hormone-refractory prostate cancer (in combination with corticosteroids).

FDA-approved Dosage

- ANLL: Induction: 12 mg/m^2 i.v. Q × 3 days (days 1, 2, 3) in combination with cytarabine; Consolidation: 12 mg/m^2 i.v. Q × 2 days (days 1, 2) in combination with cytarabine.
- Prostate cancer: 12 to 14 mg/m^2 i.v. × one dose q21d with prednisone or hydrocortisone.

Dose Modification Criteria

Hepatic: yes.

Adverse Reactions

CV: (clinical risk increases after a lifetime cumulative dose of 140 mg/m^2), CHF, tachycardia, ECG changes, chest pain; DERM: rash, alopecia, uticaria, nailbed changes; GI: N/V L3, stomatitis, mucositis, constipation, anorexia; HEMAT: myelosuppression; PULM: dyspnea; OTHER: bluish-green urine, sclera may turn bluish, phlebitis, fatigue.

Nilutamide (Nilandron)

Mechanism of Action

Antiandrogen.

FDA-approved Indications

Metastatic prostate cancer (stage D2; in combination therapy with surgical castration). Dosing should begin on same day or day after surgical castration.

FDA-approved Dosage

Give 300 mg p.o. qd × 30 days, and then 150 mg p.o. qd (with or without food).

Adverse Reactions

CNS: dizziness; CV: hypertension, angina; ENDO: hot flashes, impotence, decreased libido; GI: nausea, anorexia, increased LFTs (monitor LFTs periodically because of rare associations with cholestatic jaundice, hepatic necrosis, and encephalopathy), constipation; OCULAR: visual disturbances, impaired adaptation to dark; PULM: interstitial pneumonitis, dyspnea.

Paclitaxel (Taxol)

Mechanism of Action

Microtubule assembly stabilization.

FDA-approved Indications

- First-line: advanced ovarian cancer (in combination with cisplatin), adjuvant treatment of node-positive breast cancer (administered sequentially to standard doxorubicin-containing combination chemotherapy), non–small-cell lung cancer (in combination with cisplatin) in patients who are not candidates for potentially curative surgery and/or radiation therapy.
- Second-line: breast cancer (after failure of combination chemotherapy for metastatic disease or relapse within 6 months of adjuvant therapy); AIDS-related Kaposi's sarcoma.

FDA-approved Dosage

- Premedicate patients with dexamethasone, diphenhydramine (or its equivalent), and cimetidine or ranitidine to prevent severe hypersensitivity reactions.
- First-line ovarian cancer: 135 mg/m^2 i.v. over 24h OR 175 mg/m^2 over 3h (followed by cisplatin, 75 mg/m^2) q3wk.
- First-line breast cancer: 175 mg/m^2 i.v. over 3 hours q3wk × four cycles (administered sequentially with doxorubicin-containing chemotherapy).
- Second-line ovarian cancer: 135 or 175 mg/m^2 i.v. over 3 hours q3wk.
- Second-line breast cancer: 175 mg/m^2 i.v. over 3 hours q3wk.
- Kaposi's sarcoma: 135 mg/m^2 i.v. over 3 hours q3wk or 100 mg/m^2 i.v. over 3 hours q2wk (reduce each dexamethasone dose to 10 mg p.o.).
- NSCLC: 135 mg/m^2 i.v. over 24 hours (followed by cisplatin 75 mg/m^2) q3wk.

Dose Modification Criteria

Hepatic: yes.
Neutropenia: yes.

Adverse Reactions

CV: hypotension, bradycardia, ECG changes; DERM: alopecia; GI: N/V L2, diarrhea, mucositis; HEMAT: myelosuppression; NEURO: peripheral neuropathies; OTHER: hypersensitivity reaction, arthralgia, myalgia.

Comments

- Use non-DEHP plasticized solution containers and administration sets.
- Inline filtration (0.22-μm filter) required during administration.

Pegasparagase (Oncaspar)

Mechanism of Action

Depletes asparagine, an amino acid required by some leukemic cells.

FDA-approved Indications

Acute lymphoblastic leukemia in patients hypersensitive to native forms of L-asparaginase.

FDA-approved Dosage

- The preferred route is i.m.; i.v. administration should be over 1 to 2 hours.
- Combination or sole induction therapy: Adults and children, $\geq$ 0.6 m^2: 2,500 IU/m^2 i.m. or i.v. × one dose q14d.
- Children <0.6 m^2: 82.5 IU/kg q14d.

Adverse Reactions

CNS: malaise, confusion, lethargy, depression; CV: chest pain, hypertension, hypotension; DERM: alopecia, itching, injection-site reactions; ENDO: hyperglycemia; GI: anorexia; N/V L2, hepatotoxicity, increased LFTs, pancreatitis; GU: increased BUN and Cr; HEMAT: hypofibrinogenemia; PULM: respiratory distress, cough, epistaxis; OTHER: hypersensitivity reaction, fever, arthralgia, musculoskeletal pain, tumor lysis syndrome.

Comments

Contraindications: active pancreatitis or history of pancreatitis, serious hemorrhagic episode with native L-asparaginase, serious allergic reactions (e.g., bronchospasm) to native L-asparaginase.

Pentostatin (Nipent)

Mechanism of Action

Adenosine deaminase inhibitor.

FDA-approved Indications

Second-line (after interferon-α): hairy cell leukemia.

FDA-approved Dosage

Give 4 mg/m^2 i.v. every other week.

Dose Modification Criteria

Renal: yes; myelosuppression: yes.

Adverse Reactions

DERM: rash; GI: N/V L5, elevated LFTs; GU: mild transient rise in serum creatinine; HEMAT: leukopenia, anemia, thrombocytopenia; OTHER: fever, infection, fatigue.

Comments

• Use in combination with fludarabine is not recommended.
• Hydrate before and after pentostatin dose.

Porfimer (Photofrin)

Mechanism of Action

Photosensitizing agent.

FDA-approved Indications

Palliation of esophageal cancer (complete or partial obstruction) or photodynamic therapy of endobronchial non–small-cell lung cancer.

FDA-approved Dosage

Give 2 mg/kg i.v. × one dose followed by photodynamic therapy. Additional courses (up to three) can be administered no sooner than 30 days after prior course.

Adverse Reactions

CNS: anxiety, confusion, insomnia; CV: hypertension, hypotension, heart failure, chest pain, atrial fibrillation, tachycardia; DERM: photosensitivity; HEMAT: anemia; GI: N/V, abdominal pain, anorexia, constipation, dysphagia, esophageal edema, esophageal stricture; PULM: pleural effusion, dyspnea, pneumonia, pharyngitis, cough, respiratory insufficiency, tracheoesophageal fistula; OTHER: fever.

Comments

Patients are photosensitive (including eyes) for at least 30 days after administration.

Procarbazine (Matulane)

Mechanism of Action

Mechanism unknown.

FDA-approved Indications

First-line: (in combination with other anticancer drugs) stage III and IV Hodgkin's lymphoma.

FDA-approved Dosage

- All doses based on actual body weight unless the patient is obese or there has been a spurious weight increase, in which case lean body weight (dry weight) should be used.
- Doses may be given as a single daily dose or divided throughout the day.
- MOPP regimen: 100 mg/m^2 p.o. qd × 14 days.
- Other uses: 2 to 4 mg/kg p.o. qd × 7 days, and then 4 to 6 mg/kg p.o. qd until maximal response is obtained.
- Maintenance dose: 1 to 2 mg/kg p.o. qd.

Adverse Reactions

CNS: paresthesias, confusion, lethargy, mental depression; DERM: pruritus, hyperpigmentation, alopecia; GI: anorexia, N/V, stomatitis, xerostomia, diarrhea, constipation; HEMAT: myelosuppression; OTHER: fever, myalgia.

Comments

- Disulfiram-like reaction can occur; avoid alcoholic beverages while taking procarbazine.
- Procarbazine is a weak MAOI; avoid tyramine-rich foods, sympathomimetic drugs, and tricyclic antidepressants.

Prolifeprosan 20 with Carmustine Implant Wafer (Gliadel)

Mechanism of Action

Alkylating agent.

FDA-approved Indications

Adjuvant therapy (to surgery): recurrent glioblastoma multiforme.

FDA-approved Dosage

Each wafer contains 7.7 mg carmustine. Up to 8 wafers should be implanted at time of surgery.

Adverse Reactions

CNS: meningitis, abscess; GI: N/V L2; OTHER: abnormal healing, pain, fever.

Comments

Wafers can be broken in half. Proper handling and disposal precautions should be observed.

Rituximab (Rituxan)

Mechanism of Action

Chimeric (murine, human) monoclonal antibody directed at CD20.

FDA-approved Indications

Relapsed or refractory low-grade or follicular, CD20 positive, B-cell, non-Hodgkin's lymphoma.

FDA-approved Dosage

- Premedication with acetaminophen and/or diphenhydramine should be considered before each infusion.
- If patient experiences an infusion-related reaction, the infusion should be stopped, the patient managed symptomatically, and then the infusion should be restarted at half the rate once the symptoms have resolved.
- 375 mg/m^2 i.v. weekly × four doses (days 1, 8, 15, 22).
- First infusion: start at 50 mg/h, and then may increase by 50 mg/h every 30 minutes up to a maximum of 400 mg/h. Subsequent infusions if prior infusions tolerated: Start at 100 mg/h, and then may increase by 100 mg/h every 30 minutes up to a maximum of 400 mg/h.

Adverse Reactions

CNS: headache, dizziness; CV: hypotension, arrhythmias, peripheral edema; DERM: rash, pruritis, urticaria; GI: N/V L2, abdominal pain; HEMAT: angioedema, leukopenia, thrombocytopenia, neutropenia; INFUS: fever, chills, rigors, hypoxia, pulmonary infiltrates, adult respiratory distress syndrome, myocardial infarction, ventricular fibrillation or cardiogenic shock; OTHER: throat irritation, rhinitis, bronchospasm, hypersensitivity reaction, myalgia, back pain, tumor lysis syndrome.

Comments

- Tumor lysis syndrome has been reported within 12 to 24 hours after the infusion (high-risk: high numbers of circulating malignant cells).
- An infusion-related complex, usually reported with the first infusion (hypoxia, pulmonary infiltrates, adult respiratory distress syndrome, myocardial infarction, ventricular fibrillation, or cardiogenic shock) has resulted in fatalities.

Streptozotocin (Zanosar)

Mechanism of Action

Alkylating agent.

FDA-approved Indications

Metastatic, functional, or nonfunctional islet carcinoma of the pancreas.

FDA-approved Dosage

Give 500 mg/m² i.v. qd × 5 days q6wk, *OR* 1 g/m² i.v. qwk × 2 weeks, and then adjust based on tolerance (individual doses should be ≤ 1,500 mg/m²).

Dose Modification Criteria

Renal: yes.

Adverse Reactions

ELECTRO: hypophosphatemia; ENDO: dysglycemia, may lead to insulin-dependent diabetes; GI: N/V L5, increased LFTs, diarrhea; GU: renal tubular acidosis, increased BUN, anuria, glycosuria; HEMAT: myelosuppression.

Comments

• Vesicant.
• Renal complications are dose related and cumulative. Mild proteinuria is usually an early sign of impending renal dysfunction. Avoid other nephrotoxic agents.

Tamoxifen (Nolvadex)

Mechanism of Action

Antiestrogen.

FDA-approved Indications

Breast cancer
OR reduce the incidence of breast cancer in women at high risk for breast cancer.

FDA-approved Dosage

- Give 20 mg p.o. qd or 10 to 20 mg p.o. twice daily × 5 years. Doses greater than 20 mg/day should be given in divided doses (morning and evening).
- Breast cancer incidence reduction: 20 mg p.o. daily × 5 years.

Adverse Reactions

CV: thromboembolism; DERM: skin rash; GI: N/V L1, anorexia; GU: menstrual irregularities, hot flashes, pruritis vulvae, vaginal discharge or bleeding; HEMAT: bone marrow depression; OCULAR: vision disturbances, cataracts; PULM: dyspnea, chest pain, hemoptysis; OTHER: dizziness, headaches, tumor or bone pain; pelvic pain.

Comments

High risk is defined as women at least 35 years old with a 5-year predicted risk of breast cancer of 1.67%, as predicted by the Gail model. A Gail risk model assessment tool may be obtained by calling 1-800-456-3669, ext. 3838.

Temozolomide (Temodar)

Mechanism of Action

Alkylating agent.

FDA-approved Indications

Second-line (after a nitrosourea and procarbazine): adults with refractory anaplastic astrocytoma.

FDA-approved Dosage

Give 150 mg/m^2 p.o. qd × 5 consecutive days every 28 days.

Dose Modification Criteria

Renal: yes; Hepatic (severe): yes; myelosuppression: yes.

Adverse Reactions

CNS: depression, headache; HEMAT: bone marrow; GI: N/V L3 (reduced by taking on an empty stomach); OTHER: fatigue.

Comments

Capsules should be taken with water. Administer consistently with respect to food.

Teniposide (Vumon)

Mechanism of Action

Topoisomerase-II inhibitor.

FDA-approved Indications

Second-line (in combination with other agents): induction therapy for refractory childhood acute lymphoblastic leukemia.

FDA-approved Dosage

- In combination with cytarabine: 165 mg/m^2 i.v. over 30 to 60 minutes twice weekly × eight to nine doses.
- In combination with vincristine and prednisone: 250 mg/m^2 i.v. over 30 to 60 minutes weekly × four to eight doses.

Dose Modification Criteria

Renal: no guidelines available; hepatic: no guidelines available.

Adverse Reactions

CV: hypotension with rapid infusion; DERM: alopecia, tissue damage secondary to drug extravasation; GI: diarrhea, N/V L2, mucositis; HEMAT: myelosuppression; OTHER: anaphylaxis, hypersensitivity.

Comments

- Observe patient for at least 60 minutes after dose.
- Consider premedication with antihistamines and/or corticosteroids for retreatment (if indicated) after a hypersensitivity reaction.
- Use non-DEHP plasticized solution containers and administration sets.

Thioguanine (Tabloid)

Mechanism of Action

Antimetabolite.

FDA-approved Indications

Acute nonlymphocytic leukemias.

FDA-approved Dosage

Give 2 mg/kg p.o. qd as a single daily dose. May increase to 3 mg/kg p.o. qd as a single daily dose after 4 weeks if no clinical improvement.

Adverse Reactions

GI: anorexia, stomatitis, N/V L1, increased LFTs; HEMAT: bone marrow depression; OTHER: hyperuricemia.

Comments

Cross-resistance with mercaptopurine.

Thiotepa (Thioplex)

Mechanism of Action

Alkylating agent.

FDA-approved Indications

Superficial papillary carcinoma of the bladder, controlling intracavitary effusions secondary to diffuse or localized neoplasms of the serosal cavities, breast cancer, ovarian cancer, Hodgkin's lymphoma, non-Hodgkin's lymphoma.

FDA-approved Dosage

- i.v.: Consult current literature.
- Intravesical: dehydrate patient for 12 to 24 h before procedure.
- 60 mg in 30 to 60 mL SWFI (retain solution for 2 hours) q week × 4 weeks. May repeat for up to two more courses. Reposition patient q15min to maximize contact.
- Intracavitary: 0.6 to 0.8 mg/kg × one dose through tubing used to remove fluid from cavity. 0.3 to 0.4 mg/kg i.v. q 1 to 4 weeks.

Adverse Reactions

CNS: dizziness, headache, blurred vision, conjunctivitis; GI: anorexia, N/V, mucositis at high doses; GU: amenorrhea, reduced spermatogenesis, dysuria, chemical or hemorrhagic cystitis (intravesical); HEMAT: bone marrow depression; OTHER: fever, hypersensitivity reactions, fatigue, weakness, anaphylaxis.

Topotecan (Hycamtin)

Mechanism of Action

Topoisomerase-I inhibitor.

FDA-approved Indications

Second-line (after failure of initial or subsequent chemotherapy): Metastatic or refractory ovarian cancer, small-cell lung cancer (sensitive disease).

FDA-approved Dosage

Ovarian or lung cancer: 1.5 mg/m^2 i.v. over 30 min qd × 5 days q21d.

Dose Modification Criteria

Renal: yes; bilirubin: yes; myelosuppression: yes.

Adverse Reactions

CNS: headaches; DERM: alopecia; HEMAT: leukopenia, thrombocytopenia, neutropenia, anemia; GI: N/V L2, diarrhea, constipation, abdominal pain, stomatitis, anorexia.

Comments

Concomitant filgrastim may worsen neutropenia. If used, start filgrastim at least 24 hours after last topotecan dose.

Toremifene (Farneston)

Mechanism of Action

Nonsteroidal antiestrogen.

FDA-approved Indications

Metastatic breast cancer in postmenopausal women with estrogen receptor–positive or unknown tumors.

FDA-approved Dosage

60 mg p.o. qd.

Adverse Reactions

CNS: dizziness, depression; DERM: skin discoloration, dermatitis; ELECTRO: hypercalcemia; GI: N/V L1, constipation, elevated LFTs; GU: hot flashes, sweating, vaginal discharge, vaginal bleeding; OCULAR: ocular changes, cataracts; OTHER: sweating, tumor flare.

Comments

Do not use in patients with endometrial hyperplasia.

Trastuzumab (Herceptin)

Mechanism of Action

Humanized monoclonal antibody directed at the HER2/neu receptor.

FDA-approved Indications

- First-line (in combination with paclitaxel; no prior therapy for metastatic disease): metastatic breast cancer that overexpresses the HER2/neu protein.
- Second-line: metastatic breast cancer that overexpresses the HER2/neu protein.

FDA-approved Dosage

Initial loading dose of 4 mg/kg i.v. infused over 90 minutes. Weekly maintenance dose of 2 mg/kg i.v. infused over 30 minutes (if first dose tolerated).

Adverse Reactions

CNS: convulsions, ataxia, confusion, manic reaction, insomnia; CV: cardiomyopathy, ventricular dysfunction, congestive heart failure (incidence higher in patients receiving concurrent chemotherapy), tachycardia, hypotension; DERM: ulcerations, rash, urticaria; HEMAT: (with concurrent chemotherapy) anemia, leukopenia; GI: diarrhea, nausea, vomiting; INFUS: (first infusion) chills, fever, nausea, vomiting, pain (at tumor sites), rigors, headache, dizziness, dyspnea, rash, hypotension, asthenia; PULM: (some reactions required supplemental oxygen or ventilatory support) cough, dyspnea, rhinitis, adult respiratory distress syndrome, bronchospasm, angioedema, wheezing, pleural effusions, pulmonary infiltrates, noncardiogenic pulmonary edema, pulmonary insufficiency, hypoxia; OTHER: upper respiratory, urinary tract, and catheter infections, asthenia, allergic reactions, anaphylaxis.

Comments

- Death within 24 hours of a trastuzumab infusion has been reported. The most severe reactions seem to occur in patients with significant preexisting pulmonary compromise secondary to intrinsic lung disease and/or malignant pulmonary involvement.
- Do not administer i.v. push or i.v. bolus.
- Use *ONLY* 20 mL of supplied BWFI diluent—*DO NOT USE WHOLE DILUENT VIAL.* May use SWFI for reconstitution if patient is allergic to benzyl alcohol; product should be used immediately and unused portion discarded.

Tretinoin (Vesanoid)

Mechanism of Action

Induces maturation, cytodifferentiation, and decreased proliferation of acute promyelocytic leukemia (APL) cells.

FDA-approved Indications

Induction of remission in patients with APL FAB M3 (including the M3 variant), characterized by the t(15:17) translocation and/or the presence of the PML/RARα gene, who are refractory to or relapsed after anthracycline chemotherapy or for whom anthracycline therapy is contraindicated.

FDA-approved Dosage

Give 22.5 mg/m^2 p.o. b.i.d. (total daily dose–45 mg/m^2) until complete remission is documented. Therapy should be discontinued 30 days after complete remission is obtained or after 90 days of treatment, whichever comes first.

Adverse Reactions

CNS: dizziness, anxiety, insomnia, headache, depression, confusion, intracranial hypertension, agitation, earaches, hearing loss, pseudotumor cerebri; CV: hypertension, arrhythmias, flushing, hyperlipidemia; DERM: dry skin/mucous membranes, rash, pruritis, alopecia, mucositis; GI: N/V, diarrhea, constipation, dyspepsia; HEMAT: leukocytosis; OCULAR: visual changes; OTHER: dyspnea, fever, shivering, retinoic acid–APL syndrome (RA-APL syndrome; fever, dyspnea, weight gain, radiographic pulmonary infiltrates, and pleural or pericardial effusion).

Comments

- Teratogenic; women must use effective contraception during and for 1 month after therapy.
- RA-APL syndrome occurs in up to 25% of patients usually within first month. Early recognition and high-dose corticosteroids have been used for management. High-dose corticosteroids should be used immediately in patients with RA-APL syndrome plus leukocytosis (WBC > 50,000). Chemotherapy is sometimes added in this situation.

Valarubicin (Valstar)

Mechanism of Action

Intercalating agent. Topoisomerase-II inhibition.

FDA-approved Indications

Second-line [after bacille Calmette-Guérin (BCG) therapy]: Intravesical therapy of urinary bladder carcinoma *in situ* (CIS) in patients in whom immediate cytectomy would be associated with unacceptable morbidity or mortality.

FDA-approved Dosage

Give 800 mg intravesically qwk × 6 weeks. Patient should retain drug in bladder for 2 hours, and then void.

Adverse Reactions

GU: Irritable bladder symptoms: urinary frequency, dysuria, urinary urgency, hematuria, bladder spasm, red-tinged urine.

Comments

• Patients should maintain adequate hydration after treatment.
• Use non-DEHP plasticized solution containers and administration sets.

Vinblastine (Velban)

Mechanism of Action

Inhibits microtubule formation.

FDA-approved Indications

- Frequently responsive: testicular cancer, Hodgkin's lymphoma, non-Hodgkin's lymphoma, mycosis fungoides, Kaposi's sarcoma, histiocytic lymphoma.
- Less responsive: breast cancer, resistant choriocarcinoma.

FDA-approved Dosage

Initial (adults): 3.7 mg/m^2 i.v. weekly. May increase weekly dose up to 18.5 mg/m^2 to maintain WBC > 3000/mm^3 (see package for schema).

Dose Modification Criteria

Myelosuppression: yes; hepatic: yes.

Adverse Reactions

CNS: peripheral neuropathy, paresthesias, loss of deep tendon reflexes, SIADH; CV: hypertension; DERM: alopecia; GI: N/V L1, stomatitis, constipation, ileus; GU: urinary retention, polyuria; HEMAT: bone marrow depression; OTHER: bone pain, jaw pain, tumor pain, weakness, malaise.

Comments

- Vesicant.
- Label syringe: Administer only i.v. Fatal if given intrathecally. Label outerwrap (if used): "Do not remove covering until moment of injection. Fatal if given intrathecally. For intravenous use only."

Vincristine (Oncovin and Others)

Mechanism of Action

Inhibits microtubule formation.

FDA-approved Indications

ALL, activity in combination with other agents for Hodgkin's lymphoma, non-Hodgkin's lymphoma, neuroblastoma, Wilms' tumor, rhabdomyosarcoma.

FDA-approved Dosage

- Adults: 1.4 mg/m^2 i.v. × one dose. Can be given qwk. Sometimes doses are capped at 2 mg.
- Pediatrics: 1.5 to 2 mg/m^2 i.v. × one dose/week (sometimes individual doses are capped at 2 mg); 10 kg or less: 0.05 mg/kg i.v. qwk.

Dose Modification Criteria

Hepatic: Yes.

Adverse Reactions

CNS: peripheral neuropathy, paresthesias, numbness, loss of deep tendon reflexes, SIADH; DERM: alopecia; GI: N/V L1, stomatitis, anorexia, diarrhea, constipation, ileus; GU: urinary retention, OCULAR: ophthalmoplegia, extraocular muscle paresis; PULM: pharyngitis; OTHER: jaw pain.

Comments

- Vesicant.
- Label syringe: Administer only i.v.; Fatal if given intrathecally. Label outerwrap (if used): "Do not remove covering until moment of injection. Fatal if given intrathecally. For intravenous use only."

Vinorelbine (Navelbine)

Mechanism of Action

Inhibits microtubule formation.

FDA-approved Indications

First-line: Single agent (stage IV) or in combination with cisplatin (stage III or IV) for ambulatory patients with unresectable, advanced NSCLC.

FDA-approved Dosage

Give 30 mg/m^2 i.v. over 6 to 10 minutes every week (in combination with cisplatin, 120 mg/m^2 i.v., given on days 1 and 29, and then every 6 weeks). Flush line with 75 to 125 mL of fluid (e.g., 0.9% sodium chloride) after administration.

Dose Modification Criteria

Renal: no; neurotoxicity: yes; myelosuppression: yes; hepatic: yes.

Adverse Reactions

CNS: headache, SIADH; CV: thromboembolic events, chest pain; DERM: alopecia, vein discoloration, venous pain, chemical phlebitis; GI: N/V L2, stomatitis, anorexia, constipation, ileus, elevated LFTs; HEMAT: myelosuppression (granulocytopenia > thrombocytopenia or anemia; PULM: interstitial pulmonary changes, shortness of breath; OTHER: jaw pain, tumor pain, peripheral neuropathy, fatigue, anaphylaxis.

Comments

- Vesicant.
- Administer only i.v. Fatalities have been reported when other vinca alkaloids have been given intrathecally.

Part Two: Performance Status Scales Scores.

APPENDIX PART 2. *Performance status scales/scores: Performance status criteria*

ECOG (Zubrod)		Karnofsky		Lansky[a]	
Score	Description	Score	Description	Score	Description
0	Fully active, able to carry on all predisease performance without restriction	100	Normal, no complaints, no evidence of disease	100	Fully active, normal
		90	Able to carry on normal activity; minor signs or symptoms of disease	90	Minor restrictions in physically strenuous activity
1	Restricted in physically strenuous activity but ambulatory and able to carry out work of a light or sedentary nature (e.g., light housework, office work)	80	Normal activity with effort; some signs or symptoms of disease	80	Active, but tires more quickly
		70	Cares for self, unable to carry on normal activity or do active work	70	Both greater restriction of and less time spent in play activity
2	Ambulatory and capable of all self-care but unable to carry out any work activities. Up and about >50% of waking hours	60	Requires occasional assistance, but is able to care for most of his/her needs	60	Up and around, but minimal active play; keeps busy with quieter activities
		50	Requires considerable assistance and frequent medical care	50	Gets dressed, but lies around much of the day; no active play; able to participate in quiet play and activities
3	Capable of only limited self-care, confined to bed or chair >50% of waking hours	40	Disabled, requires special care and assistance	40	Mostly in bed; participates in quiet activities
		30	Severely disabled, hospitalization indicated. Death not imminent	30	In bed; needs assistance even for quiet play
4	Completely disabled. Cannot carry on any self-care. Totally confined to bed or chair	20	Very sick, hospitalization indicated. Death not imminent	20	Often sleeping; play entirely limited to very passive activities
		10	Moribund, fatal processes progressing rapidly	10	No play; does not even get out of bed

[a]The conversion of the Lansky to ECOG scales is intended for NCI reporting purposes only. *Karnofsky and Lansky performance scores are intended to be multiples of 10.*

Part Three: Common Toxicity Criteria (CTC).

APPENDIX PART 3. *Common toxicity criteria (CTC)*

Adverse event	0	1	2	3	4
			Grade		
Blood/bone marrow					
Bone marrow cellularity	Normal for age	Mildly hypocellular or ≤25% reduction from normal cellularity for age	Moderately hypocellular or >25–≤50% reduction from normal cellularity for age or >2 but <4 wk to recovery of normal bone marrow cellularity	Severely hypocellular or >50–≤75% reduction in cellularity for age or 4–6 wk to recovery of normal bone marrow cellularity	Aplasia or >6 wk to recovery of normal bone marrow cellularity
Normal ranges					
Children (≤18 yr)	90% cellularity average				
Younger adults (19–59)	60–70% cellularity average				
Older adults (≥60 yr)	50% cellularity average				
Note: Grade bone marrow cellularity only for changes related to treatment not disease					
CD4 count	WNL	<LLN–500/mm	200–<500/mm	50–<200/mm	<50/mm
Haptoglobin	Normal	Decreased	—	Absent	—
Hemoglobin (Hgb)	WNL	<LLN–10.0 g/dL	8.0–10.0 g/dL	6.5–<8.0 g/dL	<6.5 g/dL
		<LLN–100 g/L	80–<100 g/L	65–<80 g/L	<65 g/L
		<LLN–6.2 mM	4.9–<6.2 mM	4.0–<4.9 mM	<4.0 mM
For leukemia studies or bone marrow infiltrative/ myelophthisic processes, if specified in the protocol.	WNL	10–<25% decrease from pretreatment	25–<50% decrease from pretreatment	50–<75% decrease from pretreatment	≥75% decrease from pretreatment

	None	Only laboratory evidence of hemolysis [e.g., direct antiglobulin test (DAT, Coombs') schistocytes]	Evidence of red cell destruction and ≥2 g decrease in hemoglobin, no transfusion	Requiring transfusion and/or medical intervention (e.g., steroids)	Catastrophic consequences of hemolysis (e.g., renal failure, hypotension, bronchospasm, emergency splenectomy)
Hemolysis (e.g., immune hemolytic anemia, drug-related hemolysis, other) Also consider haptoglobin, hemoglobin					
Leukocytes (total WBC)	WNL	$<$LLN–3.0 × 10^9/L $<$LLN–3,000/mm^3	≥2.0–$<$3.0 × 10^9/L 2,000–$<$3,000/mm^3	≥1.0–$<$2.0 × 10^9/L 1,000–$<$2,000/mm^3	$<$1.0 × 10^9/L $<$1,000/mm^3
For BMT studies, if specified in the protocol.	WNL	≥2.0–$<$3.0 × 10^9/L 2,500–$<$3,000/mm^3	≥1.0–$<$2.0 × 10^9/L 1,000–$<$2,000/mm^3	≥0.5–$<$1.0 × 10^9/L 500–$<$1,000/mm^3	$<$0.5 × 10^9/L $<$500/mm^3
For pediatric BMT studies (using age, race and sex normal values), if specified in the protocol		≥75–$<$100% LLN	≥50–$<$75% LLN	≥25–$<$50% LLN	$<$25% LLN
Lymphopenia	WNL	$<$LLN–1.0 × 10^9/L $<$LLN–1,000/mm^3	≥0.5–$<$1.0 × 10^9/L 500–$<$1,000/mm^3	$<$0.5 × 10^9/L $<$500/mm^3	— —
For pediatric BMT studies (using age, race and sex normal values), if specified in the protocol		≥75–$<$100% LLN	≥50–$<$75% LLN	≥25–$<$50% LLN	$<$25% LLN
Neutrophils/granulocytes (ANC/AGC)	WNL	≥1.5–$<$2.0 × 10^9/L 1,500–2,000/mm^3	≥1.0–$<$1.5 × 10^9/L 1,000–$<$1,500/mm^3	≥0.5–$<$1.0 × 10^9/L 500–$<$1,000/mm^3	$<$0.5 × 10^9/L $<$500/mm^3
For BMT studies, if specified in the protocol	WNL	≥1.0–$<$1.5 × 10^9/L 1,000–$<$1,500/mm^3	≥0.5–$<$1.0 × 10^9/L 500–$<$1,000/mm^3	≥0.1–$<$0.5 × 10^9/L 100–$<$500/mm^3	$<$0.1 × 10^9/L $<$100/mm^3
For leukemia studies or bone marrow infiltrative/myelophthisic process, if specified in the protocol	WNL	10–$<$25% decrease from baseline	25–$<$50% decrease from baseline	50–$<$75% decrease from baseline	≥75% decrease from baseline
Platelets	WNL	$<$LLN–75.0 × 10^9/L $<$LLN–75,000/mm^3	≥50.0–$<$75.0 × 10^9/L 50,000–$<$75,000/mm^3	$<$10.0–$<$50.00 × 10^9/L ≥10,000–$<$50,000/mm^3	$<$10.0 × 10^9/L $<$10,000/mm^3
For BMT studies, if specified in the protocol	WNL	≥50.0–$<$75.0 × 10^9/L ≥50,000–$<$75,000/mm^3	≥20.0–$<$50.0 × 10^9/L 20,000–$<$50,000/mm^3	≥10.0–$<$20.0 × 10^9/L ≥10,000–$<$20,000/mm^3	$<$10.0 × 10^9/L $<$10,000/mm^3
For leukemia studies or bone marrow infiltrative/myelophthisic process, if specified in the protocol	WNL	10–$<$25% decrease from baseline	25–$<$50% decrease from baseline	50–$<$75% decrease from baseline	≥75% decrease from baseline

Continued

APPENDIX PART 3. *Continued*

Adverse event	Grade 0	Grade 1	Grade 2	Grade 3	Grade 4
Transfusion: platelets	None	—	—	Yes	Platelet transfusions and other measures required to improve platelet increment; platelet transfusion refractoriness associated with life-threatening bleeding (e.g., HLA or cross-matched platelet transfusions)
For BMT studies, if specified in the protocol	None	one platelet transfusion in 24 h	2 platelet transfusions in 24 h	≥3 platelet transfusions in 24 h	Platelet transfusions and other measures required to improve platelet increment; platelet transfusion refractoriness associated with life-threatening bleeding (e.g., HLA or cross-matched platelet transfusions)
Also consider platelets					
Transfusion; pRBCs	None			Yes	—
For BMT studies, if specified in the protocol	None	≤2 U pRBC in 24 h elective or planned	3 U pRBC in 24 h elective or planned	≥4 U prBC in 24 h	Hemorrhage or hemolysis associated with life-threatening anemia; medical intervention required to improve hemoglobin
For pediatric BMT studies, if specified in the protocol	None	≤15 mL/kg in 24 h elective or planned	>15-≤30 mL/kg in 24 h elective or planned	>30 mL/kg in 24 h	Hemorrhage or hemolysis associated with life-threatening anemia; medical intervention required to improve hemoglobin
Also consider hemoglobin					
Blood/bone marrow— other specify	None	Mild	Moderate	Severe	Life-threatening or disabling

Coagulation

Note: See the Hemorrhage category for grading the severity of bleeding events

	None	Mild	Moderate	Severe	Life-threatening or disabling
DIC (disseminated intravascular coagulation) — Also consider Platelets. Note: Must have increased fibrin split products or D-dimer to grade as DIC	Absent	—	—	Laboratory findings present with no bleeding	Laboratory findings and bleeding
Fibrinogen — For leukemia studies or bone marrow infiltrative/myelophthisic process, if specified in the protocol	WNL; WNL	≥0.75—<1.0 × LLN; <20% decrease from pretreatment value or LLN	≥0.5—<0.75 × LLN; ≥20—<40% decrease from pretreatment value or LLN	≥0.25—<0.5 × LLN; ≥40—<70% decrease from pretreatment value or LLN	<0.25 × LLN; <50 mg
Partial thromboplastin time (PTT) — Phlebitis is graded in the Cardiovascular (General) category	WNL	>ULN—≤1.5 × ULN	>1.5—≤2 × ULN	>2 × ULN	—
Prothrombin time (PT) — Thrombosis/embolism is graded in the Cardiovascular (General) category	WNL	>ULN—≤1.5 × ULN	>1.5—≤2 × ULN	>2 × ULN	—
Thrombotic microangiopathy (e.g., thrombotic thrombocytopenic purpura/TCP or hemolytic uremic syndrome/HUS)	Absent	—	—	Laboratory findings present without clinical consequences	Laboratory findings and clinical consequences, (e.g., CNS hemorrhage/bleeding or thrombosis/embolism or renal failure) requiring therapeutic intervention
For BMT studies, if specified in the protocol — Also consider Hemoglobin, Platelets, Creatinine. Note: Must have microangiopathic changes on blood smear (e.g., schistocytes, helmet cells, red cell fragments)		Evidence of RBC destruction (schisto—cytosis) without clinical consequences	Evidence of RBC destruction with elevated creatinine (≤3 × ULN)	Evidence of RBC destruction with creatinine (>3 × ULN) not requiring dialysis	Evidence of RBC destruction with renal failure requiring dialysis and/or encephalopathy
Coagulation—Other (Specify,)	None	Mild	Moderate	Severe	Life-threatening or disabling

Continued

APPENDIX PART 3. *Continued*

Adverse event	Grade				
	0	1	2	3	4
Constitutional symptoms					
Fatigue (lethargy, malaise, asthenia)	None	Increased fatigue over baseline, but not altering normal activities	Moderate (e.g., decrease in performance status by one ECOG level or 20% Karnofsky or Lansky) or causing difficulty performing some activities	Severe (e.g., decrease in performance status by ≥2 ECOG levels or 40% Karnofsky or Lansky) or loss of ability to perform some activities	Bedridden or disabling
Note: See Appendix III for performance status scales					
Fever (in the absence of neutropenia, where neutropenia is defined as AGC <1.0 × 10⁹/L)	None	38.0–39.0°C (100.4–102.2°F)	39.1–40.0°C (102.3–104.0°F)	>40.0°C (>104.0°F) for <24 h	>40.0°C (>104.0°F) for >24 h
Also consider Allergic reaction/ hypersensitivity					
Note: The temperature measurements listed above are oral or tympanic					
Hot flashes/flushes are graded in the Endocrine category					
Rigors, chills	None	Mild, requiring symptomatic treatment (e.g., blanket) or non-narcotic medication	Severe and/or prolonged, requiring narcotic medication	Not responsive to narcotic medication	—
Sweating (diaphoresis)	Normal	Mild and occasional	Frequent or drenching	—	—
Weight gain	<5%	5–<10%	10–<20%	≥20%	—
Also consider Ascites, Edema, Pleural effusion (nonmalignant)					
Weight gain associated with Veno-occlusive disease (VOD) for BMT studies, if specified in the protocol	<2%	≥2–<5%	≥5–<10%	≥10% or as ascites	≥10% or fluid retention resulting in pulmonary failure

Adverse event				
Also consider Ascites, Edema, Pleural effusion (nonmalignant). Weight loss. Also consider Vomiting, Dehydration, Diarrhea	<5%	5–<10%	10–<20%	≥20%	—
Constitutional symptoms—Other (Specify,). Amylase is graded in the Metabolic/Laboratory category		Mild	Moderate	Severe	Life-threatening or disabling
Anorexia	None	Loss of appetite	Oral intake significantly decreased	Requiring i.v. fluids	Requiring feeding tube or parenteral nutrition
Ascites (nonmalignant)	None	Asymptomatic	Symptomatic, requiring diuretics	Symptomatic, requiring therapeutic paracentesis	Life-threatening physiologic consequences
Colitis	None	—	Abdominal pain with mucus and/or blood in stool	Abdominal pain, fever, change in bowel habits with ileus or peritoneal signs, and radiographic or biopsy documentation	Perforation or requiring surgery, or toxic megacolon
Also consider Hemorrhage/bleeding with grade 3 or 4 thrombocytopenia, Hemorrhage/bleeding without grade 3 or 4 thrombocytopenia, Melena/GI bleeding, Rectal bleeding/hematochezia, Hypotension					
Constipation	None	Requiring stool softener or dietary modification	Requiring laxatives	Obstipation requiring manual evacuation or enema	Obstruction or toxic megacolon
Dehydration	None	Dry mucous membranes and/or diminished skin turgor	Requiring i.v. fluid replacement (brief)	Requiring i.v. fluid replacement (sustained)	Physiologic consequences requiring intensive care; hemodynamic collapse
Also consider Diarrhea, Vomiting, Stomatitis/pharyngitis (oral/pharyngeal mucositis), hypotension					
Diarrhea patients without colostomy	None	Increase of <4 stools/day over pretreatment	Increase of 4–6 stools/day, or nocturnal stools	Increase of ≥7 stools/day or incontinence; or need for parenteral support for dehydration	Physiologic consequences requiring intensive care; or hemodynamic collapse

Continued

APPENDIX PART 3. *Continued*

Adverse event	Grade				
	0	1	2	3	4
Patients with a colostomy	None	Mild increase in loose, watery colostomy output compared with pretreatment	Moderate increase in loose, watery colostomy output compared with pretreatment, but not interfering with normal activity	Severe increase in loose, watery colostomy output compared with pretreatment, interfering with normal activity	Physiologic consequences, requiring intensive care; or hemodynamic collapse
Diarrhea associated with graft-versus-host disease (GVHD) for BMT studies, if specified in the protocol	None	>500–≤1,000 mL of diarrhea/day	>1,000–≤1,500 mL of diarrhea/day	>1,500 mL of diarrhea/day	Severe abdominal pain with or without ileus
For pediatric BMT studies, if specified in the protocol Also consider Hemorrhage/bleeding with grade 3 or 4 thrombocytopenia. Hemorrhage/bleeding without grade 3 or 4 thrombocytopenia, Pain, Dehydration, Hypotension		*>5–≤10 mL/kg of diarrhea/day*	*>10–≤15 mL/kg of diarrhea/day*	*>15 mL/kg of diarrhea/day*	—
Duodenal ulcer (requires radiographic or endoscopic documentation)	None	—	Requiring medical management or nonsurgical treatment	Uncontrolled by outpatient medical management; requiring hospitalization	Perforation or bleeding, requiring emergency surgery
Dyspepsia/heartburn	None	Mild	Moderate	Severe	
Dysphagia, esophagitis, odynophagia (painful swallowing)	None	Mild dysphagia, but can eat regular diet	Dysphagia, requiring predominantly pureed, soft, or liquid diet	Dysphagia, requiring i.v. hydration	Complete obstruction (cannot swallow saliva) requiring enteral or parenteral nutritional support, or perforation
Note: If the adverse event is radiation related, grade either under Dysphagia–esophageal related to radiation or Dysphagia–pharyngeal related to radiation					

	Grade 0	Grade 1	Grade 2	Grade 3	Grade 4
Hepatic					
Alkaline phosphatase	WNL	>ULN–2.5 × ULN	>2.5–5.0 × ULN	>5.0–20.0 × ULN	>20.0 × ULN
Bilirubin	WNL	>ULN–1.5 × ULN	>1.5–3.0 × ULN	>3.0–10.0 × ULN	>10.0 × ULN
Bilirubin associated with graft-versus-host disease (GVHD) for BMT studies, if specified in the protocol	Normal	≥2–<3 mg/100 mL	≥3–<6 mg/100 mL	≥6–<15 mg/100 mL	≥15 mg/100 mL
GGT (γ-glutamyl transpeptidase)	WNL	>ULN–2.5 × ULN	>2.5–5.0 × ULN	>5.0–20.0 × ULN	>20.0 × ULN
Hepatic enlargement	Absent	—	—	Present	—
Note: Grade Hepatic enlargement only for treatment-related adverse event including Veno-occlusive disease					
Hypoalbuminemia	WNL	<LLN–3 g/dL	≥2–<3 g/dL	<2 g/dL	—
Liver dysfunction/failure (clinical)	Normal	—	—	Asterixis	Encephalopathy or coma
Portal vein flow	Normal	—	Decreased portal vein flow	Reversal/retrograde portal vein flow	—
SGOT (AST) (serum glutamic oxaloacetic transaminase)	WNL	>ULN–2.5 × ULN	>2.5–5.0 × ULN	>5.0–20.0 × ULN	>20.0 × ULN
SGPT (ALT) (serum glutamic pyruvic transaminase)	WNL	>ULN–2.5 × ULN	>2.5–5.0 × ULN	>5.0–20.0 × ULN	>20.0 × ULN
Hepatic—Other (Specify)	None	Mild	Moderate	Severe	Life-threatening or disabling
Infection/febrile neutropenia					
Catheter-related infection	None	Mild, no active treatment	Moderate, localized infection, requiring local or oral treatment	Severe, systemic infection, requiring i.v. antibiotic or antifungal treatment or hospitalization	Life-threatening sepsis (e.g., septic shock)
Febrile neutropenia (fever or unknown origin without clinically or microbiologically documented infection) (ANC <1.0 × 10^9/L, fever ≥38.5°C) Also consider Neutrophils Note: Hypothermia instead of fever may be associated with neutropenia and is graded here	None	—	—	Present	Life-threatening sepsis (e.g., septic shock)
Infection (documented clinically or microbiologically) with grade 3 or 4 neutropenia	None	—	—	Present	Life-threatening sepsis (e.g., septic shock)

Continued

643

APPENDIX PART 3. *Continued*

Adverse event	Grade				
	0	1	2	3	4
(ANC <1.0 × 10⁹/L) Also consider Neutrophils Notes: Hypothermia instead of fever may be associated with neutropenia and is graded here In the absence of documented infection, grade 3 or 4 neutropenia with fever is graded as Febrile neutropenia					
Infection with unknown ANC	None	—	—	Present	Life-threatening sepsis (e.g., septic shock)
Note: This adverse event criterion is used in the rare case when ANC is unknown					
Infection without neutropenia	None	Mild, no active treatment	Moderate, localized, infection requiring local or oral treatment	Severe, systemic infection requiring i.v. antibiotic or antifungal treatment or hospitalization	Life-threatening sepsis (e.g., septic shock)
Also consider Neutrophils Wound-infectious is graded in the Dermatology/Skin category Infection/Febrile Neutropenia— Other (Specify)					
Metabolic/laboratory					
Acidosis (metabolic or respiratory)	Normal	pH <normal, but ≥7.3	—	pH <7.3	pH <7.3 with life-threatening physiologic consequences
Alkalosis (metabolic or respiratory)	Normal	pH >normal, but ≤7.5	—	pH >7.5	pH >7.5 with life-threatening physiologic consequences

Adverse Event	WNL/None	Mild	Moderate	Severe	Life-threatening or disabling
Amylase	WNL	>ULN–1.5 × ULN	>1.5–2.0 × ULN	>2.0–5.0 × ULN	>5.0 × ULN
Bicarbonate	WNL	<LLN–16 mEq/dL	11–15 mEq/dL	8–10 mEq/dL	<8 mEq/dL
CPK (creatine phosphokinase)	WNL	>ULN–2.5 × ULN	>2.5–5 × ULN	>5–10 × ULN	>10 × ULN
Hypercalcemia	WNL	>ULN–11.5 mg/dL >ULN–2.9 mM	>11.5–12.5 mg/dL >2.9–3.1 mM	>12.5 mg/dL >3.1–3.4 mM	>13.5 mg/dL >3.4 mM
Hypercholesterolemia	WNL	>ULN–300 mg/dL >ULN–7.75 mM	>300–400 mg/dL >7.75–10.34 mM	>400–500 mg/dL >10.34–12.92 mM	>500 mg/dL >12.92 mM
Hyperglycemia	WNL	>ULN–160 mg/dL >ULN–8.9 mM	>160–250 mg/dL >8.9–13.9 mM	>250–500 mg/dL >13.9–27.8 mM	>500 mg/dL >27.8 mM or acidosis
Hyperkalemia	WNL	>ULN–5.5 mM	>5.5–6.0 mM	>6.0–7.0 mM	>7.0 mM
Hypermagnesemia	WNL	>ULN–3.0 mg/dL >ULN–1.23 mM	—	>3.0–8.0 mg/dL >1.23–3.30 mM	>8.0 mg/dL >3.30 mM
Hypernatremia	WNL	>ULN–150 mM	>150–155 mM	>155–160 mM	>160 mM
Hypertriglyceridemia	WNL	>ULN–2.5 × ULN	>2.5–5.0 × ULN	>5.0–10 × ULN	>10 × ULN
Hyperuricemia	WNL	>ULN–≤10 mg/dL ≤0.59 mM without physiologic consequences	—	>ULN–≤10 mg/dL ≤0.59 mM with physiologic consequences	>10 mg/dL >0.59 mM
Also consider Tumor lysis syndrome, Renal failure, Creatinine, Hyperkalemia					
Hypocalcemia	WNL	<LLN–8.0 mg/dL <LLN–2.0 mM	7.0–<8.0 mg/dL 1.75–<2.0 mM	6.0–<7.0 mg/dL 1.5–<1.75 mM	<6.0 mg/dL <1.5 mM
Hypoglycemia	WNL	<LLN–55 mg/dL <LLN–3.0 mM	40–55 mg/dL 2.2–<3.0 mM	30–<40 mg/dL 1.75–<2.2 mM	<30 mg/dL <1.7 mM
Hypokalemia	WNL	<LLN–3.0 mM	—	2.5–<3.0 mM	<2.5 mM
Hypomagnesemia	WNL	<LLN–1.2 mg/dL <LLN–0.5 mM	0.9–<1.2 mg/dL 0.4–<0.5 mM	0.7–<0.9 mg/dL 0.3–<0.4 mM	<0.7 mg/dL <0.3 mM
Hyponatremia	WNL	<LLN–130 mM	—	120–<130 mM	<120 mM
Hypophosphatemia	WNL	<LLN–2.5 mg/dL <LLN–0.8 mM	≥2.0–<2.5 mg/dL 0.6–<0.8 mM	≥1.0–<2.0 mg/dL 0.3–<0.6 mM	<1.0 mg/dL <0.3 mM
Hypothyroidism is graded in the Endocrine category					
Lipase	WNL	>ULN–1.5 × ULN	>1.5–2.0 × ULN	>2.0–5.0 × ULN	>5.0 × ULN
Metabolic/Laboratory—Other (Specify, ____)	None	Mild	Moderate	Severe	Life-threatening or disabling

APPENDIX 4. *WHO and RECIST criteria for response*

Characteristic	WHO	RECIST
Measurability of lesions at baseline	1. Measurable, bidimensional (product of LD and greatest perpendicular diameter)[a] 2. Nonmeasurable/evaluable (e.g., lymphangitic pulmonary metastases, abdominal masses)	1. Measurable, unidimensional (LD only, size with conventional techniques ≥20 mm; spiral computed tomography ≥10 mm) 2. Nonmeasurable: all other lesions, including small lesions. Evaluable is not recommended
Objective response	1. Measurable disease (change in sum of products of LDs and greatest perpendicular diameters, no maxium number of lesions specified) CR: disappearance of all known disease, confirmed at ≥4 wk PR: >50% decrease from baseline, confirmed at ≥4 wk PD: >25% increase of one or more lesions, or appearance of new lesions NC: neither PR or PD criteria met 2. Nonmeasurable disease CR: disappearance of all unknown disease, confirmed at ≥4 wk; PR: estimated decrease of ≥50%, confirmed at ≥4 wk PD: estimated increase of ≥25% in existent lesions of appearance of new lesions NC: neither PR or PD criteria met	1. Target lesions [change is sum of LDs, maximum of 5 per organ up to 10 total (more than one organ)] CR: disappearance of all target lesions, confirmed at ≥4 wk PR >30% decrease from baseline, confirmed at 4 wk PD: ≥20% increase over smallest sum observed, or appearance of new lesions SD: neither PR or PD criteria met 2. Nontarget lesions CR: disappearance of all target lesions and normalization of tumor markers, confirmed at ≥4 wk PD: unequivocal progression of nontarget lesions, or appearance of new lesions Non-PD: persistence of one or more nontarget lesions and/or tumor markers above normal limits
Overall response	1. Best response recorded in measurable disease 2. NC in nonmeasurable lesions will reduce a CR in measurable lesions to an overall PR 3. NC in nonmeasurable lesions will not reduce a PR in measurable lesions	1. Best response recorded in measurable disease from treatment start to disease progression or recurrence 2. Non-PD in nontarget lesions(s) will reduce a CR in target lesions(s) to an overall PR 3. Non-PD in nontarget lesion(s) will not reduce a PR in target lesions(s)

Duration of response	1. CR
	   From: date CR criteria first met
	   To: date PD first noted
	2. Overall response
	   From: date of treatment start
	   To: date PD first noted
	3. In patients who only achieve a PR, only the period of overall response should be recorded
		1. Overall CR
		   From: date CR criteria first met
		   To: date recurrent disease first noted
		2. Overall response
		   From: date CR or PR criteria first met (whichever status came first)
		   To: date recurrent disease or PD first noted
		3. SD
		   From: date of treatment start
		   To: date PD first noted

WHO, World Health Organization; RECIST, Response Evaluation Criteria in Solid Tumors; LD, longest diameter; CR, complete response; PR, partial response; PD, progressive disease; NC, no change; SD, stable disease.

aLesions that can be measured only unidimensionally are considered measurable (e.g., mediastinal adenopathy, malignant hepatomegaly).

From *J Natl Cancer Inst* 2000;92:179–181, with permission.

APPENDIX 5: BODY SURFACE AREA

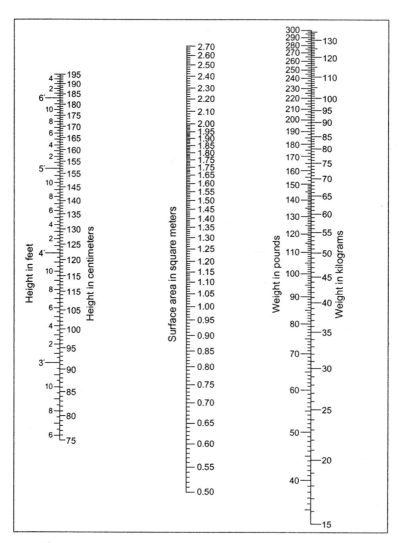

Reprinted by permission of the publishers from Functional Endoc
Birth Through Adolescence by Nathan B. Talbot et al., Cambridge
Harvard University Press, Copyright c 1952 by the Commonwealth

Amputees (approximate surface area of amputated part):

Hand and 5 fingers	3%	Foot	3%
Arm, lower	4%	Leg, lower	6%
Arm, upper	6%	Leg, thigh	12%

Subject Index